D1312229

Corticothalamic Projections and Sensorimotor Activities

Editors:

Tamas L. Frigyesi, M.D.

Department of Neurology

College of Physicians & Surgeons of Columbia University

Eric Rinvik, M.D.

Department of Anatomy, University of Oslo

Melvin D. Yahr, M.D.

Department of Neurology,

College of Physicians & Surgeons of Columbia University

Raven Press, Publishers ■ New York

ISBN number 0-911216-35-9
Library of Congress Catalog Card number 74-181303

Preface

"In the thalamus, that large neuronal mass at the rostral end of the mesencephalon, it is said, lies the key to the secrets of the cerebral cortex." This was the opening statement by Earl Walker at the First International Symposium sponsored by the Parkinson's Disease Research Center held in 1964. Since then, the Center has sponsored three additional symposia, all of which had the stated objectives of reporting on those areas of neurobiological research in which significant advances had been made in the study of sensorimotor control systems, and determining which new analytical approaches might be expected to expand the understanding of neural mechanisms underlying abnormal functions in these systems.

These meetings attested to the fact that the thalamus occupies the penultimate position in the hierarchy of subsystems which constitute the senorimotor organization. The constant adaptation of mammals to alterations in the environment is effected by changes in the external and internal milieus which, in turn, elicit responses mediated via the motor pathways, the only output, except for hormone release, of the mammalian central nervous system. Since all sensory systems converge on the thalamus, its hodology, structural properties and functional characteristics appear to be essential to an understanding of how central, high order mechanisms operate on signals from the external and internal milieus and affect responses to environmental changes.

During the last three decades, the thalamus has been regarded primarily as the last link in projection systems from, mainly, the lower neuraxisto the cerebral cortex. In addition, the thalamus has been considered to be an "*inter*neuronal machine" (Purpura, this volume), i.e., intrathalamic complex interneuronal networks may execute "integrative processes" in the thalamic relays on a multitude of converging pathways from the lower neuraxis and the retina. During these 30 years, attention was focused principally on structure-function relations of intrathalamic and *thalamo-cortical* systems.

The concept that the reverse systems are equally important is not new, as is apparent from Mettler's historical overview in this volume. For nearly a century, morphologists and physiologists have been concerned with the *corticothalamic* pathways and their functions. As early as in 1903, S. Ramón y Cajal advanced the hypothesis, remarkable for its time, that neocortical influences operate on the dorsal thalamus by way of corticothalamic fibers, and that these projections provide the morphological basis for our capacity to limit conscious experiences to a particular and restricted region of the sensory fields.

Based on observations made a few years later on human clinical material, Head and Holmes (1912) corroborated the concept of cortical control of thalamic activities. In their view, cortico-thalamic projection activities form an *inhibitory system* which filters the excessive sensory stimuli funneling through the dorsal thalamus. These suppositions introduced the notion that the neo-cortex, via corticothalamic projection activities, is capable of regulating its own input at the thalamic level of the neuraxis.

The experiments of Dusser de Barenne and McCulloch (1938) represented a major step forward in the elaboration of corticothalamic projection activities. They demonstrated that reciprocal connections operate between particular thalamic regions and specific neocortical fields. These experiments have introduced the notion of regional specificity of the neocortical control over discrete thalamic regions related to specific sensory modalities.

A major extension of the Dusser de Barenne–McCulloch experiments was effected by Jasper (1949) who demonstrated that specific neocortical fields are capable of activating certain dorsal thalamic nuclei which, in turn, exert generalized effects upon other areas of the neocortex in both hemispheres.

During the last three decades, a period heralded by the classical studies of Dempsey and Morrison (1942), so much attention has been devoted to the study of thalamocortical relations that problems of corticothalamic relations have been all but neglected. During recent years, however, an upsurge has occurred in the number of publications dealing with anatomical and physiological aspects of corticothalamic relations, which indicates a renewed interest in this problem. Therefore, it was deemed desirable to hold a conference to survey the new data and concepts which have evolved from this renaissance, especially as they relate to normal and abnormal sensorimotor activities. The proceedings of this meeting are recorded herein. Perusal of this volume should reveal that the meeting was held at a relatively early state of redevelopment of this field. This is indicated by the fact that much of the material is based on heretofore unpublished data. These proceedings also substantiate Cajal's foresight; corticothalamic projections are more abundant than previously suspected and the activities transmitted by them are of functional importance comparable to those mediated by thalamocortical projections.

The Editors trust that this volume will be of interest to all concerned with current knowledge related to normal and abnormal sensorimotor function.

Our special thanks go to three individuals to whom we are greatly indebted for their invaluable assistance in publishing this volume: Mrs. Eli Ginzberg for her judicious editorial assistance and advice; Miss Ethel Wilson for composing the pages and typesetting the entire volume in a remarkably short period of time, thus facilitating the early publication of this volume; and Mr. Robert Schwartz for his tireless and imaginative assistance at every step, from the organization of the meeting to the publication of this volume. Finally, the cooperation and support of Dr. Alan Edelson of Raven Press is gratefully acknowledged.

Tamas L. Frigyesi, M.D.
Eric Rinvik, M. D.
Melvin D. Yahr, M.D.

New York and Oslo, June, 1972.

Contents

List of Contributors

ALBE-FESSARD, D.—Physiologie des Centres Nerveux, Université de Paris, France

AMASSIAN, V. E.—Department of Physiology, Albert Einstein College of Medicine, New York City

ASANUMA, H.—Department of Physiology, New York Medical College, New York City

CARPENTER, M. B.—Department of Anatomy, College of Physicians and Surgeons, Columbia University, New York City

COHEN, B.—Department of Neurology, Mount Sinai School of Medicine, New York City

COOPER, I. S.—Department of Neurologic Surgery, St. Barnabas Hospital, Bronx, N.Y. and Department of Anatomy, New York Medical College, New York City

COURVILLE, J.—Department of Physiology, Faculty of Medicine, University of Montreal, Quebec, Canada

CROSBY, E. C.—Department of Anatomy, University of Alabama, Birmingham, Alabama

EDWARDS, S. B.—Department of Anatomy, University of Pennsylvania, Philadelphia, Pa.

EVARTS, E. V.—Laboratory of Neurophysiology, National Institute of Mental Health, Bethesda, Maryland

FOX, C. A.—Department of Anatomy, Wayne State University, Detroit, Michigan

FRIGYESI, T. L.—Parkinson's Disease Research Center, Department of Neurology, College of Physicians and Surgeons, Columbia University, New York City

GILMAN, S.—Department of Neurology, College of Physicians and Surgeons, Columbia University, New York City

GRUNDFEST, H.—Department of Neurology, College of Physicians and Surgeons, Columbia University, New York City

HASSLER, R.—Max-Planck-Institut für Hirnforschung, Neurobiologische Abteilung, Frankfurt/Main, Germany

HOLLÄNDER, H.—Max-Planck-Institut für Psychiatrie, München, Germany

JASPER, H. H.—Centre de Reserches en Sciences Neurologiques, Département de Physiologie, Université de Montréal, Québec, Canada.

KUYPERS, H. G. J. M.—Department of Anatomy, Rotterdam Medical Faculty, Rotterdam, The Netherlands

LAMARRE, Y.—Centre de Recherches en Sciences Neurologiques, Université de Montréal, Québec, Canada

MASSION, J.—Laboratoire de Neurophysiologie Générale, INP-CNRS, Marseille, France

METTLER, F. A.—Departments of Anatomy and Neurology, College of Physicians and Surgeons, Columbia University, New York City

NOBACK, C. R.—Department of Anatomy, College of Physicians and Surgeons, Columbia University, New York City

PETRAS, J. M.—Walter Reed Army Institute of Research, Washington, D.C.

PRIBRAM, K. H.—Department of Psychology, Stanford University, Palo Alto, California

PURPURA, D. P.—Department of Anatomy and the Rose F. Kennedy Center for Research in Mental Retardation and Human Development, Albert Einstein College of Medicine, Yeshiva University, Bronx, New York

RINVIK, E.—Department of Anatomy, University of Oslo, Norway

SAX, D. S.—Veterans Administration Hospital, Boston, Massachusetts

SCHEIBEL, A. B.—Departments of Anatomy and Psychiatry, and Brain Research Institute of the University of California at Los Angeles, Center for the Health Sciences, Los Angeles, California

SCHEIBEL, M. E.—Departments of Anatomy and Psychiatry, and Brain Research Institute of the University of California at Los Angeles, Center for the Health Sciences, Los Angeles, California

SCHWARTZ, D.—Toronto, Ontario, Canada

SPRAGUE, J. M.—Department of Anatomy, and Institute of Neurological Sciences, University of Pennsylvania, Philadelphia, Pa.

STERIADE, M.—Laboratoire de Neurophysiologie, Département de Physiologie, Faculté de Médicine, Université Laval, Québec, Canada

STRICK, P. L.—Department of Anatomy, School of Medicine; Department of Animal Biology, School of Veterinary Medicine; and Institute of Neurological Sciences, University of Pennsylvania, Philadelphia, Pa.

SZABO, J.—Department of Anatomy, University of Ottawa, Ontario, Canada

YAHR, M. D.—Department of Neurology, College of Physicians and Surgeons, Columbia University, New York City

YAKOVLEV, P. I.—Elmer E. Southard Research Laboratory of Normal and Pathological Anatomy and Development of the Brain, Walter E. Fernald State School, Waltham, Mass.

YORK, D. H.—Department of Physiology, Queen's University, Kingston, Ontario, Canada

Corticothalamic Projections and Sensorimotor Activities
T. Frigyesi, E. Rinvik, and M.D. Yahr, editors. © 1972
Raven Press, New York.

The Corticothalamic Projection: the Structural Substrate for the Control of the Thalamus by the Cerebral Cortex

Fred A. Mettler

Prior to the transformation of the concept of neuronal composition into a body of generally accepted fact (in the last decade of the nineteenth century) it was supposed that the neurocytes in the cerebral cortex, as well as those located elsewhere including the thalamus, were interconnected by means of a generalized syncytial arrangement. In such a frame of reference efforts to search for specific corticothalamic fibers* (Wernicke, 1881) would have had little relevance since no one could be certain that everything was not potentially connected with everything else. During the eighties, the climate of opinion gradually shifted away from the concept of a diffuse reticulum. (For a review of early concepts of the reticular formation see Soury (1899, p. 1740 *et seq.*), and for one of later reticular theory see Mettler, 1964). This recognition of individual neuronal identity implied not only morphologic precision but also the attractive possibility of elucidating physiology in terms of specific pathways which retain their functional identity even after the afferents have entered the neuraxis.

Flechsig's studies of differential myelination made it clear that certain prominent afferent pathways not only developed as distinct entities but that they were connected to the thalamus and, through this, to particular cortical loci which he considered "gateways" to the brain. In addition, he was able to define a powerful descend-

----

* As noted below we are concerned here only with fibers which have their origin in the cerebral cortex and proceed to the dorsal thalamus. Space will not allow us to explore cortical projections to the hypothalamus and other parts of the ventral thalamus which have been of considerable interest since Gustave Roussy first called attention, in his thesis of 1907, to the neurovegetative accompaniments of the so-called Dejerine-Roussy syndrome. (The corticifugal connections of the cortex with the hypothalamus have been reviewed by a number of writers (Gellhorn, 1953) and a *precis* appears on pages 435-6 of Peele's 1961 publication.)

ing efferent mechanism, also arising from a particular cortical locus. The basis for this appears to have been the work of his associate von Tchisch (1886). Between these entrances and exits lie regions which came to be called associational. There was considerable discussion as to whether the primary receptive and emissive loci were involved in higher cerebral functioning or whether this was a unique function of the association areas. Later, when it was found that the association as well as primary receptive regions gave rise to projection fibers it would be argued (Poliak, 1932, p. 213) that their function could not be exclusively of the "higher process" type.

In the meanwhile (in the first decade of the present century), one of the first orders of business was the necessity of determining what the connections (and, derivatively, functions) might be of those thalamic masses* whose functions could not easily be surmised on the basis of obvious connections. Among those who directed their

----

*The nomenclature of the thalamus is further discussed below. For the moment it will suffice to say that, as in horticulture and entomology, work on the thalamus has always been hampered by difficulties due to nomenclature. Comparative neurologists have long been aware of this problem but clinicians are generally unprepared for the fact that lower forms do not possess diencephalic arrangements which can conveniently be designated by any terminology developed for the human brain. The thalamic regions of carnivores, rodents and avians all have distinctive terminologies which cannot be applied outside the form without doing some violence to important concepts. It is only by generalizing, in a broader sense than many specialists are willing to allow that one can employ the same terms across species lines. The first satisfactory treatment of this subject occupied the major efforts of the comparative anatomist, James Papez, over a long period of years (Papez and Aronson, 1934; Aronson and Papez, 1934). In this historical sketch we employ a modification (Mettler, 1948) of that system of terminology. The knowledgeable reader will perceive that the speakers in the present symposium illustrate the still confused state of thalamic terminology. It is obvious, for example, that what is called VL by one investigator is not identical with the VL of another. Professor Jasper has animadverted upon the use of the expression "non-specific" as applied to those thalamic nuclei which are not the primary relay in the principal afferent systems. That expression is an outgrowth of physiologic preconceptions attached to the revival, in the late 1940's, of the non-specific concept of reticular function, a concept concerning which Mettler animadverted in 1964 in a critical review of reticular "systems" and "non-specific" functions. It has not been possible, in this symposium (as it was in the ARNMD symposium on the hypothalamus) to obtain any agreement among the speakers as to terminology and the resolution of this subject is still far from obvious. The reader is warned that when one participant employs a particular structural connotation it may not be in the same sense that another participant does and, in particular, when a non-anatomist uses a structural designation he may not be referring to any anatomically recognizable entity but to the hypothetical substrate of a physiological function.

attention to this subject was Monakow who was particularly interested in the distribution of the fiber systems passing through the upper mesencephalic tegmentum (1895). Since it was known that particular thalamic regions degenerated when restricted cortical areas were damaged, he was able to correlate these two levels topographically. (This material was reviewed by Soury*, op. cit., p. 643 et seq.) The early development of electrophysiology, and of methods of preparing stained serial sections of the neural system was, at that early date, still unable to provide any conclusive information as to which of the fibers that coursed between the diencephalon and cortex were ascending and which, descending. Comparative physiology and neuropathology reenforced the imperfect knowledge that some parts of the cortex were predominantly receptive and others predominantly motor, but this threw very little light upon the relative importance of possible corticothalamic projections. It was apparent to Monakow that the specificity of the relations between the thalamus and the cortex, on the one hand, and those of the large sensory systems to the thalamus, on the other, could be used as a clue to the nature of the functions of the cortex and consequently he focussed his attention upon a series of studies which eventuated in 1914 in his classic book on cerebral localization.

During World War I, the subject of cerebral localization was further extended by the employment of electrical stimulation, and by the perfection of neurosurgical techniques which, in the post-war period, were applied to the investigation and treatment of the convulsive disorders and cerebral tumors, activities which provided an abundance of information about motor function. This work can be followed in the various publications of Otto Foerster (1923, et seq.) and later by his associate, Penfield (Penfield and Erickson, 1941, Penfield and Jasper, 1954). During the twenties, a corollary to work on the motor system was developed by Dusser de Barenne who applied strychnine to various portions of the sensory apparatus with a view to throwing its maximum extent into relief. To the outlying parts of the sensory receptive mechanism (especially those in the cerebral cortex), Dusser de Barenne applied the term "secondary" sensory mechanism (1924). For obvious technical reasons, anatomical studies of the thalamus rarely concern themselves with the issue of the existence of relative abundance of corticothalamic fibers. Such studies are more often descriptions of the form and disposition of the cell bodies which compose the constituent "nuclei" of the thalamus than of fiber connections. When they are of the latter type they deal usually with thalamofugal fibers or with the endings of easily defined systems, such as tractus opticus basalis (O'Leary, 1940) (or, in the case of chiroptera-anterior accessory optic tract, Gillilan, 1941). It is to studies of the cortex that we must go in order to locate the sources of most of our information upon the morphology of corticothalamic connections, and in such work the investigators have been more concerned with location of origin than with the precise spot and manner of termination.

The first clear demonstration of the validity of the assumption that the cerebral

----

* Soury was a classicist, not a physician. For biographic notes on this severely neurotic scholar see Schiller (Haymaker and Schiller, 1970, p. 573).

cortex projected back upon the thalamus was an outgrowth of histologic studies of stained degenerating fibers which suggested that among the abundant corticifugal systems, some of the fibers did not pass beyond the thalamus. The second volume (1901) of Dejerine's magnificent treatise on the anatomy of the nervous system contains a summary (p. 370) of existing opinion on this subject at the turn of the century. Meynert, Flechsig, Bechterew and Edinger believed that most of the fibers in the corona radiata were corticothalamic; von Monakow held the opposite point of view. The intermediate position was taken by Koelliker, who thought that the relative abundance of fibers of particular types of polarity was a necessary reflection of the function of the connection, the fibers running between the lateral geniculate and occipital cortex, for example, being predominantly thalamocortical. In a number of pathologic cases, with relatively large lesions, Dejerine used the Marchi method to demonstrate the existence of degenerated fibers coursing between the cortex and thalamus. For example, a perirolandic lesion was found to be accompanied by widespread degeneration throughout the thalamus. Although corticipetal as well as corticifugal fibers degenerated under such conditions, and he could not be certain of polarity, he delineated (1901, fig. 249) a corticifugal connection from the occipital cortex to the lateral geniculate body. By 1906 the principle was generally accepted, even at clinical levels, that the thalamus contained "the terminal arborizations of neuraxones of cells lying in the cortex" as well as "in the sensory cranial and spinal nuclei below" (Mettler, 1906). Although the Marchi method (Marchi and Algeri 1885) was well established at that time, it should not be assumed that this enabled the workers of the times to determine the polarity of the degenerated fibers they were examining since most of their material came from necropsies of cases that had lived long enough to have permitted retrograde degeneration to occur. (A significant critique of the Marchi technique was published by De Lange in 1908, see his p. 115.)

At the present time it is difficult to appreciate what a relatively small role experimentation played in the investigative efforts of the turn of the century. It was not until the late twenties (D'Hollander, 1922; Allen, 1923; Kingsbury and Johannsen, 1927; Duncan, 1931; Mettler, 1932) that a sufficiently large body of properly timed, experimental Marchi material was available to form comprehensive judgments about polarity. The earliest papers specifically devoted to corticothalamic projections, and which fulfilled this requirement were those of D'Hollander (1922), Biemond (1930), Poliak (1932), Hirasawa and Kato (1935), Mettler (1935-6), Koikegami and Imogawa (1936) and Levin (1936). A valuable review of the material of this and the immediately succeeding period is available in Knook (1965).

Even before functionally oriented, experimental, anatomopathologic studies were going on, independent evidence for the existence of corticothalamic fibers had, however, been developed by the pure morphologic investigations of Cajal, Golgi, Koelliker and others.

For Cajal, corticothalamic fibers may be either of a "descending motor," or "descending sensory" nature (Ramon Cajal, 1911, II; 876, fig. 548, item a). In the latter case they end in a "sensory nucleus," such as the medial or lateral geniculate. The silver impregnated material Cajal drew upon for these conclusions was obtained from new-born rodents and lagomorphs and, in fortunately situated fibers, was small enough to visualize their entire length. He states that corticothalamic fibers arise from sensomotor (i.e., central) cortex and delineated them as originating from gigantopyramids.

Diencephalic terminology. We have already indicated that a major obstacle to experimental work on the thalamus arises from the difficulty of determining what parts of the thalamus of experimental animals, such as the rat and cat, correspond with one another, and with the parts of the simpler primate and human thalamus. Even before such comparisons can be made, it is necessary (Clark, 1932) to come to some agreement as to what to call the parts of the latter.

Anatomically speaking, the thalamus is a part of the diencephalon, which comprises all the material in the caudal part of the embryologic prosencephalon (forebrain); the rostral part of the prosencephalon being the telencephalon. The diencephalon, in turn, is divided into the epithalamus (pineal body and habenular region), thalamus and metathalamus (which taken together were formerly called "optic thalamus" and are now often spoken of as dorsal thalamus, or thalamus "proper"), and ventral thalamus (which includes the septal and preoptic regions, the hypothalamus and the subthalamus, which is the rostral continuation of the mesencephalic tegmentum). Officially, the epithalamus and dorsal thalamus compose the thalamencephalon.

In official anatomic terminology (histologic as well as gross), designation of the components of the thalamencephalon remain admittedly controversial (Mitchell, 1968). At this point it is necessary to anticipate some comments I made in my summary of the first morning's session with respect to the terms dorsal and ventral thalamus.

Examination of the medial wall of the human thalamus generally discloses a rather definite hypothalamic sulcus extending from the anterior commissure caudally to the iter. This roughly indicates the division not only between the "dorsal thalamus" above it, and the hypothalamus below, but also between the former and nuclear masses which lie rostral and caudal to the hypothalamus proper. These are, proceeding from before backward, the septal region, and preoptic region, in front of the hypothalamus and, behind it, the subthalamus, tegmentum and mesencephalon (Mettler, 1948, pp. 396-400). The attention of most writers on the "thalamus" has been focussed upon the "dorsal thalamus," and the essential feature of the terminology at present is one or another modification of its division into three nuclear groups—anterior, lateral and medial.

During the early part of the century there were two converging, but still independent, schools of diencephalic taxonomy with respect to the dorsal thalamus. One of these had been developed by clinical neurologists who had a need to describe the location of areas in which they encountered morbid changes in the brains of persons who had died after suffering from some particular disorder. The other descriptive idiom had arisen as the result of work by comparative anatomists who were influenced by both embryologic and comparative studies. In 1909 these two terminologies were represented respectively by the nomenclature of Monakow (1895) (anterior tubercle, lateral nucleus, medial nucleus, ventral nucleus and posterior nucleus) and that of Koelliker (1896) (anterior nucleus, anteromedial nucleus, mediomiddle nucleus, ventral reticular nucleus, lateral reticular nucleus, dorsal reticular nucleus, nucleus of the midline, lateral nucleus, ventral nucleus, lateral posterior nucleus, habenular nucleus and posterior nucleus). Münzer and Wiener and Haller and others used still different terms. Each of the larger sub-divisions named above encompassed subsidiary units, the names of many of which had been taken over from earlier terminologies. Thus Monakow's medial nucleus was subdivided into parts a, b and c, of which b was Luy's classical centre median. A consistent effort to reconcile these divergent terminologies was made in publications issuing from Obersteiner's Institut für Anatomie und Physiologie des Centralnervensystems which was, appropriately enough, a synonym of the Neurologischen Institut an der Wiener Universität. Ernest Sachs, one of the early workers on the thalamus in Obersteiner's laboratory, subsequently removed to Sir Victor Horsley's laboratory and gave (1909) the following version of Obersteiner and Marburg's synthesis of Koelliker's terminology: n. anterior, n. disseminati, n. medius, n. lateralis, n. lateralis ventralis, centre median, n. arcuatus, external and internal geniculate bodies.

At the time Sachs was active in Obersteiner's and Horsley's laboratories it was conceded that the thalamus served as a relay in the optic and somatosensory (as represented by the medial lemniscus) systems to the cerebral cortex. It was also believed that the same relationship existed for the auditory and probably other sensory modalities. It is, of course, now evident that this assumption was not entirely justified with respect to pain, olfaction, gustation and vestibular function. Sachs seems to have been the first to notice that the "inner" (medial) and "outer" (lateral) divisions of the thalamus are relatively independent organizations even though he was in error in concluding that the medial mass projected to the caudate nucleus.

Gradually it became apparent that there were more nuclear masses in the thalamus than could be accounted for on the basis of the assumption that each nucleus was the relay station in the course of a particular ascending primary afferent system. Le Gros Clark (1932) introduced a concept of "upper" and "lower" level nuclei in the thalamus in order to rationalize some of the observed differences between the morphology of human and infraprimate thalami. "A distinctive feature of the mammalian thalamus is the development of an upper level (topographically and functionally speaking) which is not represented in submammalian forms. This occupies the dorsal part of the thalamus above the ventral nucleus, from which it is more or less separated by transversely disposed intralaminar nuclei, and comprises such nuclear masses as the lateral nucleus and the dorsomedial nucleus. These upper levels receive no significant afferent connections from lower sensory centres except by relays through the lower levels of the thalamus. They are related rather to the 'association' areas of the cortex, whereas the nuclei of lower thalamic levels are connected with the sensory projection areas, and they exhibit a progressive increase in relative size and elaboration in higher mammalian types culminating in the primates where the association areas of the cortex attain to their fullest development."

Clark was not aware of a report by Dusser de Barenne and Sager (1931) who had injected strychnine into the thalamus and had been able to enhance bilaterally the effect of tactile, painful and thermal stimulation of the skin. Since this occurred not only when the lateral nuclear group was injected but also after injections into the medial nucleus, mammillary body, and lateral geniculate (strychnine "generally causes dif-

fuse discharges when introduced into the central nervous system." Fulton, 1949, p. 372), it is doubtful whether Clark would have seen in it any support for his nomenclature for the thalamus, which was:
"A. - Lower levels of the thalamus. (1) Ventral group of nuclei, including the main ventral nucleus of the thalamus and its subdivisions, and the nucleus medialis ventralis. (2) Anterior group of nuclei. (3) Nuclei related to the optic tract, including the dorsal and ventral nuclei of the lateral geniculate body, the large-celled nucleus of the optic tract, and the pretectal nucleus. (4) Medial geniculate body.
B. - Upper levels of the thalamus. (1) Lateral group of nuclei, including the pars principalis, or main part of the lateral nucleus and its subdivisions, the pars posterior of the lateral nucleus, and the nucleus suprageniculatus. (2) The centre median nucleus. (3) The dorso-medial nucleus."

While Clark's concept of a separate type of function for the dorsomedial nucleus was a valuable one, he went awry in placing the centromedian nucleus in the same category with the dorsomedial. He recognized "that the dorsomedial nucleus is not represented by any nuclear homologue in the sub-mammalian thalamus" and found fibers passing in both directions between it and the frontal cortex. With respect to the "ventral thalamus" (see preceding definition) he says, "While the ventral part of the diencephalon is ... essentially concerned with the internal environment of the organism, the dorsal part (which includes the thalamus proper and the epithalamus) forms an elaborate sensory correlation centre for the reception of impulses which owe their origin to changes in the external environment. It is through the pars dorsalis diencephali that the organism is enabled to develop an awareness of objective phenomena."

About this time, Fulton and Ingraham (1929) had observed that prechiasmatic lesions altered emotional behavior and Clark saw in this experiment* confirmation of his belief that "the dorso-medial nucleus provides a mechanism whereby the highest functional levels of the brain are enabled to control the more primitive elements of mental activity, such as are represented in emotional reactions, instinctive impulses, etc."

It has been mentioned that it is possible to divide the dorsal thalamus into three large nuclear groups, anterior, medial and lateral and, in order to provide a background for the subsequent discussions, it will be useful to bear in mind that of these

----

* This experiment should not be confused with Fulton and Jacobsen's 1935 report on a frontally lobotomized chimpanzee. In the first report, on a cat, the authors specifically excluded neopallial severance as the factor responsible for the familiar rage reactions they described. In the latter they attributed the change to cortical ablation. Corticothalamic connections were not directly involved in their speculations as to the emotional changes which were considered a confirmation of physiologic opinions on frontal lobe function dating back to Bianchi and earlier. For the role Fulton and Jacobsen's report had in activating Egas Moniz to initiate frontal lobotomy, for the treatment of psychoses in humans, see Freeman and Watts (1950, p. XVI).

masses (the following terminology is from Mettler, 1948), the anterior group projects upon the cingulate part of the limbic lobe, the medial group upon that part of the frontal lobe rostral to area 6 and the lateral group upon parts of the rest of the cerebral mantle, with the front of the lateral nuclear group projecting upon area 6 and the back projecting upon the temporal and occipital primary receptive areas.

The terminology of what are here called medial and lateral groups requires some explication. Between these two groups lies an intralaminar group of nuclei which can be classified with either or considered a separate group. Included in it are several nuclear masses of which the classic centre median is the most prominent. This centromedian nucleus projects to the striatum, especially the putamen.

The lateral nuclear group can be divided into a lateral nuclear group proper and a ventral nuclear group. The correspondence between these in terms of common terminologies is:

Lateral part of lateral group	Lateral nuclear group
Lateral or dorsal nucleus	Lateral dorsal nucleus
Pulvinar	Pulvinar
Metathalamus	Metathalamus
Ventral part of lateral group	Ventral nuclear group
Anterior portion VA	Ventral anterior nucleus
Intermediate portion VL	Ventral lateral nucleus
Posterior portion VP	Ventral posterior nucleus

Of these, VA receives fibers from the pallidum and projects to area 6. VL receives the brachium conjunctivum, as well as fibers from the pallidum, and projects to the precentral gyrus. VP receives somatosensory afferents and projects to the postcentral gyrus and adjacent cortex.

Each of these nuclear groups can be further subdivided and these show topographically localized variations in the distribution of their cortical projections.

Summary of corticothalamic connections. The situation with regard to corticothalamic fibers in the early thirties, just before the application of the high-gain, amplification techniques which made modern electroneurophysiologic investigations possible, may be summarized as follows, according to region of fiber origin. In this summary it must be borne in mind that, in addition to conflicting data obtained in different animal forms, there was a certain amount of variation reported even for the same form. In rats, Clark (1932) thought all of the cortex projected to the ventral part of the lateral nuclear group but in higher forms such generalized connections were not always found and Clark himself did not believe they existed in primates.

Occipital region. In addition to Dejerine's striogeniculate connection, noted above, Kurzveil (1909) had traced a bundle from the canine region to the medial anterior part of the pulvinar. Tschermak (1909) accepted striogeniculate (to the lateral geniculate) and striopulvinar projections in his general treatise on the physiology of the human brain. Striogeniculate connections of one type or another have been confirmed by all investigators (Clark, 1932, Mettler, 1935, etc.) and for many species

(Nauta and Bucher, 1954, for the rat, and so on). In the monkey, Mettler (1935, pg. 236) was able to confirm the projection of the extramacular part of the primate striate cortex upon the lateral geniculate body. This striogeniculate projection did not appear to follow any very rigid somatotopic organization. In addition to it, and a striopulvinar projection, he also traced fibers from the upper lip of the calcarine fissure to the caudal two-thirds of the lateral thalamic nucleus (LPN) itself. Since projections from the striate (as contrasted with the para- and peristriate) cortex to the lateral geniculate body have been denied by a number of responsible investigators (Fulton, 1949, p. 278, f.n.) the exact nature of this connection is critical to the validity of the principle of reciprocal connection so widely accepted. There are several obstacles to arriving at an easy decision. In the first place the exact homologies of the striate cortex (area 17) are not clear from a comparative anatomical point of view. In the second place, area 17 is difficult to ablate without interfering in one way or another, if even only by postoperative pressure and vascular changes and glial invasion. In the monkey, where area 17 lies on the lateral surface of the occipital operculum, Mettler (1935-6) found a very small lesion to be followed by degeneration proceeding to the lateral geniculate, but Poliak questioned whether such degeneration might not be retrograde which seems unlikely in view of the 11-day survival time of Mettler's animals. An area 17-lateral geniculate projection was subsequently once again verified by Drooglever-Fortuyn (1938) for the rabbit. Another problem is the precise location of ending in the lateral geniculate (the optic system ends chiefly in the dorsal nucleus). Mettler could not recognize any special pattern of localization, but localization in the ventral nucleus has been described following a lesion which encroached upon area 18 and 19 (Knook, 1965, p. 99). At the present time most authorities cite a projection from area 17 to the lateral geniculate (Krieg, 1963, Truex and Carpenter, 1969).

Temporal region. Temporogeniculate (medial geniculate) fibers were described by Dejerine (1901), Thompson (1900-1901) and many others (Clark, 1932, for example), although Krieg (1963, his page 371) did not find any. In connection with Rinvik's presentation (in this symposium) it is interesting to observe that Thompson enunciated a "law of bilateral association." According to this, any cortical area projecting to a gray mass on one side of the brain is also connected to the corresponding site on the other side. It is to be noted that Thompson's cortical lesions were restricted to the temporal region, which is the one locus which regularly sends fibers through the anterior commissure which is the route Rinvik found his crossed fibers to take. Landau (1919), who considered the claustrum related to the amygdala, was unable to trace any fibers to it from the insular cortex. According to Mettler (1935), the superior temporal gyrus sends fibers to the medial geniculate body, and the remainder of the temporal region (especially the dorso-posterior part) projects to the pulvinar and lateral nucleus. He also described fibers which passed from the superior temporal gyrus to the lateral hypothalamic nucleus.

Limbic region. There is good agreement that the cingulate cortex projects upon the anterior group of nuclei but not on the exact topographic relations of this connection. Clark and Boggon (1933) found it limited to the dorsolateral part of the principal anterior nucleus (the anteroventral nucleus) but, in the guinea pig, Gerebtshoff and Wauters (1941–1943) found that the rostral cingulate cortex projected to the ventromedial part of the principal anterior nucleus (nuc. anteromedialis), the posterior cingulate to the accessory anterior nucleus (nucleus anterodorsalis) and the retrosplenial area to the region which Clark and Boggon reported was the only one to receive cingulate fibers. Pribram (Pribram and Fulton, 1954) also found fibers passing from the cingulate cortex to the anterior nucleus. Mettler's conclusions (1943) that, in the monkey, the principal anterior nucleus (anteroventral and anteromedial) projects to the cingulate cortex but that the projection of the accessory anterior (anterodorsal nucleus) is unclear (although it distributes to the cortex) is probably in better agreement with Clark and Boggon than with Gerebtshoff and Wauters.

Frontal region. E. Sachs, Sr. (1909) found a projection from the precentral gyrus to the caudal part of the lateral nuclear group, but Bianchi (1922) felt that this region projects to the rostral part of the lateral nuclear group. In carnivores, Riese (1925) had traced fibers from the motor region to the ventral part of the lateral nuclear group and, while Biemond (1930) verified these in the rabbit, he could not find them in monkeys. In 1954 and 1963, Krieg found that corticothalamic fibers from area 4 end in the ventral part of the lateral nuclear group (ventralis lateralis) and, to a lesser extent in ventralis posterior inferior, and perhaps also in paracentral nucleus and nucleus medialis. According to him, these corticothalamics can be distinguished from the thalamocorticals by virtue of their finer calibre. He also felt he had excluded the possibility that they might be collaterals of the pyramidal projection. Carpenter, (Truex and Carpenter, 1969, p. 579) has called attention to an observation by Olszewski (1952), who noticed that precentral corticothalamics run to both the pars oralis and pars caudalis of the ventral lateral nucleus. As Carpenter points out, the cerebellum projects to the pars oralis only.

Descriptions of fibers from the frontal cortex to the medial nucleus appear in the earliest literature on the subject (for a review, see Clark, 1932, p. 466) but were questioned by users of Dusser de Barenne's "physiologic neuronographic" technique, discussed elsewhere. Mettler (1935) was among those confirming a frontomedial connection from premotor cortex rostral to the location where the motor cortex projects to the lateral nuclear group. Others who verified it were Murphy and Gellhorn (1945), Clark (1948) and Meyer (1949). A projection from area 6 to ventralis posterior inferior was described by Krieg (1963, p. 347) who (1954) stated that the projection of area 6 is to the same region as that from 4. "The same points are shared by motor and premotor area." A projection from the frontal region to the submedial nucleus was described by Clark (1948). A projection from the frontal region to the laminary nuclear group has been described by Petras (1964). According to him, area 4 communicates with the centromedian nucleus, and area 6 with the parafascicular and paracentral nuclei.

The frontal cortex has another characteristic projection which runs to the striatum. Since the striatum may be regarded as a precursor of the neopallial mantle, this connection is of considerable interest to psychologists and psychiatrists, as well as to the theoretically-inclined neurophysiologist (see the presentation by Pribram in this symposium). According to Cajal, collaterals of the pyramidal tract reach the caudate nucleus and putamen and this connection has been repeatedly verified. In 1935 Mettler described frontostriate fibers originating in the cortex rostral to area 4. Some of these travel through the subcallosal fasciculus. Frontostriatal connections from cortex rostral to the Betz cell area have since been repeatedly confirmed (Sachs, Brendler and Fulton, 1949, Showers, 1958). Mettler (1945) was of the opinion that area 6 was one of the contributors of these fibers but, according to Krieg (1954), none arise from area 6.

Fibers from the frontal cortex to the globus pallidus were described and denied by many authors. The difficulty is not whether such fibers are present but whether they merely pass through (Mettler, 1945, frontal and temporal regions) or actually end (Mettler, 1945, area 6) in the globus pallidus. This is the sort of question which required to be reinvestigated by bouton degeneration or, better still, electrophysiologic (Stoll, Ajmone-Marsan and Jasper, 1951) techniques.

Parietal region. Many investigators felt that the psychophysiologic requirements of somatosensation demanded a powerful and widely distributed feedback system from the cortex to the thalamus. By the thirties this idea had to undergo some modification, parietothalamic fibers not having been consistently encountered (Minkowski, 1923-4). Poliak (1932, p. 71) stated that the situation in the monkey was as follows: "The existence of an extensive descending cortico-thalamic fiber system, which according to some investigators plays an important role in normal and in pathological somatosensory function (Head, Wallenberg, see also Long, Mellus, Ramon y Cajal, Probst, Hollander, Villaverde and my paper, 1926), cannot definitely be denied, although fibers of this character are somewhat more numerous only in the most ventral zone of the ventro-lateral nucleus."

It will be noticed that according to Poliak the somatosensory receptive cortex is distributing not primarily to the thalamic area which projects to it but to that part of the thalamus which projects to the motor cortex. According to this view the primary thalamic feedback is not reciprocal but complements the intracortical associational system. However, truly reciprocal connections have since been described by many observers. For example, Krieg (1963, p. 347) reported an abundant projection from the simian postcentral gyrus to all parts of posterior portion of the ventral part of the lateral group (VPL, VPM and VPI). According to Clark (1932), the rodent's parietal area projects not only to the thalamus but also emits a pretectal projection.

The reticular thalamic nucleus represents a special morphologic problem. In Mettler's experience, it undergoes complete retrograde degeneration when all the cortex is removed (Scheibel and Scheibel, 1966, however, could not find any fibers in their Golgi sections that they could trace from this nucleus to the cerebral cortex), but it is difficult to detect somatotopically organized loss in it when restricted cortical areas are removed. One gets the impression (Mettler, 1943) that particular parts of the reticular nucleus project to rather widely distributed portions of the pre- and postcentral gyri. This impression is strengthened by the observations of Carman, Cowan and Powell (1964) that it receives fibers from practically all of the cerebral cortex. Because of this extensive corticoreticular system and also because the reticular nucleus is traversed by so many fiber systems it is difficult to draw any conclusions as to what portions of the cortex project upon it, and to what part of the nucleus. Thus it is hard to use it as a test for the reciprocal connection hypothesis.

The intralaminary nuclei also present special problems, not only because they do not disappear entirely when the cerebral cortex is removed and therefore do not project to the cerebral cortex in the usual sense, but because the most easily studied of these, the centromedian, is more particularly related to the corpus striatum (Papez and Rundles, 1937, Walker, 1938, Mettler, '43, '45, '48 see fig. 341 *et seq.*, Freeman and Watts, '50, pg. 287) than to the cerebral cortex; its projections passing to the striatum (especially the putamen) itself and, to some extent, to the medial segment of the pallidum. If we recall that the striatum can be regarded as the precursor of the cerebral cortex, such a relationship provides us with a valuable clue to the reorganization of Clark's principle of phylogenetic hierarchy in the thalamus and permits us to point out the peculiar nature of the centromedian nucleus to be referred to again below.

Function of corticothalamic fibers. In general, practical clinical writers have been more interested in corticothalamic connections than have experimental theorists. In his *Design for a Brain*, Ashby (1952) managed to get along without them and Eccles (1953) was also able to dispose of the neurophysiological basis of mind without ever mentioning such connections. According to Cajal (1903), the corticothalamics discharge the necessary function of purposefully ordering sensory impressions in order to allow the development of attention. This suggestion was expanded by Tilney (Tilney and Riley, 1923, p. 780) in the following speculation. "These fibers ... may conduct impulses from the frontal cortex concerned with the regulation and control of thalamic functions." If uncontrolled, "the emotional impulses arising in the thalamus would undoubtedly create much confusion in the expression of volitional motion. The sensory combinations entering into primitive feeling tone and the emotive expressions arising out of them must therefore be subjected to the control of intelligence and experience, or else the complex social adjustments imposed by civilization would not be properly made. For this reason the cerebral pallium ... directly concerned in the correlation" of experience and the constitution of intelligence might well exert a modifying influence upon primitive emotional reactions. The cortico-thalamic connection, accordingly, appears not only to subject the primordial feeling tone to the dictates of the will, restraining emotive expression in order to meet the demands of social adjustment, but quite as much reflects upon the thalamus the psychic activities of the frontal lobe for the purpose of calling into play the proper emotional responses."

Tilney, a clinical associate of the morphologist, Oliver Strong, and the paleontologist, William Gregory (at Columbia University and the American Museum of Natural History), stood at the intellectual boundary (characterized by psychologic inference from comparative anatomy) which, at that time, divided introspective psychology from experimental behaviorism. Explanations were accepted by Clark (1932, p. 467) and by Fulton (1949, p. 283) but discounted by Penfield and Jasper (1954, p. 167). The unique features of Tilney's speculation were derived from observations made by him of cases of pseudobulbar palsy.

Recent speculations about the function of the corticothalamic link have added little to the reasonable conjecture of the turn of the century that a reciprocal signalling system would have obvious utility (later expressions of this are to be found in McCulloch, 1944, King, Naquet and Magoun, 1957 and others) or the inferences derived from Roussy's emphasis upon the affective release engendered by thalamic destruction (i.e., that the affective phenomena, succeeding upon thalamic discharge are inhibited, as expressed by Tilney, as already noted). Clark's emphasis upon the essentially different character of the medial and lateral thalamic nuclear groups indicated that such an activatory versus inhibitory dichotomy was much too simple since the functions of the corticothalamic fibers, whatever their nature and functions may be, would probably be different in the case of these two different categories of nuclei. That this was a step in the proper direction became apparent by the growth of a considerable literature which has been devoted to the dubious antinomy of specific versus non-specific nuclei (as Jasper has pointed out, in his discussion of the proceedings of the first afternoon of this symposium). Here again we deal not only with a simplistic dichotomy but also with a questionable characterization since the medial nuclear group is not really any less "specific" than the lateral. That the emphasis has been placed upon an irrelevant feature has become increasingly evident in the course of this symposium. While one is not required to accept Frigyesi and Schwartz's theoretical elaboration, it is clear from their data, and from Jasper's remarks, that the application of the term "non-specific" to any portion of the thalamus may be rather misleading, the confusion arising from the fact that the terms specific and unspecific were unfortunately introduced as synonyms for primary cortical relay versus nuclei with other types of connections. As a matter of fact, the entire hierarchy of thalamic nuclei is very specifically and intricately organized (Frigyesi and Machek, 1970, p. 205) depending upon what one is looking for. The detailed and elaborate nature of this organization argues for a high degree of importance for the factors of order and timing of impulses in reception and transmission, and which must enter into whatever activity patterns develop.

Returning to our previous comments on the centromedian nucleus one may wonder why Clark placed it in the same category as the dorsomedial since many persons at that time considered it a relay in the trigeminothalamic system (Papez and Rundles, 1937). Clark admits (1952, p. 463) that his view is at variance with established opinion, but he based it upon the phylogenetic consideration that the classical *centre median* of Luys is a unique primate characteristic which evolves from rather unimpressive intralaminary elements, such as are seen in *Tupaia minor*. He concluded that it is "an integrating mechanism related to" other parts of the primate thalamus.

Morphologic studies never satisfactorily solved the problem of the function of the centromedian nucleus. The trigeminothalamic fibers which run to it seem to go beyond as so also do cerebellar and pallidal efferents. A large corticofugal projection from area 4 passes to it but, since the major outflow of the centromedian nucleus is to the striatum, why should the cortex which itself is already directly connected with the striatum require an additional relay through the centromedian? Electrophysiologic data (Purpura and Cohen, 1962, and the following papers in this symposium suggest that the explanation for this lies in the provision of a timing mechanism which introduces a high degree of sophistication into the manner in which the ancient striatal outflow is coordinated with the highly specialized discharges required by the learned behavior of primates.)

Neurophysiologic techniques. The critical limitation of the histologic techniques in use in the thirties was not artifactual, as has frequently been stated. Competent workers know their artifacts and make allowances for them. The difficulty was uncertainty as to where axons ended. It has already been indicated that Poliak (1932) felt that many of the degenerated fibers which can be found in the pulvinar were corticotectal *fibres en passant*. Surely, there are corticotectal fibers, but does their presence negate the possibility of corticopulvinar elements? Although the Bielschowsky and Rio Hortega techniques provided adequate methods for studying the morphology of degenerating synaptic mechanisms relatively few workers were willing to apply these time-consuming methods to highly variable experimental material. In the meanwhile the writers who were unwilling to speculate had to be content with a reportorial position—such as, following parastriate lesions, "degenerated fibers could be found in the pulvinar." However, during the interim, vacuum tube amplification had opened new possibilities for the detection of the polarity of nerve conduction in buried regions and short fibers of small diameter. This new line of work showed morphologists where it would be profitable to invest the time and effort necessary to employ silver stains for the study of bouton degeneration. Although the electrophysiologic apparatus available at that time was very cumbersome, expensive, and plagued with artifacts, it offered considerable promise that the techniques which were being used to study the Weaver-Bray effect, and other monitored afferent inputs, might soon clear up this question of fiber termination. In the meanwhile the technical obstacles which electrophysiology faced were very considerable, especially in the measurement of short time intervals (for which the d'Arsonval galvanometer-rotating mirror-cinematograph hook-up was too inert for the measurement of significantly short intervals).

It was at this stage of affairs that Dusser de Barenne (1916, 1924, *et seq.*) came forward with the strychninization technique, already mentioned, and which he called "physiologic neuronography." We have previously quoted from Poliak's 1932 monograph, in which he comments on the long recognized, theoretical desirability of a corticothalamic feedback system for somatosensation. Dusser de Barenne and McCulloch (1938, 1941) felt that their particular approach provided physiologic evidence for the system Poliak could not find morphologically. How reliable the strychnine ("physiological neuronograph") technique was is open to question. Penfield and Jasper (1954, p. 177) concluded, on the basis of that literature, that corticifugal fibers from the frontal cortex must be rather sparse but, as we have seen above, there is now good concurrence among morphologists on the existence of a significant projection of this type.

Lack of concordance between histologic and electrophysiologic data. We have already stated that, in spite of the years of effort devoted to the morphologic study of corticothalamic relationships, substantial discrepancies remain within the morphologic literature itself. While some of these are due to the differences in types of data afforded by different histologic techniques, and to variations between species, and to the peculiar circumstances of particular experiments, as well as to terminologic confusion, many points—such as the precise nature of the thalamo-cortical-corticothalamic feedback circuits—remain moot.

When we consider that the electrophysiologic literature enjoys its own complement of disconcerting discrepancies, within its own particular frame of reference, it is not surprising if these two literatures not only fail to agree in many respects but that many apparent agreements may be merely coincidental. One must not place too much confidence in concordances between morphologic and electrophysiologic conclusions until one has examined both rather critically. In some instances, as in Jasper and Droogleever-Fortuyn's (1947) and Chang's (1950) conclusions, that nuclear masses projecting to particular areas of the cortex are also reciprocally connected, we have repeatedly mentioned that, while this seems to be generally true (the doubt of Krieg about the medial geniculate and the shaky foundation of area 17 projection will be recalled), the anatomic data show considerable variation in the extent to which different afferent systems are reciprocally connected and whether they are really connected with the same cells that receive the primary afferent input. Data of these types are difficult to evaluate by either morphologic and electrophysiologic techniques.

As electrophysiologic equipment improved, it became possible to explore the powerful discharges generated by the application of strychnine to nerve cells (electrical recording apparatus was still not sufficiently refined to stimulate discrete cellular units and to pick up small potentials in deep tissue, in the presence of much artifactual background noise) but the inability to correlate a generalized disturbance caused by an ongoing chemical process led to constant efforts to refine technique. Ultimately, reliable methods of localizing the region stimulated, of measuring time intervals, and picking up from very restricted loci, opened the way for the development of an enormous literature, including extensive reviews of the far from consistent data supplied by preceding morphologic investigators. One of the principal difficulties in comparing the morphologically and electrophysiologically developed data is an extension of the terminologic problem to physiologists who were not familiar with its nature or basis. We have seen that morphologists still have not come to complete agreement on a terminology and, when the physiologist is forced to describe his results in morphologic terms, the underlying confusion becomes enormously magnified. This is unfortunate, and efforts such as this symposium must be energetically pursued to minimize it since the obvious limitation of morphologic investigation is its inability to shed satisfactory light on function. Without the assistance of electrophysiologic techniques, it would have been impossible to disentangle the functions of the corticothalamic fibers from those of the cortex on the one hand and those of the thalamus on the other. It is only when temporally meaningful sequences of the detailed events of neuronal transmission became available that the concepts of presynaptic and postsynaptic inhibition could be developed and the latter applied to the cerebral cortex and thalamus.

REFERENCES

1 ALLEN, W.F. 1923 Origin and distribution of the tractus solitarius in the guinea pig. J. Comp. Neur. 35: 171-204.

2 ARONSON, L.R. and PAPEZ, J.W. 1934 Thalamic nuclei of Pithecus (Macaca) rhesus. Dorsal thalamus. Arch. Neurol. & Psych. 32: 27-44.

3 ASHBY, W.R. 1952 Design for a Brain. Wiley. New York.

4 BIANCHI, L. 1922 Mechanism of the Brain and the Function of the Frontal Lobes. Wood. N.Y.

5 BIEMOND, A. 1930 Experimentell-anatomische Untersuchungen über die corticifugalen optischen Verbindungen bei Kaninchen und Affen. Ztschr. f.d.ges. Neurol. u. Psych. 129: 65-127.

\- CAJAL. See RAMON y CAJAL.

6 CARMAN, J.B., COWAN, W.M. and POWELL, T.P.S. 1964 The cortical projections upon the claustrum. J. Neurol., Neurosurg. and Psych. 27: 46-51.

7 CHANG, H.T. 1950 The repetitive discharges of corticothalamic reverberating circuit. J. Neurophysiol. 13: 235-257.

8 CLARK, W.E. LeGROS 1932 The structure and connections of the thalamus. Brain, 55: 406-470.

9 CLARK, W.E. LeGROS and BOGGON, R.H. 1933 On the connections of the medial cell groups of the thalamus. Brain 56: 83-99.

10 CLARK, W.E. LeGROS 1948 The connexions of the frontal lobe in the brain. Lancet, 1: 353-356.

11 DEJERINE, J. 1895-1901 Anatomie des centres nerveux. Paris. J. Rueff.

12 DeLANGE, S.J. 1908 La methode de Marchi. Le Nevraxe. 10: 83-116.

13 D'HOLLANDER, F. 1922 Recherches anatomiques sur les couches optiques. Arch. Biol., Paris, 32: 249-344.

\- DROOGLEEVER-FORTUYN. See FORTUYN.

14 DUNCAN, D. 1931 Marchi method; discussion of some sources of error and value of this method for studying primary changes in myelin sheath. Arch. Neurol. and Psych. 25: 327-355.

15 DUSSER de BARENNE, J.G. 1916 Experimental researches on sensory localizations in the cerebral cortex. Quart. J. Exptl. Physiol. 9: 355-390.

16 DUSSER de BARENNE, J.G. 1924 Experimentelle untersuchungen über die Lokalisation des sensiblen Rindensebietes im Grosshirnrind des Affen (Macacus). Deutsch Ztschr. f. Nervenh. 83: 273-301.

17 DUSSER de BARENNE, J.G. and McCULLOCH, W.S. 1938 The direct functional interrelation of sensory cortex and optic thalamus. J. Neurophysiol. 1: 176-186.

18 DUSSER de BARENNE, J.G. and McCULLOCH, W.S. 1941 Functional interdependence of sensory cortex and thalamus. J. Neurophysiol. 4: 304-310.

19 DUSSER de BARENNE, J. and SAGER, O. 1931 Ueber die sensiblen Functionen des Thalamus opticus der Katze (Untersucht mit der Methode der örtlichen Strychninvergiftung.) Zeitschr. f.d. ges. Neurol. u. Psych. 133: 231-272.

20 ECCLES, J.C. 1953 The Neurophysiological Basis of Mind. Oxford Univ. Press. New York.

21 FOERSTER, O. 1923 Die Topik der Hirnrinde in ihrer Bedeutung für die Motilität. Deut. Zeitschr. F. Nervenheilh. 77: 124-139.

22 FOERSTER, O. 1926 Zur operativen Behandlung der Epilepsie. Deutsche. Ztschr.

Nervenheilk. 89: 137-147.
23 FORTUYN, J. DROOGLEEVER 1938 Experimteel-anatomisch onderzoek over de verbindingen van de hersenschors naar de thalamus opticus van het konign. Thesis. Amsterdam.
24 FREEMAN, W. and WATTS, J.W. 1950 Psychosurgery. Thomas. Springfield, Illinois.
25 FRIGYESI, T.L. and MACHEK, J. 1970 Basal ganglia-diencephalon synaptic relations in the cat. Brain Res. 20: 201-217.
26 FULTON, J.F. and INGRAHAM, F.D. 1929 Emotional disturbances following experimental lesions of the base of the brain. J. Physiol. XXVII-XXVIII.
27 FULTON, J.F. and JACOBSEN, C.F. 1935 The functions of the frontal lobes. Adv. in mod. Biol. 4: 113-123.
28 GELLHORN, E. 1953 Physiological Foundations of Neurology and Psychiatry. Univ. of Minn. Press, Minneapolis.
29 GEREBTSHOFF, M.A. and WAUTERS, A. 1941-3 Recherches sur l'écorce cérébrale et le thalamus du cobaye. La Cellule. 49: 5-70.
30 GILLILAN, L.A. 1941 The connections of the basal optic root (posterior accessory optic tract) and its nucleus in various animals. J. Comp. Neur. 74: 376-408.
31 HAYMAKER, W. and SCHILLER, F. 1970 The Founders of Neurology. Thomas, Springfield.
32 HIRASAWA, K. and KATO, K. 1935 Fasern, insbesondere die corticalen extrapyramidalen aus den Areae 8 und 9 der Grosshirnrinde beim Affen. Folia Anat. japon. 13: 189-217.
33 JASPER, H.H. and DROOGLEEVER-FORTUYN, J. 1947 Experimental studies on the functional anatomy of petit mal epilepsy. Res. Pub. Assoc. Res. Nerv. & Ment. Dis., 26: 272-298.
34 KAPPERS, C.U.S., HUBER, G.C.and CROSBY, E. The Comparative Anatomy of the Nervous System. Macmillan, New York.
35 KING, E.E., NAQUET, R. and MAGOUN, H.W. 1957 Alterations in somatic efferent transmission through the thalamus by central mechanisms and barbiturates. J. Pharmacol. Exptl. Therap. 119: 48-62.
36 KINGSBURY, B. and JOHANNSEN, O.A. 1927 Histological Technique. Wiley, New York.
37 KNOOK, H.L. 1965 The Fibre-Connections of the Forebrain. Van Gorcum. Leiden.
38 KOELLIKER, A. 1896 Handbuch der Gewebelehre des Menschen. Leipzig. Engelmann.
39 KOIKEGAMI, H. and IMOGAWA, M. 1936 Über die Fasern, insbesondere die korticalen extrapyramidalen aus der Area 19a der Grosshirnrinde beim Affen. Morph. Jb. 77: 587-604.
40 KRIEG, W.J.S. 1954 Connections of the Frontal Cortex of the Monkey. Thomas, Springfield.
41 KRIEG, W.J.S. 1963 Connections of the cerebral cortex. Brain Books, Evanston.
42 KURZVEIL, F. 1909 Beitrag zur Lokalisation der Sehsphäre des Hundes. Pflüger's

Arch. 129: 607-625.
43 LANDAU, E. 1918-1919 The comparative anatomy of the nucleus amygdalae, the claustrum and the insular cortex. J. Anat. 53: 351-360.
44 LEVIN, P.M. 1936 The efferent fibers of the frontal lobe. J. Comp. Neur. 63: 369-420.
45 MARCHI, V. and ALGERI, G. 1885 Sulle degenerazioni discendenti consecutive a lesioni della corteccia cerebrale. Revista sperim. di freniat. e med. leg. 11: 492-4.
46 McCULLOCH, W.S. 1944 The functional organization of the cerebral cortex. Physiol. Rev. 24: 390-407.
47 METTLER, FRED A. 1932 Marchi method for demonstrating degenerated fiber connections within the central nervous system. Stain Tech. 7: 95-106.
48 METTLER, FRED A. 1935-6 Corticifugal fiber connections of Macaca mulatta. J. Comp. Neurol. 61: 1-37, 509-542; 62: 263-291; 63: 25-47.
49 METTLER, FRED A. 1943 Extensive unilateral cerebral removals in the primate: physiologic effects and resultant degeneration. J. Comp. Neurol. 79: 185-245.
50 METTLER, FRED A. 1945 Fiber connections of the corpus striatum of the monkey and baboon. J. Comp. Neur. 82: 169-204.
51 METTLER, FRED A. 1948 Neuroanatomy. Mosby, St. Louis.
52 METTLER, FRED A. 1964 Anatomic structures and physiologic systems. Psych. Quart. 38: 203-247.
53 METTLER, LEE H. 1906 Diseases of the nervous system. Cleveland Press, Chicago, pg. 692.
54 MEYER, M. 1949 Study of efferent connexions of the frontal lobe in the human brain after leucotomy. Brain, 72: 265-296.
55 MINKOWSKI, M. 1923-4 Étude sur les connexions anatomiques des circonvolutions rolandiques, parietales et frontales. Schweiz. Arch. f. Neurol. u. Psych. 12: 71, 227; 14: 255; 14: 97.
56 MONAKOW, C. v. 1895 Experimentelle und pathologish-anatomische Untersuchungen über die Haubenregion. Arch. f. Psych. 27: 1-128, 386-478.
57 MONAKOW, C. v. 1914 Die Lokalisation im Grosshirn. Bergmann, Wiesbaden.
58 MURPHY, F.O. and GELLHORN, E. 1945 Further investigations on diencephalic-cortical relations and their significance for the problem of emotion. J. Neurophysiol. 8: 431-447.
59 NAUTA, W.J.H. and BUCHER, V.M. 1954 Efferent connections of the striate cortex in the albino rat. J. Comp. Neurol. 100: 257-285.
60 O'LEARY, J.L. 1940 A structural analysis of the geniculate nucleus of the cat. J. Comp. Neur. 73: 405-430.
61 OLSZEWSKI, J. 1952 The Thalamus of the Macaca Mulatta, Karger, Basel.
62 PAPEZ, J.W. and ARONSON, L.R. 1934 Thalamic nuclei of Pithecus (Macacus) rhesus; ventral thalamus. Arch. Neurol. & Psych. 32: 1-26.
63 PAPEZ, J.W. and RUNDLES 1937 The dorsal trigeminal tract and the centre median nucleus of Luys. J. Nerv. and Ment. Dis. 85: 505-519.
64 PEELE, T.L. 1961 The Neuroanatomic Basis for Clinical Neurology. McGraw Hill, New York.

65 PENFIELD, W. and ERICKSON, T. 1941 Epilepsy and Cerebral Localization. Thomas, Springfield.
66 PENFIELD, W. and JASPER, H. 1954 Epilepsy and the functional anatomy of the human brain. Little, Brown & Co., Boston.
67 PETRAS, J.M. 1964 Some fiber connections of the precentral cortex (areas 4 and 6). Anat. Rec. 148: 322.
68 POLIAK, S. 1932 The main afferent fiber systems of the cerebral cortex in primates. Univ. Calif. Press, Berkeley.
69 PRIBRAM, K.H., and FULTON, J.F. 1954 An experimental critique of the effects of anterior cingulate ablations in monkeys. Brain, 77: 34-44.
70 PURPURA, D.P. and COHEN, B. 1962 Intracellular synaptic activities of thalamic neurons during evoked recruiting responses. Proc. 22nd Intnl.Congr. Physiol.Sc.Excerpta Med. Internl. Congr. Sr. 48, Leiden.
71 RAMON y CAJAL S. 1903 Plan de estructura del talamo optico. Rev. med. cir. pract. Madrid, Mayo.
72 RAMON y CAJAL, S. 1909-11 Histologie du Système Nerveux. Maloine, Paris.
73 RIESE, W. 1925 Beitrage zur Faseranatomie der Stammganglien. J. f. Psychiat. u. Neurol. 31: 81-122.
74 SACHS, E. 1909 On the structure and functional relation of the optic thalamus. Brain, 32: 95-186.
75 SACHS, E., Jr., BRENDLER, S.J. and FULTON, J.F. 1949 The orbital gyri, Brain, 72: 227-240.
76 SHOWERS, M.J. 1958 Correlation of medial thalamic nuclear activity with cortical and subcortical neuronal areas. J. Comp. Neurol. 109: 261-315.
77 SCHEIBEL, M.E. and SCHEIBEL, A.B. 1966 The organization of the nucleus reticularis, thalami: A Golgi study. Brain Res. 1: 43-62.
78 SOURY, J. 1899 Système Nerveux Central. Masson, Paris.
79 STOLL, J., AJMONE-MARSAN, C. and JASPER, H.H. 1951 Electrophysiological studies of subcortical connections of anterior temporal region in cat. J. Neurophysiol. 14: 305-316.
80 THOMPSON, W.H. 1900-01 Degenerations resulting from lesions of the cortex of the temporal lobe. J. Anat. & Physiol. 35: 147-165.
81 TILNEY, F. and RILEY, H.A. 1923 The Form and Functions of the Central Nervous System. Hoeber, N.Y.
82 TSCHERMAK, A. 1909 Physiologie des Gehirns. In W.A. Nagel's Handbuch der Physiologie des Menschens. Band 4.
83 TSCHISCH, W. v. 1886 Untersuchungen zur Anatomie der Grosshirnganglien des Menschen. Ber. ü.d. Verh. d. kön. säch Gesellach. d. Wissensch. zu Leipzig. 38: 95-101.
84 TRUEX, R.C. and CARPENTER, M.B. 1969 Human Neuroanatomy. Williams and Wilkins. Baltimore.
85 WALKER, E. 1938 The Primate Thalamus. Univ. Chicago Press. Chicago.
86 WERNICKE, C. 1881 Lehrbuch der Gehirnkrankheiten, Kassel, Fischer.

Corticothalamic Projections and Sensorimotor Activities
T. Frigyesi, E. Rinvik, and M.D. Yahr, editors. © 1972
Raven Press, New York.

Synaptic Mechanisms in Coordination of Activity in Thalamic Internuncial Common Paths

Dominick P. Purpura

INTRODUCTION

"Thalamic neurones form a path upon which the dorsal-column-fillet and spino-cerebellar-peduncular paths converge. Each internuncial path is therefore usually, to some extent, a common path, just as usually the receptive neurone, i.e., private path, itself is common to a small number of receptors. Since each instance of convergence of two or more afferent neurones upon a third, which in regard to them is efferent, affords an opportunity for coalition or interference of their actions, each structure at which it occurs is a mechanism for co-ordination. Whatever may be the intimate nature of the mechanism which gives co-ordination by the formation of a common path from tributary paths, such common paths exist in extraordinary profusion in the architecture of the gray-centered nervous system of vertebrates."

The Integrative Action of the Nervous System
Sir Charles S. Sherrington, 1906 (p. 145)

The convergence of internuncial common paths onto thalamic neurons amply attests to the importance of the thalamus as a "mechanism for co-ordination" in the Sherringtonian sense. But having said this in no way brings us closer to the truth of what is co-ordinated in the thalamus or how the mechanisms for co-ordination derive from physiological processes. As to the question, "What is actually co-ordinated in the thalamus?", the answer is invariably, "Sensorimotor activities". The same answer is applicable to questions relating to internuncial systems throughout the neuraxis as Sherrington long recognized. What confers primacy upon the thalamus in this regard is the magnitude of the convergent input from spinal cord, brain stem, cerebellum, corpus striatum and cerebral cortex; the extraordinary diversity of neuronal elements upon which the input is funnelled; and the massive projections from internuncial common paths of the thalamus to the cerebral cortex and basal ganglia. As regards neurophysiological correlations of behavior, however, the generalization that the thalamus plays a major role in the integration of sensorimotor activities rests more on what surely must be the case, than what has actually been demonstrated. This is not to ignore those separate lines of inquiry, that have led to the characterization of input-output functions of thalamic neurons with private line operations on the one hand, and analysis of thalamic neurons with more generalized operations on the other. But despite the large volume of extant research on the structure and function of the thalamus little is known concerning the physiological basis for sensorimotor co-ordination in the thalamus or for that matter, how convergent inputs, irrespective of their overt functional significance, are distributed in thalamic interneuronal common paths. This state of events is not likely to be altered without considerably more information on the synaptic organization of thalamic neuronal subsystems activated by different inputs and further analysis of the manner in which diverse synaptic mechanisms contribute to the processing of this convergent input.

Several aspects of the foregoing problems have been investigated in the author's laboratories for the past decade in attempts to provide additional information on the nature and organization of synaptic systems constituting the 'common path' of different convergent and reciprocally related thalamic projection pathways. The present survey attempts to highlight major findings in these investigations that relate to problems of the organization of intrathalamic interneuronal systems operated by different inputs and the diversity of synaptic processes that contribute to these differences. Suffice it to say that these problems are relevant to many of the reports included in this volume.

Intrathalamic Organization of Internuclear Synaptic Systems.

Medial and intralaminar nuclear groups of the thalamus comprise a heterogeneous system of synaptically interrelated neurons whose activation by repetitive, low-frequency stimulation is capable of influencing the discharge characteristics of neurons in widespread parts of the thalamus (Fig. 1A) (40, 46). This system has been referred to variously as the nonspecific, or generalized thalamocortical projection system as well as the thalamic reticular system (10, 23, 24, 29, 30). Electrical stimulation almost anywhere within this system will result in evoked cortical responses which typically increase in amplitude during initial phases of a continuous train of 6-12/sec stimuli as illustrated in Fig. 1 (10, 29). Depending upon the site of cortical registration evoked responses may exhibit different latencies and waveforms with prominent surface-negativities recorded maximally in rostral cortical locations.

The organizational features of the interneuronal pathways set into operation by medial thalamic (MTh) stimulation can be discerned by examination of the patterns of postsynaptic potentials (PSPs) elicited in neurons located in different nuclear groups of the thalamus (40, 46). The most frequently encountered synaptic events are summarized in Fig. 1A. The first MTh stimulus, which elicits very little activity in cortex nonetheless evokes a short-latency, prolonged inhibitory postsynaptic potential (IPSP) in many elements. Successive stimuli evoke similar long duration IPSPs which are generally preceded by EPSPs of variable duration and effectiveness. Neurons of intralaminar nuclei may exhibit high-frequency bursts of discharges superimposed on

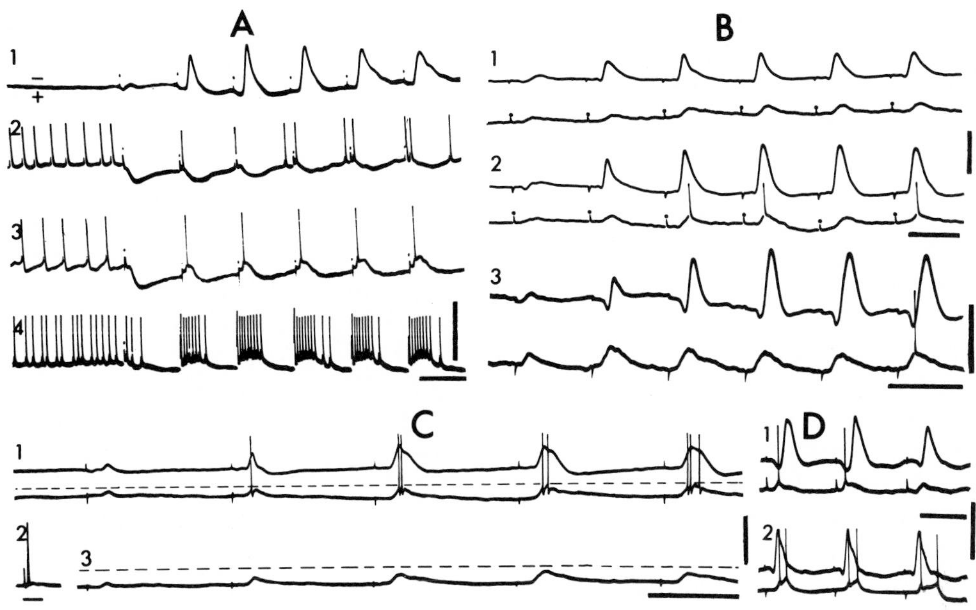

FIG. 1. Patterns of evoked synaptic activities observed in intracellular recordings from different types of neurons during thalamocortical synchronization induced by low-frequency (7-10/sec) stimulation of medial nonspecific thalamic nuclei. Calibrations throughout, 50 mv for intracellular records; 100 msec.

A: 1, example of surface-negative cortical recruiting response. 2-4, EPSP-IPSP sequences recorded in thalamic neurons in different nuclei during recruiting responses. IPSPs, prominent in thalamic elements during this type of activity, play a major role in synchronizing thalamic neuronal discharges. (From: Purpura and Shofer, (46).

B: Upper channel records, recruiting responses from motor cortex; lower channel records, intracellular activities of caudate neurons. 1, threshold stimulation elicits prominent EPSPs in a caudate neuron. 2, increase in stimulus strength produces cell discharges. 3, cell discharges are rare in caudate neurons despite large amplitude EPSPs during recruiting responses. IPSPs are not common in contrast to findings in thalamic neurons. (From: Purpura and Malliani, (43).

C: Characteristics of EPSPs elicited in a pyramidal neuron of motor cortex during recruiting response. 1, EPSP builds up with repetitive stimulation. 2, antidromically evoked response (cal. 10 msec). 3, slow increase in membrane potential reduces the effectiveness of EPSPs. Dashed line through "firing level" as indicated in 1.

D: PSP patterns and associated cell discharges in two cortical interneurons. These elements generally exhibit a larger number of spike discharges than large pyramidal cells during recruiting responses. (From: Purpura, Shofer and Musgrave, (47).

EPSPs (Fig. $1A_4$). In other neurons IPSPs may tend to summate, thereby driving the membrane potential to relatively hyperpolarized levels, and limiting discharges to periods between successive IPSPs when EPSPs can attain the firing level. The net effect of such EPSP-IPSP sequences is to synchronize neuronal discharges in widespread parts of the thalamus. Indeed so effective is the control of thalamic neuronal activity by internuclear interneuronal pathways arising in nonspecific nuclei that in favorable experiments the PSP patterns observed in widely separated neurons may be remarkably similar in over characteristics (Fig. 2) (42).

Distinguishing features of the IPSPs observed in thalamic neurons during MTh-stimulation are their latency and time-course. While latencies as short as 4-6 msec have been observed in some ventroanterior and ventrolateral thalamic neurons, for the most part IPSP latencies range from 10-40 msec. IPSP durations of 100-200 msec have commonly been observed, with summation of IPSPs occurring when stimuli are timed to occur prior to the termination of an IPSP (Fig. 2). There can be no question but that these prolonged IPSPs reflect the operation of chemically transmitting inhibitory synapses which activate specific ionic conductances. Evidence supporting this conclusion is illustrated in Fig. 3 from an experiment in which membrane resistance was monitored in a thalamic neuron during the MTh-evoked IPSPs (16). Under these conditions the

---

FIG. 2. Temporal relations of EPSP-IPSP sequences in neurons located in different thalamic regions during motor cortex recruiting responses (upper channel records) evoked by 7/sec stimulation of medial thalamic nonspecific nuclei. The three unidentified neurons were impaled at different depths from the dorsolateral surface of the exposed thalamus during a single penetration of the microelectrode. Depths as follows: (A) 2.0 mm; (B) 4.5 mm; (C) 6.5 mm. Timing of the first three spike discharges elicited by EPSPs is synchronized in the three elements. IPSP latencies and duration are similar except during late phases in B. Note IPSP summation leading to progressive hyperpolarizing shift of membrane potential during continued stimulation. Broken lines drawn through "firing levels" determined by first synaptically evoked response of each series. (From: Purpura et al., (42).

FIG. 3. Relative membrane resistance changes in a thalamic neuron during low-frequency (5 c/sec) stimulation of medial thalamus (MTh). Neuron located in VA-VL regions of the thalamus. 1, marker channel indicating time and duration of transmembrane current injection. 2, cortical surface recording of evoked recruiting responses. 3, intracellular record showing membrane potential changes produced by 25 c/sec, 20 msec duration, 2 nA inward current pulses. A, Control. Neuron exhibits several 50 mV spontaneous spike discharges followed by a quiescent phase. B, MTh stimulation is initiated at first arrowhead (Δ) during a burst of spontaneous spikes. Increase in membrane polarization begins 30-40 msec after the stimulus and exhibits variations in relation to subsequent stimuli (Δ) in C and D. Recruiting responses exhibit 'alternation' characteristics (C_2, D_2). Membrane resistance decrease follows the time course of the evoked membrane potential increase. E, several seconds after cessation of stimulation. (From: Feldman and Purpura, (16).

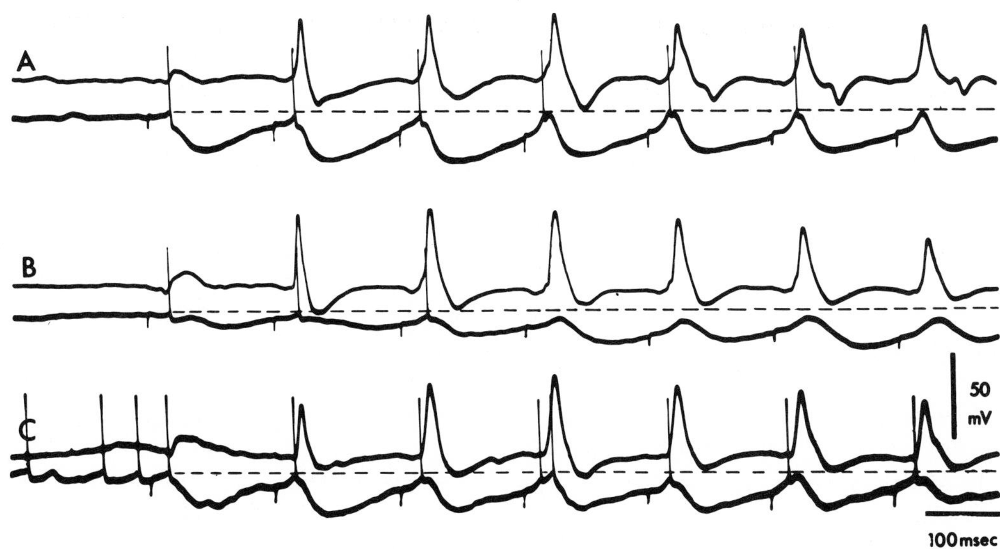

FIG. 2

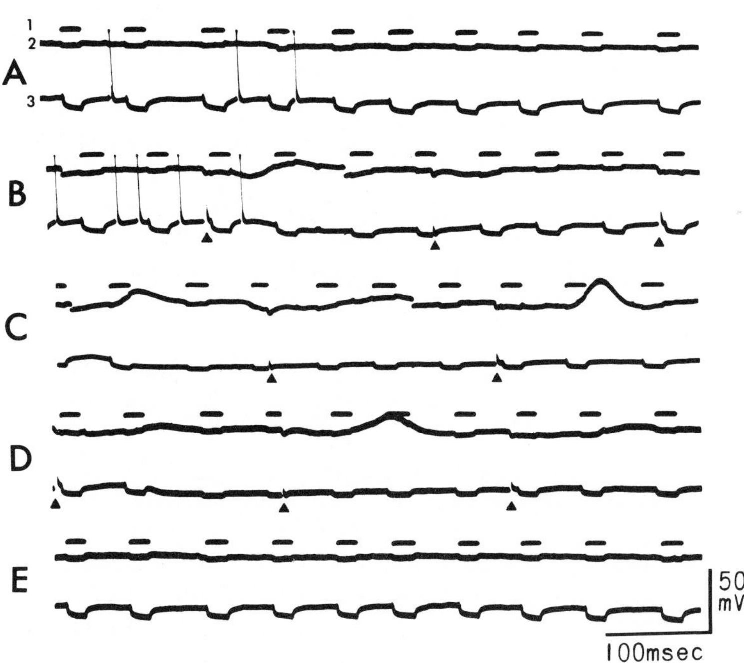

FIG. 3

increase in membrane polarization during the depression of neuronal discharge is associated with a marked and persisting increase in membrane conductance. Thus the generalized synchronizing effects produced by MTh stimulation on thalamic neurons are adequately accounted for in terms of EPSP-IPSP sequences. There would appear to be no necessity to invoke additional processes, such as postanodal exaltation (1) in the mechanism of neuronal synchronization (35, 36). This conclusion has been affirmed by recent studies of others (5).

The synaptic effects observed in thalamic neurons during MTh-stimulation are not distributed equipotently in different nuclear organizations. Prominent effects are particularly noted throughout ventrolateral, rostral and dorsolateral thalamic nuclear groups (19, 21, 38). Most important from the standpoint of the control exerted by nonspecific-specific internuclear interneuronal synaptic pathways on thalamocortical projection activity is the fact that MTh-induced EPSP-IPSP sequences are invariably observed in VL neurons interposed in the cerebello-thalamocortical projection pathway (8, 20, 42, 45). Depending upon the temporal relations between brachium conjunctivum- and MTh-evoked responses in VL relay cells, such PSP sequences may result in complete suppression (Fig. 4) or facilitation of VL relay activity (44). Thus the nonspecific-specific internuclear pathway provides a powerful mechanism for "gating" or modulating the input-output functions of the major afferent system to the motor cortex and its corticofugal projection systems (36, 42).

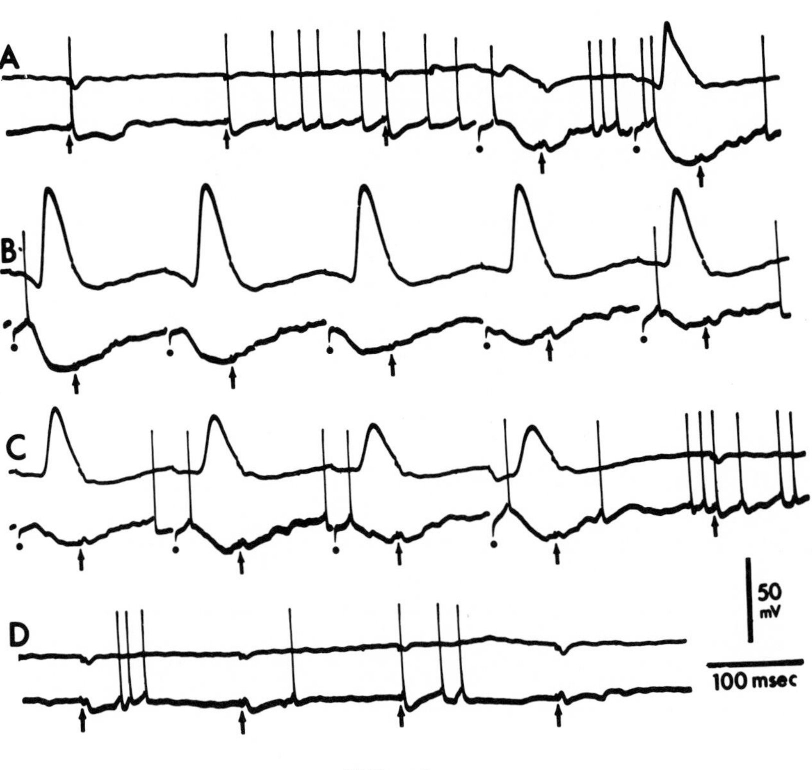

FIG. 4

In striking contrast to the effects observed in VL neurons during MTh-stimulation it has not been possible to detect a significant influence of MTh-stimulation on relay neurons of the ventrobasal complex (27). However, although VB neurons exhibiting monosynaptic EPSPs to medial lemniscus stimulation fail to respond to medial thalamic stimulation this is not the case for VB neurons activated multisynaptically by lemniscal volleys (27). Evidently electrical stimulation of medial and intralaminar thalamic nuclei is not capable of activating those neuronal subsystems impinging upon VB relay cells which participate in spontaneous synchronizing activities such as are observed during spontaneous 6-12/sec spindle bursts (Fig. 5). This emphasizes the multiplicity of neuronal organizations involved in different varieties of "synchronizing" activities in different thalamic nuclear groups (1-5). More to the point is the conclusion from observations of the differential effects of MTh-stimulation on VL and VB relay cells that nonspecific-specific internuclear pathways appear to operate preferentially in relation to relay and associative thalamic neurons in which preservation of place and modality specificity is not an essential feature of the transformation process.

Reciprocal Interactions

It was not appreciated until recently that the internuclear synaptic pathways linking medial and ventrolateral thalamic nuclei (45) are reciprocal in nature (11, 13). However, it is not to be inferred from this that the reciprocal pathways are functionally equivalent in overt operation, since striking differences have been noted in the latencies of IPSPs evoked in medial thalamic neurons following VA-VL stimulation in comparison to the IPSP latencies observed in VA-VL neurons following medial thalamic stimulation. Examples of very short (1-1.5 msec) latency prolonged IPSPs intracellularly recorded from medial thalamic neurons in response to single stimuli delivered to VA-VL areas of the thalamus are illustrated in Fig. 6. Such IPSPs are among the shortest latency inhibitory events observed in thalamic neurons in the course of an extensive series of investigations of internuclear relations (11, 12, 13, 18, 19, 21).

The complex transactions taking place in specific-nonspecific internuclear synaptic pathways are illustrated by the results shown in Figs. 7 and 8. Repetitive low-

---

FIG. 4. Inhibition of VL cell discharges evoked by 7/sec brachium conjunctivum (BC) stimulation (at arrows) during concomitant 7/sec medial thalamic stimulation (indicated by dots under shock artifacts). Medial thalamic stimulation precedes BC stimulation by 70 msec during the interaction. (A-D) Continuous record: Medial thalamic stimulation elicits a typical long-latency surface-negative recruiting response in motor cortex. A sequence of small EPSPs and more prominent prolonged IPSPs are observed in the VL cell. (A-C) Inhibition of BC-evoked discharges occurs during the thalamocortical recruitment. (D) Cessation of medial thalamic stimulation reveals persisting but variable inhibition of BC-evoked discharges. (From: Purpura et al., (45).

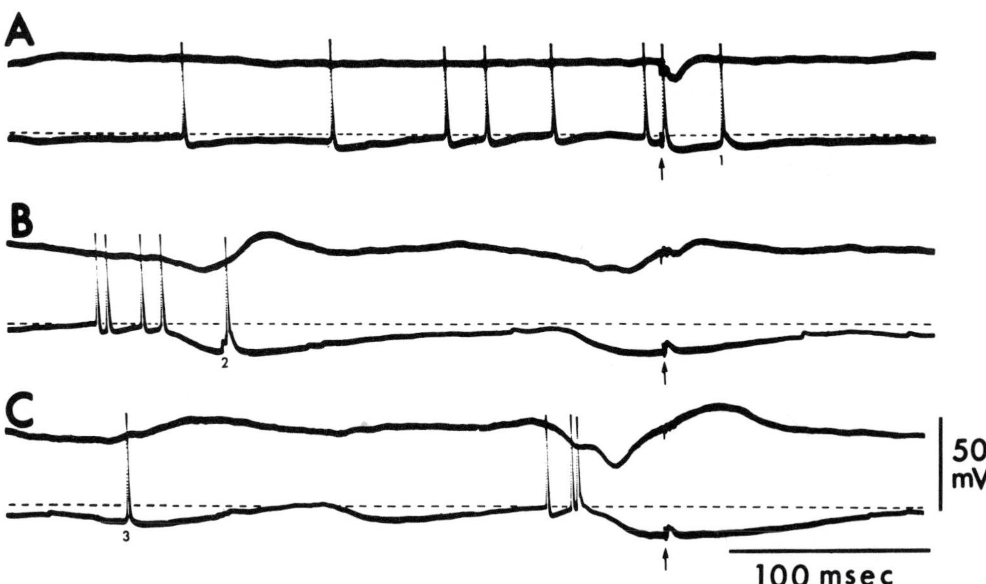

FIG. 5. Membrane potential changes in an identified VB relay cell during spontaneously developing cortical spindle waves. Horizontal dashed lines are drawn through baseline membrane potential levels to emphasize magnitude and duration of membrane hyperpolarizations during different phases of electrocortical waves. A–C: from a continuous record in which segments have been removed to permit alignment of monosynaptic responses to medial lemniscus (ML) stimulation (at arrows). During spontaneous IPSPs relay discharges are blocked revealing the ML-evoked EPSP in isolation. Spontaneous spike discharges are modulated in frequency during IPSPs. Some of these spikes arise from a level of increased membrane polarization (1 and 3) and one exhibiting multiple brief depolarizations (cf. Maekawa and Purpura, (26) is shown in B (2). (From: Maekawa and Purpura, unpublished.)

frequency stimulation of VA-VL regions of the thalamus elicits primary and augmenting responses in motor cortex. Simultaneous recordings of cortically evoked responses and intracellular activities of a medial thalamic neuron reveal that both the primary and augmenting responses are associated with short-latency IPSPs in the thalamic neurons. But the augmenting response is associated with an alteration in IPSP latency and an interruption, probably caused by an EPSP, which tends to reduce the early phase of the IPSP and shift the latency of its second component (Fig. 7).

A much more dramatic alteration in synaptic drives observed during repetitive VA-VL stimulation is shown in Fig. 8. In these recordings from a medial thalamic neuron the first stimulus of the repetitive train elicits a long latency, prolonged IPSP where-

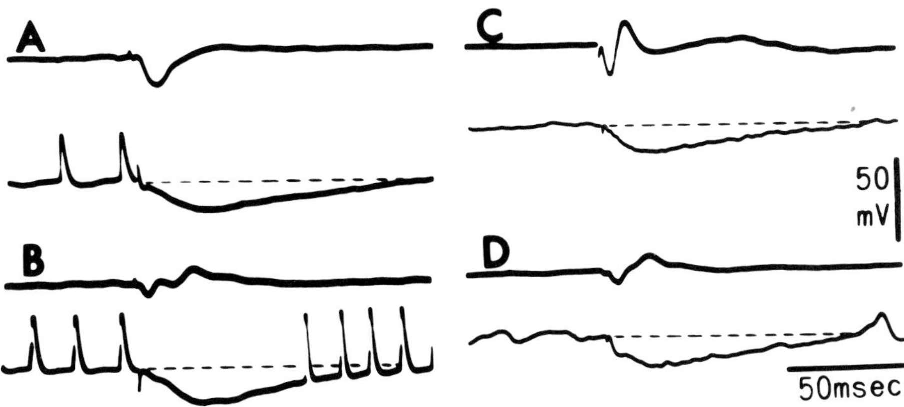

FIG. 6. Examples of intracellular recordings (lower channel records) obtained with 2 M potassium citrate filled micropipettes from medial thalamic neurons in 4 different preparations. Specific responses to VL stimulation recorded monopolarly from motor cortex are shown in upper channel records (negative upwards). Amplitudes of cortical surgace responses ranged from 200-250 μV. A and B, cells exhibiting 30-40 mV spike potentials prior to VL stimulation and short-latency IPSPs immediately following stimulation. C and D, cells partially depolarized following impalements. In these elements, as well as in A and B, IPSPs are not preceded by EPSP. Dashed horizontal lines drawn through baseline membrane potential. Note that the IPSP characteristics in medial thalamic neurons are independent of the characteristics of primary evoked responses recorded in motor cortex. (From: Desiraju et al., (11).

as successive stimuli evoke powerful EPSPs with bursts of spike potentials. These EPSPs arise from a baseline of sustained membrane hyperpolarization resulting from summation of IPSPs.

The foregoing studies highlight the intrathalamic organization of synaptic pathways linking neurons in specific and nonspecific nuclei. They emphasize the fact that despite the obvious complexity of these pathways, as judged in part, by the variable latencies of synaptic events initiated by stimulation in specific or nonspecific nuclei, relatively few PSP patterns underlie the physiological operations in this interneuronal system. The regularity of the EPSP-IPSP sequence pattern is particularly noteworthy in both specific and nonspecific elements irrespective of the site of stimulation within the system of reciprocal interconnections. This speaks in favor of some degree of uniformity in the intrinsic organization of excitatory and inhibitory interneuronal elements constituting the internuclear projection pathway. Such differences that do exist in PSP patterns in different nuclei may be accounted for by local variations in intrinsic

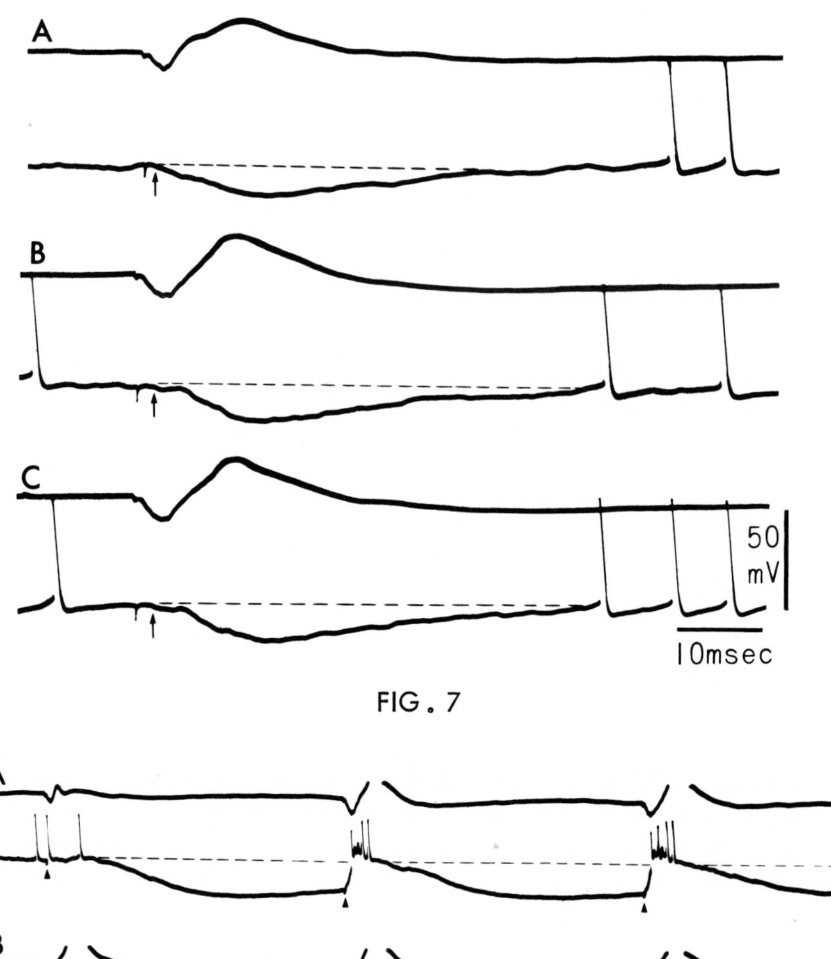

FIG. 7

FIG. 8

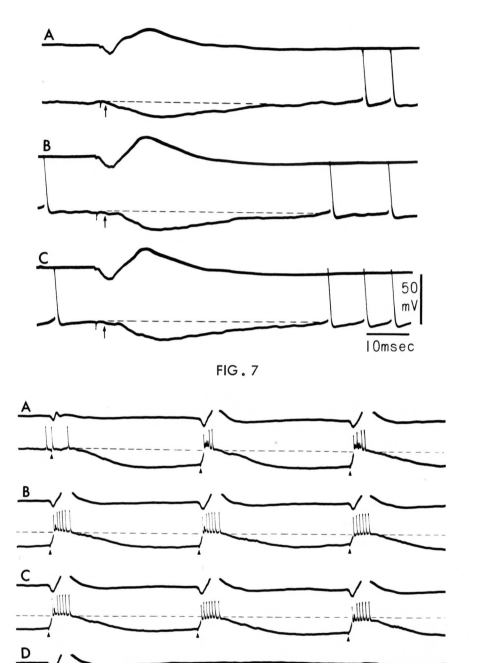

synaptic organization (38). Viewed in this fashion it is not surprising that local variations in synaptic organizations may, under appropriate conditions give rise to patterns of synchronizing activities that are different in different parts of the thalamus, particularly when functional coupling via internuclear pathways is minimal or absent. To the extent that the mechanisms underlying the evoked synchronizing activities illustrated in Figs. 1-8 are related to the spontaneous spindles in unanesthetized decorticate preparations or animals with cortical and spinal lesions (3, 4, 5) it follows that the variations in spindle characteristics observed in the latter studies may be largely related to the factors noted above.

A problem of no little concern is how electrical stimulation, which obviously activates all elements indiscriminately within the vicinity of effective stimulating currents, can elicit the stereotype PSP patterns in neurons randomly impaled in different nuclear groups of the thalamus. One explanation is possible if it is assumed

---

FIG. 7. Alterations in characteristics of IPSPs elicited in a neuron of the medial thalamus (MTh) during repetitive stimulation (6 c/sec) of n. ventralis lateralis (VL). Upper channel records are surface evoked responses (negativity upwards) recorded from motor cortex. A-C, first 3 responses to VL stimulation at 6 c/sec. A, first stimulus elicits a typical positive-negative primary response in motor cortex. Intracellular recording from a MTh neuron located at a depth of 4.5 mm from the surface of the thalamus reveals a 1.5-2.0 msec latency IPSP (at arrow). B, the second stimulus occurring 140 msec after the first produces an 'augmented' surface evoked response. This is associated with a 2 msec increase in latency of the IPSP which may have been interrupted by a small EPSP. The IPSP is increased in duration and is succeeded by a more prominent EPSP that elicits a spike potential. C, the third stimulus evokes essentially similar cortical surface and intracellular synaptic events as the second stimulus. Baseline membrane potential is indicated by the dashed lines. (From: Desiraju and Purpura, (13).

FIG. 8. Dramatic enhancement of short-latency prolonged EPSPs superimposed on long-duration IPSPs in a medial thalamic (MTh) neuron (depth, 5.5 mm) during 5 c/sec VA-VL stimulation. Arrow heads indicate stimulus artifacts. A, the first stimulus elicits a spike discharge on a short-latency EPSP that is not well illustrated. A prolonged IPSP with a latency of 30-40 msec follows the initial synaptic events. The second and subsequent stimuli delivered during the residual membrane hyperpolarization of the prolonged IPSP evokes a polysynaptic 'giant' EPSP, with superimposed high-frequency spikes and partial spikes. A-C, continuous recording. Two sec. strip of record removed between C and D. In D, the last stimulus of the repetitive train elicits a smaller EPSP with delayed discharges. The terminal IPSP exhibits a superimposed spontaneous EPSP and spike discharge before return to baseline membrane potential level as indicated throughout by the horizontal dashed lines. (From: Desiraju and Purpura, (13).

that stimulation anywhere within the thalamic interneuronal system activates elements which project to a common pool of inhibitory neurons and which, in turn, project widely and diffusely back upon the interneuronal system. Recent studies (50, 51) including those summarized elsewhere in this volume, have suggested a possible role of elements in n. Reticularis in the distribution of this inhibitory activity. A second possibility is that excitatory and inhibitory elements are locally organized in different parts of the thalamus in such a fashion as to permit, through their relations with other neurons, the EPSP-IPSP sequences observed in target neurons. Unfortunately there is no direct evidence that the prolonged IPSPs shown in Figs. 1-8 reflect the high-frequency repetitive activity of inhibitory interneurons since prolonged transmitter action alone might explain the prolonged conductance increases demonstrable in thalamic neurons during the synchronizing IPSPs (16, 35). For present purposes it seems prudent to relegate the EPSP-IPSP sequences to the activity of subsets of excitatory and inhibitory interneurons, organized in some reciprocally related fashion. While the hazards are obvious in this, particularly insofar as the present formulation suggests a *deus ex machina*, it has the advantage of sparing the reader from being subjected to improbable wiring diagrams of interconnected black and white circles and arrows. The obvious problem with such circuit diagrams is that any one of a large number of possible constructions may be equally valid!

Common Path Convergence onto Thalamic Relay Cells and Interneurons.

Neurons of the ventrolateral and ventroanterior nuclei of the thalamus constitute a projection field for convergent inputs from the cerebellum via the brachium conjunctivum and from the lentiform nucleus via the ansa lenticularis (31, 32, 39). Examination of the mode of distribution of postsynaptic activities generated in VL elements by these input systems and the relationship of these activities to PSP patterns elicited by stimulation of nonspecific-specific internuclear pathways provides information on the organization of the VL projection field (12).

Stimulation of motor cortex or corona radiata permits identification of antidromically evoked VL relay cells as shown in Fig. 9A. A significant proportion of such VL relay cells also exhibit monosynaptically evoked EPSPs following brachium conjunctivum (Fig. 9B) and ansa lenticularis stimulation (Fig. 9C). Similar results are shown in Fig. 10A-D from another VL relay cell. However, it should be noted that whereas ansa lenticularis stimulation elicits only a monosynaptic EPSP in the VL relay cell (Fig. 10E), brachium conjunctivum stimulation evokes a monosynaptic EPSP that is succeeded by an IPSP (Fig. 10F). Delayed IPSPs following monosynaptic EPSPs in VL cells activated by brachium conjunctivum stimulation have been noted previously (45). This contrasts with the effects observed in VL relay cells activated by lenticulofugal projections which rarely elicit IPSPs succeeding the monosynaptic EPSPs. Thus although lenticulofugal and cerebellofugal convergent projections may exert monosynaptic excitatory actions on some VL relay cells cerebello-thalamic projections gain access to inhibitory neurons which are not immediately accessible to lenticulofugal projections to the same VL relay cells (38, 39).

Both types of stimulation also activate populations of interneurons in which dispersion of activity generated by convergent projections is evident in medium latency PSPs. Such interneurons influenced by brachium conjunctivum and ansa lenticularis stimulation may exhibit reciprocally related PSPs as shown in Fig. 10G and H. This convergent influence does not, however, occur throughout the interneuronal fields of the VL nucleus. For while it is not possible to induce the prolonged EPSP-IPSP se-

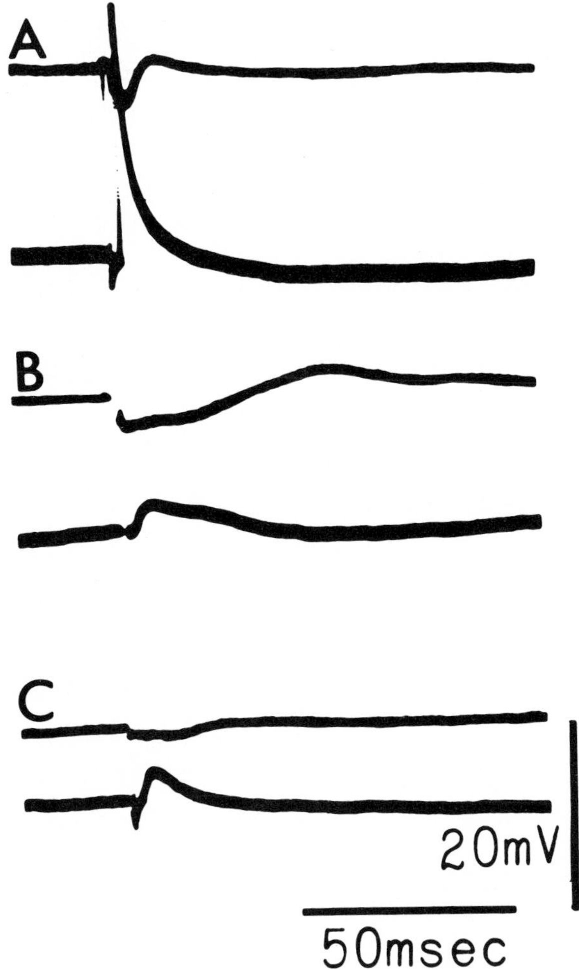

FIG. 9. Convergent excitatory synaptic activation of a VL-relay neuron. A, antidromic spike potential elicited in the VL neuron following corona radiata stimulation in region of motor cortex. B, subthreshold monosynaptic EPSP with additional PSP components evoked by brachium conjunctivum stimulation. C, monosynaptic EPSP evoked by ansa lenticularis stimulation. (From: Desiraju and Purpura, unpublished.)

quences characteristic of widespread synchronization of thalamic interneurons (Fig. 1-8) by repetitive stimulation of the brachium conjunctivum, such PSP patterns are commonly observed following ansa lenticularis or entopeduncular nucleus stimulation. Indeed it is not unusual to find interneurons in VA-VL regions of the thalamus that exhibit EPSP-IPSP sequences following repetitive n. entopeduncularis stimulation which are similar to the PSP patterns evoked by repetitive MTh-stimulation (Fig. 10 I-L). Interneurons may also be found which respond to MTh-stimulation but fail to show responses to ansa lenticularis or entopeduncular stimulation. The converse of this has been observed in only a few instances. It is noteworthy that the most frequently encountered patterns of convergent interaction between lenticulofugal and other types of stimulation is that shown in Fig. 10 I-L. This suggests that a much more

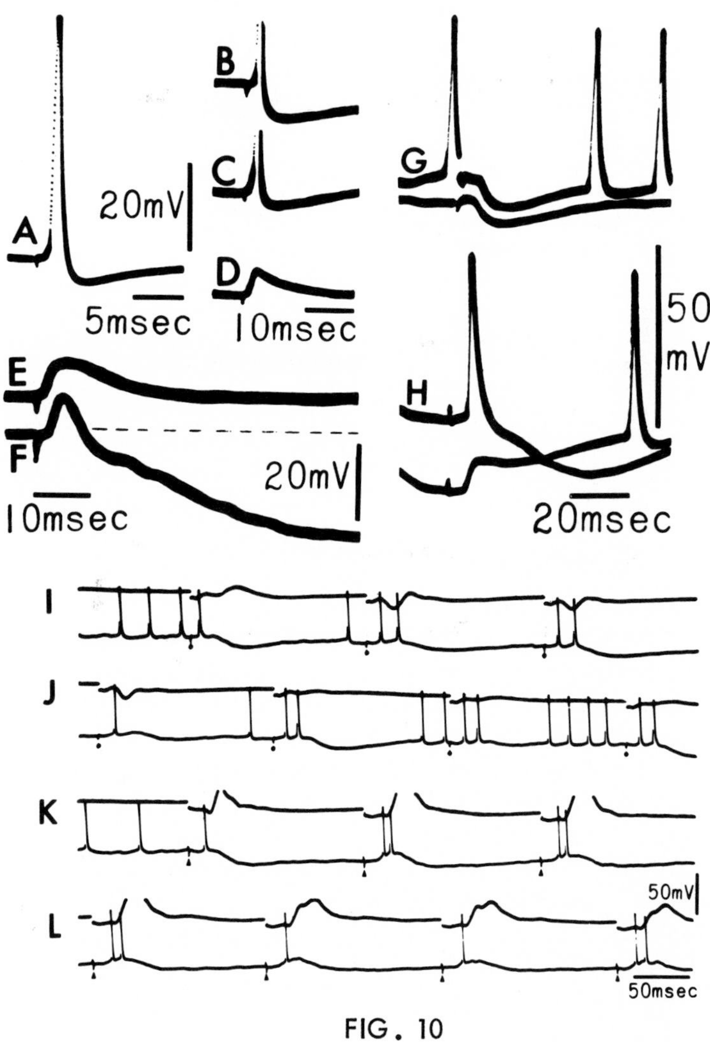

FIG. 10

potent effect is exerted by lenticulofugal inputs upon interneurons in the intrathalamic internuclear projection system than upon VL relay cells in the direct cerebello-thalamocortical projection pathway. Further extrapolation of the data summarized in Fig. 10 permits the conclusion that the outflow pathways of the corpus striatum to the thalamus preferentially influence the interneuronal system activated by nonspecific-specific internuclear pathways (39). Thus the similarities in effects observed in VL cells by repetitive stimulation of striopallidal and nonspecific thalamic nuclei (12, 18, 19, 20, 21) may be explained by the capacity of these common paths to engage similar interneuronal organizations.

The functional significance of the complex distribution of lenticulofugal, cerebellofugal and internuclear synaptic pathways within different domains of thalamic interneuronal organizations can not be assessed from the insufficient data at hand. What seems clear for the present is that the internuncial system of the thalamus, which has been examined in part here, constitutes the major interface between these thalamopetal convergent common paths and relay cells with projections to cortex (36). Additional complexities are introduced into the organizational picture of this interneuronal interface by the fact that corticothalamic projections also inject their input into this internuncial system (18).

Examples of the effects of repetitive stimulation of the corona radiata or internal capsule on relay neurons of the ventrobasal (VB) complex (27) and on a neuron located

---

FIG. 10. Intracellular recording of convergent monosynaptic excitation of a ventrolateral neuron by ansa lenticularis (A, C and D) and brachium conjunctivum (B) stimulation. Spikes in B and C truncated for display purposes. Note minimal latency differences of EPSPs in B and C. Ansa lenticularis-evoked EPSP is shown in isolation in D. E and F: Records obtained from a different ventrolateral neuron following ansa lenticularis (E), and brachium conjunctivum (F) stimulation. Only the brachium-evoked EPSP is succeeded by a prolonged IPSP, the early phase of which exhibits low-amplitude oscillations. G and H: Example of convergent but reciprocal synaptic effects observed in a ventrolateral neuron following ansa lenticularis (G), and brachium conjunctivum (H) stimulation. Responses in each case were elicited at two levels of membrane polarization. G: Upper record obtained during spontaneous discharges, lower record during a phase of increased membrane polarization in which spontaneous discharges were eliminated. In each instance, ansa lenticularis stimulation evokes a 4 to 6 msec IPSP. H: Lower record of the pair obtained during a spontaneous long-duration IPSP. Brachium conjunctivum stimulation elicits a 4-6 msec latency EPSP and spike discharge. The EPSP is revealed in isolation during the spontaneous IPSP. I-L: Example of similar long-latency EPSP-IPSP sequences elicited in a ventrolateral neuron by repetitive stimulation in the region of n. entopeduncularis (I and J: continuous recording) and stimulation of MTh (K and L: continuous recording). Upper channel records obtained from motor cortex. Note prominent long-latency surface-negative recruiting response evoked by MTh stimulation. (From: Desiraju and Purpura, (12).

in the medial thalamus are illustrated in Fig. 11 and 12, respectively. Stimulation of the internal capsule evokes activities in the thalamic relay cells which are compounded of antidromic-"recurrent" synaptic events and orthodromic (corticothalamic) activation of VB cells. In the series of responses shown in Fig. 11A, the first capsular stimulus elicits a partial antidromic response which is followed by a prolonged IPSP. Successive stimuli introduced during the late phases of the IPSP evoke full antidromic spikes probably as a consequence of the restoration of membrane potential associated with the IPSP. Of particular interest, however, is the fact that successive stimuli produce progressively longer latency IPSPs, a phenomenon that is clearly inconsistent with the view that such IPSPs are generated by a disynaptic recurrent pathway, (1, 2). The EPSP-IPSP sequences evoked by repetitive internal capsule stimulation in VB relay cells, and the effects which evoked prolonged IPSPs exert on relay transmission (Fig. 11 B-D) are similar in many respects to the synaptic events generated in thalamic neurons by stimulation of nonspecific-specific internuclear synaptic pathways. A point of some importance is that while VB relay cells are usually not strongly influenced by nonspecific-specific internuclear pathways (27) corticothalamic afferents readily gain access to the interneuronal system which can be set into operation during spontaneous spindle waves.

In the case of neurons of the medial thalamus, corona radiata or internal capsule stimulation can effectively elicit rhythmical EPSP-IPSP sequences which mimic but do not identically mirror the PSP patterns evoked by stimulation of specific-non-

---

FIG. 11. Inhibitory effects of internal capsule stimulation (indicated by dots) on identified VB relay cells. Records are from three different cells impaled during a single experiment. A, internal capsule stimulation elicits a partial antidromic spike with first stimulus and full spike with successive stimuli of 6/sec sequence. IPSP is of short latency initially, then develops with longer latency during increase in membrane potential associated with summation of successively evoked prolonged IPSPs. B, conditioning stimulus is delivered to the site in capsule about 1 mm anterior to stimulation site in A. ML stimulation is delivered 80 msec after capsule stimulus. Note that only an occasional blockade of ML evoked response occurs during late phases of the IPSP. C and D, continuous records, capsular stimulation at same site as in B. Prominent IPSPs are evoked by capsular stimulation which are more effective in suppressing ML evoked discharges. Maximum inhibitory interactions are observed with 40-60 msec intervals between conditioning (capsule) and testing (ML) stimulation (D). (From: Maekawa and Purpura, (27).

FIG. 12. Intracellular recordings from the same medial thalamic neuron studied in Figure 8. A-E, continuous record during low-frequency stimulation of the corona radiata of pericruciate cortex (at arrow heads). Note that the first stimulus triggers a repetitive series of EPSP-IPSP sequences which resemble the PSP patterns evoked by VA-VL stimulation in Figure 8. Dashed lines indicate membrane potential baseline level in the absence of stimulation. (From: Desiraju and Purpura, unpublished.)

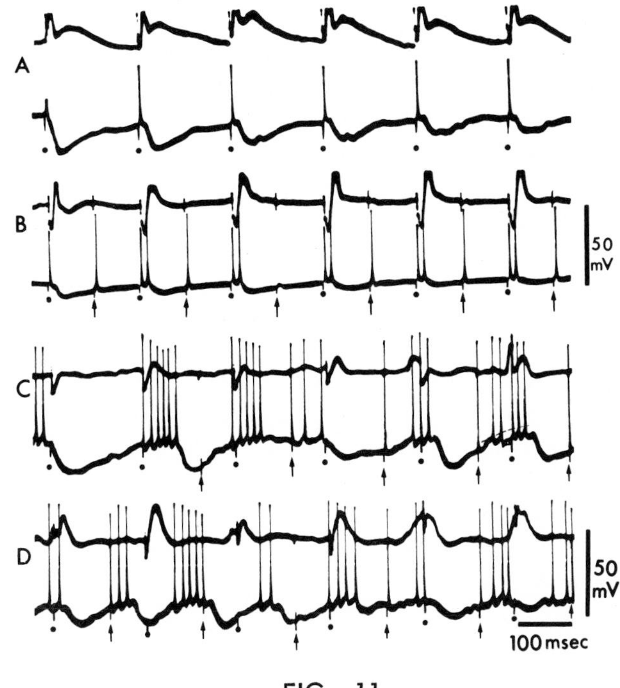

FIG. 11

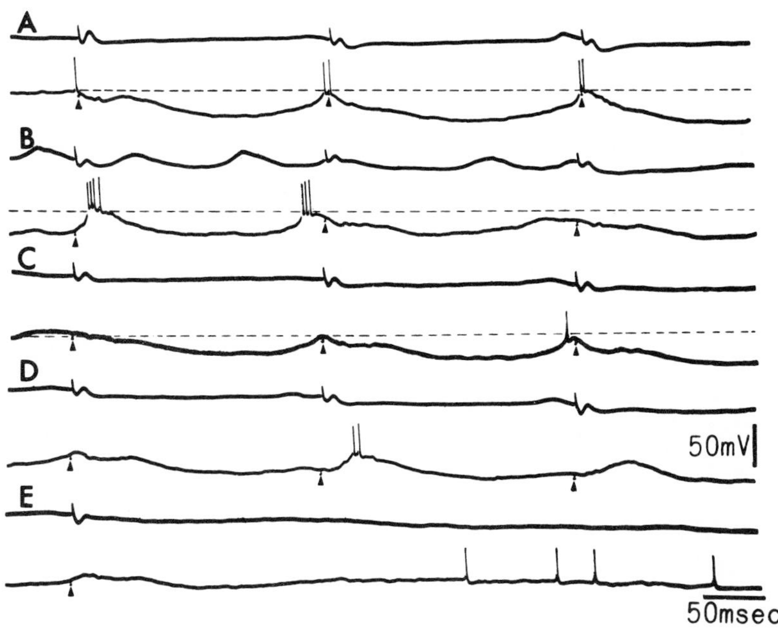

FIG. 12

specific internuclear projection pathways (Fig. 8). The first stimulus in both instances elicits a prolonged multiphasic IPSP, but whereas successive stimuli delivered to VA-VL regions are effective in triggering powerful EPSPs (Fig. 8), such stimuli to the corona radiata cannot influence the rhythmical EPSP-IPSP sequences triggered by the first corona radiata stimulus (Fig. 12). Additional studies have confirmed the wide variety of EPSP-IPSP patterns that can be elicited in thalamic neurons by cortical or internal capsule stimulation (18).

The foregoing results taken together with observations on the convergence of striatothalamic, cerebellothalamic and reciprocal nonspecific-specific projections to interneuronal elements of the thalamus serve to reinforce the concept developed here of multiple entry pathways into the interneuronal machinery regulating the discharge characteristics of a large proportion of thalamic neurons. The intracellular data provide essential evidence in support of the Sherringtonian view of the thalamic internuncial system as a target for convergent activities originating in diverse common paths. Inasmuch as input specificity is lost within this interneuronal network it follows that the signal value of discrete patterns of discharges in individual common paths must be of minor importance in the transactions carried out in the thalamic internuncial system, in contrast to the relay elements monosynaptically activated by lemniscal, spinothalamic, optic tract and thalamopetal auditory projections. It remains an open question as to how transactions in the thalamic internuncial system provide the "mechanisms for co-ordination" essential in the control of sensorimotor behavior. Suffice it to say that this problem is probably beyond the operational capabilities of present day intracellular recording techniques for obvious reasons.

Diversity of Synaptic Events and Functional Properties of Thalamic Neurons

Thalamic neurons have not been studied with intracellular recording and stimulating techniques as extensively as spinal motoneurons and cortical neurons. Consequently few attempts have been made to examine the range of functional diversity which these elements may exhibit under different conditions of activation. Brief "all-or none" EPSPs (26)as well as smoothly summating EPSPs may occur in the same elements. The former are considered to be generated by impulses in single presynaptic axons, usually specific projection fibers. Smoothly summating EPSPs and IPSPs as typically observed in the vast majority of thalamic neurons examined, are illustrated in Figs. 1-12. Their prolonged temporal characteristics dominate the recordings from thalamic neurons following activation of different input systems. For the most part the PSP patterns observed in thalamic neurons do not differ from the patterns of synaptic events recorded from neurons at other neuraxial sites (38).

Recently a new pattern of PSPs has been detected in intracellular recordings from principal cells of the dorsal lateral geniculate nucleus in the cat (17). In addition to typical 'all-or-none' EPSPs (or S-potentials) (6, 28) some neurons exhibit brief EPSPs which are interrupted by IPSPs (Fig. 13). For convenience such PSP patterns have been designated diphasic-PSP (17). Diphasic-PSPs exhibit summation patterns in a manner similar to S-potentials observed in isolation. However, the con-

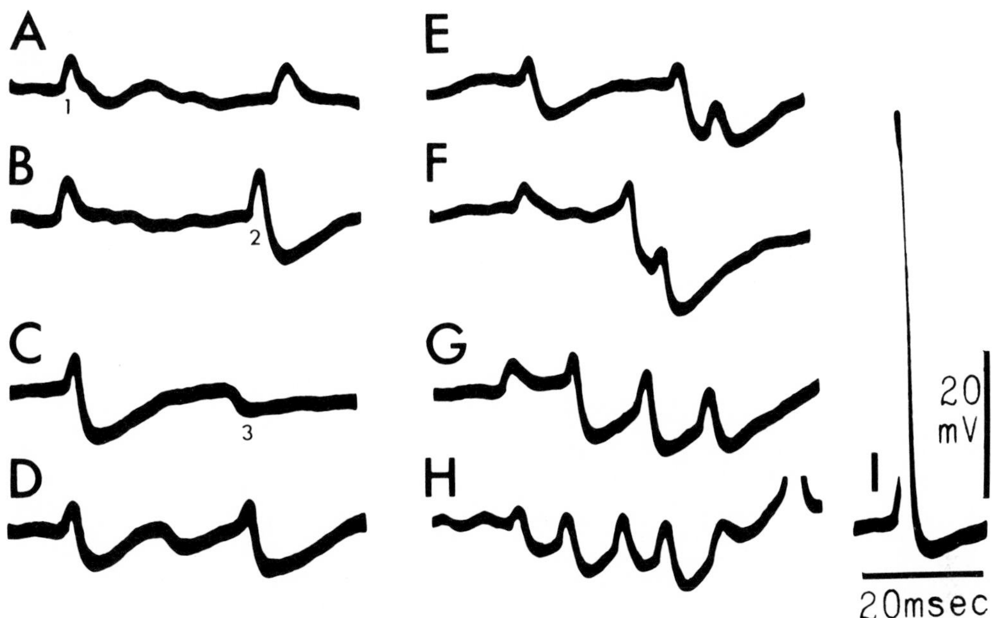

FIG. 13. Examples of individual EPSPs (S-potentials) and diphasic-PSPs recorded from an LGN neuron during resting maintained activity in the dark. The sample records are portions of a continuous recording during which several hundred PSPs occurred during the resting discharge. A, two S-potentials one of which (1) is succeeded by a small delayed IPSP. B, an S-potential and a diphasic-PSP (2). C, a diphasic-PSP and a slow IPSP (3). D, two diphasic-PSPs are separated by a slow IPSP. E-H, summation characteristics of the diphasic-PSPs. Note in H that after a burst of 4 summating diphasic-PSPs an S-potential triggers a spike discharge on a delayed depolarization. I, example of a spike potential elicited by the EPSP component of a diphasic-PSP. (From: Fertziger and Purpura, (17).

sequence of this is to produce a step-wise increase in membrane polarization and reduction in the spontaneous discharge frequency of LGN neurons. In view of the close temporal relations of the EPSP and IPSP components of the diphasic-PSPs, the IPSP component may limit the effectiveness of the prior S-potential. When the EPSP component of the diphasic-PSP triggers a spike discharge in many instances the spike may be partially short-circuited by the conductance increase associated with the succeeding IPSP (Fig. 14). This indicates that the IPSP component of the diphasic-PSP is generated before cell discharge induced by the EPSP is completed. In other words there would appear to be insufficient time for the IPSP-component of the diphasic-PSP to be generated by an impulse in the impaled neuron that activates a recurrent inhibitory pathway (7). Cells exhibiting such diphasic-PSPs constitute a small frac-

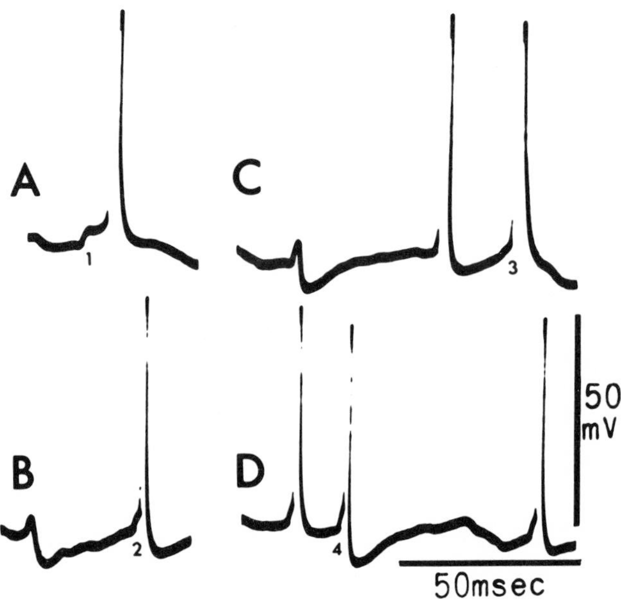

FIG. 14. Effects of diphasic-PSPs on spike potentials during different phases of dark discharge of an LGN neuron. A, a typical S-potential (1) initiates a spike potential that is preceded by a delayed depolarization. B, a spike potential (2) initiated at the peak of the EPSP component of the diphasic-PSP is succeeded by the IPSP phase of the latter. Compare the spike duration in A and B. C, spikes are initiated by fast and slow (3) EPSPs. D, the occurrence of a spike in relation to the IPSP component of a diphasic-PSP (4) results in marked reduction of spike amplitude and spike duration by the conductance increase associated with the IPSP. (From: Fertziger and Purpura, (17).

tion of the principal neurons of the lateral geniculate nucleus with a resting dark discharge. During the prolonged IPSPs observed in "off-cells" of this type the diphasic-PSPs are suppressed (Fig. 15). It is inferred from this that the diphasic-PSPs are generated in LGN neurons by retino-geniculate afferents. Stimulation of optic radiations or brainstem reticular regions is ineffective in eliciting diphasic-PSPs. Since optic tract axons terminate preferentially in relation to dendrites of LGN principal neurons, it may be that the diphasic-PSPs reflect the operation of reciprocal dendro-dendritic synapses between principal neurons and interneurons of the LGN (17). This suggestion derives from observations on the olfactory bulb in which reciprocal dendro-dendritic synapses between mitral and granule cell dendrites are believed to constitute the morphological substrate for the EPSP-IPSP sequence observed in mitral cells (48). Dendo-dendritic synapses have been identified in the lateral geniculate nucleus (15) as well as elsewhere in the thalamus in cat (49). If such dendro-dendritic synapses represent reciprocally related excitatory and inhibitory elements then a mechanism

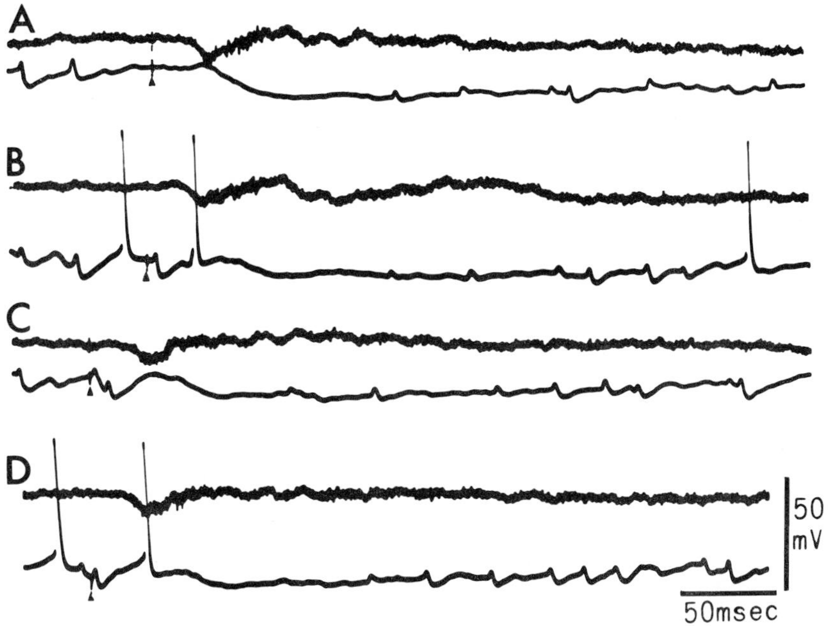

FIG. 15. Examples of the effect of stroboscopic flash stimulation on diphasic-PSPs in an LGN neuron. The evoked potential monopolarly recorded from the surface of the LGN is shown in the upper channel. Photic stimulation indicated by the arrow head below the stimulus artifact. A, two diphasic-PSPs precede photic stimulation which elicits a small long latency EPSP and a succeeding prolonged IPSP. S-potentials and diphasic-PSPs are eliminated during the initial 100 msec of the IPSP. B-D, same as in A. Note that the diphasic-PSPs and spikes seen immediately after the photic stimulation artifact were not evoked by the stimulus. (From: Fertziger and Purpura, (17).

would be provided for effecting EPSP-IPSP sequences in the absence of cell discharge, as illustrated in Figs. 13-15.

The demonstration of diphasic-PSPs in thalamic neurons illustrates the necessity for caution in assuming that all the possible types of synaptic interaction between thalamic neurons have been catalogued to date. The diversity of arrangement of different synaptic complexes in the thalamus argues against this on morphological grounds. In fact it remains to determine the properties of synaptic interactions between extremely small neurons of the thalamus which are probably rapidly destroyed by impalement with micropipettes employed in present day intracellular studies.

The suggestion that dendritic synaptic interactions may occur between thalamic neurons raises the question as to the role of heterogeneous properties of dendrites (34, 37) in some of the changes in excitability observed in relay and non-relay cells of the thalamus under different conditions of activation. It has been argued elsewhere that the high degree of synaptic security of lemniscal VB relays is due in part to the capac-

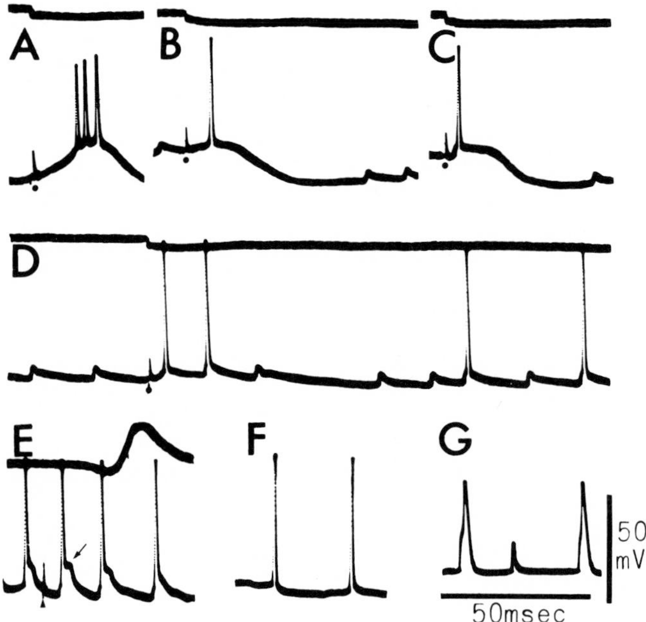

FIG. 16. Sequential changes in intracellular responses of a neuron in the ventro-lateral nucleus of the thalamus during and after prolonged low frequency (6/sec) stimulation of pallidal entopeduncular (lenticular) projections. Upper channel, monopolar recordings from motor cortex. A: Response recorded several seconds after impalement of the neuron. Lenticular stimulation elicited no response in cortex but did evoke a short latency EPSP in the thalamic neuron. B and C: Examples of recordings made 20 sec after onset of stimulation. Note appearance of small, all-or-none, depolarizing potentials. D: 40 sec after onset of stimulation, frequency of partial responses has increased and some of these fast prepotentials (FPPs) trigger large amplitude spikes. E: Immediately after cessation of lenticular stimulation, which lasted approximately 90 sec; stimulus in E was delivered to medial thalamic region which evoked a prominent negative wave in cortex but did not influence activity of thalamic neuron. Spikes recorded during post-lenticular stimulation exhibited FPPs and delayed depolarization (at arrow). F: 20 sec after E. Note absence of pre- and post-spike depolarizations. G: Examples of spike decomposition during early cell depolarization which revealed initial segment-soma components. (From: Purpura et al., (41).

ity of lemniscal afferents to initiate partial or full spikes in VB cell dendrites (26). Other lines of evidence indicate that "dendritic excitability" may fluctuate dramatically during prolonged synaptic excitatory bombardment as illustrated in Fig. 16 in recordings from a thalamic VL neuron during long duration stimulation of lenticulofugal projections. The alteration in "dendritic excitability" is inferred from the appearance of bursts of rapid depolarizing potentials or partial responses which exhibit "all-or-none" characteristics (41). The persistence of partial dendritic responses following cessation of stimulation may be taken as evidence for a short-term alteration in the functional properties of dendrites subsequent to their prolonged activation. It goes without saying that such alterations may provide a mechanism for facilitation of synaptic pathways which places greater emphasis on postsynaptic events than has been considered heretofore.

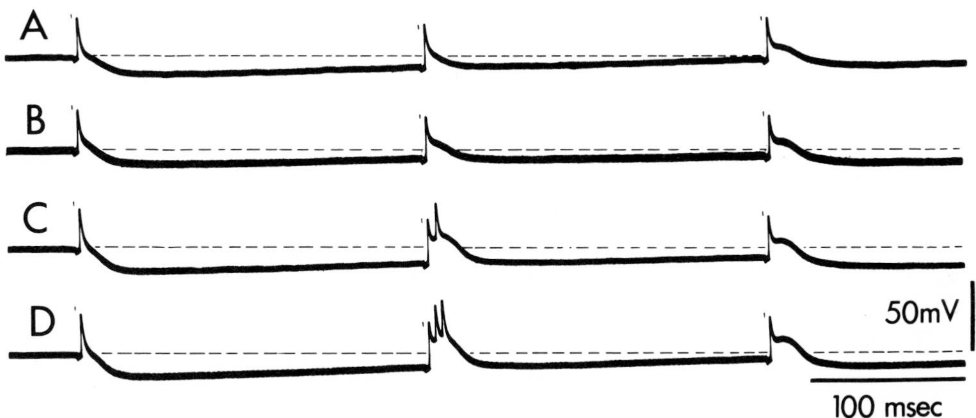

FIG. 17. Development of delayed depolarizations and associated spike discharges during repetitive antidromic activation of a VL-relay neuron. A-D, four series of stimuli each recorded several seconds apart. The first stimulus in each series evokes antidromic spikes and succeeding prolonged IPSPs. Successive antidromic spikes at this stimulus frequency arise from levels of increased membrane polarization. Note progressive enhancement of delayed depolarizations and associated spike discharges. (From: Desiraju and Purpura, (14) and unpublished.)

The contribution of excitability changes in dendrites to the responses of thalamic neurons to orthodromic stimulation (Fig. 16) may be seen also in some unusual events observed in thalamic relay cells during their antidromic activation (14). These events depend upon relay cells exhibiting prolonged IPSPs following initial antidromic invasion. (Whether such IPSPs are generated by a recurrent pathway or orthodromic stimulation of corticothalamic projections is not at issue here.)

Examples of the progressive development of prolonged delayed depolarizing potentials following antidromic spikes in a VL relay cell are shown in Fig. 17. Samples of responses from four separate series of repetitive stimulations of the corona radiata illustrate that the prolonged delayed depolarizations may be associated with one or more spikes in a high-frequency burst. That the delayed depolarization is not a late EPSP is clearly shown by the findings that if antidromic invasion does not occur the delayed depolarization is not seen (Fig. 18A 1-2). Fig. 18 also illustrates the observation that partial depolarization of the element during a traumatic disturbance produced by the intracellularly located micropipette results in loss of the delayed depolarization following the antidromic spike. Recovery of membrane potential results in the progressive return of the delayed depolarizations. The sequence of changes in antidromically evoked responses to the first six corona radiata stimuli is shown in greater detail in Fig. 19. The increase in membrane potential during the IPSP subsequent to the first stimulus is shown by the separation of the base lines of the records 1 and 2 in Fig. 19A. During the maximum phase of the IPSP initiated by stimulus, 1, which also elicited an antidromic spike, the second stimulus fails to evoke an antidromic response.

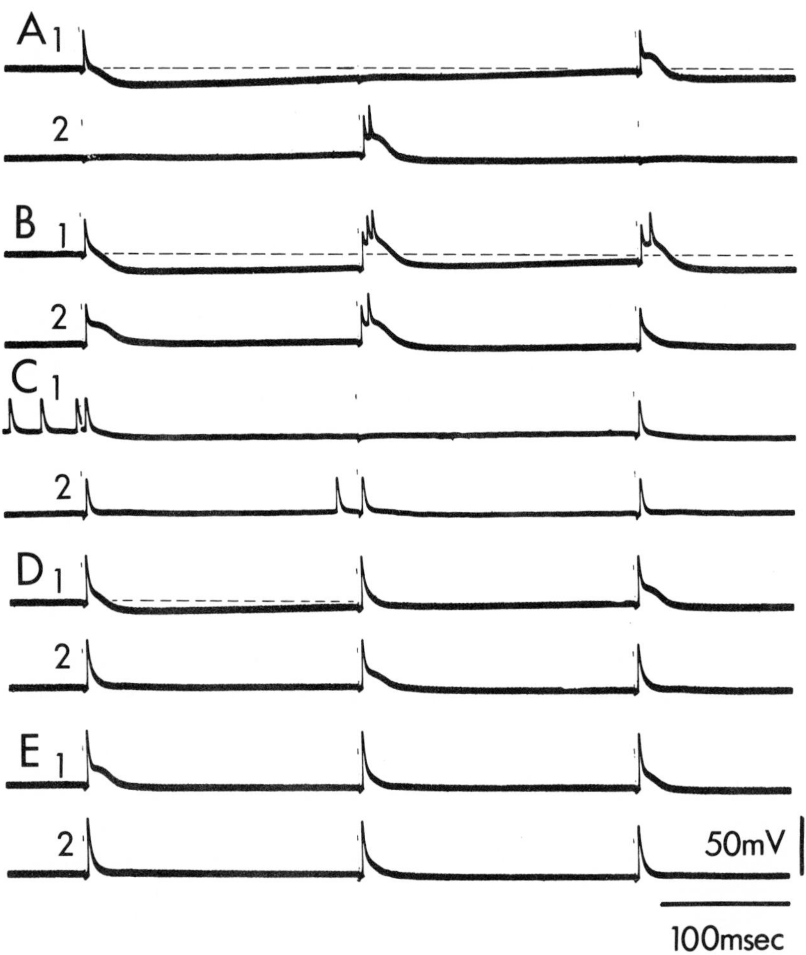

FIG. 18

Subsequent stimuli evoke both antidromic spikes and variable delayed depolarizations (Fig. 19 B and C). Multiple spikes are triggered in an all-or-none fashion at the peak of the delayed depolarization (Fig. 19B 3).

Several interpretations may be placed on the observations of Figs. 17-19. The most plausible explanation is that the increase in membrane polarization of the soma-dendritic membrane produced during the IPSP permits the antidromic spike to invade the dendrites in a graded fashion. The persisting depolarization of distal dendritic tree would then act as a stimulus for triggering repetitive discharges from the soma and possible proximal dendritic regions of the neuron. Viewed in this fashion the delayed depolarization is attributed to current flowing into the cell body from dendrites subsequent to the spike invasion as described elsewhere (9, 22, 25, 33).

The extent to which the different response characteristics of different types of thalamic neurons may be referable to the properties of their dendrites remains to be determined. There have been too few intracellular studies of thalamic neurons reported to date to warrant any comments concerning the generality of the observations illustrated in Figs. 16-19. However, it hardly seems likely that these observations represent unusual processes which are not met with in the 'normal' operation of thalamic neurons. For the present it seems useful to admit the possibility of a wide spectrum of properties of thalamic neurons, which is consistent with the remarkably morphological heterogeneity of these elements.

COMMENT

The Sherringtonian view of the thalamus as a mechanism for co-ordination is entirely supported by the studies summarized above which indicate an extraordinary convergence of several common paths onto internuncial networks that dominate the synaptic transactions in the thalamus as a whole. To be sure the entry pathways into these internuncial networks maintain some degree of anatomical and segration which allows

---

FIG. 18. Further analysis of the relationship between the development of antidromic spikes and delayed depolarizations in a VL-relay cell at different membrane potential levels. In A-E, records 1 and 2 are continuous. A, alternation of antidromic spike invasion. Failure of antidromic spikes fails to elicit a delayed depolarization, indicating that the latter is not synaptically generated. B, each stimulus of the repetitive train evokes an antidromic spike and succeeding delayed depolarization, with variable superimposed discharges. C, the micropipette is dislodged from its prior position and an injury discharge is produced. Antidromic stimulation evokes spikes which are not followed by delayed depolarization. D and E, recovery of recording conditions as in A and B. The increase in spike potentials is attributable to attainment of a more secure intracellular positioning of the microelectrode and partial restoration of membrane potential. In E the delayed depolarization is seen clearly for the first time after the initial antidromic spike. (From: Desiraju and Purpura, (14) and unpublished.)

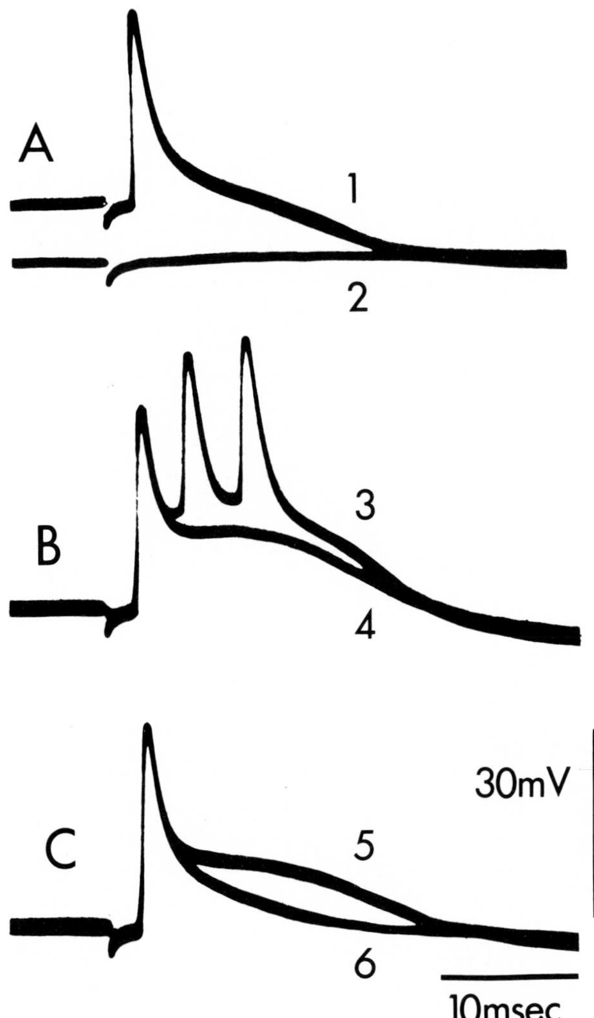

FIG. 19. Details of the sequential changes in antidromic responses of a VL relay cell during the first six responses of a repetitive train of stimuli as in Figs. 17 and 18. A, The first stimulus elicits an antidromic spike with a minimal delayed depolarization and an IPSP. The separation between records 1 and 2 represents the increase in membrane potential produced by the prolonged IPSP. The second stimulus during the IPSP fails to evoke an antidromic spike. B, The third stimulus elicits an antidromic spike and repetitive spikes superimposed on the delayed depolarization. The fourth stimulus evokes a delayed depolarization that is subthreshold for spike generation. C, Progressive attenuation of the delayed depolarizations occurs with the fifth and sixth stimulus. (From: Desiraju and Purpura, (14) and unpublished.)

their recognition as discrete input systems in the usual morphological sense. But the consequences of this input when translated into physiological events encompass a wide range of interneuronal activities distributed in space and time beyond the confines of the locus of entry of a particular input pathway. The preferential activation of a population of thalamic neurons by a specific input system does not contradict this view. What this says in effect is that certain private line operations have a high degree of synaptic security. But it does not follow from this that the relay elements interposed in the private line are not available for recruitment into the operations of the internuncial network under appropriate conditions.

This view of the thalamus as an "interneuronal machine" obviously runs counter to more traditional approaches to thalamic organization which have emphasized the definition of discrete input-output pathways and functions related to modality and/or place specific neuronal observations. The evidence for such operations is too strong to be abjured. Still the question may be raised as to whether these operations can be safely divorced from more general intrathalamic transactions which must surely relate to operations in other systems. Unfortunately very little is known about the functional significance of these intrathalamic transactions to warrant even the most tenuous speculations. At best such speculations are not likely to imply anything more than that these transactions are important in thalamic "integrative processes"—which merely substitutes one vague generalization for another, i.e., "co-ordination".

The range of synaptic events demonstrable in thalamic neuronal operations argues against any simplistic construction of neuronal circuitry that would satisfy the physiological basis for any of the intrathalamic operations summarized here and elsewhere (35, 36, 38, 39). On the other hand this should not detract from the heuristic value of constructions based upon clear morphophysiological correlations whenever these can be effected. The reader must judge for himself the extent to which these criteria are met in reports elsewhere in this volume in which the data obtained have prompted such constructions.

Many aspects of the intracellular data reviewed here are applicable to the analysis of corticothalamic relations, which have been noted only briefly in this survey. Apart from the orthodromic synaptic effects observed in relay and other closely related neurons activated by corticothalamic afferents, mention has been made of the influence of corticofugal inputs on the intrathalamic, interneuronal organizations activated by other thalamopetal projection systems. Until more is known concerning the relative effectiveness and distribution of the corticofugal input to the interneuronal machinery of the thalamus it is not possible to specify the unique contribution of this input to the totality of afferent drives on thalamic neurons in different functional states. Insofar as this subject is of vital importance for our adequate understanding of thalamic operations its treatment in many of the succeeding reports should breach this hiatus in knowledge.

ACKNOWLEDGMENTS.

Work summarized in this survey was supported in part by a grant from the National Institute of Neurological Diseases and Stroke, NS-07512.

REFERENCES

1 ANDERSEN, P. and ANDERSSON, S.A. Physiological Basis of the Alpha Rhythm, Appleton-Century-Crofts, New York, 1968.

2 ANDERSEN, P., ECCLES, J.C. and SEARS, T.A. The ventro-basal complex of the thalamus: Types of cells, their responses and their functional organization, J. Physiol., 174 (1964b) 370-399.

3 ANDERSSON, S.A., HOLMGREN, E. and MANSON, J.R. Synchronization and desynchronization in the thalamus of the unanesthetized decorticate cat, Electroenceph. clin. Neurophysiol., 31 (1971) 335-346.

4 ANDERSSON, S.A., HOLMGREN, E. and MANSON, J.R. Localized thalamic rhythmicity induced by spinal and cortical lesions, Electroenceph. clin. Neurophysiol., 31 (1971) 347-356.

5 ANDERSSON, S.A. and MANSON, J.R. Rhythmic activity in the thalamus of the unanesthetized decorticate cat, Electroenceph. clin. Neurophysiol., 31 (1971) 21-34.

6 BISHOP, P.O., BURKE, W., and DAVIS, R. The interpretation of the extracellular response of single lateral geniculate cells, J. Physiol. (Lond.), 162 (1962) 451-472.

7 BURKE, W. and SEFTON, A.J. Discharge patterns of principal cells of lateral geniculate nucleus of rat, J. Physiol., 187 (1966) 213-229.

8 COHEN, B., HOUSEPIAN, E.M. and PURPURA, D.P. Intrathalamic regulation of activity in a cerebello-cortical projection system, Exptl. Neurol., 6 (1962) 492-506.

9 CRILL, W.E. Unitary multiple-spiked responses in cat inferior olive nucleus, J. Neurophysiol., 33 (1970) 199-209.

10 DEMPSEY, E.W. and MORISON, R.S. The production of rhythmically recurrent cortical potentials after localized thalamic stimulation, Amer. J. Physiol., 135 (1942) 293-300.

11 DESIRAJU, T., BROGGI, G., PRELEVIC, S., SANTINI, M. and PURPURA, D.P. Inhibitory synaptic pathways linking specific and nonspecific thalamic nuclei, Brain Research, 15 (1969) 542-543.

12 DESIRAJU, T. and PURPURA, D.P. Synaptic convergence of cerebellar and lenticular projections to thalamus, Brain Research, 15 (1969) 544-547.

13 DESIRAJU, T. and PURPURA, D.P. Organization of specific-nonspecific thalamic internuclear synaptic pathways, Brain Research, 21 (1970) 169-182.

14 DESIRAJU, T. and PURPURA, D.P. Antidromic responses and 'recurrent' IPSPs of thalamic VL neurons, Fed. Proc., 29 (1970) Abs. 444.

15 FAMIGLIETTI, E.V. Jr. Dendro-dendritic synapses in the lateral geniculate nucleus of the cat, Brain Research, 20 (1970) 181-191.

16 FELDMAN, M.H. and PURPURA, D.P. Prolonged conductance increase in thalamic neurons during synchronizing inhibition, Brain Research, 24 (1970) 329-332.

17 FERTZIGER, A.P. and PURPURA, D.P. Diphasic-PSPs during maintained activity of cat lateral geniculate neurons, Brain Research, 33 (1971) 463-467.

18 FRIGYESI, T.L. and MACHEK, J. Basal ganglia-diencephalon synaptic relations in the cat. I. An intracellular study of dorsal thalamic neurons during capsular and basal ganglia stimulation, Brain Research, 20 (1970) 201-217.

19 FRIGYESI, T.L. and MACHEK, J. Basal ganglia-diencephalon synaptic relations in the cat. II. Intracellular recording from dorsal thalamic neurons during low-frequency stimulation of the caudato-thalamic projection systems and the nigrothalamic pathway, Brain Research, 27 (1971) 59-78.

20 FRIGYESI, T.L. and PURPURA, D.P. Functional properties of synaptic pathways influencing transmission in the specific cerebello-thalamocortical projection system, Exptl. Neurol., 10 (1964) 305-324.

21 FRIGYESI, T.L. and RABIN, A. Basal ganglia-diencephalon synaptic relations in the cat. III. An intracellular study of ansa lenticularis lenticular fasciculus and pallidosubthalamic projection activities, Brain Research, 35 (1971) 67-87.

22 FUJITA, Y. Activity of dendrites of single Purkinje cells and its relationship to so-called inactivation response in rabbit cerebellum, J. Neurophysiol., 31 (1968) 131-141.

23 JASPER, H.H. Diffuse projection systems: The integrative action of the thalamic reticular system, Electroenceph. clin. Neurophysiol., 1 (1949) 405-420.

24 JASPER, H.H. Functional properties of the thalamic reticular system. In J.F. Delafresnaye (Ed.), Brain Mechanisms and Consciousness, Blackwell, Oxford, England, 1954, pp. 374-401.

25 KERNELL, D. The delayed depolarization in cat and rat motoneurones, Prog. Brain Res., 12 (1964) 42-55.

26 MAEKAWA, K. and PURPURA, D.P. Properties of spontaneous and evoked synaptic activities of thalamic ventro-basal neurons, J. Neurophysiol. 30 (1967) 360-381.

27 MAEKAWA, K. and Purpura, D.P. Intracellular study of lemniscal and nonspecific synaptic interactions in thalamic ventro-basal neurons, Brain Research, 4 (1967) 308-323.

28 McILWAIN, J.T. and CREUTZFELDT, O.D. Microelectrode study of synaptic excitation and inhibition in the lateral geniculate nucleus of the cat, J. Neurophysiol., 30 (1967) 1-21.

29 MORISON, R.S. and DEMPSEY, E.W. A study of thalamo-cortical relations, Amer. J. Physiol., 135 (1942) 281-292.

30 MOUNTCASTLE, V.B. Sleep, wakefulness, and the conscious state: intrinsic regulatory mechanisms of the brain. In V.B Mountcastle (Ed.), Medical Physiology, Vol. II, Mosby, St. Louis, 1968, pp. 1315-1342.

31. NAUTA, W.J.H. and MEHLER, W.R. Projections of the lentiform nucleus in the monkey, Brain Research, 1 (1966) 3-42.

32 NAUTA, W.J.H. and MEHLER, W.R. Fiber connections of the basal ganglia. In G. Crane and R. Gardner, Jr. (Eds.), Psychotropic Drugs and Dysfunctions of the Basal Ganglia, Public Health Service Publ. No. 1938, U.S. Gov't. Printing Office, Washington, D.C., 1969, pp. 68-72.

33 NELSON, P.G. and BURKE, R.E. Delayed depolarization in cat spinal moto-

neurons, Exptl. Neurol., 17 (1967) 16-26.

34 PURPURA, D.P. Comparative physiology of dendrites. In G.C. Quarton, T. Melnechuk and F.O. Schmitt (Eds.), The Neurosciences: A Study Program, Rockefeller Univ. Press, New York, 1967, pp. 372-393.

35 PURPURA, D.P. Interneuronal mechanisms in synchronization and desynchronization of thalamic activity. In M.A.B. Brazier (Ed.), The Interneuron, UCLA Forum in Medical Sciences, 1969, pp. 467-496.

36 PURPURA, D.P. Operations and processes in thalamic and synaptically related neural subsystems. In The Neurosciences II, Rockefeller Univ. Press, New York, 1970, pp. 458-470.

37 PURPURA, D.P. Dendrites: Heterogeneity in form and function. In A. Remond (Editor-in-Chief), Hand. Electroenceph. clin. Neurophysiol., Vol. 1, Elsevier, Amsterdam, 1971, pp. 1B-3 to 1B17.

38 PURPURA, D.P. Intracellular studies of synaptic organizations in the mammalian brain. In G.D. Pappas and D.P. Purpura (Eds.), Structure and Function of Synapses, Raven Press, New York, 1972, pp. 257-302.

39 PURPURA, D.P. Electrophysiological properties of basal ganglia synaptic relations. In Int. Encyclo. Pharmacol. Therapeut., 1972, (in press).

40 PURPURA, D.P. and COHEN, B. Intracellular recording from thalamic neurons during recruiting responses, J. Neurophysiol., 25 (1962) 621-635.

41 PURPURA, D.P., DESIRAJU, T., PRELEVIC, S. and SANTINI, M. Excitability changes in dendrites of thalamic neurons during prolonged synaptic activation, Brain Research, 10 (1968) 457-458.

42 PURPURA, D.P., FRIGYESI, T.L., McMURTRY, J.G. and SCARFF, T. Synaptic mechanisms in thalamic regulation of cerebello-cortical projection activity. In D.P. Purpura and M.D. Yahr (Eds.), The Thalamus, Columbia Univ. Press, New York, 1966, pp. 153-170.

43 PURPURA, D.P. and MALLIANI, A. Intracellular studies of the corpus striatum. I. Synaptic potentials and discharge characteristics of caudate neurons activated by thalamic stimulation, Brain Research, 6 (1967) 325-340.

44 PURPURA, D.P., McMURTRY, J.G. and MAEKAWA, K. Synaptic events in ventrolateral thalamic neurons during suppression of recruiting responses by brain stem reticular stimulation, Brain Research, 1 (1966) 63-76.

45 PURPURA, D.P., SCARFF, T. and McMURTRY, J.G. Intracellular study of internuclear inhibition in ventrolateral thalamic neurons, J. Neurophysiol., 28 (1965) 487-496.

46 PURPURA, D.P. and SHOFER, R.J. Intracellular recording from thalamic neurons during reticulocortical activation, J. Neurophysiol., 26 (1963) 494-505.

47 PURPURA, D.P., SHOFER, R.J. and MUSGRAVE, F.S. Cortical intracellular potentials during augmenting and recruiting responses. II. Patterns of synaptic activities in pyramidal and nonpyramidal tract neurons, J. Neurophysiol., 27 (1964) 133-151.

48 RALL, W., SHEPARD, G.M., REESE, T.S. and BRIGHTMAN, M.W. Dendrodendritic synaptic pathway for inhibition in the olfactory bulb, Exp. Neurol., 14 (1966) 44-56.

49 RALSTON, H.J. and HERMAN, M.M. The fine structure of neurons and synapses in the ventrobasal thalamus of the cat, Brain Research, 14 (1969) 77-98.
50 SCHEIBEL, M.E. and SCHEIBEL, A.B. Anatomical basis of attention mechanisms in vertebrate brains. In G.C. Quarton, T. Melnechuk and F.O. Schmitt (Eds.), The Neurosciences: A Study Program, Rockefeller Univ. Press, New York, 1967, pp. 577-602.
51 SCHLAG, J. and WASZAK, M. Characteristics of unit responses in nucleus reticularis thalami, Brain Research, 21 (1970) 286-287.

DISCUSSION

KUYPERS:

You talked about the medial thalamic and nonspecific areas. I would like to know what did you mean by those.

PURPURA:

In the past decade we have used the term "medial thalamic region" to refer to the composite of nuclear groups situated 2 mm. from the midline and extending in a rostral-caudal direction from the anterior pole of the thalamus to the caudal border of the CM-Pf complex. Stimulation almost anywhere within this region elicits cortical surface recuriting responses which vary somewhat in latency and configuration depending upon placement of stimulating electrodes. The recruiting response or evoked-synchronization is very readily obtained and constitutes an electrophysiological "signature" of activation of this medial thalamic system. Stimulation more lateral in the thalamus introduces complexities in the responses which are compounded of both short and long latency activities or admixtures of specific and nonspecific projection activities in the classical sense of designation of these responses. It is of course well known that small movements of the stimulating electrodes can result in very dramatically different types of rhythmically recurrent responses in cortex. This leads to many complications of interpretations but it must be allowed that this technique has also led to important historical developments in the field of thalamocortical relations.

KUYPERS:

What I am wondering about specifically is whether your findings pertain to the dorsomedial nucleus or to the intralaminar nuclei. You feel, you are in the lateral part of the dorsal medial nucleus?

PURPURA:

It has long been known that stimulation in the lateral part of the dorsomedial nucleus can also result in recruiting responses in rostral cortex.

KUYPERS:

I assume then that we are dealing with a part of the dorsal medial and with the interlaminar nuclei. I think on the basis of electrophysiology one would call this a non-specific area.

PURPURA:

I think the designation of these nuclei as "nonspecific" is unfortunate.

KUYPERS:

Oh, I am sorry but I think that you are accustomed to do so though. Anyhow, this non-specific area I think is specific in the way that the motor cortex projects somatotopically to the centremedian and the intralaminar nuclei (Petras, Trans. Am. Neur. Ass., 1965; Kuypers and Pandya, The Thalamus, Columbia Univ. Press, 122, 1966; Kuypers and Lawrence, Brain Res. 4: 151, 1967). This is the basis for my objection against using the term non-specific in respect to the centremedian and perhaps also the intralaminar nuclei.

PURPURA:

Look, Henricus, you are entitled to your objections about the way I use the word. But I don't think you should object to the designation from the physiological standpoint. It is known that in the designation of specific nuclei, such as VL, elements can be identified by orthodromic and antidromic activation. There is a good correspondence between morphological and electrophysiological data in respect to specific input-output relations. However, the situation is quite different physiologically when one goes beyond the trajectory of the monosynaptic input and engage interneurons polysynaptically linked to neurons that are not on the direct projection pathways. Under these conditions, one is dealing with possibilities of interactions in interneuronal pools with elements 2, 3, 4 or more synapses removed from the specific pathway. While these interneurons are not immediately related to cerebellofugal inputs, they may still be within the domain of cerebellar influences. The territories of these interneuronal domains are within the synaptic sphere of elements arising in CM-Pf and in VL. It is likely that it is within these interneuronal networks the major business is transacted of what's really important—not at the monosynaptic input level. After all most of the functions of the brain are really concerned with interneuronal operations. What are you objecting to?

KUYPERS:

What I am still objecting to is that I don't know really which anatomical structures you are dealing with—that is my shortcoming.

PURPURA:

No, it's not your shortcoming.

KUYPERS:

The area which I'm talking about...

PURPURA:

I believe you are making the point that in any study of nuclear relations we must define the input and output. This is fine when the situation permits it. But bear in mind that the whole field of spinal cord physiology is now addressing the issue of 'how do interneurons operate?' This is true even in the Aplysia abdominal ganglia which are veritable interneuronal machines. In the thalamus the same applies. I think we are in agreement with the obvious, i.e., we should know where the afferents are ending in a particular nucleus. But beyond the first synapse, morphology is lost. When I say a cell is activated by stimulation in the medial thalamus it may also be activated by corticothalamic volleys and other inputs. Such an element must be engaged in many operations involving VA-VL nuclear activities.

STERIADE:

In the first series of your papers you showed powerful inhibitory sequences in VL neurons following low-rate stimulation of the medial thalamic nuclei. Later, in the paper with Maekawa, you specified that less potent inhibitory projections arising in the medial thalamus are distributed to VB neurons. Now, you find that the same type of stimulation eliciting recruiting responses, is associated with no inhibitory effect in the LGB. Your findings on powerful IPSPs triggered in VL neurons either during recruiting by medial thalamic stimuli or during spontaneously developing spindles have been well corroborated by our own experiments conducted on chronically implanted cats and showing virtual disappearance of the monosynaptically relayed VL activity during behavioral sleepiness with EEG spindles, in spite of the unchanged presynaptic spike. But this is a finding common to the VB and LGB, at which levels slow sleep in behaving preparations or spontaneously occurring EEG spindles in paralyzed animals are constantly associated with a striking diminution of the monosynaptically relayed activity evoked by stimulating the medial lemniscus and the optic tract, respectively. This can also be seen by looking at the first (presynaptic) deflection in the specific cortical response to either VB or LGB stimuli, and reflecting the thalamic output, which is undoubtedly diminished until disappearance during periods of sleep with EEG spindles. This resulted from experiments done in the laboratory of the late Dr. Cordeau on the visual system (Exptl. Neurol., 1965, 11: 90-103) and in my own laboratory on the somesthetic specific thalamo-cortical responses (J. Neurophysiol., 1969, 32: 251-265). Reticular or natural arousal induces recovery of this inhibition of synaptic transmission not only in the VL, but also in the VB and LGB (these data are reviewed in Int. Rev. Neurobiol., 1970, 12: 87-144). This implies that a diffuse inhibition is exerted in all these specific nuclei during slow sleep and especially during periods of EEG spontaneous spindles or recruiting responses. How do you explain this homogenous picture in all the thalamic relay nuclei, likely exerted through nonspecific-specific thalamic links, in view of your present description of different effects in each of them by setting in motion the same system?

PURPURA:

What happens during electrical stimulation and during slow wave sleep are obviously very different things. Nevertheless the effects of medial thalamic stimulation on VL and VB relay cells are quite different. But the question implies something else. Perhaps what transpires during slow wave sleep involves much more than activity confined to the nonspecific system of the thalamus, although the nonspecific nuclei may be involved. There are, after all, many different kinds of spindle waves and these can be reproduced by stimulation of different sites in the thalamus. Similarly slow wave processes in cortex during behavioral sleep may involve different kinds of thalamic neuronal organizations which may have little effect on some relay neurons. Recall that cutaneous receptor fields of thalamic VB neurons do not seem to be affected by alterations in sleep-wakefulness behavior.

AMASSIAN:

I have two questions, first, the very interesting difference between the two kinds of EPSP in the lateral geniculate cells. I think many years ago, Kuffler and his collaborators (Kuffler, S.W., FitzHugh, R. and Barlow, H.B. Maintained activity in the cat's retina in light and darkness. J. Gen. Physiol. 40 (1957) 683-702) looking at the output of individual ganglion cells, found that the interval distribution resembled a gamma process. You might expect, given the rates of discharge in these cells and consequently the rates of occurrence of the two kinds of EPSPs, that on a random basis you would get a certain frequency of superposition. Do you in fact ever get the types one and two EPSPs sitting on top of one another.

PURPURA:

Yes we do.

AMASSIAN:

You do, fine. That's a point in favor of one of your interpretations. Now, the second question, unfortunately,gets back to medial thalamus again. Do you really have an answer to the problem of electrical stimulation not only exciting orthodromic pathways but also causing antidromic invasion of fiber systems with complicated distributions within thalamus and so on. Could the effects you describe depend upon such antidromic distribution of the activity?

PURPURA:

Insofar as one is going to use electrical stimulation anywhere in the neuraxis, this is a problem we face interminably, whether its stimulation of the cortex or stimulation anywhere else. I think that anytime electrical stimulation is utilized within the neuraxis from the spinal cord on, this criticism must be faced. I can only say that when one records intracellularly from thalamic or striatal neurons and looks very carefully for antidromic invasion, the remarkable thing is how infrequently antidromic invasion is observed. So that's no criterion. I don't know what the reason is for this. But, I think you are right. I think what we have to do is try to get away from electrical stimulation. I'm not too worried by the fact that I may be activating systems antidromically and via collaterals if I do find that I have discovered new ways in which collateralization may have become important in the brain.

KUYPERS:

I want to bring up a different point. In respect to the electrophysiological studies, I am always bothered by the fact that they tend to deal merely with the behavior of cells while we ultimately are interested in the behaviour of the organism. However, the electrophysiological data of Dr. Purpura may be directly related to behavioral data obtained by Vanderwolf (Psychological Review, 78: 83-113, 1971). He destroyed the medial thalamus, which would seem to correspond with the non-specific area of Dr. Purpura. After such medial thalamus lesions, Dr. Vanderwolf found that the initiation of active avoidance movements was strongly impaired. These and Dr. Purpura's data in part might pertain to one and the same thing. They might be interpreted as to show that the medial thalamic area plays an essential part in getting the lateral thalamic area rolling. If this is correct it would represent a meeting ground of physiological and psychological concepts.

PURPURA:

I think that apart from the question of looking at neurons as neurons, obviously the system is important. The question is to what extent is it absolutely essential. There have been studies reported on initiation of movement, in which attempts were made to develop conditioned reflex activities when lesions really significantly interfere with performance. But the point is this is a system that is geared for parallel processing of information in many areas.

HASSLER:

I am afraid that this problem of unspecific influence becomes even more complicated if we include the pallidum and the pallidal system as you showed. I think you are quite correct in saying that only few thalamic cells have convergence of dentate and pallidal fibers. But then you also said that this is the way "the cerebellum comes into discussion with the basal ganglia." I don't believe that this is correct because the main efferent pathway of the internal pallidum (of the entopeduncular nucleus is its homologue in the cat) is going to the anterior part of VL, (V.o.a.) and then they both project to the motor cortex; there is no doubt about this. V.o.a. projects to some special part of area 6 and V.o.p. (or the posterior part of VL) projects to area 4. Perhaps you saw the paper of Sasaki and Diekman which showed that one can activate the cortex from the pallidum unspecifically but one can also do it from the internal segment of the pallidum which is really a specific pathway. Pallidal evoked recruiting responses and field potentials are seen exclusively in area 6 and not in area 4. So I think the problem becomes even more difficult if one does not accept the nucleus VL as a functional unit. Actually VL is not one nucleus; it has two completely different afferent systems, namely the dentate system and the pallidal system.

PRIBRAM:

The word nonspecific was originally coined to mean non-sensory specific and all the discussion here plus the work of Dr. Albe-Fessard, Busser and many others has indicated that the motor systems are indeed nonspecific systems in the sense of non-sensory specific systems. That doesn't mean that there is not a discrete anatomical organization to these systems. Perhaps if we could accept the term "nonspecific" to mean "non-sensory specific" and not "non-discrete," we could have a meeting of minds.

JASPER:

I cannot agree with you, Dr. Pribram, because motor systems can be specific too, with specific topographical relationships. It's on the basis of such topographic relationships in either sensory or motor systems that we classify them as specific or nonspecific. But I am ready to throw out the term completely. I do not believe that there is anything that is nonspecific in the thalamus—that is an expression of our ignorance—just like the use of idiopathic in medicine when the cause of a disease is unknown. Microelectrode studies show a remarkable specificity of function in thalamic cells—some with complex relations to sensory and motor functions, others with still more complex functions, such as "novelty detectors," etc. But it is likely that those which seem not to be influenced by our manipulations of the patients merely have other complex functions which we have not as yet been able to ascertain.

Corticothalamic Projections and Sensorimotor Activities
T. Frigyesi, E. Rinvik, and M.D. Yahr, editors. © 1972
Raven Press, New York.

Organization of Thalamic Connections from Motor and Somatosensory Cortical Areas in the Cat

Eric Rinvik

It has been known for a long time that reciprocal connections exist between the thalamus and the cerebral cortex. The thalamocortical connections representing the last link in the relay of impulses of different sensory modalities have naturally attracted the main attention of morphologists as well as physiologists. In the last decade, however, there has been a steadily increasing interest in the mechanisms underlying the central nervous control and modulation of sensory impulses. In this connection it has been well established that the cerebral cortex can influence the transmission of impulses in the spinal cord, dorsal column nuclei and trigeminal nuclei (3, 4, 22, 23, 33, 38, 41, 98). However, to date, few investigators have undertaken a more systematic and detailed analysis of the influence exerted by the cerebral cortex on the transmission of impulses in the various thalamic sensory relay nuclei. This may be due partly to the emphasis that has been put so far on the thalamocortical projection systems.

Over the years, a substantial number of investigators have described corticothalamic fibers from the frontal and parietal lobe in animals and man, in papers dealing more generally with corticofugal fibers (for refs. see 84). Most of these investigators used the Marchi method for tracing degenerating myelinated fibers. With the introduction of the silver impregnation methods for the tracing of degenerating unmyelinated as well as myelinated axons (30, 66, 67), and spurred by the increasing interest in central nervous control of sensory activity, more detailed studies on the corticothalamic projections have recently been undertaken by several investigators. The following account will present some of the findings that have been made in our laboratory on the projections from motor and somatosensory cortical areas in the cat. The light microscopical observations from silver-impregnated experimental material will be described first. This will be followed by the presentation of some preliminary electron microscopical findings on the corticothalamic projections in the cat. Finally some aspects of the synaptology of the normal nucleus ventralis lateralis thalami (VL) will be presented.

PROBLEMS CONNECTED WITH THE USE OF THE METHOD OF ANTEROGRADE DEGENERATION IN THE STUDY OF CORTICOTHALAMIC FIBER PROJECTIONS

The following description of the organization of corticothalamic fiber projections is based on the evaluation of the degeneration picture seen in silver-impregnated sections (30, 67) from the thalamus of adult cats with small cortical lesions. This method of studying anterograde degeneration has been successfully used in the investigations of fiber connections in the central nervous system. However, some particular problems arise when this method is used for the investigation of corticothalamic connections. Following a lesion of the cerebral cortex, one must consider the possibility of the occurrence of "indirect Wallerian degeneration" (8, 32, 34-37, 77), that is, degeneration proceeding centrifugally from the soma of damaged thalamocortical axons. For a detailed account of the many aspects of this problem, the reader is referred to the recent review by Grant (35). In the present context only a few relevant points will be emphasized.

It is important to recall that the speed of axonal degeneration in the central nervous system varies considerably among different species and even from one fiber system to another in the same species. Following lesions of the cingular cortex in the adult rabbit, the earliest signs of "indirect Wallerian degeneration" of thalamocortical fibers in the anterior nuclei of the thalamus are seen after 10 days (77). On the other hand, a very prominent cell shrinkage is seen in the cells in the lateral geniculate body (GL) 3 days after a lesion is made in the visual cortex in the same animal (19). In the adult cat the speed of fiber degeneration does not appear to be as quick as in the rabbit, and most authors agree that the degenerating fibers which are seen in silver-impregnated sections from the adult cat's thalamus following cortical lesions represent genuine corticothalamic axons if the survival time is between 3 and 7 days (26, 31, 42, 84-86). It is wise to recall, however, that chromatolysis is seen in 50% of the cells in the adult cat's GL 3 days following lesions of the visual cortex (19) and degenerating thalamocortical axons might be present in such cases. It is therefore of the greatest importance to evaluate carefully Nissl-stained sections for possible signs of an early retrograde cellular degeneration in the thalamic areas when degenerating fibers are seen in silver-impregnated material following similarly placed cortical lesions. The corticothalamic projections which are reported on below are interpreted as genuine corticothalamic fibers since evidence of retrograde cellular changes could not be detected in the relevant thalamic nuclei in Nissl-stained sections after similar cortical lesions and following survival times of less than one week.

CORTICOTHALAMIC FIBERS FROM THE FIRST SOMATOSENSORY CORTICAL AREA (SI) IN THE CAT

It appears to be difficult to distinguish physiologically the primary "sensory" and "motor" areas in the cat's cerebral cortex, as particularly stressed by Livingston and Phillips (48), Buser (15) and Brooks et al. (13, 14). In recent years physiolo-

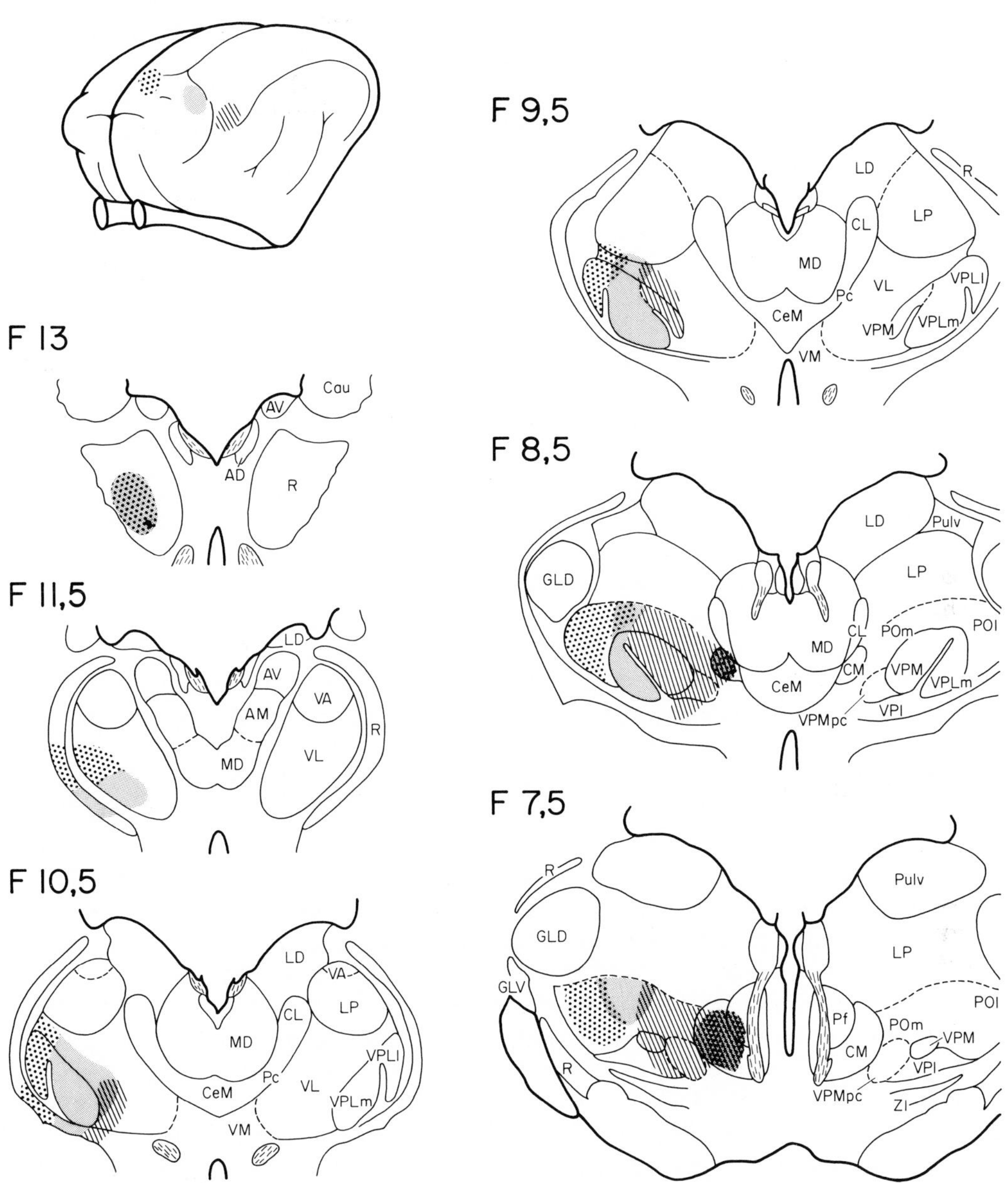

FIG. 1. Diagram summarizing the areas of termination in the thalamus of fibers arising in different parts of the posterior sigmoid gyrus caudal to the postcruciate dimple (SI). The density of corticothalamic fibers to various thalamic nuclei is not indicated.

gists have expressed the view that the postcruciate dimple marks the border between the "motor" and the "sensory" cortices. This would fit with the cyto- and myeloarchitectonic map of the cat's cerebral cortex presented by Hassler and Muhs-Clement (39). These authors have reported that frontal agranular cortex with a well-developed lamina V containing large pyramidal cells extends caudally almost to the postcruciate dimple, but that there exist individual variations in this respect.

The corticothalamic projections which are to be reported here have all been observed following cortical lesions limited to the posterior sigmoid gyrus caudal to the postcruciate dimple and to the caudal half of the coronal gyrus.

Following such lesions there is ample degeneration in several ipsilateral thalamic nuclei (Fig. 1). The degeneration is most profuse in the ventrobasal complex (VB) (Fig. 6), here defined as comprising the medial and lateral nucleus ventralis posterior (VPM and VPL, respectively). These two nuclei are clearly separated from each other by a medullated fiber bundle (83). A similar medullated lamina also divides VPL into a medial (VPLm) and a lateral (VPLl) sections (83).

There is a distinct somatotopical organization in the projection from SI upon VB: medial (hindlimb area) and lateral (forelimb area) parts of the posterior sigmoid gyrus, caudal to the postcruciate dimple, send fibers to VPLl and VPLm, respectively. The caudal coronal gyrus (face area) projects upon VPM, mainly the dorsolateral part of the nucleus (84) (Fig. 1).

This somatotopical organization in the projection from SI upon VB in the adult cat has been described by several authors (42, 47, 84). The corticofugal fibers to VB from SI terminate throughout the whole rostrocaudal extent of the nuclear complex. However, the silver-impregnation methods used in this study do not permit conclusions concerning the organization of the field of termination of the corticothalamic fibers, as has been shown with the Golgi method by Scheibel and Scheibel (92, 96 and elsewhere in this volume). Although care must be taken in evaluating the caliber of degenerating axons in silver-impregnated material, the corticothalamic fibers to VB appear to be rather thick as they enter VB, but their caliber then seems to diminish quickly within the nuclear complex itself.

Significant terminal degeneration is seen in the posterior group of thalamic nuclei (PO) following lesions of the cat's SI (42, 84) (Fig. 1). The term PO in the cat was introduced by Rose and Woolsey (91), and it has been largely accepted by several authors working on cats or other animals and on man (2, 10, 26, 40, 42, 46, 58-60, 62, 72, 83, 100, 101).

Considerable confusion exists in the literature concerning the delimitation of this thalamic region; in the present study it follows the outline given for the cat by Rose and Woolsey (91) and Poggio and Mountcastle (76), as it has been reported in more detail elsewhere (83). It is particularly important to realize that the rostral part of PO merges with the caudal part of VPLl, and that the ventral part of caudal LP is also included in PO. In agreement with most authors (5, 10, 11, 40, 42, 46, 58-60, 76, 91), the magnocellular part of the medial geniculate body (MGmc) is included in PO as well.

Following a lesion to the medial part of the posterior sigmoid gyrus caudal to the postcruciate dimple, or to the caudal coronal gyrus, the ensuing terminal degenerations are mainly localized within the lateral (POl) and medial (POm) parts of PO, respectively. Corticofugal fibers to PO from the lateral part of the postcruciate gyrus terminate mainly in the transitional area between POl and POm (Fig. 1). The finding of a topographical organization in the corticofugal projection from SI upon PO as well as VB is rather unexpected on the basis of the physiological data of the properties of single units in PO. It has been shown that the majority of the neurons are place and modality unspecific, that is, sensory information from all parts of the body converge upon this area (16, 22, 76, 100, 101).

In the present context, another point deserves particular attention. Although reciprocal connections between SI and VB are well established, they do not appear between PO and the cerebral cortex. Heath and Jones (40) have studied the anterograde degeneration following stereotactically placed lesions in various parts of PO in the adult cat. A minor part of PO (MGmc and nucleus suprageniculatus, Sg) projects upon the cerebral cortex, but not to SI. A large part of PO that receives corticofugal fibers from SI thus does not appear to project back upon the cerebral cortex at all. Heath and Jones (40) have tentatively suggested that the non-cortical projecting part of PO can be regarded as a caudal extension of the thalamic intralaminar system.

Following lesions of SI, terminal degeneration has consistently been found in the nucleus ventralis lateralis (VL) (84), although this connection is not mentioned by Chandler (18) or Jones and Powell (42) in their anatomical studies. Kusama et al. (47), on the other hand, described a few degenerating fibers in VL following lesions of the cat's SI. Degeneration in VL following lesions of SI is never as profuse as that in VB or PO, but neither is it sparse either (Fig. 9). The degeneration is restricted to that part of VL which borders on VB. Moreover, there is a clear topographical organization in the projection from SI upon VL: medial and lateral parts of the postcruciate gyrus send fibers to areas of VL lying immediately dorsal to VPLl and VPLm, respectively, while the caudal coronal gyrus projects upon a small area of VL lying immediately rostral to the oral pole of VPM. This is interesting since evoked potentials following polysensory stimulation in the cat have been recorded in the ventral part of VL (55, 56).

In a recent extensive physiological study on the regulation of VL units by sensory activity, Massion (54) has described effects upon VL neurons following stimulation of the cat's SI. However, he obtained a bilateral effect upon VL following stimulation of SI in one hemisphere. This observation is not reconcilable with the anatomical data which clearly show a unilateral projection upon VL from SI (47, 84). Moreover, from Massion's thesis (54), it appears that the cortical influence on VL is exerted on the whole nucleus. From the available anatomical data (84), however, it appears that the intensity of the degeneration in VL following a lesion of SI diminishes rather quickly from the dorsal border of VPL towards the internal medullary lamina.

A more detailed knowledge of the latencies of the responses of cells in ventral and dorsal parts of VL following stimulation of SI may help to clarify the discrepancies between the anatomical and physiological findings.

It is not clear whether the cells in VL project upon the primary somatosensory cortical area. Reports in the literature of studies on retrograde cellular degeneration do not seem to indicate such a cortical connection for VL. Recently, Smaha et al. (97) have found evidence of a projection from VL upon SI in the adult cat in an anterograde degeneration study following electrolytic lesions in VL. It is not clear from their paper, however, how large their lesions were, and the possibility of fibers passing through the area of the lesion from other thalamic nuclei is not considered.

More details on the organization of cortical efferents to VL will be discussed after the fibers to this nucleus from the motor cortical areas have been described.

The cat's SI projects upon several other thalamic structures in addition to the fibers to VL. A large number of degenerating fibers are seen in the reticular nucleus of the thalamus (R). Although a majority of these fibers obviously are merely passing through on their way to other thalamic nuclei, the author concluded from the degeneration picture in the light microscope that some fibers actually terminate in R (84). This was in agreement with other investigators who have described corticofugal fibers to R, using silver impregnation techniques in the cat (7, 42, 68). Degenerating fibers appear to terminate in the rostral cap of R as well as in those regions of R that lie close to the areas of termination in VB and VL. It was emphasized, however, that electron microscopical investigations are needed to provide a final answer to the problem of whether the degenerating fibers actually end in R (84) (see below).

It has also been shown that SI projects upon the nucleus centrum medianum (CM) (84). In the same paper, it was stated that corticofugal fibers from SI were said to terminate in a large-celled part of the nucleus parafascicularis (Pf) lying lateral to the fibers of the habenulo interpeduncular tract. A careful re-examination of the material and of Nissl-stained serial sections through the normal cat's thalamus, however, has convinced the author that the region in question is the caudalmost extension of nucleus centralis lateralis (CL), as stated by Mehler (57). This area of termination of the corticofugal fibers from SI appears to correspond to the area of termination of spinothalamic fibers, as recently described in the cat (10).

The degenerating corticofugal fibers from SI to CM and caudal CL are much thinner than the fibers to VB, VL and PO, and they are easily missed during the impregnation procedure if the suppression times are too long. No evidence was found which could indicate a somatotopical organization in the cortical projection upon CM.

CORTICOTHALAMIC PROJECTIONS FROM THE SECOND SOMATOSENSORY CORTICAL AREA (SII) IN THE CAT

The second somatosensory cortical area (SII) of the cat lies in the anterior ectosylvian gyrus (103, 104). This gyrus has been divided into 3 zones (A, B and C) by Carreras and Andersson (17) according to a pattern of vessels crossing the anterior ectosylvian gyrus, and based upon the properties of single neurons in the gyrus.

Zone A lies at the transition area between the second auditory area (AII) and SII, while zones B and C are located well within the confines of the latter sensory area (17).

Following lesions restricted to the anterior ectosylvian gyrus in the cat, ample terminal degeneration is seen in the ipsilateral VB as well as in restricted parts of PO (Fig. 2) (25, 42, 85). There are, however, some differences between the projections from SI and SII to VB and PO. The density of the terminal degeneration in PO following lesions of SII exceeds that in VB (Figs. 10,11) (25, 85), while the reverse obtains in animals with lesions of SI (42, 85). Following lesions of SII, terminal degeneration is present throughout the rostrocaudal extent of VPL (42, 85). DeVito (25), on the other hand, found only few degenerating fibers in rostral VPL following similar lesions.

There is a distinct somatotopical organization of the corticofugal projections from SII upon VB (42, 47, 85). Rostral parts of SII (zone C) project upon VPLm and VPM, while fibers originating in Carreras and Andersson's zone B (17) terminate in VPLl (Fig. 2). A similar organization is seen in the projection to PO (85) (Fig. 2). On the other hand, when the cortical lesion is limited to the most caudal part of the anterior ectosylvian gyrus (zone A), no degenerating fibers are found in VB, but are found mainly in POl and MGmc. These anatomical findings are of particular interest when related to the physiological data of Carreras and Andersson (17). These authors found that about 20% of the neurons in SII were modality and place unspecific and thus very much resemble the cells in PO(76). Such cells are found more commonly as the recording electrode is moved posteriorly and superiorly along the axis of the anterior ectosylvian gyrus, and they are particularly numerous in the narrow zone between AII and SII (zone A).

It should be emphasized that SI and SII both project upon VB as well as PO. The termination in PO of fibers from SI lies within the area of termination of fibers from SII (42, 84, 85), but the latter field of termination appears to exceed that of the former (84, 85). In this connection it again is of interest to recall that Heath and Jones (40) found no evidence of a projection from PO upon SII, except for a restricted connection from MGmc and Sg upon Carreras and Andersson's zone A (17).

The area of terminal degeneration in PO following lesions in SI and in SII appears to coincide with the area shown to receive fibers from the cat's spinal cord (10, 58, 59). It is important, however, that this area is less extensive than the total posterior group as defined by several authors (26, 40, 42, 60, 76, 83, 91). This fact, and the evidence for a topographical or even somatotopical organization in the projection from SI and SII upon PO, are indicative that this region may not be as heterogeneous as originally stated by Poggio and Mountcastle (76).

Although all authors agree that VB and PO receive the majority of cortical afferents from SII, opinions differ concerning the projection from this cortical area to other thalamic nuclei. Chandler (18) describes a bilateral projection to CM in the cat, and other investigators have also seen degeneration (terminal ?) in CM following lesions of SII (25, 47). The author (85) found some degenerating terminal fibers in

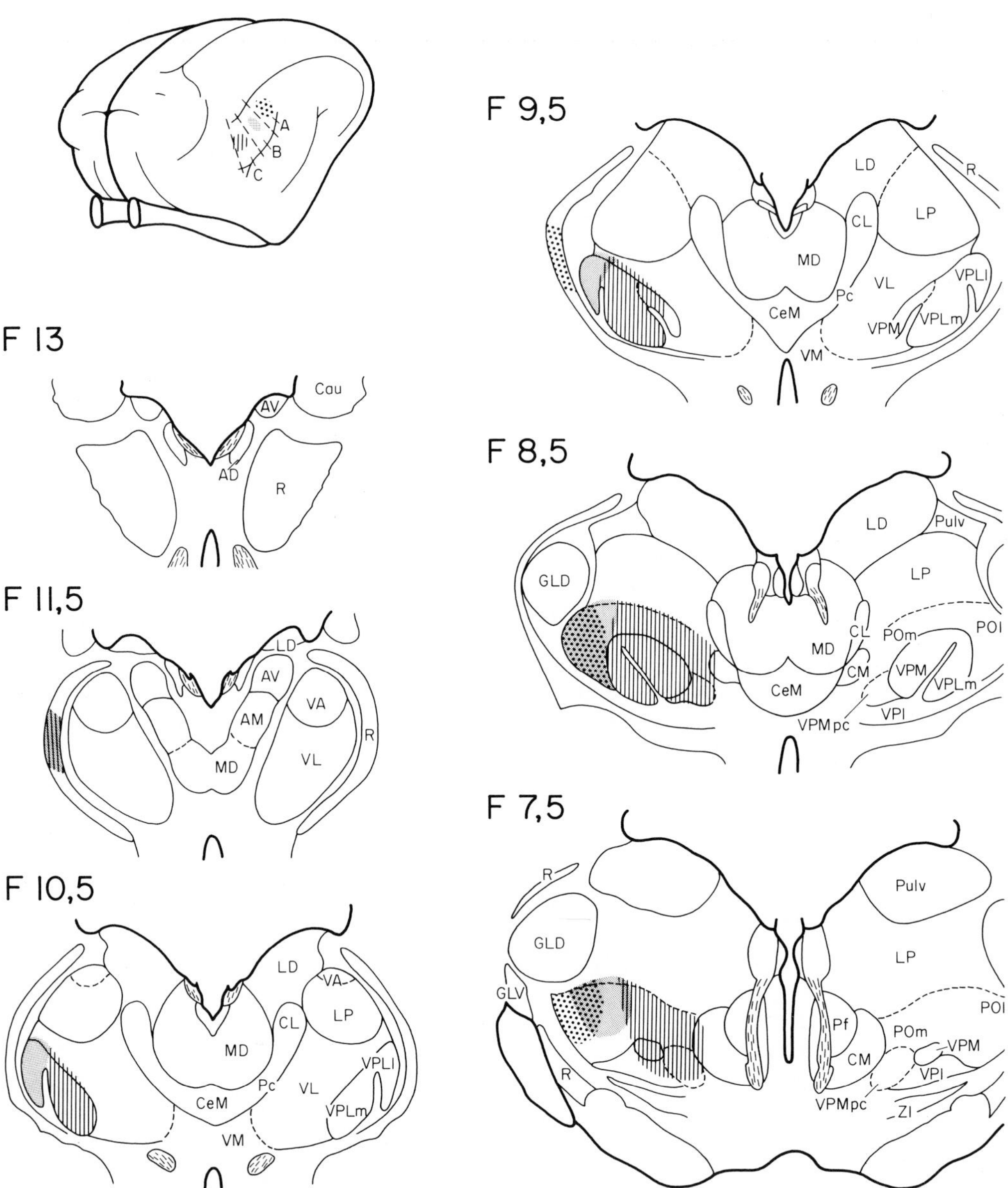

FIG. 2. Diagram summarizing the areas of termination in the thalamus of fibers arising in different parts of the anterior ectosylvian gyrus (SII). The density of corticothalamic fibers to various thalamic nuclei is not indicated.

CM only following lesions of the rostral part of SII (Carreras and Andersson's zone C), (17) but not following lesions of the remaining part of SII. Jones and Powell (42) do not describe fibers from SII to CM at all.

Most authors seem to agree that some corticofugal fibers from SII end in restricted parts of R (25, 42: Fig. 9, but not in text, 85).

Degenerating fibers are seen coursing through parts of nucleus ventralis anterior (VA) and VL on their way to caudal thalamic structures (85). Although Kusama et al. (47) mention that corticofugal fibers from SII actually terminate in the ventrolateral corner of VL, other investigators who have studied the thalamic projections from the cat's SII have found no evidence of an unequivocal terminal degeneration in any part of VL (25, 42, 85). Thus there appears to be a difference in the projection upon the thalamus from SI and SII, since the former cortical area sends fibers to restricted parts of VL (Figs. 1, 9).

CORTICOTHALAMIC FIBERS FROM THE PRIMARY MOTOR CORTICAL AREA (MI) IN THE CAT

As mentioned earlier, there seem to be some discrepancies in the literature concerning the delimitation of the cat's primary motor cortical area. According to the cyto- and myeloarchitectonic studies of Hassler and Muhs-Clement (39), the cat's homologue of the simian area 4 is situated in the posterior sigmoid gyrus rostral to the postcruciate dimple, and it extends across the cruciate sulcus onto the lateral part of the anterior sigmoid gyrus. Area 6 is found on the medial part of the anterior cruciate gyrus and the rostral part of the entire gyrus.

Following lesions of these areas (4 and 6) in the cat, profuse degeneration is seen in the ipsilateral VL (Figs. 3, 8). There is a gradual increase in the density of terminal degeneration in VL as the lesions are placed at successively more rostral levels from the postcruciate dimple. The cruciate sulcus itself marks a rather abrupt increase in the number of corticofugal fibers to VL; the greatest number of such fibers come from the medial as well as the lateral parts of the precruciate gyrus (84) (Fig. 3). On the other hand, Kusama et al. (47) found very little degeneration in VL after lesions of the medial part of the anterior sigmoid gyrus.

The areas of termination of corticofugal fibers from the anterior and posterior sigmoid gyri differ in VL. Corticofugal fibers from the rostral part of the latter gyrus (area 4) end in the same parts of VL and show the same topographical organization as do fibers to VL from the caudal part of the same gyrus (SI) (see above). However, the density of the terminal degeneration appears to be higher following lesions limited to area 4. On the other hand, fibers to VL from the anterior sigmoid gyrus (area 6) show no clear topographical arrangement. The majority of these fibers terminate throughout the rostrocaudal extent of VL in a rather broad zone lying just medial to VB. This area coincides generally with the terminal field of the cortical efferents from the gyrus coronalis. Furthermore, whether the lesions are confined to the anterior or posterior sigmoid gyri or extend to the coronal gyrus, the density of the terminal degeneration in VL diminishes towards the internal medullary lamina. Thus, two patterns are

Corticothalamic Projections from MI

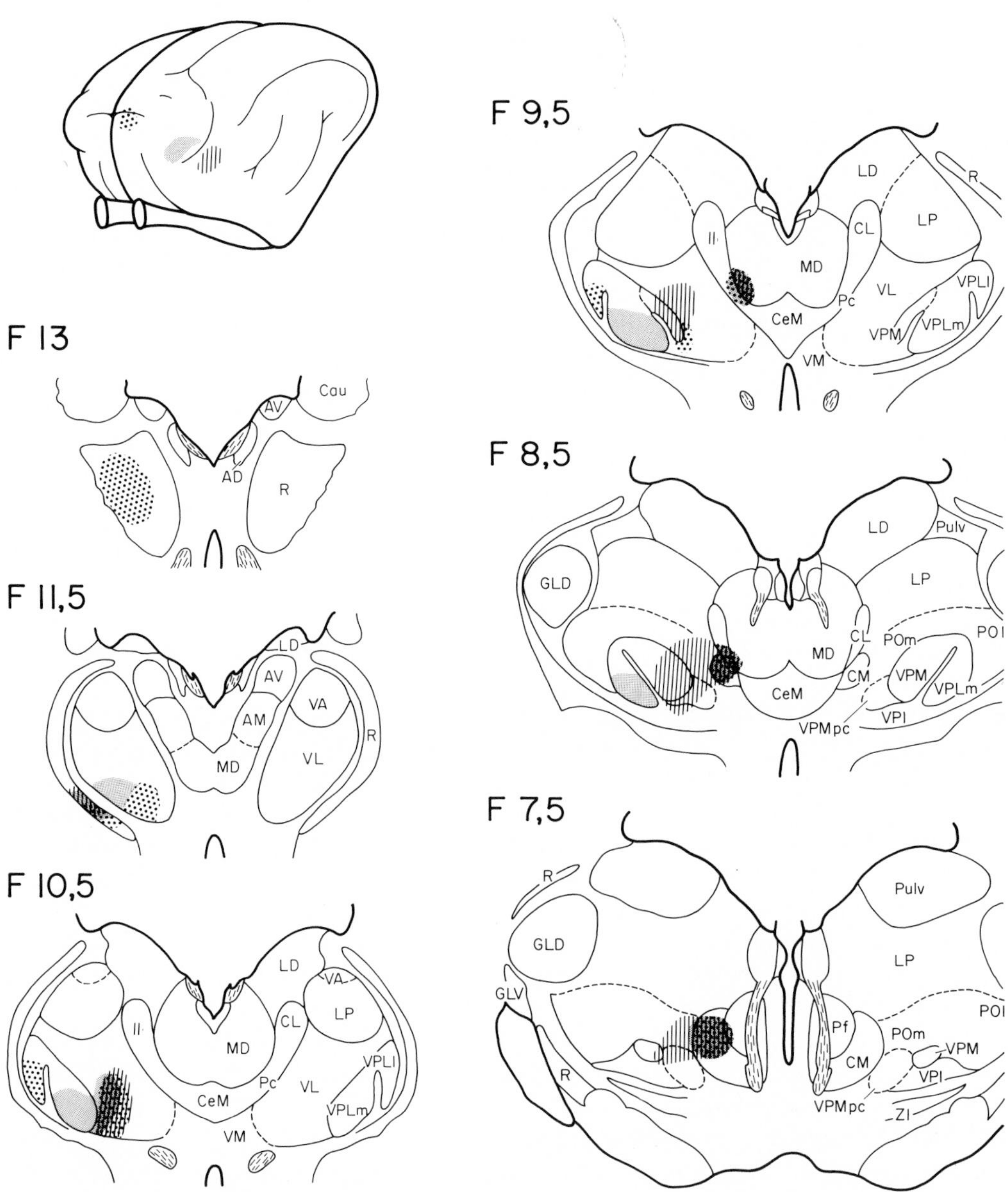

FIG. 3. Diagram summarizing the areas of termination in the thalamus of fibers arising in different parts of the posterior sigmoid gyrus anterior to the postcruciate dimple and from the anterior sigmoid gyrus (MI, Areas 4 and 6). The density of corticothalamic fibers to various thalamic nuclei is not indicated.

apparent in the cortical projections from SI and MI upon VL in the cat. First, only the projection from the posterior sigmoid gyrus, rostral and caudal to the post-cruciate dimple (area 4 and SI) shows a clear tendency toward a topographical arrangement in the distribution of fibers from its medial and lateral parts. Second, although the density of terminal degeneration in VL is highest following lesions restricted to the anterior sigmoid gyrus (mainly area 6) (39), these corticothalamic fibers show topical arrangement only to a limited extent, and overlap throughout the rostrocaudal extent of VL in a zone which is located just medial to VB.

These observations are of interest when compared with the physiological findings of Massion (54 , and elsewhere in this volume), and Rispal-Padel and Massion (87). These authors have reported that the cat's trunk and axial musculature is "represented" in medial parts of VL, which in turn project upon area 6. The extremities are "represented" more laterally within VL in a zone that projects upon area 4, that is, the posterior sigmoid gyrus rostral to the postcruciate dimple (54, 87).

Furthermore, following lesions of MI, unequivocal terminal degeneration in VB is also seen (Fig. 7). The density of the terminal degeneration in VPL decreases as the lesion is placed at successively more rostral levels from the post-cruciate dimple. When the lesion is confined within area 6 (39), only occasional degenerating fibers are seen in VPL. This may explain why Kusama et al. (47) did not find degeneration in VPL following lesions of the medial part of the anterior sigmoid gyrus, while the author (84) did. In these studies, the lesions involved the depth of the cruciate sulcus, and thus encroached upon area 4 (39, 84).

A topographical organization similar to the one described for the projection from SI upon VPL is recognized in the connections from area 4. There is, however, one point of difference. Whereas corticofugal fibers from SI terminate throughout the whole extent of VPL, the density of the terminal degeneration following lesions within area 4 is higher in the ventral parts of VPLl and VPLm, while more scattered degenerating fibers are seen in the middle and dorsal parts of the nuclei. This is interesting since the impulses from the extremities are relayed through cerebellum and VL to area 4 (54, 87) and neurons which receive somatic sensory impulses from the distal parts of the limbs in the cat, rabbit, monkey and man, have been localized to the ventral part of VPL (1, 63, 64, 89).

Lesions limited to the rostral part of the coronal gyrus result in terminal degeneration in the ventromedial parts of VPM and also in the adjoining parts of the parvocellular part of VPM (VPMpc). It should be recalled that area 3 of the cat's somatosensory cortex extends rostrally along the coronal gyrus (39). As mentioned earlier, the caudal half of the coronal gyrus projects primarily upon the more dorsolateral parts of VPM. In a careful retrograde cellular study in the macaque, Roberts and Akert (88) found that the medial and basal VPM projects upon granular precentral opercular cortex, while the dorsal and lateral part sends fibers to the lower one third of the postcentral gyrus.

The density of the terminal degeneration in VPMpc and in nucleus ventralis posterior inferior (VPI) in the cat is higher following lesions in the caudal part of the coronal gyrus than when the lesion is situated more rostrally. Physiological studies have provided evidence that the gustatory impulses are mediated through the medial and caudal parts of VPM in the cat and monkey (6, 9, 24, 28, 71). Though none of these authors uses the terms VPMpc and VPI, it appears from their figures that this is indeed the region in question.

Thus, in the cat, following lesions restricted to area 4, terminal degeneration is limited to VL, and degenerating fibers are also found in the somatosensory relay nuclei (VB). In this connection it appears relevant to recall that Chow and Pribram (20) in a retrograde cellular study in the monkey observed that VPL projects upon both banks of the central fissure. Similar observations have been made by LeGros Clark and Boggon (21).

The cat's MI sends fibers to thalamic nuclei other than VL and VB, but their number appears quite small compared to the projections upon VL and VB. Following lesions of the cat's motor cortex, and particularly area 6, terminal degeneration as judged from light microscopical studies has been seen in R, CM and PF as well as caudal CL (7, 68, 84), in caudal nucleus paracentralis (Pc) (7, 84), and in the ventrolateral corner of caudal nucleus medialis dorsalis (MD) (68, 84). The evidence does not suggest that the cortical projections to CM in the cat are similar to those, somatotopically organized, in the monkey and chimpanzee (75; Petras, elsewhere in this volume).

It appears from these observations that the cat's motor cortex influences not only somatosensory and motor relay nuclei of the thalamus, but also several other nuclei whose cortical connections appear to be more widespread (53, 65), or whose connections with the cerebral cortex are, at best, doubtful but which probably project upon parts of the basal ganglia (12, 50-52, 57, 78, 92, 93, 95).

THE CORTICOTHALAMIC PROJECTION FROM THE SUPPLEMENTARY MOTOR AREA (MII) IN THE CAT

No detailed physiological investigations have been undertaken to map out the cat's homologue of the supplementary motor area (MII) in monkey and man. However, Woolsey (103, 104) has tentatively suggested that this area in the cat is situated on the medial wall of the rostral hemisphere. Moreover, anatomical investigations have shown similarities between the subcortical projections from MI and those from the medial wall of the cat's rostral hemisphere. Following lesions within the latter area, degenerating terminal fibers have been found in the spinal grey matter (69), the dorsal column nuclei and the spinal trigeminal nucleus (Rinvik, unpublished observations). Furthermore, in such cases degenerating fibers have been traced to VB and VL as well as to several other thalamic nuclei, including VA, CM, Pf, CL and lateral MD (86) (Fig. 4).

There is, however, one notable difference between the corticothalamic projections from MII and those from MI, SI and SII. While the latter projections are strictly ipsilateral, the fibers from the medial wall of the cat's rostral hemisphere are bilaterally distributed to the thalamic nuclei (86). The density of the terminal degeneration in the thalamus, ipsilateral to a lesion in MII, is always superior to that seen contra-

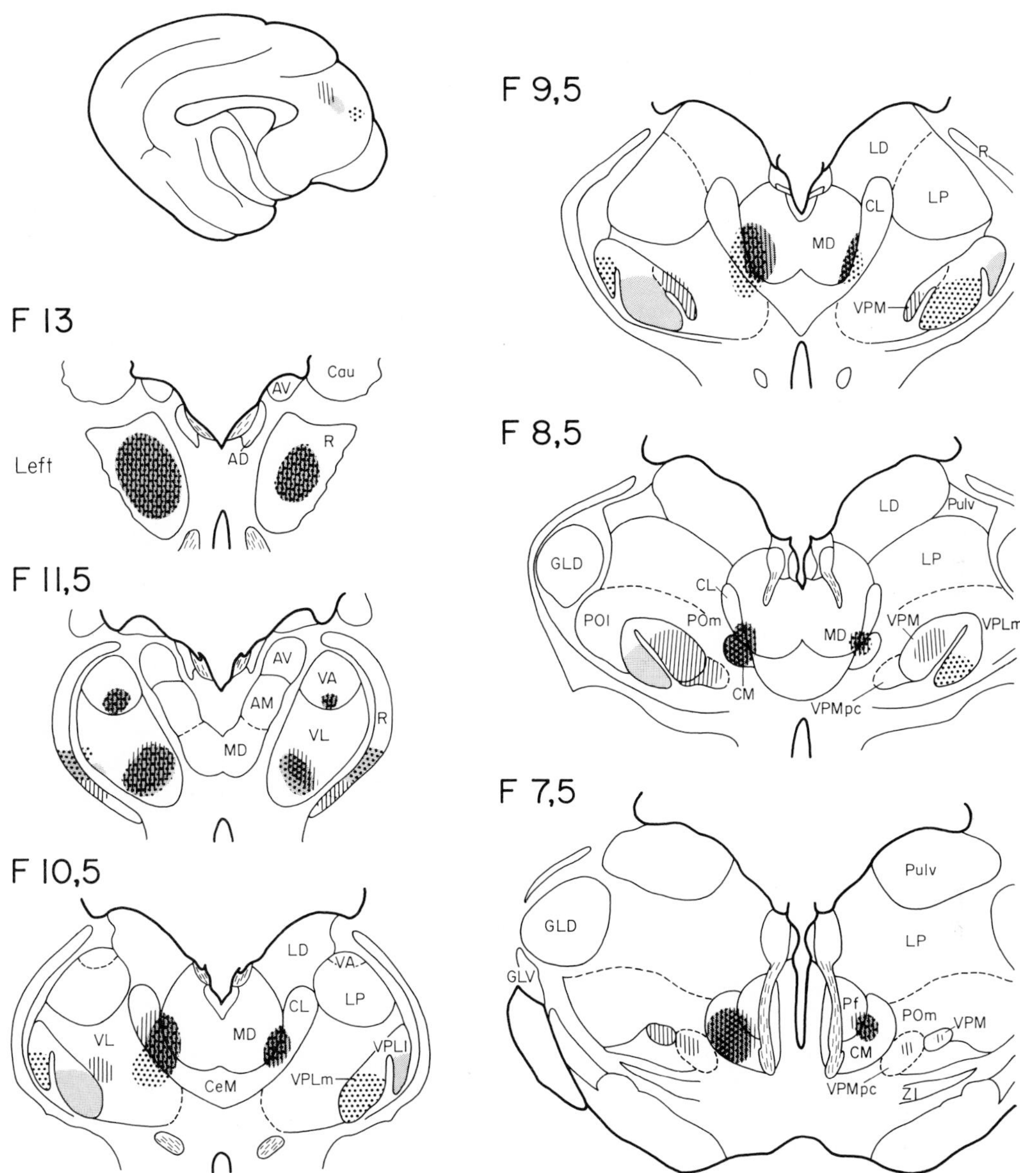

FIG. 4. Diagram summarizing the areas of termination in the thalamus of fibers arising in different parts of the medial wall of the rostral hemisphere ("supplementary motor area", MII). The density of corticothalamic fibers to various thalamic nuclei is not indicated.

laterally.

Two points deserve mention in this connection. When the lesion is placed quite dorsally on the medial wall or on the medial convexity of the precruciate gyrus, very few and scattered degenerating fibers are seen in the contralateral VL and VB. By placing the lesion successively more ventral on the medial wall, the density of contralateral degeneration in these nuclei increases (86). Since the precentral agranular cortex extends over the convexity of the precruciate gyrus and, for a short distance, on the dorsal aspect of the medial wall of this gyrus in the cat (39, 90), a bilateral projection to VL and VB appears to be a characteristic feature of frontal granular cortex on the medial wall of the rostral hemisphere.

The degeneration in VL following lesions of MII is restricted to the medial parts of the rostral half of the nucleus and to the areas of VL which border on the regions of VB, which also show terminal degeneration. The degeneration in VL following lesions of MII, however, is never as profuse as that seen in the nucleus following lesions of MI.

Furthermore, it has been possible to discern a somatotopical organization in the bilateral projection from this cortical area upon VB and also to show that this organization appears to be a diagonal one. Thus, in cases where terminal degeneration is seen in the hindlimb region of VB (VPLl), on the side of the lesion, the terminal degeneration on the contralateral side is limited to the forelimb area of VB (VPLm) (Figs. 4, 12). When the ipsilateral degeneration is seen in VPLm, it is limited to VPLl on the contralateral side. On the other hand, the projection to VPM is always symmetrical on both sides.

The terminal degeneration in VB following a lesion of the medial wall of the rostral hemisphere is not evenly distributed throughout the nuclei, but appears to be more concentrated in the ventral parts of VPLl and VPLm. This distribution of terminal degeneration within VPL is similar to that seen following lesions of area 4 on the convexity of the hemisphere, notwithstanding the fact that the cytoarchitectonic characteristics of the two cortical areas in question differ markedly; one is agranular, while the other has the characteristics of koniocortex.

THE COURSE OF THE CORTICOTHALAMIC FIBERS

The course followed by the corticothalamic fibers varies according to their area of termination and, to some extent, according to their area of origin (84–86). Generally it appears that the corticothalamic fibers from the sensorimotor cortical areas of the cat can follow three major pathways (Fig. 5). 1. A fair number of corticofugal fibers to VL and VB leave the internal capsule at rostral telencephalic levels and pierce the rostral cap of R. They then course through VA and parts of VL before they terminate in more or less restricted regions in the latter nucleus and in VB. Fibers coursing through R and VA have been described by Chandler (18) in the cat and by Scheibel and Scheibel (93, 94) in Golgi material. 2. The majority of the corticofugal fibers to VL and VB, however, leave the internal capsule at slightly more caudal levels and enter R and the external medullary lamina. They course in a caudal and medial direc-

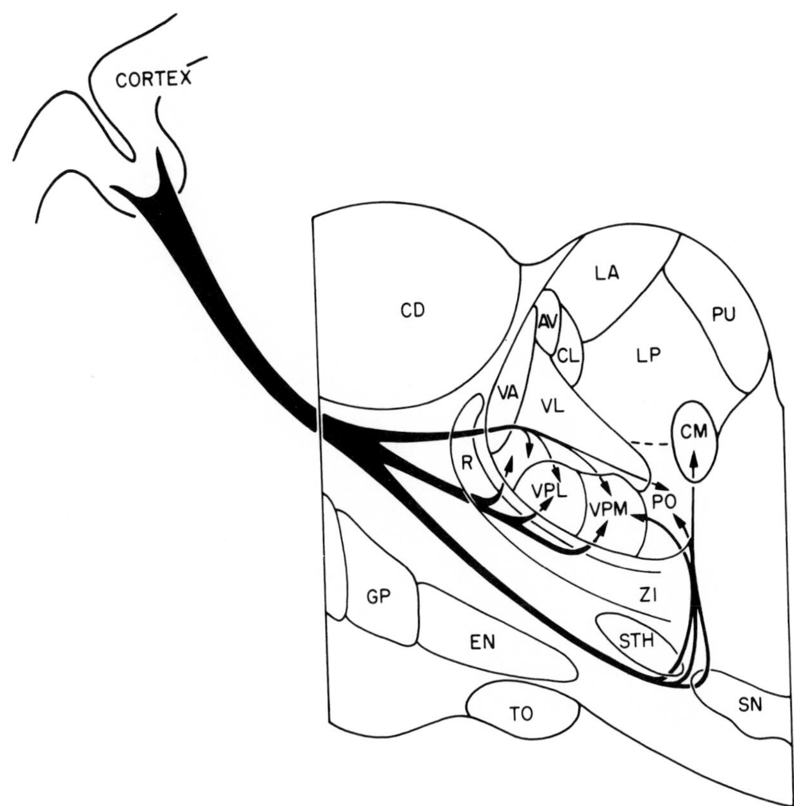

FIG. 5. Diagram summarizing the 3 major pathways followed by the corticothalamic fibers from SI, SII, MI and MII. For details see the text and Rinvik (84-86).

tion in these structures and are distributed to restricted areas in VL and VB at successively more caudal levels. 3. The third major pathway taken by the corticothalamic fibers is more circuitous. At the mesodiencephalic junction, corticothalamic fibers leave the cerebral peduncle and course in a rostrodorsal direction towards the basal and inferior thalamic regions. They traverse the zona incerta, and may even traverse the rostral part of the substantia nigra. Most corticofugal fibers to VPM, VPMpc and VPI seem to follow this route. This also applies to cortical efferents which are destined for POm, CM, Pf, caudal parts of CL and Pc, and the lateral part of caudal MD. Scheibel and Scheibel (95) have described a similar course of corticofugal fibers in Golgi material, and Jones and Powell (42) have followed such fibers to posterior thalamic regions in Nauta sections in the cat.

The corticothalamic fibers to PO follow different routes according to their area

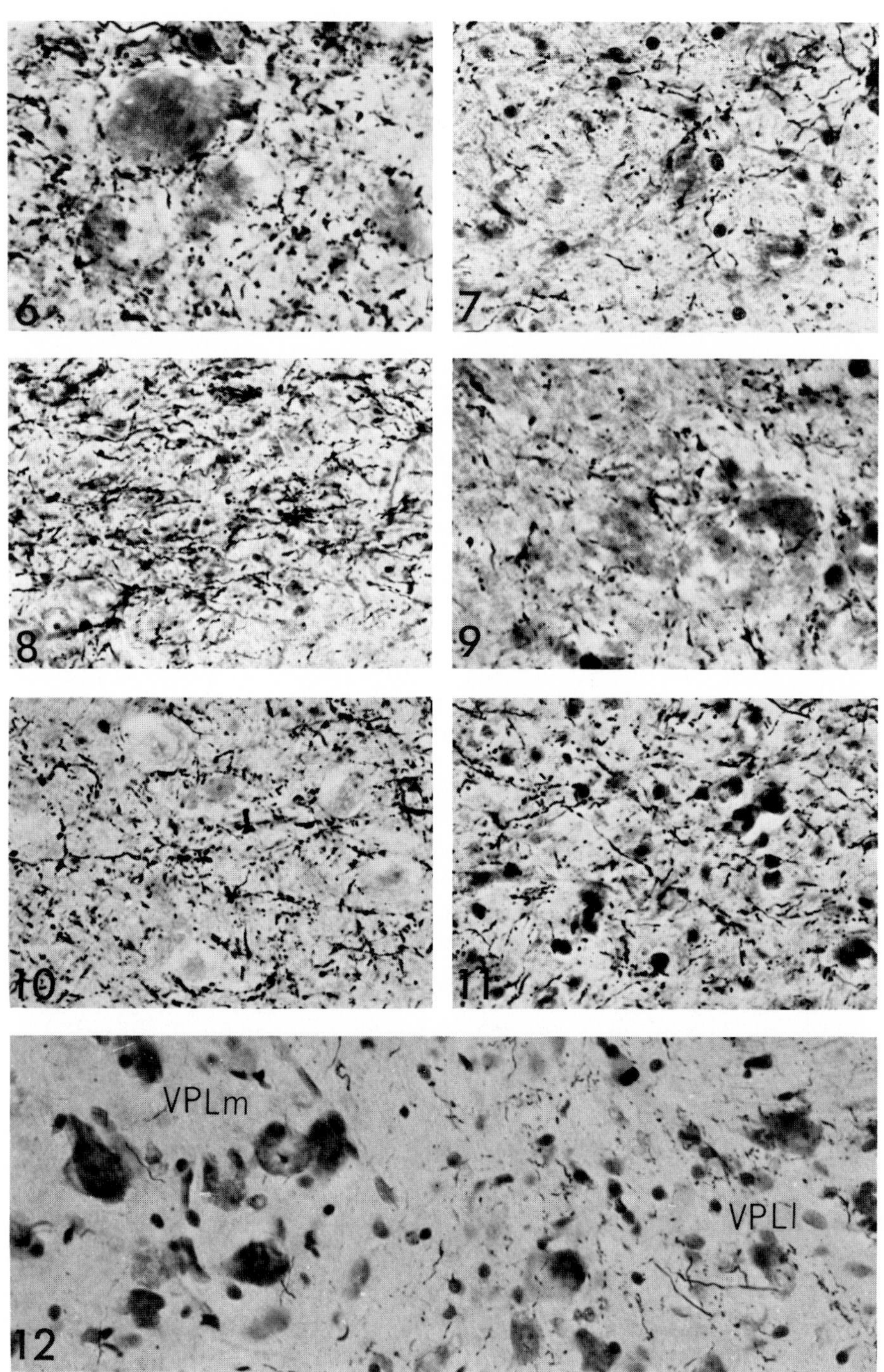

FIGS. 6-12

FIG. 6. Degenerating fibers in VPLm, 7 days following a lesion in the lateral part of the caudal postcruciate gyrus (SI). Nauta. Magnification: X 585.

FIG. 7. Degenerating fibers in VPLl, 7 days following a lesion of the medial part of the anterior sigmoid gyrus and the wall of the cruciate sulcus (MI). Compare to Fig. 6. Nauta. Magnification: X 345.

FIG. 8. Degenerating fibers in VL, 7 days following a lesion of the rostral part of the coronal gyrus. Nauta. Magnification: X 345.

FIG. 9. Degenerating fibers in VL in the same animal depicted in Fig. 6. Nauta. Magnification: X 585.

FIG. 10. Degenerating fibers in POm, 7 days following a lesion of the anterior ectosylvian gyrus (SII). Nauta. Magnification: X 345.

FIG. 11. Degenerating fibers in VPM in the same animal as in Fig. 10. Nauta. Magnification: X 345.

FIG. 12. Degenerating fibers in ipsilateral VPLl following a lesion located ventrally and rostrally in the medial wall of the cat's rostral hemisphere. Note the absence of degenerating fibers in VPLm. Nauta, impregnated and counterstained with cresyl-violet. Magnification: X 315.

of termination. Most destined for POm seem to course by way of the "cerebral peduncle loop." The fibers which end in POl, however, course largely through R and the external medullary lamina, or they pierce the rostral pole of R and traverse VA and VL before ending in POl. This different course may explain the relatively scanty overlap between the areas of terminal degeneration in POl and POm (see above).

The course taken by the corticothalamic fibers should be borne in mind when electrolytic lesions are made in the diencephalon. A lesion in VA or VL is almost certain to damage corticothalamic fibers to more caudally situated structures. On the other hand, a lesion placed in the medial part of the mesodiencephalic junction will inevitably involve corticofugal fibers to VPM, VPMpc, VPl, CM, Pc, POm and the lateral part of caudal MD.

Following a lesion of MII on the medial wall of the cat's rostral hemisphere, the degenerating fibers are grouped medially in the anterior limb of the internal capsule. Many of them cross in the dorsal part of the anterior commissure and reach the contralateral internal capsule. From here some of the degenerating fibers reach contralateral subcortical structures, including the thalamus (86). These findings indicate that the anterior commissure not only represents a commissural system, but also serves as a pathway for crossed fiber projections from the cerebral cortex to subcortical structures.

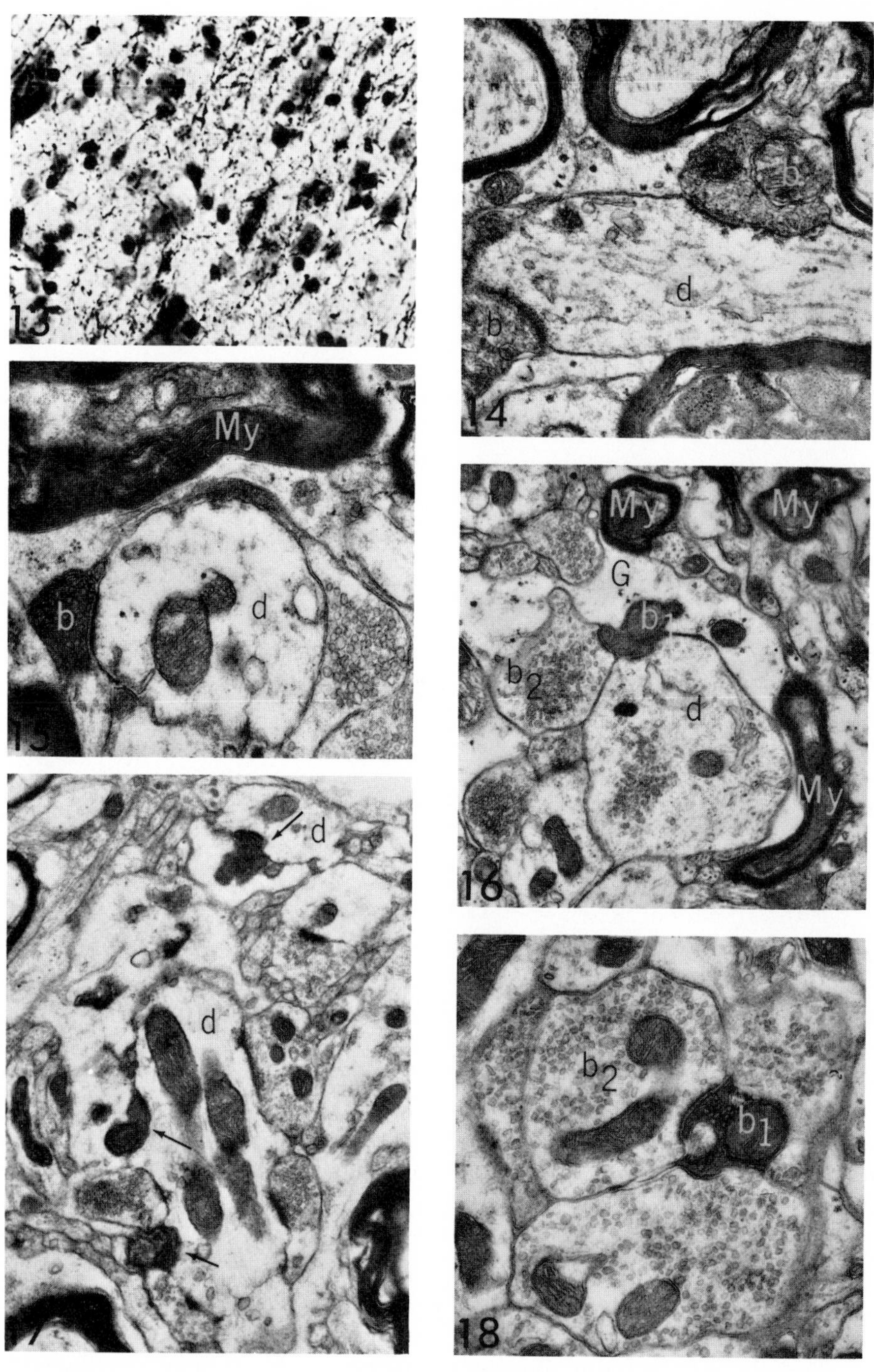

FIGS. 13-18

FIG. 13. Degenerating fibers in R, 7 days following a lesion of the posterior sigmoid gyrus. Nauta and cresyl-violet. Magnification: X 585.

FIG. 14. Degenerating boutons (b) on a dendrite (d) in R, 8 days following a lesion of the pericruciate gyri of the cat. Magnification: X 24,000.

FIG. 15. Degenerating bouton (b) on a dendrite (d) in VPLm, 4 days and 17 hours following a lesion of the pericruciate gyri. My: degenerating myelinated fiber. Magnification: X 24,000.

FIG. 16. Degenerating bouton (b1) in VPLm, presynaptic to an apparently normal bouton (b2) and to a dendrite (d) containing a cluster of vesicles. My: degenerating myelinated axons. Notice the prominent glial profile (G). See text. Same animal as in Fig. 15. Magnification: X 15,200.

FIG. 17. Several degenerating boutons (arrows) contacting dendrites (d) in VL in same animal depicted in Fig. 15. Magnification: X 15,000.

FIG. 18. Degenerating bouton (b1) engaged in asymmetrical contact with apparently normal bouton (b2) in VL in the same animal as in Figs. 15-17. Magnification: X 24,000.

ELECTRON MICROSCOPICAL INVESTIGATIONS ON CORTICOTHALAMIC CONNECTIONS.

In any light microscopical investigation using silver impregnation methods for the study of anterograde axonal degeneration, it is often rather difficult to distinguish with certainty the passing degenerating fibers from the "terminal" degeneration (84). This is a particular problem in the thalamus where so many degenerating corticofugal fibers pass through several thalamic nuclei before reaching their area of termination. Do some of the degenerating fibers end in the nuclei, or are they merely fibers passing through? Even when the degenerating fibers can no longer be followed on serial sections, it can be argued that the use of shorter survival times or of other impregnation methods (84, 86, 99) might reveal that they actually terminate in another field. These problems are particularly relevant when the light microscopical degeneration picture in the reticular nucleus of the thalamus (R) following cortical lesions is evaluated. Although a large number of degenerating fibers merely pass through this nucleus on their way to other thalamic nuclei (Fig. 13), several investigators have concluded from light microscopical studies of silver-impregnated material that some corticofugal fibers actually terminate in the cat's R (7, 42, 68, 84, 86). However, it was cautiously emphasized (84) that only electron microscopical investigations could conclusively show whether corticofugal fibers actually end in R. A series of normal and experimental electron microscopical investigations of the cat's thalamus is in progress by the author in collaboration with I. Grofova. Some preliminary ultrastructural findings, supporting the light microscopical observations, will be briefly mentioned.

In several animals, lesions were made in the pericruciate and coronal gyri, and the animals were allowed to survive for 3—34 days. The brains were cut in the stereotactic frontal plane after perfusion-fixation for electron microscopical investigations. Great care was taken in sampling blocks from animals with similar lesions and survival times from those thalamic areas where terminal degeneration was expected according to light microscopical examination of silver-impregnated material. In the ultra-thin sections from animals who survived 4—5 days after a lesion of the cruciate gyri, we found degenerating boutons of the dark type in the cat's VB, in agreement with the findings of Jones and Powell (44) (Figs. 15, 16). Furthermore, in the thalamus from the same animals where degenerating boutons are seen in VB, we have seen degenerating boutons in R (Fig. 14), VL (Figs. 17, 18) and POm (Fig. 19), in precisely those areas where the degeneration picture was considered "terminal" in the light microscopical investigations (84). Furthermore, in both VB (Fig. 16), VL (Fig. 18) and PO (Fig. 19), degenerating boutons are seen which are presynaptic to apparently normal boutons.

It can, of course, be argued that some of the degenerating boutons which are seen in the ultra-thin sections from various thalamic nuclei following cortical lesions belong not to corticothalamic axons, but to intrathalamic collaterals of thalamocortical axons that have undergone "indirect Wallerian degeneration" (vide supra). As stated earlier, it therefore is important to correlate the electron microscopical findings with light microscopical studies of Nissl-stained sections from the same thalamic regions following similar cortical lesions. In none of our animals who survived 4—5 days following lesions of the sensorimotor cortical areas, have we seen cellular changes in the Nissl-stained material from those thalamic regions where degenerating fibers are seen in the silver-impregnated material.

DENDRO-DENDRITIC AND DENDRO-SOMATIC SYNAPSES IN THE CAT'S VL

Several chapters in this volume present data on functional properties of neurons in the cat's VL and their central role in the regulation of motor activities. It therefore seems relevant to present some preliminary findings on the normal ultrastructure of this thalamic nucleus. The data to be presented here will be confined to one particular aspect of VL synaptology.

Recently a reluctant but steadily increasing interest has been devoted to the possible existence of dendro-dendritic synapses in the vertebrate central nervous system, that is, specializations where both the pre- and postsynaptic elements are considered dendrites by all conventional criteria (73). In vertebrates dendro-dendritic synapses have been described in such specialized central nervous regions as the retina (27), and in the olfactory bulb (79, 80). More recently, however, Ralston and Herman (82) have described similar structures in the cat's VB. Furthermore, the existence of dendro-dendritic synapses has been reported in the cat's lateral geniculate body (29, 102) and medial geniculate body (61). In all instances the pre-

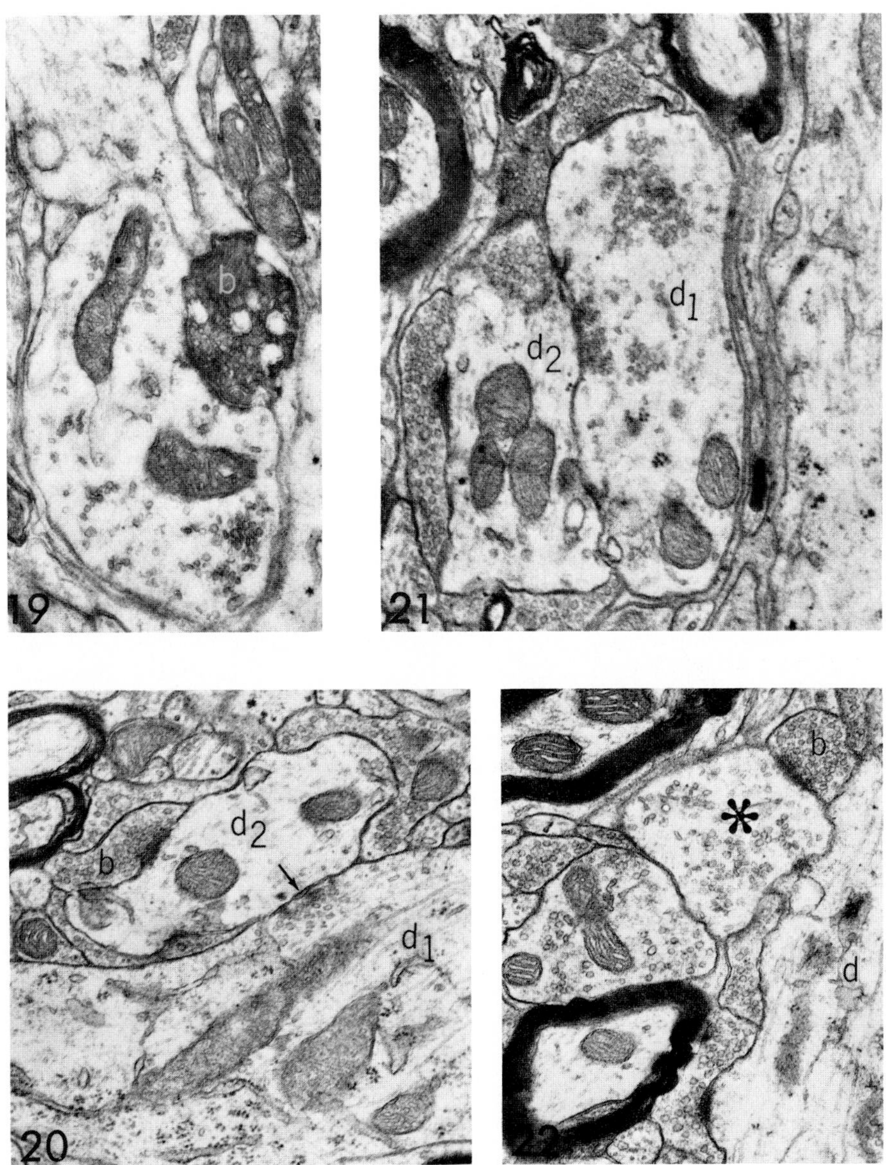

FIGS. 19-22

synaptic structure shows all the criteria generally attributed to dendrites (73). They are considerably larger than ordinary unmyelinated axons, and have a highly irregular course and irregular contours. They contain isolated ribosomes, polysomes or even rough-surfaced endoplasmic reticulum. They do not have the morphological charac-

FIG. 19. Degenerating bouton (b) in POm, presynaptic to a structure containing clusters of vesicles (dendrite ? axon ? see text !). Same animal as in Fig. 15. Magnification: X 24,000.

FIG. 20. Dendro-dendritic specialization (arrow) on a random section from VL. The larger dendritic profile (d1), containing rough-surfaced endoplasmic reticulum, free ribosomes and a small cluster of vesicles, appears to be "presynaptic" to a smaller dendrite (d2), which in turn is contacted by a bouton (b). See text. Magnification: X 24,000.

FIG. 21. Dendro-dendritic specialization on a random section from VL. Notice clusters of vesicles in d1. Both dendrites (d1 and d2) are contacted by boutons. (For details see text.) Magnification: X 24,000.

FIG. 22. One bouton (b) in VL which is presynaptic to a structure containing vesicles. Is the latter a bouton or a dendrite? Compare with the longitudinally cut dendrite (d) and with Figs. 20 and 21. See text.) Magnification: X 24,000.

teristics of axon initial segments (45, 70, 74), and they are finally contacted by a varying number of boutons. In a few cases such dendrites have been followed from the cell soma (49) or from a major, proximal dendritic trunk (29). The only feature that distinguishes these structures from "ordinary" dendrites is that they contain "synaptic" vesicles which aggregate at membrane specializations towards other dendrites. At such specializations there is a clear widening of the extracellular space between the apposed membranes, and the membranes show thickenings which have the characteristics of synapses.

Such dendro-dendritic synapses have been observed in the cat's VL (Figs. 20, 21, 26). They are quite common, and they are seen throughout the rostrocaudal extent of the nucleus. On random as well as serial sections, it is clear that the pre- as well as postsynaptic dendritic elements are contacted by boutons. These boutons are of varying size and they contain either round or pleomorphic vesicles. On the other hand, the vesicle population in the presynaptic dendrite is always of the mixed type (material fixed in formaldehyde/glutaraldehyde and post-osmicated).

On serial sections it also appears that the presynaptic dendrites have irregular swellings along their course and thus appear to be beaded. This is particularly evident in Figs. 23-25, which show a dendrite making synaptic contact with a cell soma as well as with a dendrite. At the swellings the dendrite contains smaller or larger clusters of vesicles and it is contacted by several boutons along its course.

One conclusion emanating from these observations is that it has become very difficult to state with certainty whether axo-axonic synapses encountered in random sections in the cat's VL are really axo-axonic synapses, or only axo-dendritic ones where the postsynaptic dendrite contains vesicles (Fig. 22). It would not be surprising if several axo-axonic synapses which have been reported in some thalamic nuclei

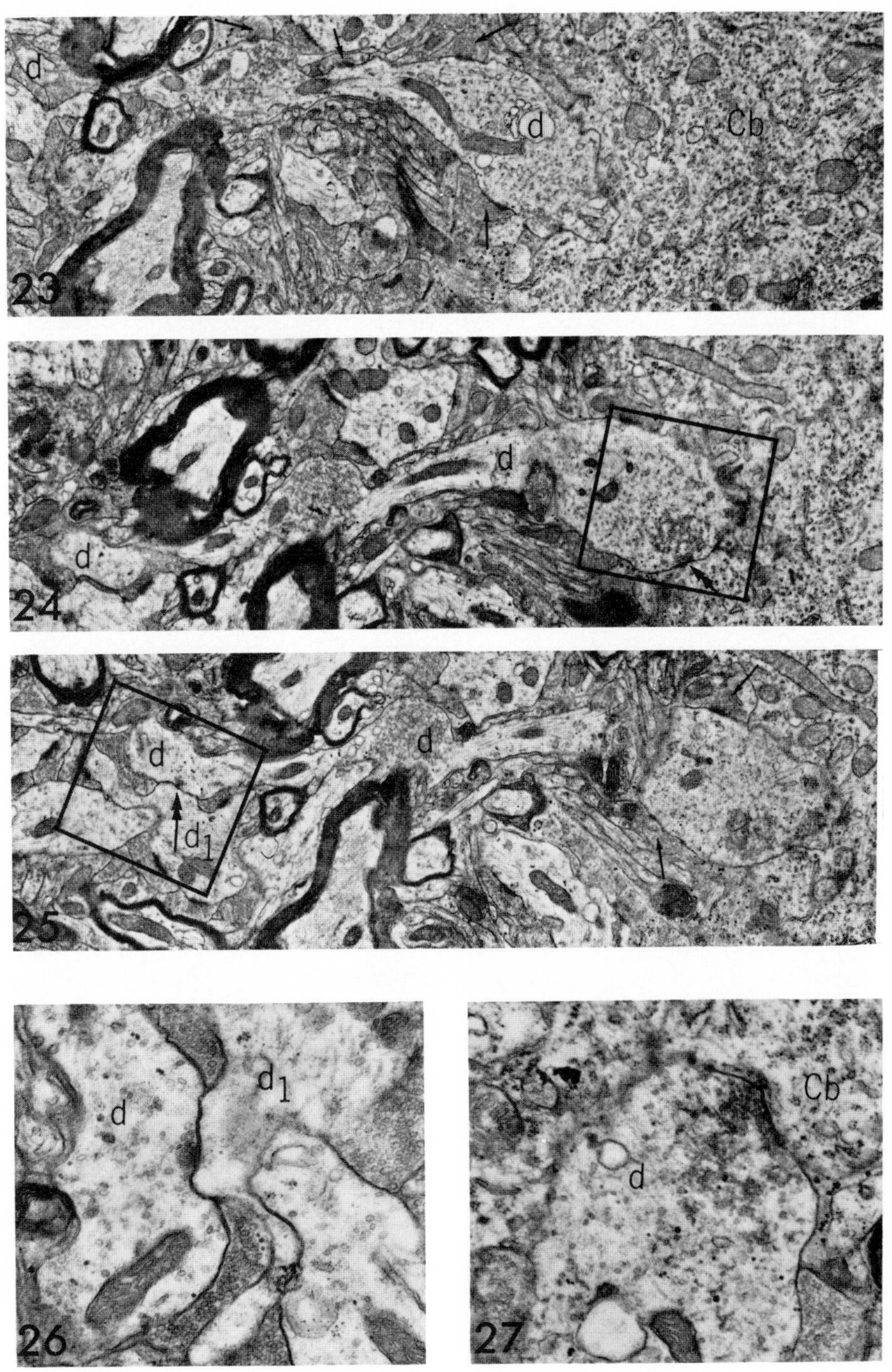

FIGS. 23-27

FIGS. 23-25. Three sections from a series through VL in the cat showing a dendrite (d), with irregular contours, being contacted by several boutons (single-headed arrows). At several places the dendrite contains clusters of vesicles and appears to make contact (double-headed arrow) with a cell soma (Cb) and with a dendrite (dl). Magnification: X 9,000.

FIG. 26. Detail of the square area in Fig. 25 showing the dendro-dendritic specialization between d and dl. Notice the widening of the extracellular space at the vesicle aggregation in d. Magnification: X 24,000.

FIG. 27. Detail of the area indicated with a square in Fig. 24, actually taken from the neighboring section in the series. Notice the widening of the apposed membranes between the dendrite (d) and the cell body (Cb). Magnification: X 18,000.

(and other central nervous structures) in reality are axo-dendritic synapses where the dendrite contains vesicles.

The functional significance of such dendro-dendritic and dendro-somatic synapses remains enigmatic (see (81)). Of particular interest, however, are the recent observations of Morest (61) on the cat's medial geniculate body. From his large experience on this thalamic nucleus based on light microscopical investigations of Golgi material, he states firmly that the dendrites, which in the electron microscope are seen to contain vesicles and establish synaptic contacts with other dendrites, belong to Golgi type II neurons. More data are needed before this statement can be generally accepted or rejected, but it certainly opens new vistas about the functioning of Golgi type II neurons if future investigations disclose a similar relationship of Golgi II neurons in dendro-dendritic synapses in VB and VL (Fig. 16), that would tentatively indicate that the cerebral cortex can directly influence Golgi II neurons. The observations made by Morest (61) on the medial geniculate body will undoubtedly spur an intensive search for the possibility of a similar relationship for the Golgi type II neurons in other thalamic and non-thalamic structures.

ABBREVIATIONS

AII	second auditory area
AD	nucleus anterior dorsalis thalami
AM	nucleus anterior medialis thalami
AV	nucleus anterior ventralis thalami
Cau.,CD	nucleus caudatus
CeM	nucleus centralis medialis thalami
CL	nucleus centralis lateralis thalami
CM	nucleus centrum medianum thalami
EN	nucleus entopeduncularis

GL	corpus geniculatum laterale
GLD	corpus geniculatum laterale dorsalis
GLV	corpus geniculatum laterale ventralis
GP	globus pallidus
LA	nucleus lateralis anterior thalami
LD	nucleus lateralis dorsalis thalami
LP	nucleus lateralis posterior thalami
MD	nucleus medialis dorsalis thalami
MGmc	corpus geniculatum medialis, magnocellular part
MI	primary motor cortical area
MII	supplementary motor area
Pc	nucleus paracentralis thalami
Pf	nucleus parafascicularis thalami
PO	posterior group of thalamic nuclei
POl	lateral part of PO
POm	medial part of PO
PU, Pulv.	pulvinar
R	nucleus reticularis thalami
SI	primary somatosensory cortical area
SII	second somatosensory cortical area
SN	substantia nigra
STH	nucleus subthalamicus
TO	tractus opticus
Sg	nucleus supra geniculatus
VA	nucleus ventralis anterior thalami
VB	ventrobasal complex
VL	nucleus ventralis lateralis thalami
VM	nucleus ventralis medialis thalami
VPI	nucleus ventralis posterior inferior thalami
VPL	nucleus ventralis posterior lateralis thalami
VPLl	lateral part of VPL
VPLm	medial part of VPL
VPM	nucleus ventralis posterior medialis thalami
VPMpc	parvocellular part of VPM
ZI	zona incerta

REFERENCES

1 ALBE-FESSARD, D., ARFEL, G., et GUIOT, G., Activités électriques charactéristiques de quelques structures cérébrales chez l'homme, Ann. Chir., 17 (1963) 1185-1214.

2 ALBE-FESSARD, D., and BOWSHER, D., Responses of monkey thalamus to somatic stimuli under chloralose anaesthesia, Electroenceph. clin. Neurophysiol., 19 (1965) 1-15.

3 ANDERSEN, P., ECCLES, J.C., SCHMIDT, R.F., and YOKOTA, T., Depolarization of presynaptic fibers in the cuneate nucleus, J. Neurophysiol. 27 (1964) 92-106.

4 ANDERSEN, P., ECCLES, J.C., and SEARS, T.A., Cortically evoked depolarization of primary afferent fibers in the spinal cord, J. Neurophysiol., 27 (1964) 63-77.

5 ANDERSON, F.D., and BERRY, C.M., Degeneration studies of long ascending fiber systems in the cat brain stem, J. comp. Neurol., 111 (1959) 195-230.

6 APPELBERG, B., and LANDRGEN, S., The localization of the thalamic relay in the specific sensory path from the tongue of the cat, Acta physiol. scand., 42 (1958) 342-357.

7 AUER, J., Frontal lobe efferents to diffusely thalamic projecting nuclei. In J.A. Kappers (Ed.), Progress in Neurobiology I, Amsterdam, 1956, pp. 315-316.

8 BERESFORD, W.A., A discussion on retrograde changes in nerve fibres. In M. Singer and J.P. Schade (Eds.), Degeneration Patterns in the Nervous System, Progress in Brain Research, Vol. 14, Elsevier, Amsterdam, 1965, pp. 33-56.

9 BLOMQUIST, A.J., BENJAMIN, R.M., and EMMERS, R., Thalamic localization of afferents from the tongue in squirrel monkey (Saimiri sciureus), J. comp. Neurol., 118 (1962) 77-88.

10 BOIVIE, J., The termination of the spinothalamic tract in the cat. An experimental study with silver impregnation methods, Exp. Brain Res., 12 (1971) 331-353.

11 BOWSHER, D., The termination of secondary somatosensory neurons within the thalamus of Macaca mulatta. An experimental degeneration study, J. comp. Neurol., 117 (1961) 213-227.

12 BOWSHER, D., Some afferent and efferent connections of the parafascicular-center median complex. In D.P. Purpura & M.D. Yahr (Eds.), The Thalamus, Columbia Univ. Press, 1966, pp. 99-108.

13 BROOKS, V.B., RUDOMIN, P., and SLAYMAN, C.L., Sensory activation of neurons in the cat's cerebral cortex, J. Neurophysiol., 24 (1961) 286-301.

14 BROOKS, V.B., RUDOMIN, P., and SLAYMAN, C.L., Peripheral receptive fields of neurons in the cat's cerebral cortex, J. Neurophysiol., 24 (1961) 302-325.

15 BUSER, P., Observations sur l'organisation fonctionelle du cortex moteur chez le chat, Bull. schweiz. Akad. med. Wiss., 16 (1960) 355-397.

16 CALMA, I., Observation on the activity of the posterior group of nuclei of the thalamus, J. Physiol. (Lond.), 172 (1964) 47 P.

17 CARRERAS, M., and ANDERSSON, S.A., Functional properties of neurons of the anterior ectosylvian gyrus of the cat, J. Neurophysiol., 26 (1963) 100-126.

18 CHANDLER, C. RUTH, Thalamic termination of corticofugal fibres from somatic sensory areas I and II in the cat. An experimental degeneration study. Thesis, Liverpool, 1964, 103 p. + bibliography.

19 CHOW, K.L., and DEWSON, J.H. III, Numerical estimates of neurons and glia in the lateral geniculate body during retrograde degeneration, J. comp. Neurol., 128 (1966) 63-73.

20 CHOW, K.L., and PRIBRAM, K.H., Cortical projection of the thalamic ventrolateral nuclear group in monkeys, J. comp. Neurol., 104 (1956) 57-75.

21 CLARK, W.E.LeG., and BOGGON, R.H., The thalamic connections of the parietal and frontal lobes of the brain in the monkey, Phil Trans. B., 224 (1935) 313-359.

22 DARIAN-SMITH, I., Cortical projections of thalamic neurons excited by mechanical stimulation of the face of the cat, J. Physiol. (Lond.), 171 (1964) 339-360.

23 DARIAN-SMITH, I., and YOKOTA, T., Corticofugal effects on different neuron types within the cat's brain stem activated by tactile stimulation of the face, J. Neurophysiol., 29 (1966) 185-206.

24 DELL, P., Corrélations entre le système végétatif et le système de la vie de relation. Mesencéphale, diencéphale et cortex cerebral, J. Physiol. (Paris), 44, (1952) 471-557.

25 DeVITO, J.L., Thalamic projection of the anterior ectosylvian gyrus (somatic area II) in the cat, J. comp. Neurol., 131 (1967) 67-78.

26 DIAMOND, I.T., JONES, E.G., and POWELL, T.P.S., The projection of the auditory cortex upon the diencephalon and brain stem in the cat, Brain Research, 15, (1969) 305-340.

27 DOWLING, J.E., and BOYCOTT, B.B., Organization of the primate retina: electron microscopy, Proc.roy.Soc. B., 166 (1966) 80-111.

28 EMMERS, R., Localization of thalamic projection of afferents from the tongue in the cat, Anat. Rec., 148 (1964) 67-74.

29 FAMIGLIETTI, E.V. Jr., Dendo-dendritic synapses in the lateral geniculate nucleus of the cat, Brain Research, 20 (1970) 181-191.

30 FINK, R.P., and HEIMER, L., Two methods for selective silver impregnation of degenerating axons and their synaptic endings in the central nervous system, Brain Research, 4 (1967) 369-374.

31 GAREY, L.J., JONES, E.G., and POWELL, T.P.S., Interrelationships of striate and extrastriate cortex with the primary relay sites of the visual pathway, J. Neurol. Neurosurg. Psychiat., 31 (1968) 135-157.

32 GEHUCHTEN, A. VAN, La dégénérescence dite rétrograde ou dégénérescence wallérienne indirecte, Névraxe, V (1903) 1-107.

33 GORDON, G., and JUKES, M.G.M., Descending influences on the exteroceptive organization of the cat's gracile nucleus, J. Physiol. (Lond.), 291 (1964) 291-319.

34 GRANT, G., Silver impregnation of degenerating dendrites, cells and axons central to axonal transection. II. A Nauta study on spinal motor neurones in kittens. Exp. Brain Res., 6 (1968) 284-293.

35 GRANT, G., Neuronal changes central to the site of axon transection. A method for the identification of retrograde changes in perikarya, dendrites and axons by silver impregnation. In W.J.H. Nauta and S.O.E. Ebbesson (Eds.), Contemporary research methods in neuroanatomy, Springer Verlag, Berlin-Heidelberg-New York, 1970, pp. 173-183.

36 GRANT, G., and ALDSKOGIUS, H., Silver impregnation of degenerating dendrites, cells and axons central to axonal transection. I. A Nauta study on the hypoglossal nerve in kittens, Exp. Brain Res., 3 (1967) 150-162.
37 GRANT, G., and WESTMAN, J., The lateral cervical nucleus in the cat. IV. A light and electron microscopical study after midbrain lesions with demonstration of indirect Wallerian degeneration at the ultrastructural level, Exp. Brain Res., 7 (1969) 51-67.
38 HAGBARTH, K.-E., and KERR, D.I.B., Central influences on spinal afferent conduction, J. Neurophysiol., 17 (1954) 295-307.
39 HASSLER, R., und MUHS-CLEMENT, K., Architektonischer Aufbau des sensorimotorischen und parietalen Cortex der Katze, J. Hirnforsch., 6 (1964) 377-420.
40 HEATH, C.J., and JONES, E.G., An experimental study of ascending connections from the posterior group of thalamic nuclei in the cat, J. comp. Neurol., 141 (1971) 397-426.
41 JABBUR, S.J., and TOWE, A.L., Cortical excitation of neurons in dorsal column nuclei of cat, including an analysis of pathways, J. Neurophysiol., 24 (1961) 499-509.
42 JONES, E.G., and POWELL, T.P.S., The projections of the somatic sensory cortex upon the thalamus in the cat, Brain Research, 10 (1968) 369-391.
43 JONES, E.G., and POWELL, T.P.S., The cortical projection of the ventroposterior nucleus of the thalamus in the cat, Brain Research, 13 (1969) 298-318.
44 JONES, E.G., and POWELL, T.P.S., An electron microscopic study of the mode of termination of cortico-thalamic fibres within the sensory relay nuclei of the thalamus, Proc.roy.Soc.B., 172 (1969) 173-185.
45 JONES, E.G., and POWELL, T.P.S., Synapses on the axon hillocks and initial segments of pyramidal cell axons in the cerebral cortex, J. Cell Sci., 5 (1969) 495-508.
46 JONES, E.G., and POWELL, T.P.S., Connexions of the somatic sensory cortex of the rhesus monkey. III. Thalamic connexions, Brain, 93 (1970) 37-56.
47 KUSAMA, T., OTANI, K., and KAWANA, E., Projections of the motor, somatic sensory, auditory and visual cortices in cats, In T. Tokizane and J.P. Schade (Eds.) Progress in Brain Research, Vol. 21A, Elsevier, Amsterdam, 1966, pp. 292-322.
48 LIVINGSTON, A., and PHILLIPS, C.G., Maps and thresholds for the sensorimotor cortex of the cat, Quart.J.exp.Physiol., 42 (1957) 190-205.
49 LUND, R.D., Synaptic patterns of the superficial layers of the superior colliculus of the rat, J.comp.Neurol., 135 (1969) 179-208.
50 MACCHI, G., Organizzazione morfologica delle connessioni talamo-corticali, Monit. Zool. Ital., suppl. 66, (1958) 25-121.
51 MACCHI, G., CARRERAS, M., and ANGELERI, F., Ricerche sulle connessioni talamo-corticali. II. Sulle proiezioni dei nuclei della linea mediana e intralaminari: il problema delle connessioni talamo-rinencefaliche (Studio sperimentale nel gatto), Arch.ital.Anat.Embriol., 60 (1955) 413-440.
52 MACCHI, G., and De RISIO, G., Ricerche sulle connessioni talamo-corticali, Arch.ital.Anat.Embriol., 59 (1954) 431-456.

53 MACCHI, G., MARCHESI, G.F., and QUATTRINI, A., Nuovi contributi allo studio delle connessioni efferenti dei nuclei della linea mediana e intralaminari del talamo, Boll.Soc.ital.Biol.sper., 43 (1967) 1414-1417.
54 MASSION, J., Étude d'une structure motrice thalamique, le noyau ventrolatéral, et de sa régulation par les afferences sensorielles. Thesis, Paris, 1968, 134 pp.
55 MASSION, J., ANGAUT, P., et ALBE-FESSARD, D., Activités evoquées chez le chat dans la région du nucleus ventralis lateralis par diverses stimulations sensorielles. I. Étude macro-physiologique, Electroenceph. clin. Neurophysiol., 19 (1965) 433-451.
56 MASSION, J., ANGAUT, P., et ALBE-FESSARD, D., Activités evoquées chez le chat dans la région du nucleus ventralis lateralis par diverses stimulations sensorielles. II. Étude micro-physiologique, Electroenceph. clin. Neurophysiol., 19 (1965) 452-469.
57 MEHLER, W.R., Further notes on the center median nucleus of Luys. In D.P. Purpura and M.D. Yahr (Eds.), The Thalamus, Columbia University Press, 1966, pp. 109-122.
58 MEHLER, W.R., The posterior thalamic region in man, Confin. neurol. (Basel), 26 (1966) 18-29.
59 MEHLER, W.R., FEFERMAN, M.E., and Nauta, W.J.H., Ascending axon degeneration following antero-lateral cordotomy. An experimental study in the monkey, Brain, 83 (1960) 718-750.
60 MOORE, R.Y., and GOLDBERG, J.M., Ascending projections of the inferior colliculus in the cat, J.comp.Neurol., 121 (1963) 109-136.
61 MOREST, D.K., Dendrodendritic synapses of cells that have axons: the fine structure of the Golgi type II cell in the medial geniculate body of the cat, Z.Anat.Entwickl.Gesch., 133 (1971) 216-246.
62 MORRISON, A.R., HAND, P.J., and O'DONOGHUE, J., Contrasting projections from the posterior and ventrobasal thalamic nuclear complexes to the anterior ectosylvian gyrus of the cat, Brain Research, 21 (1970) 115-121.
63 MOUNTCASTLE, V., and HENNEMAN, E., Pattern of tactile representation in thalamus of cat, J. Neurophysiol., 12 (1949) 85-100.
64 MOUNTCASTLE, V., and HENNEMAN, E., The representation of tactile sensibility in the thalamus of the monkey, J.comp.Neurol., 97 (1952) 409-440.
65 MURRAY, M., Degeneration of some intralaminar thalamic nuclei after cortical removals in the cat, J.comp.Neurol., 127 (1966) 341-368.
66 NAUTA, W.J.H., Über die sogenannte terminale Degeneration im Zentralnervensystem und ihre Darstellung durch Silberimpregnation, Schweiz. Arch. Neurol. Psychiat., 66 (1950) 353-376.
67 NAUTA, W.J.H., Silver impregnation of degenerating axons. In W.F. Windle (Ed.), New research techniques of neuroanatomy, Thomas, Springfield, Ill., 1957, pp. 17-26.
68 NIIMI, K., KISHI, S., MIKI, M., and FUJITA, S., An experimental study of the course and termination of the projection fibers from cortical areas 4 and 6 in the cat, Folia psychiat. neurol. jap., 17 (1963) 167-216.

69 NYBERG-HANSEN, R., Corticospinal fibres from the medial aspect of the cerebral hemisphere in the cat. An experimental study with the Nauta method, Exp. Brain Res., 7 (1969) 120-132.

70 PALAY, S.L., SOTELO, C., PETERS, A., and ORKAND, P.M., The axon hillock and the initial segment, J.Cell Biol., 38 (1968) 193-201.

71 PATTON, H.D., Ruch, T.C., and WALKER, A.E., Experimental hypogeusia from Horsley-Clarke lesions of the thalamus in Macaca mulatta, J.Neurophysiol., 7 (1944) 171-184.

72 PERL, E.R., and WHITLOCK, D.G., Somatic stimuli exciting spinothalamic projections to thalamic neurons in cat and monkey, Exp. Neurol., 3 (1961) 256-296.

73 PETERS, A., PALAY, S.L., and WEBSTER, H. de F., The Fine Structure of the Nervous System. Hoeber, New York, 1970, 198 pp.

74 PETERS, A., PROSKAUER, C.C., and KAISERMAN-ABRAMOF, I.R., The small pyramidal neuron of the rat cerebral cortex. The axon hillock and initial segment, J.Cell Biol., 39 (1968) 604-619.

75 PETRAS, J.M., Some fiber connections of the precentral and postcentral cortex with the basal ganglia, thalamus and subthalamus, Trans.Amer.neurol.Ass., (1965) 274-275.

76 POGGIO, G.F., and MOUNTCASTLE, V.B., A study of the functional contributions of the lemniscal and spinothalamic systems to somatic sensibility. (Central nervous mechanisms in pain), Bull.Johns Hopk.Hosp., 106 (1960) 266-316.

77 POWELL, T.P.S. and COWAN, W.M., A note on retrograde fibre degeneration, J.Anat. (Lond.), 98 (1964) 579-585.

78 POWELL, T.P.S., and COWAN, W.M., The interpretation of the degenerative changes in the intralaminar nuclei of the thalamus, J.Neurol.Neurosurg. Psychiat., 30 (1967) 140-153.

79 PRICE, J.L., The synaptic vesicles of the reciprocal synapse of the olfactory bulb, Brain Research, 11 (1968) 697-700.

80 RALL, W., SHEPHERD, G.M., REESE, T.S., and BRIGHTMAN, M.W., Dendrodendritic synaptic pathway for inhibition in the olfactory bulb, Exp. Neurol. 14 (1966) 44-56.

81 RALSTON, H.J. III, Evidence for presynaptic dendrites and a proposal for their mechanism of action, Nature, 230 (1971) 585-587.

82 RALSTON, H.J., and HERMAN, M.M., The fine structure of neurons and synapses in the ventrobasal thalamus of the cat, Brain Research, 14 (1969) 77-98.

83 RINVIK, E., A re-evaluation of the cytoarchitecture of the ventral nuclear complex of the cat's thalamus on the basis of the corticothalamic connections, Brain Research, 8 (1968) 237-254.

84 RINVIK, E., The corticothalamic projection from the pericruciate and coronal gyri in the cat. An experimental study with silver-impregnation methods, Brain Research, 10 (1968) 79-119.

85 RINVIK, E., The corticothalamic projection from the second somatosensory cortical area in the cat. An experimental study with silver impregnation methods,

Exp. Brain Res., 5 (1968) 153-172.

86 RINVIK, E., The corticothalamic projection from the gyrus proreus and the medial wall of the rostral hemisphere in the cat. An experimental study with silver impregnation methods, Exp. Brain Res., 5 (1968) 129-152.

87 RISPAL-PADEL, L., and MASSION, J., Relations between the ventrolateral nucleus and the motor cortex in the cat, Exp. Brain Res., 10 (1970) 331-339.

88 ROBERTS, T.S. and Akert, K., Insular and opercular cortex and its thalamic projection in Macaca mulatta, Schweiz.Arch.Neurol.Neurochir.Psychiat. 92 (1963) 1-43.

89 ROSE, J.E., and MOUNTCASTLE, V.B., The thalamic tactile region in rabbit and cat, J.comp.Neurol., 97 (1952) 441-489.

90 ROSE, J.E., and WOOLSEY, C.N., Structure and relations of limbic cortex and anterior thalamic nuclei in rabbit and cat, J. comp. Neurol., 89 (1948) 279-348.

91 ROSE, J.E., and WOOLSEY, C.N., Cortical connections and functional organization of the thalamic auditory system of the cat. In H.F. Harlow and C.N. Woolsey (Eds.), Biological and Biochemical Bases of Behavior, Univ. of Wisconsin Press, 1958, pp. 127-150.

92 SCHEIBEL, M.E., and SCHEIBEL, A.B., Patterns of organization in specific and nonspecific thalamic fields. In: The Thalamus, Eds. D.P. Purpura and M.D. Yahr, Columbia Univ. Press, 1966, pp. 13-46.

93 SCHEIBEL, M.E. and SCHEIBEL, A.B., The organization of the nucleus reticularis thalami. A Golgi study, Brain Research, 1 (1966) 43-62.

94 SCHEIBEL, M.E., and SCHEIBEL, A.B., The organization of the ventral anterior nucleus of the thalamus. A Golgi study, Brain Research, 1 (1966) 250-268.

95 SCHEIBEL, M.E., and SCHEIBEL, A.B., Structural organization of nonspecific thalamic nuclei and their projection towards cortex, Brain Research, 6 (1967) 60-94.

96 SCHEIBEL, ME., and SCHEIBEL, A.B., Elementary processes in selected thalamic and cortical subsystems—the structural substrates. In F.O. Schmitt (Ed. in chief), The Neurosciences: second study program, Rockefeller Univ. Press. New York, 1970, pp. 443-457.

97 SMAHA, L.A., KAELBER, W.W., and MAHARRY, R.R., Efferent projections of the nucleus ventralis lateralis. An experimental study in the cat, J.Anat. (Lond.), 104 (1968) 33-40.

98 TOWE, A.L., and JABBUR, S.J., Cortical inhibition of neurons in dorsal column nuclei of cat, J.Neurophysiol., 24 (1961) 488-498.

99 WALBERG, F., Does silver impregnate normal and degenerating boutons? A study based on light and electron microscopical observations of the inferior olive, Brain Research, 31 (1971) 47-65.

100 WHITLOCK, D.G., and PERL, E.R., Afferent projections through ventrolateral funiculi to thalamus of cat, J.Neurophysiol., 22 (1959) 133-148.

101 WHITLOCK, D.G., and PERL, E.R., Thalamic projections of spinothalamic pathways in monkey, Exp.Neurol., 3 (1961) 240-255.

102 WONG, M.T.T., Somato-dendritic and dendro-dendritic synapses in the

squirrel monkey lateral geniculate nucleus, Brain Research, 20 (1970) 135-139.

103 WOOLSEY, C.N., Organization of somatic sensory and motor areas of the the cerebral cortex. In H.F. Harlow and C.N. Woolsey (Eds.), Biological and Biochemical Bases of Behavior, Univ. of Wisconsin Press, 1958, pp. 63-81.

104 WOOLSEY, C.N., Cortical localization as defined by evoked potential and electrical stimulation studies. In G. Schaltenbrand and C.N. Woolsey (Eds.), Cerebral Localization and Organization, Univ. of Wisconsin Press, 1964, pp. 17-32.

DISCUSSION

CROSBY:

This and certain preceding papers by Dr. Rinvik report corticothalamic fibers to the dorsal thalamus of the cat and present evidence for a much wider distribution of such fascicles than has previously been recognized. The corticothalamic fibers described arise from the gyrus proreus (which includes the motor cortex or area 4, the premotor area or area 6 and probably certain primary association areas) and from the pericruciate areas (in which are represented SI, SII, an associated vestibular area and apparently some primary somesthetic association cortex). The demonstration of such numerous corticothalamic fibers has depended largely upon the experimenter's technical skill and on careful timing of the material.

Dr. Rinvik's results show a marked overlap in the distribution of the corticothalamic fibers from the gyrus proreus as compared with that of comparable fibers from the fronto-orbital regions. The differences in distribution of corticothalamic fibers from these two areas are seen particularly in the additional projection of fascicles from the fronto-orbital cortex to the posterior thalamic region and to the nucleus ventralis posterolateralis. Moreover, when the combined distribution of fibers from the gyrus proreus and the fronto-orbital cortex is compared with that from the pericruciate and coronal areas, again there is a striking overlap in the thalamic terminations of the two groups, although the latter areas discharge additionally to various other thalamic centers such as certain intralaminar nuclei and an increased territory in the posterior part of the dorsal thalamus. A small area associated with (or perhaps a part of) the somesthetic cortex, from which several observers have been able to pick up recordings following stimulation of parts of the peripheral vestibular apparatus, sends fibers to the medial geniculate nucleus.

It appears highly probable, as Dr. Rinvik has pointed out, that, in spite of the wide distribution and great overlap of the corticothalamic fibers, in some thalamic nuclei at least, the fibers from the motor and the sensory cortices do not terminate in like amounts in the same portions of a thalamic nucleus, for example in nucleus ventralis posterior. Differences in termination of the corticothalamic fibers in a thalamic nucleus should be significant implying specificity of the connections. Certainly, the numerous overlapping corticothalamic fibers must be important in thalamic regulation of cortical responses.

The experiments reported by Dr. Rinvik indicate a relation between the somatotopic patterns demonstrable at motor and sensory cortical levels and those obtainable from the nuclei in the ventrolateral thalamus. It is quite certain that other thalamic nuclei—such as the nucleus dorsomedialis—also have somatotopic patterns that are reflected in the relations of special parts of the cortex with specific parts of the thalamic nucleus considered. Such relations provide for stimulation or inhibition of a limited portion of a thalamic nucleus in response to a localized cortical excitation.

Impulses are also relayed by way of intralaminar, parafascicular and perhaps other thalamic nuclei over the so-called "non-specific" corticothalamic fibers to the cortex. They carry impulses brought forward to thalamic levels over the ascending reticular paths which are regarded as having an arousal effect on the cortex and so related to the rhythmic cortical discharges. According to some observers, certain thalamocortical systems are inhibitory over cortical activity. The return paths, or corticothalamic fibers, to the various thalamic nuclei, whether components of specific or non-specific arcs, may well be a part of the mechanism for regulation of cortical activity and for increasing or decreasing or in general regulating the cortical rhythmic discharges. Undoubtedly, some of the corticothalamic neurons relay impulses which are inhibitory; it seems highly probable that other corticothalamic fibers are excitatory over thalamic neurons.

Using the electron microscope to study terminations of some fibers of this system in relation to the cells of the ventrobasal nuclear area, Dr. Rinvik has established clearly the presence of inhibitory terminations on fibers of this type. This, of course, does not ensure that all terminations of such corticothalamic fibers in this ventrobasal complex or in other thalamic nuclei to which they distribute are of this type. Certainly, many more preparations must be studied before the question of the amount and distribution of inhibitory versus excitatory fibers in these nuclei can be settled. Dr. Rinvik has suggested that some corticothalamic fibers may serve as supportive rather than as essential fibers. Would inhibition of the activity of a neuron be regarded as a supportive function? Or should such a term be applied only when there are possible excitatory effects?

The role of, and in fact the existence of, dendrodendritic synapses in this general pattern of corticothalamic interrelations is at present unclear. It is being discussed elsewhere in this volume by others with adequate preparations which are not available to the present reviewer and, therefore, will not be considered further here. Nevertheless, one remembers rather wistfully the definition of a dendrite as the process which conducted toward the cell body, and that of an axon as the process which conducted away from the cell body regardless of the length or branching or other morphological features of the process in question.

What functions these corticothalamic fibers have in ordinary behavior is as yet uncertain. Whether or not it would be possible to eliminate them without destroying paths which are essential for the projection of sensory impulses to the cortex or pyramidal or extrapyramidal discharges from it, is at present undetermined. Behavioral studies, observations on the effects of specific lesions and further ultramicroscopic experimental procedures will be necessary before these questions can be answered. Like many other good research papers, this contribution by Dr. Rinvik not only presents valuable information but it also raises many questions which cannot yet be answered. Therein lies a considerable part of its value.

Corticothalamic Projections and Sensorimotor Activities
T. Frigyesi, E. Rinvik, and M.D. Yahr, editors. © 1972
Raven Press, New York.

Fastigial Cerebellar Projections to the Ventrolateral Nucleus of the Thalamus and the Organization of the Descending Pathways

J. Kievit and H. G. J. M. Kuypers

The descending pathways from the cerebral cortex and the brain stem represent the main instrument by which the brain controls movements. The cerebellum which is also involved in motor control is connected with these descending pathways by way of its efferent fibers to the brain stem and the thalamus (5, 16, 18, 41, 56, 67, 72, 73, 74). The cerebellar fibers to the brain stem are distributed mainly to cell groups which give rise to the descending brain stem pathways. The fibers to the thalamus bear a special relationship to the descending cortical pathways since they are mainly distributed to the ventrolateral (VL) nucleus of the thalamus, which projects to the frontal motor cortex (1, 59, 74) whence the majority of the corticospinal fibers arises (27, 28, 31).

The descending pathways from the cerebral cortex and the brain stem may be grouped into different categories, according to their patterns of termination in the spinal gray matter (29, 32). The aim of the present study was to determine whether in the rhesus monkey the projections from the different cerebellar nuclei to both the brain stem and the thalamus are preferentially directed to the different categories of descending pathways. In order to clarify this point, first the organization of the descending pathways will be reviewed.

The pathways from the brain stem terminate mainly in the spinal intermediate zone (32, 46, 49). Those from the cerebral cortex terminate in the intermediate zone, the dorsal horn and in some species also in the motoneuronal cell groups of the ventral horn (13, 22, 28, 50). The fibers to the dorsal horn modulate mainly sensory transmission while those to the intermediate zone influence mainly motoneurons (2, 19, 37, 43).

----

* J. Kievit, med. cand., is a student-assistant in the Department of Anatomy of the Rotterdam Medical Faculty.
** The paper was presented by H.G.J.M. Kuypers.

The pathways from the brain stem may be subdivided into two groups on the basis of their spinal termination patterns. One group of fibers terminates in the ventromedial part of the intermediate zone bilaterally (32, 46, 49). These fibers will be referred to as the ventromedial brain stem pathway. The other group of fibers terminates in the lateral bulbar reticular formation (29, 32, 38) and in the dorsolateral part of the spinal intermediate zone unilaterally (29, 32, 46, 49) and will be referred to as the lateral brain stem pathway.

The fibers of the ventromedial brain stem pathway are derived from (29, 32, 46, 49) the vestibular complex, the superior colliculus, interstitial nucleus of Cajal and the bulbar medial reticular formation. The bulk of the fibers of the lateral brain stem pathway originates in the contralateral mesencephalon, in particular in the red nucleus (29, 33, 38, 46, 49). In cat these rubral fibers are derived from both the parvicellular and the magnocellular portions of the nucleus while in the monkey they are derived mainly from the magnocellular portion (33, 53). The cell groups of the ventromedial brain stem pathway are extensively interconnected. However, their efferent fibers avoid the pars magnocellularis of the red nucleus which gives rise to the lateral brain stem pathway.

The distribution of the cortical fibers in the spinal gray matter differs between these species. In cat virtually no cortical fibers terminate in the motoneuronal cell groups and the fibers to the intermediate zone terminate mainly in its dorsolateral part contralaterally (12, 46), i.e., in the same area as the fibers of the lateral brain stem pathway. In contrast, in the rhesus monkey a considerable number of cortical fibers terminate in the motoneuronal cell groups of distal extremity muscles (13, 28, 51). Further the fibers to the intermediate zone terminate in its dorsolateral part contralaterally and in its ventromedial part bilaterally (13, 28, 31). Thus, in the rhesus monkey the terminal distribution of these cortical fibers in the intermediate zone overlaps with that of both the lateral and the ventromedial brain stem pathways.

The cortical fibers to the spinal intermediate zone and the motoneuronal cell groups in the rhesus monkey originate mainly in the precentral gyrus and the most caudal part of the premotor area (± FB) (31), i.e., in the precentral motor cortex described by Woolsey and his collaborators (76). The fibers to the ventromedial part of the intermediate zone are derived from the rostral part of this motor cortex and from a portion of its caudal part between the hand and foot representation areas (31). However, the latter areas themselves project their fibers almost exclusively to the dorsolateral part of the intermediate zone and to motoneurons of distal extremity muscles (31) (Fig. 1).

FIG. 1. A illustrates the origin of the frontal projections to the medial reticular formation of the brain stem (thin lines) and to the pars magnocellularis of the red nucleus (heavy lines). B illustrates the origin of the precentral projections to the different parts of the spinal intermediate zone. The areas shown in solid black distribute their fibers primarily to the dorsolateral part of the intermediate zone contralaterally. The shaded area distributes fibers to the ventromedial parts of the intermediate zone bilaterally. Reprinted from Kuypers and Brinkman, Brain Research, 24 (1970) 29-48 with permission.

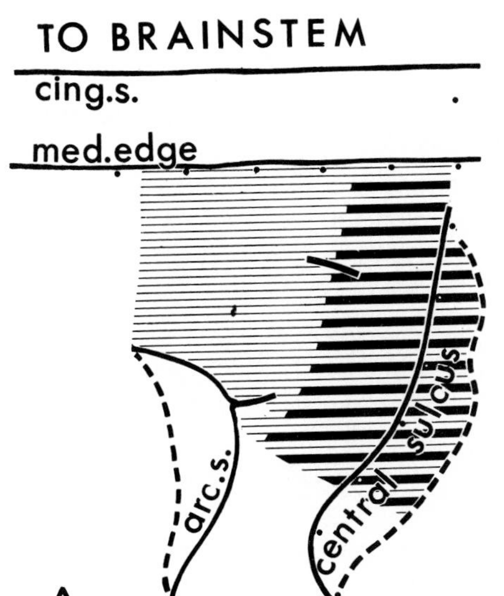
TO BRAINSTEM
cing.s.
med.edge
arc.s.
central sulcus
A

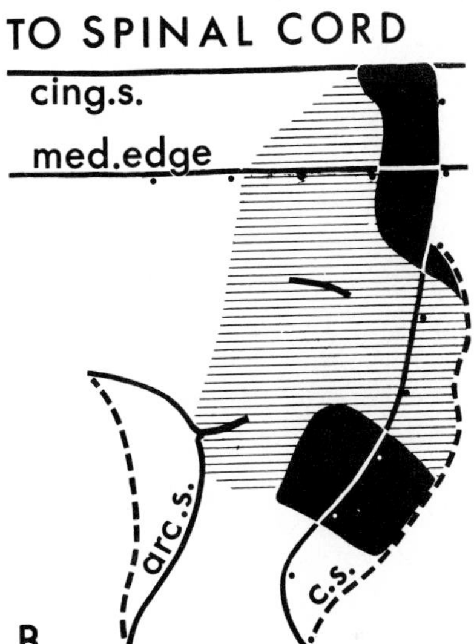
TO SPINAL CORD
cing.s.
med.edge
arc.s.
c.s.
B

FIG. 1

All cells in the intermediate zone, where many of the descending pathways terminate, send their main axons into the funiculi (7, 61, 66). In cat these propriospinal fibers in the ventral funiculi of both enlargements are distributed mainly to the ventromedial parts of the intermediate zone and to motoneurons of axial and proximal limb muscles (60, 64). Those in the dorsal and intermediate portions of the lateral funiculi are distributed mainly to the dorsal and lateral parts of the intermediate zone and to motoneurons of distal extremity muscles and intrinsic extremity flexors (60, 64). With respect to the origin of these propriospinal fibers, a contrast appears to exist in that cells in the most lateral portion of the intermediate zone send their fibers into the lateral funiculus while cells in the most ventral portion send theirs into the ventral funiculus (7, 39, 40, 64, 65). In the cat the former cells would be mainly influenced by the corticospinal and the lateral brain stem pathways, the latter mainly by the ventromedial brain stem pathway. This suggests that the corticospinal and the lateral brain stem pathways in the cat differ from the ventromedial brain stem pathway in that the former by their connection with propriospinal elements would influence especially distal extremity muscles and intrinsic extremity flexors while the latter would influence especially axial and proximal extremity muscles. If the propriospinal connections in the monkey are arranged in the same way as in the cat, the same two groups of pathways may be distinguished. However, in the monkey the pathways to the ventromedial part of the intermediate zone,which would influence especially axial and proximal limb muscles, encompass both the ventromedial brain stem pathway and corticospinal elements. The functional implications of these anatomical data are in general agreement with several physiological findings (6, 52, 55, 62, 75) and are strongly supported by the differences in motor defects observed following interruption of the various descending pathways (29, 34, 35).

We have pointed out that in the rhesus monkey cortical fibers to the spinal intermediate zone are derived mainly from the area of the precentral motor cortex described by Woolsey and his collaborators (76). However, the frontal cortex also distributes fibers to the cell groups of the descending brain stem pathways (33). In the rhesus monkey, these fibers come from a much wider area than those to the spinal cord and are derived from both the precentral gyrus (FA) and the premotor area (FB, FC, caudal FD). The premotor area, which is taken to include the cortex within the concavity of the

---

FIG. 2. Schematic diagram illustrating some ascending and descending connections from the deep cerebellar nuclei in the monkey. The diagram shows that the bulk of the ascending fibers from the fastigial nucleus (solid black) to the contralateral VL nucleus of the thalamus decussates within the cerebellum, while the ascending fibers from the interpositus and dentate nuclei (- - -) decussate in the mesencephalon. In the cat a few fastigial fibers (—?—) ascend with the interpositus and dentate fibers through the ipsilateral brachium conjunctivum (cf. 69, 70). Note further that fastigial fibers (represented unilaterally) are also distributed to brain stem cell groups which project to the ventromedial portion of the spinal intermediate zone. This portion also receives cortical fibers from specific parts of the precentral motor cortex (stippled area in left hemisphere).

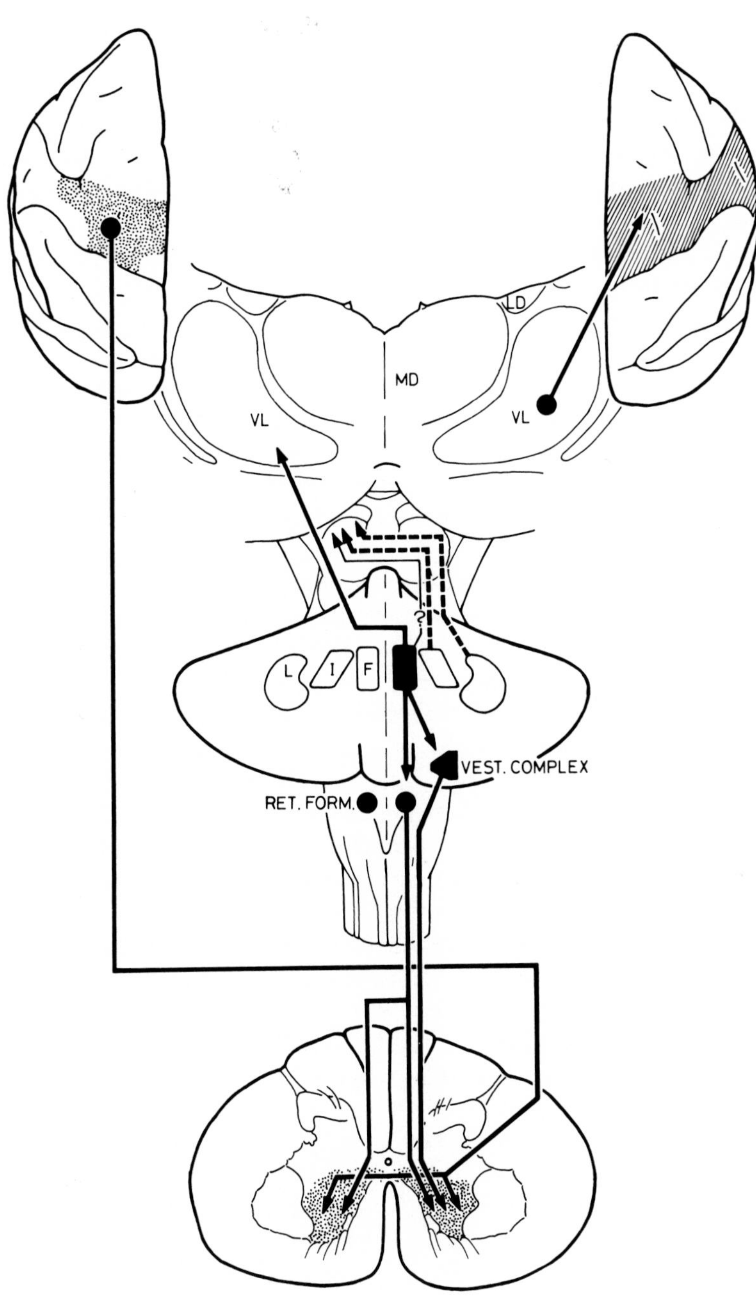

FIG. 2

arcuate sulcus, distributes its fibers to cell groups of the ventromedial brain stem pathway (Fig. 1). This implies that the premotor area is mainly concerned with body and limb-body movements; this hypothesis is in keeping with many physiological observations (25, 71). The precentral area distributes fibers to the magnocellular red nucleus (33), the main origin of the lateral brain stem pathway (Fig. 1). This suggests that the precentral area influences individual movements of the extremities, especially their distal parts. This is supported by the fact that stimulation of this area elicits individual extremity movements (76) even in the absence of the pyramidal tracts (36).

The cerebellum is closely related to the descending motor pathways and its efferent fibers establish connections with the cells of origin of both the brain stem pathways and the corticospinal pathways. The connections with the cells of origin of the corticospinal pathways are established by way of the ventrolateral nucleus of the thalamus.

In the cat, the cerebellar fibers to the cell groups of the two respective brain stem pathways tend to come from different cerebellar nuclei. The fastigial-vermal complex distributes its fibers to cell groups of the ventromedial brain stem pathway (16, 67, 69, 72, 73). The interpositus nucleus also distributes fibers to some of these cell groups, but in addition projects to the magnocellular red nucleus (4, 18, 69) which gives rise to the bulk of the lateral brain stem pathway. In other words, the fastigial-vermal complex in the cat influences the brain stem pathway to the ventromedial parts of the intermediate zone and would therefore be involved in control of body and limb-body movements. The interpositus nucleus, on the other hand, influences also the pathway to the dorsolateral part of the intermediate zone and for this reason would be involved in the control of individual movements of the limbs, especially their distal parts. This is in keeping with the original findings of Chambers and Sprague (14, 15).

It seems reasonable to assume that the ascending projections from the interpositus and the fastigial nuclei to the thalamus would follow this same pattern and by way of the VL would lead to cortical areas which are related to the dorsal and the ventromedial parts of the spinal intermediate zone respectively. It appears, then, that in the cat the interpositus and fastigial projections influence the caudal and the rostral parts of the motor cortex (58) by way of the lateral and ventromedial parts of the VL (3, 4, 5, 57) respectively. However, this concept may be tested most fruitfully in the rhesus monkey since the termination of the cortical fibers in the intermediate zone of this animal is more extensive than in the cat and coincides with the termination areas of both the lateral and the ventromedial brain stem pathways (Fig. 2).

The cortical fibers to the ventromedial part of the intermediate zone in the rhesus monkey are mainly derived from the rostral part of the motor cortex and from a portion of its caudal part* between the hand and foot representation areas (31). As a consequence, both the fibers from these parts of the motor cortex and those of the ventro-

----

* Electrical stimulation of these parts of the motor cortex elicits mainly body and limb-body movements (76).

medial brain stem pathway converge on neurons in the same part of the intermediate zone. The distribution of the fastigial projections to the brain stem suggests that the fastigial fibers terminate preferentially in cell groups which project to the ventromedial part of the intermediate zone. This would imply that the ascending fastigial projections to the contralateral thalamus in the rhesus monkey would terminate in those parts of the VL nucleus which project to the rostral part of the motor cortex and to the portion of its caudal part between the hand and foot representation areas. In the rhesus monkey the rostral part of the motor cortex—and part of the adjoining premotor area—receives thalamic projections from the medial portion of the VL nucleus while the caudal part receives them mainly from the lateral and ventral portions (1, 59) (Fig. 3). In view of this, the fastigial projections in the rhesus monkey were expected to be more extensive than in the cat and to terminate in the medial part of the VL nucleus and in a portion of its lateral part.

This hypothesis was tested in four cats (C1-C4) and in four rhesus monkeys (M1-M4) by transecting the ascending fastigial projections and comparing the distribution of the degenerating fibers and terminals in the thalami of these animals. The majority of the fastigial fibers to the contralateral thalamus in cat and monkey decussate within the cerebellum (9, 21, 22, 23, 69), while the ascending fibers from the interpositus and the dentate nuclei decussate outside the cerebellum in the mesencephalon. In order to transect fastigial projections selectively, the cerebellum was bisected in all eight animals in the mid-sagittal plane (Fig. 2). In addition, in one of the cats and one of the monkeys one brachium conjunctivum was also transected. In some of the animals (M2, M3, M4, C1, C4), one of the fastigial nuclei was damaged.

All animals survived the operation for seven days.* The cerebellum and the lower brain stem were cut in celloidin sections and stained according to the Kluver Barrera technique (26). The mesencephalon and diencephalon were cut transversally in frozen sections, in some cases (M3, M4 and C2, C3, C4) according to the Horsely Clark stereotactic plane. The sections were impregnated with silver according to the Fink-Heimer technique (20) and the degeneration was charted with the help of an X-Y plotter.

In the cats with only a cerebellar bisection, the bilaterally ascending degeneration in the mesencephalon and the diencephalon was distributed symmetrically (Fig. 4). At the level of the superior colliculus, degenerating fiber bundles ascended in the central tegmentum adjoining the central gray. From these bundles degenerating fibers were distributed to the deep layers of the superior colliculus, the nucleus of the posterior commissure, the central gray and the medial mesencephalic reticular formation. The ascending bundles continued into the diencephalon through the dorsal por-

----

* In other experiments in our department (Dr. D.G. Lawrence) the thalamic degeneration was studied in cats following transection of the brachium conjunctivum after survival periods of 3, 5 and 7 days respectively. In these cases the degeneration was found to be most pronounced after a survival of 7 days which made us choose this survival period.

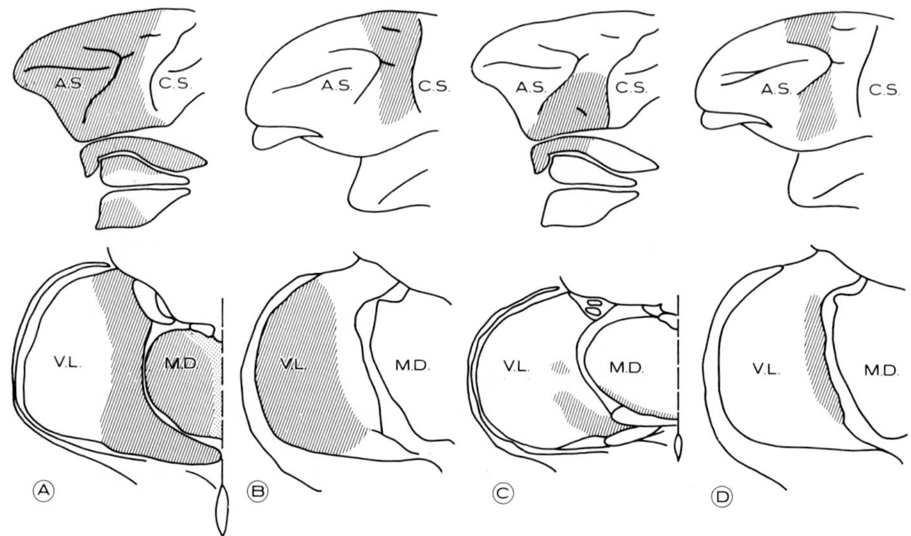

FIG. 3

tion of the prerubral field and the ventral portion of the area of the centre median. From these bundles degenerating fibers were distributed to the zona incerta and to the VM, VL and VA nuclei of the thalamus. A limited number of degenerating fibers was distributed also to the centre median and the intralaminar nuclei. The fibers to the VM, VL and VA terminated in specific areas. In the VM dense terminal degeneration occurred only in its lateral part. In the caudal portion of the VL dense terminal degeneration occurred mainly in its ventromedial part, adjoining the intralaminar nuclei. Further rostrally, degeneration was present also in its dorsomedial part and continued in diminishing density into the dorsomedial part of the caudal VA. Laterally in the VL a few clusters of degenerating fibers and terminals were present, medial to the rostral portion of the VPL nucleus. Some clusters were present also in the ventrolateral part of the VA. Rostrally, this degeneration was more prominent than the degeneration in the dorsomedial part of the VA.

In case C1, the inferior collicular commissure and the central gray at the caudal entrance of the aqueduct were slightly damaged. In this case bilateral degeneration also occurred in the inferior colliculus and its brachium, the medial geniculate body, the nucleus lateralis dorsalis of the thalamus and the mammillary bodies.

The distribution of the degeneration in our cases is very similar to that described by Angaut and Bowsher (5), after lesions of the fastigial nuclei. However, Angaut and Bowsher (5) did not report clusters of degeneration in the lateral parts of the VL and VA. The presence of these clusters in our material probably resulted from a more extensive destruction of fastigio-thalamic fibers than may be achieved by small lesions of the nucleus.

In the three monkeys with a cerebellar bisection, the bilateral degeneration in the mesencephalon and the diencephalon was distributed symmetrically (Fig. 4). The ascending bundles of degenerating fibers were present in the dorsal portion of the prerubral field around the habenulo-interpeduncular tract and in the ventral portion of the area of the centre median. From these bundles a few degenerating fibers terminated in the zona incerta, the centre median-parafascicular complex and the intralaminar nuclei. The bulk of the ascending fibers terminated in the VIM (the pars oralis of the VPL of Olszewski (48)) and in the VL. A few fibers terminated also in the VA. The fibers to these nuclei reached their destination along a medial and a lateral trajectory; i.e., through the centre median and through the lateral part of the VPL nucleus. In the VL a diffuse terminal degeneration occurred medially in the caudal half of the area X of Olszewski. In addition, in the VIM and the VL a great many clusters of degener-

---

FIG. 3. Distribution of the retrograde changes in the VL nucleus of the thalamus after lesions of different parts of the precentral and premotor areas. A and C are from Figs. 8 and 12 of T.S. Roberts and K. Akert, Schweiz. Arch. f. Neurol. Neurochir. u. Psychiat., 92 (1963) 1-43. Used with permission. B and D are from Fig. 18, 3 of Comparative anatomy of frontal cortex and thalamocortical connections by K. Akert in: The Frontal Granular Cortex and Behavior, McGraw Hill, Inc., 1964. Used with permission of McGraw Hill Book Company.

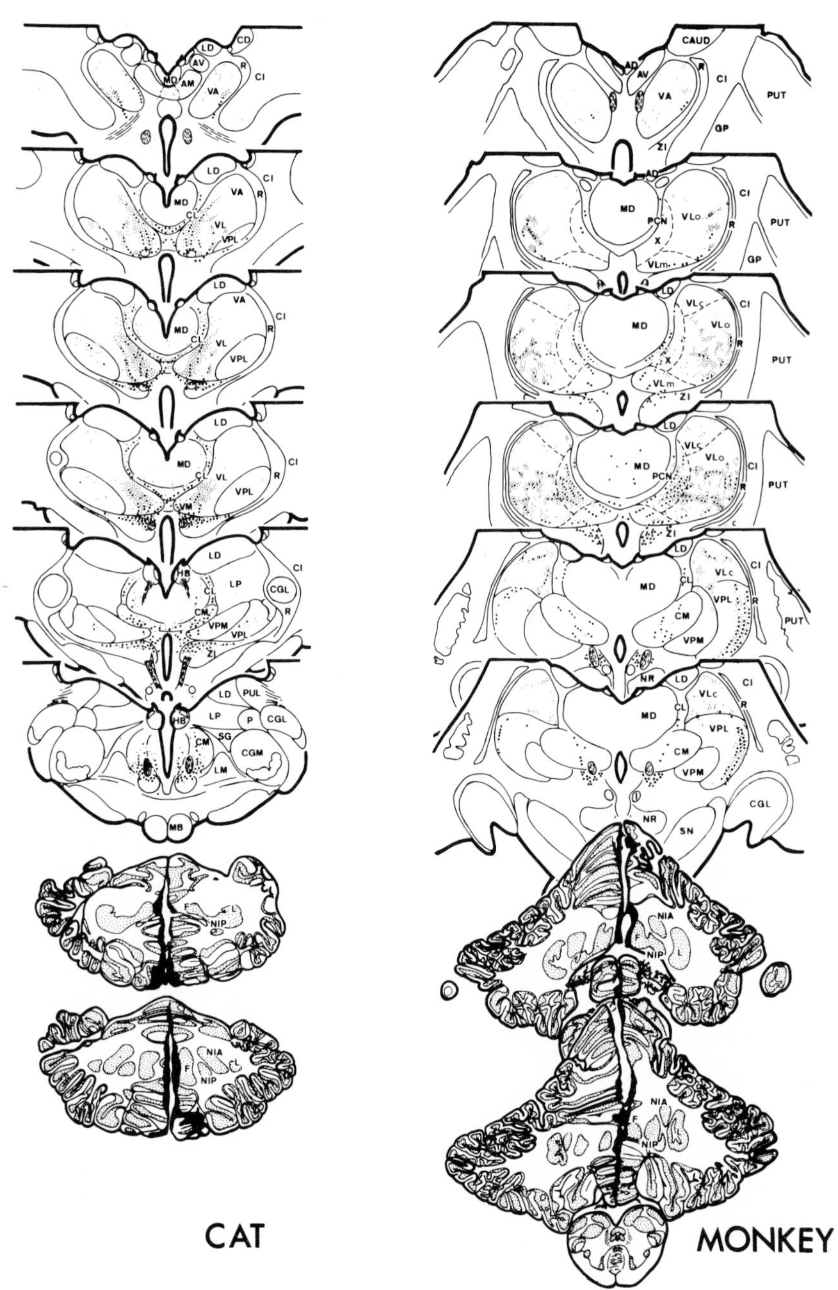

FIG. 4

ating elements were present, which were arranged in a curved band extending from medial to ventrolateral across the nucleus. These clusters which were interconnected by strands of degenerating fibers were present in the ventral portion of the VL caudalis (48), but were most prominent in the VL oralis. In the lateral part of the VL the clusters extended into the most rostral portion of the nucleus and thus continued further rostrally than the terminal degeneration in its medial part (area X (48)).

These findings demonstrate that in the monkey the distribution of the crossed fastigial fibers in the VL is more extensive than in cat. Further they support the original hypothesis that the fastigial fibers in the monkey are distributed to the medial part of the VL and to a portion of its lateral part.

In cat C3 and in monkey M4 the cerebellar bisection was combined with a transection of the right brachium conjunctivum (Fig. 5). In both these animals the distribution of the degenerating elements in the right VL and VA—ipsilateral to the transected brachium— was virtually the same as observed in the previous cases. Some degeneration also occurred in the right medial geniculate body and in the medial part of the right VPM (cf. 23) (case M4). This degeneration probably resulted from damage to the ipsilateral inferior colliculus (42, 44, 45, 54) and to fibers from the ipsilateral principal nucleus of the trigeminus (10, 68).

The degeneration in the left thalami, i.e.,contralateral to the transected brachium conjunctivum, was considerably more widespread than in the right (Fig. 5). In the cat (C3) some fibers were distributed to the centre median-parafascicular complex and the intralaminar nuclei. The bulk of the fibers, however, was distributed to the ventrolateral part of the VM, throughout the VL,and to the VA, especially its lateral part (cf. 4, 5, 16, 67). Further, some degenerating fibers were distributed to the zona incerta and thence to the caudal part of the reticular nucleus. In the monkey (M4) contralateral to the transected brachium a similar distribution pattern was found as in the cat (C3) (cf. 41). Some degenerating fibers were distributed to the intralaminar nuclei and the pars multiformis of the dorsomedial nucleus (cf. 41). The bulk of the degenerating fibers was distributed in varying density throughout the VIM (pars oralis of VPL of Olszewski (48)), the VL and the VA. The fibers reached the nuclei by way of a lateral trajectory through the lateral part of the VPL and a medial one through the centre median. Some degenerating fibers were distributed also to the zona incerta and thence to the reticular nucleus of the thalamus (Fig. 5).

The degeneration in the thalamus of cases C3 and M4 ipsilateral to the transected brachium was of the same quantity and distribution as that in cases C1, 2, 4 and in

---

FIG. 4. Semidiagrammatic representation of the distribution of the ascending degeneration in the diencephalon of cat C2 and monkey M3 after cerebellar bisection. Bundles of degenerating fibers are indicated by large dots. Terminal degeneration is indicated by fine stippling. Note in monkey M3 the degeneration in the medial part of the VL and the clusters of degeneration in the lateral part. The terminal degeneration in the right VPL of monkey M3 was related to a small infarct in the caudal part of the nucleus gracilis.

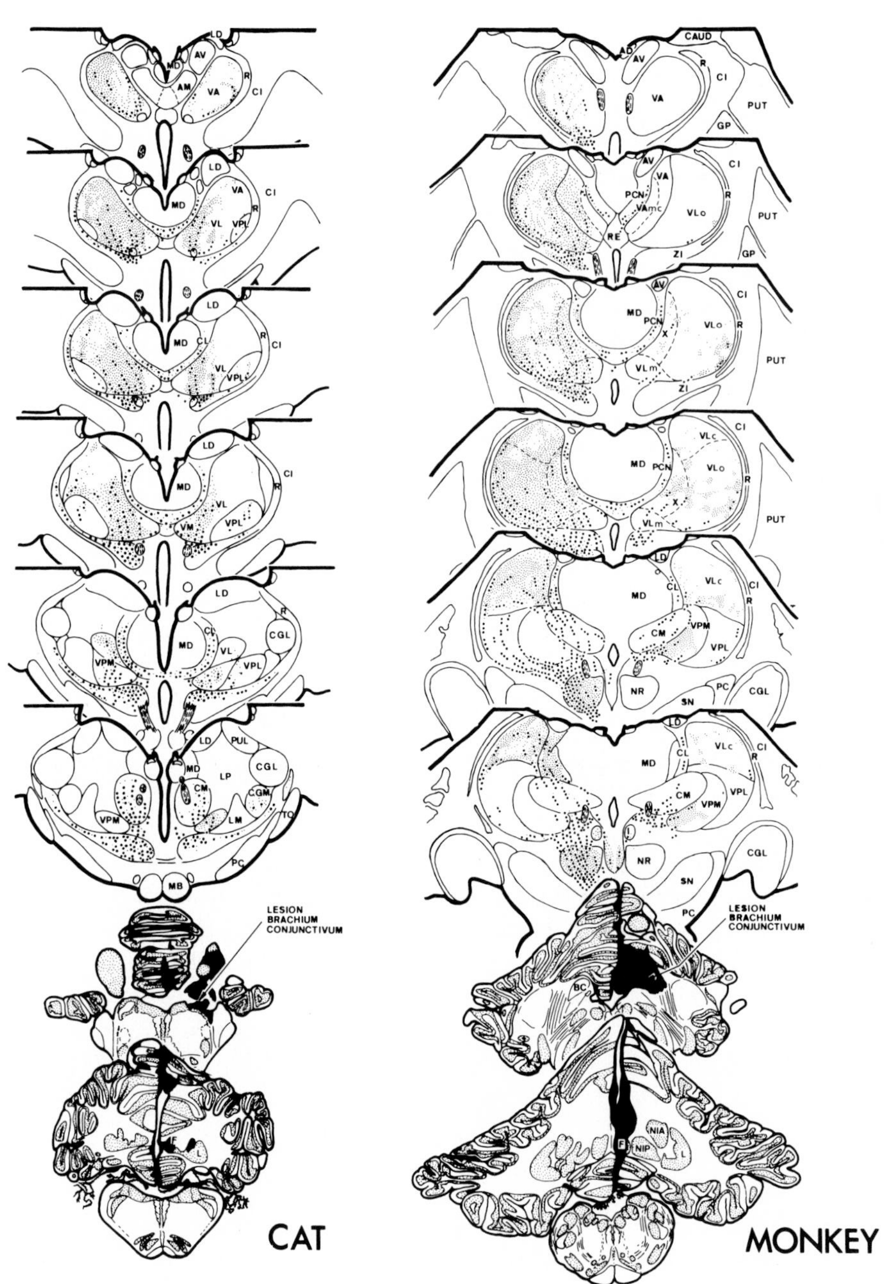

LD
AV
MD
AM
VA
R
CI
VL
VPL
CL
VM
CGL
VPM
PUL
LP
CM
CGM
LM
TO
PC
MB
LESION BRACHIUM CONJUNCTIVUM
CAT
CAUD
AD
PUT
GP
PCN
VAmc
VLo
RE
ZI
X
VLm
VLc
NR
SN
BC
NIA
NIP
F
L
MONKEY

FIG. 5

cases M1, 2, 3 respectively, following only a bisection of the cerebellum. This further supports the idea that among the cerebello-thalamic fibers only fastigial elements decussate within the cerebellum. However, observations in the cat (69, 70) indicate that a few fastigial fibers from the lateral portion of the nucleus do not decussate within the cerebellum and travel in the most medial portion of the ipsilateral brachium conjunctivum (Fig. 2). In order to determine the thalamic distribution of these fibers in cat C5, the most medial portion of the brachium conjunctivum was transected without damaging the cerebellar nuclei (Fig. 6).

The bulk of the ascending fibers in this case (C5) crossed in the mesencephalon and terminated in the VL-VA complex of the contralateral thalamus. Only few degenerating elements occurred in the ipsilateral thalamus, mainly in the VPM and in the VL-VA complex. This degeneration probably resulted from damage to the ascending fibers from the ipsilateral principal nucleus of the trigeminus (10, 11) and to the uncinate tract overlaying the brachium conjunctivum (9, 16, 56, 67, 69) respectively. The degeneration in the contralateral VL-VA complex was distributed in largely the same fashion as following bisection of the cerebellum (cases C1, 2, 4). However, the degeneration in case C5 tended to be less dense than in cases C1, 2, 4 but was somewhat more pronounced in the rostrolateral part of the VL-VA complex than in these cases.

These findings suggest that the fastigial fibers (and possibly some of the interpositus posterior fibers (69, 70)), which ascend in the extreme medial portion of the brachium conjunctivum, tend to be distributed to the same parts of the contralateral VL-VA complex as the fastigio-thalamic fibers which decussate within the cerebellum. The relatively more pronounced degeneration in the rostrolateral part of the VL-VA complex (Fig. 6) in case C5 as compared to the other cases probably results from the interruption of fibers from the N.I.P. which projects to this area. To our knowledge no data are available concerning the presence of the former group of fastigio-thalamic fibers in the rhesus monkey.

The findings in this study support the original hypothesis and demonstrate that in the rhesus monkey the crossed fastigial fibers to the VL nucleus have a wider distribution than in the cat and terminate in its medial portion which projects to the rostral part of the motor cortex (1, 59) and in an area in its lateral portion which projects to the caudal part (1, 59). However, it remains to be shown that at least some of the recipient cells of the crossed fastigial fibers in the lateral portion of the VL do project

---

FIG. 5. Semidiagrammatic representation of the distribution of the ascending degeneration in the diencephalon of cat C3 and monkey M4 following cerebellar bisection and transection of the right brachium conjunctivum. Symbols as in Fig. 4. Note that in both animals the distribution of the degeneration in the VL and VA ipsilateral to the transected brachium is identical with that following cerebellar bisection (cf. Fig. 4). The additional degeneration in the VPM and the CGM is probably related to damage to the inferior colliculus and to ascending fibers from the principal nucleus of the trigeminus ipsilaterally.

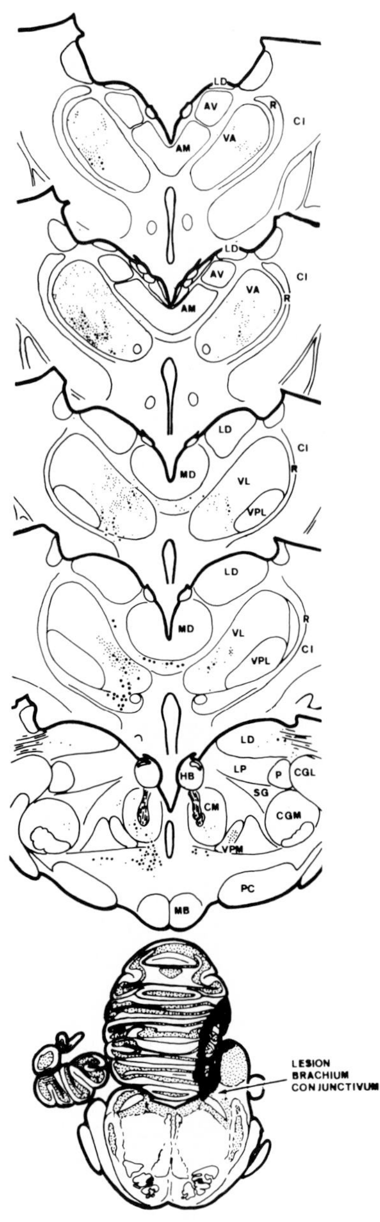
LD
AV
R
CI
AM
VA
MD
VL
VPL
HB
LP
P
CGL
SG
CM
CGM
VPM
PC
MB
LESION
BRACHIUM
CONJUNCTIVUM

CAT

FIG. 6

to the caudal precentral territory between the hand and foot representation areas.

With respect to the present findings two additional points may be noted. In the cat the border between the VL and the VA nuclei (24) is difficult to determine on the basis of cytoarchitecture. In addition, the distribution of the cerebellar projections disregards the traditional VL-VA border and extends without interruption from the VL into the lateral parts of the traditional VA. This holds true for both the distribution of the contralateral brachium conjunctivum as well as for the distribution of the fastigial fibers which cross in the cerebellum (Figs. 4, 5). This arrangement suggests that the ventrolateral part of the traditional VA may represent the most rostral outpost of the VL. In that case the VA in the cat would replace the VL from medially rather than from dorsally, i.e., in the same way as in the rhesus monkey (48). Because of these uncertainties in the cat no definite border line has been drawn between the VL and the VA in our illustrations.

Our findings combined with those of others (11, 17, 41, 47) indicate that in the VL nucleus a contrast exists between the distribution of the fastigial cerebellar fibers and that of the fibers from the globus pallidus and the substantia nigra. The fibers from the latter two sources terminate in the lateral and ventral parts of the nucleus which project to the caudal part of the motor cortex. In contrast the medial part of the VL nucleus which projects to the rostral part of the motor cortex receives no fibers from either the globus pallidus or the substantia nigra but receives many fastigial fibers (Fig. 4). The selective distribution of fibers from the globus pallidus to the centre median (47) may be in keeping with this pattern since the cortical fibers to the centre median come mainly from the precentral gyrus and not from the premotor area which projects to the nucleus parafascicularis (30, 33, 50).

SUMMARY

On the basis of the distribution of the corticospinal fibers, it was expected that fastigial projections to the VL nucleus of the contralateral thalamus would be more widespread in the rhesus monkey than in the cat. In the monkey this projection was expected to be distributed not only to the medial part of the VL as in the cat but also to a portion of its lateral part. This hypothesis was supported by the distribution of the degenerating elements found in the thalami of four cats and four rhesus monkeys, in which the crossed fastigio-thalamic fibers were transected by a bisection of the cerebellum in the mid-sagittal plane. In the cat a few fastigial fibers ascend in the most medial portion of the ipsilateral brachium conjunctivum. Our additional findings indicate that these fibers, after crossing in the mesencephalon, terminate largely in the same thalamic areas as the fastigial fibers which cross within the cerebellum.

FIG. 6. Semidiagrammatic representation of the distribution of the ascending degeneration in the diencephalon of cat C5 following transection of the extreme medial tip of the right brachium conjunctivum without damage to the cerebellar nuclei. Symbols as in Fig. 4. Note that the degeneration in the contralateral VL-VA complex is distributed in largely the same fashion as following cerebellar bisection (cf. Fig. 4).

ACKNOWLEDGMENTS

This study was in part supported by Grant No. 13-31-12 (1971) of the Dutch Organization for Fundamental Research in Medicine (FUNGO). The authors wish to thank Mr. E. Dalm, Mr. J.P.M. Schoelitsz and Miss C.M. Biemond for their technical help and Mr. W. v.d. Oudenalder and Miss P.C. Delfos for their photographic help. They are also grateful to Miss J. Brinkman for her help with one of the illustrations, to Miss A.M.B. Wessels for typing the manuscript and to Drs. D.G. Lawrence and J.S.G. Miller for reading it.

ABBREVIATIONS

AD	N. Anterior dorsalis
AM	N. Anterior medialis
AV	N. Anterior ventralis
BC	Brachium conjunctivum
CAUD	N. Caudatus
CGL	Corpus geniculatum laterale
CGM	Corpus geniculatum mediale
CI	Capsula interna
CL	N. Centralis lateralis
CM	N. Centrum medianum
F	N. Fastigii
GP	Globus pallidus
HB	Corpus Habenulare
I	N. Interstitialis
L	N. Lateralis
LD	N. Lateralis dorsalis
LM	Lemniscus medialis
LP	N. Lateralis posterior
MB	Corpus mammillare
MD	N. Medialis dorsalis
NIA	N. Interpositus anterior
NIP	N. Interpositus posterior
NR	N. Ruber
P	N. Posterior
PC	Pedunculus cerebri
PCN	N. Paracentralis
PUL	Pulvinar
PUT	Putamen
R	N. Reticularis
RE	N. Reuniens
SG	N. Suprageniculatus

SN	Substantia nigra
TO	Tractus opticus
VA	N. Ventralis anterior
VAmc	N. Ventralis anterior pars magnocellularis
VL	N. Ventralis lateralis
VLc	N. Ventralis lateralis pars caudalis
VLm	N. Ventralis lateralis pars medialis
VLo	N. Ventralis lateralis pars oralis
VM	N. Ventralis medialis
VPL	N. Ventralis posterior lateralis
VPM	N. Ventralis posterior medialis
X	Zona X
ZI	Zona incerta

REFERENCES

1 AKERT, K. Comparative anatomy of frontal cortex and thalamofrontal connections. In J.M. Warren and K. Akert (Eds), The Frontal Granular Cortex and Behavior, McGraw Hill Inc., New York, 1964, pp. 372-394.

2 ANDERSEN, P., ECCLES, J.C., and SEARS, T.A. Cortically evoked depolarization of primary afferent fibers in the spinal cord, J. Neurophysiol., 27 (1964) 63-77.

3 ANGAUT, P. Etude Anatomique Experimental des Efferences Cerebelleuses Ascendantes. Analyse Electro-anatomique des Projections Cerebelleuses sur le Noyau Ventral-lateral du Thalamus. Thesis, Paris, 1969.

4 ANGAUT, P. The ascending projections of the nucleus interpositus posterior of the cat cerebellum: An experimental anatomical study using silver impregnation methods, Brain Research, 24 (1970) 377-394.

5 ANGAUT, P., and BOWSHER, D. Ascending projections of the medial cerebellar (fastigial) nucleus: An experimental study in the cat, Brain Research, 24 (1970) 49-68.

6 BROOKHART, J.M. A study of corticospinal activation of motoneurons, Res. Public. Ass. nerv. ment. Dis., 30 (1952) 157-173.

7 CAJAL, Ramon y, S. Histologie du Système Nerveux de l'Homme et des Vertebres, Consejo Superior de Investigaciones Cientificas Instituto Ramon y Cajal, Madrid, 1952, I p. 986, II p. 993.

8 CARPENTER, M.B. The dorsal trigeminal tract in the rhesus monkey, J. Anat. (Lond.), 91 (1957) 82-93.

9 CARPENTER, M.B. Lesions of the fastigial nuclei in the rhesus monkey, Amer. J. Anat., 104 (1959) 1-33.

10 CARPENTER, M.B., and STEVENS, G.H. Structural and functional relationships between the deep cerebellar nuclei and the brachium conjunctivum in the rhesus monkey, J. Comp. Neurol., 107 (1957) 109-163.

11 CARPENTER, M.B., and STROMINGER, N.L. Efferent fibers of the subthalamic nucleus in the monkey. A comparison of the efferent projections of the sub-

thalamic nucleus, substantia nigra and globus pallidus, Amer. J. Anat., 121 (1967) 41-71.

12 CHAMBERS, W.W., and LIU, C.N. Corticospinal tract of the cat. An attempt to correlate the pattern of degeneration with deficits in reflex activity following neocortical lesions, J. Comp. Neurol., 108 (1957) 23-55.

13 CHAMBERS, W.W., and LIU, C.N. An experimental study of the corticospinal system in the monkey (Macaca mulatta), J. Comp. Neurol., 123 (1965) 257-284.

14 CHAMBERS, W.W., and SPRAGUE, J.M. Functional localization in the cerebellum I, J. Comp. Neurol., 103 (1955) 105-129.

15 CHAMBERS, W.W., and SPRAGUE, J.M. Functional localization in the cerebellum II, Arch. Neurol. Psychiat. (Chicago), 74 (1955) 653-680.

16 COHEN, D., CHAMBERS, W.W., and SPRAGUE, J.M. Experimental study of the efferent projections from the cerebellar nuclei to the brain stem of the cat, J. Comp. Neurol., 109 (1958) 233-259.

17 COLE, M., NAUTA, W.J.H., and MEHLER, W.R. The ascending efferent projections of the substantia nigra, Trans. Amer. Neurol. Ass., 89 (1964) 74.

18 COURVILLE, J. Somatotopical organization of the projection from the nucleus interpositus anterior of the cerebellum to the red nucleus. An experimental study in the cat with silver impregnation methods, Exp. Brain Res., 2 (1966) 191-215.

19 FETZ, E.E. Pyramidal tract effects on interneurons in the cat lumbar dorsal horn, J. Neurophysiol., 31 (1968) 69-80.

20 FINK, R.P., and HEIMER, L. Two methods for selective silver impregnation of degenerating axons and their synaptic endings in the central nervous system, Brain Research, 4 (1967) 369-374.

21 FLOOD, S., and JANSEN, J. The efferent fibers of the cerebellar nuclei and their distribution on the cerebellar peduncles in the cat, Acta. Anat., 63 (1966) 137-166.

22 JANE, J.A., CAMPBELL, C.B.G., and YASHON, D. Pyramidal tract. A comparison of two prosimian primates, Science, 147 (1965) 153-155.

23 JANSEN, J., and JANSEN, J. Jr. On the efferent fibers of the cerebellar nuclei in cat, J. Comp. Neurol., 102 (1955) 607-632.

24 JASPER, H.H., and AJMONE-MARSAN, C. A Stereotaxic Atlas of the Diencephalon of the Cat, Natl. Res. Council of Canada (Ottawa), 1954.

25 KENNARD, M.A., and ECTORS, L. Forced circling movements in monkeys following lesions of the frontal lobes, J. Neurophysiol., 1 (1938) 45-54.

26 KLUVER, H., and BARRERA, E. A method for the combined staining of cells and fibers in the nervous system, Neuropath. Exp. Neurol., 12 (1953) 400-403.

27 KUYPERS, H.G.J.M. Some projections from the peri-central cortex to the pons and lower brain stem in monkey and chimpanzee, J. Comp. Neurol., 110 (1958b) 221-256.

28 KUYPERS, H.G.J.M. Central cortical projections to motor and somatosensory cell groups, Brain, 83 (1960) 161-184.

29 KUYPERS, H.G.J.M. The descending pathways to the spinal cord, their anatomy and function. In J.C. Eccles and J.P. Schade (Eds.), Organization of the

Spinal Cord, Progress in Brain Research, Vol. 11, Elsevier, Amsterdam, 1964, pp. 178-200.

30 KUYPERS, H.G.J.M. Cortical projections to the center median of Luys and the red nucleus. In D.P. Purpura and M.D. Yahr (Eds.), The Thalamus, Columbia University Press, New York, 1966, pp. 122-126.

31 KUYPERS, H.G.J.M., and BRINKMAN, J. Precentral projections to different parts of the spinal intermediate zone in the rhesus monkey, Brain Research, 24 (1970) 29-48.

32 KUYPERS, H.G.J.M., FLEMING, W.R., and FARINHOLT, J.W. Subcorticospinal projections in the rhesus monkey, J. Comp. Neurol., 118 (1962) 107-137

33 KUYPERS, H.G.J.M., and LAWRENCE, D.G. Cortical projections to the red nucleus and the brain stem in the rhesus monkey, Brain Research, 4 (1967) 151-188.

34 LAWRENCE, D.G., and KUYPERS, H.G.J.M. The functional organization of the motor system in the monkey. I. The effects of bilateral pyramidal lesions, Brain, 91 (1968a) 1-14.

35 LAWRENCE, D.G., and KUYPERS, H.G.J.M. The functional organization of the motor system in the monkey. II. The effects of lesions of the descending brain stem pathways, Brain, 91 (1968b) 15-36.

36 LEWIS, R. and BRINDLEY, G.S. The extrapyramidal cortical motor map, Brain 88 (1965) 397-406.

37 MARCHIAVAFA, P.L., and POMPEIANO, O. Pyramidal influence on spinal cord during desynchronized sleep, Arch. ital. Biol., 102 (1964) 500-529.

38 MARTIN, G.F., and DOM, R. Rubrobulbar projections of the opossum (Didelphis virginiana), J. Comp. Neurol., 139 (1970) 199-214.

39 MATSUSHITA, M. Some aspects of the interneuronal connections in the cat's spinal gray matter, J. Comp. Neurol., 136 (1969) 57-80.

40 MATSUSHITA, M. The axonal pathways of spinal neurones in the cat. J. Comp. Neurol., 138 (1970) 391-418.

41 MEHLER, W.R. Idea of a new anatomy of the thalamus, J. Psychiat. Res., 8 (1971) 203-217.

42 MOORE, R.Y., and GOLDBERG, J.M. Projections of the inferior colliculus in the monkey. Exp. Neurol., 14 (1966) 429-438.

43 MORRISON, A.R., and POMPEIANO, O. Pyramidal discharge from somatosensory cortex and cortical control of primary afferents during sleep, Arch. ital. Biol., 103 (1965) 538-568.

44 MOUNTCASTLE, V.B., and HENNEMAN, E. Pattern of tactile representation in thalamus of cat, J. Neurophysiol., 12 (1949) 85-100.

45 MOUNTCASTLE, V.B., and HENNEMAN, E. The representation of tactile sensibility in the thalamus of the monkey, J. Comp. Neurol., 97 (1952) 409-439.

46 NYBERG-HANSEN, R. Functional organization of descending supraspinal fiber systems to the spinal cord. Anatomical observations and physiological correlations, Ergeb. Anat. Entw. Gesch., 39 (1966) 6-48.

47 NAUTA, W.J.H., and MEHLER, W.R. Projections of the lentiform nucleus in

the monkey, Brain Research, 1 (1966) 3-42.

48 OLSZEWSKI, J. The Thalamus of the Macaca Mulatta, S. Karger, Basel, 1952.

49 PETRAS, J.M. Cortical, tectal and tegmental fiber connections in the spinal cord of the cat, Brain Research, 6 (1967) 275-324.

50 PETRAS, J.M. Some fiber connections of the motor and somatosensory cortex of simian primates and felid, canid, and procyonid carnivores, Ann. New York Acad. Sc., 167 (1969) 469-505.

51 PHILLIPS, C.G. The Ferrier Lecture 1968, Motor apparatus of the baboon's hand, Proc. Roy. Soc. B., 173 (1969) 141-174.

52 POMPEIANO, O. Analisi degli effetti della stimolazione elettrica del nucleo rosso del gatto decerebrato, R.C. Accad. naz. Lincei Cl. Sci. fis., mat., nat., Ser. VIII, 22 (1957) 100-103.

53 POMPEIANO, O., and BRODAL, A. Experimental demonstration of a somatotopical origin of rubrospinal fibers in the cat, J. Comp. Neurol., 108 (1957) 225-252.

54 POWELL, E.W., and HATTON, J.B. Projections of the inferior colliculus in cat, J. Comp. Neurol., 136 (1969) 183-192.

55 PRESTON, J.B., SHENDE, M.C., and UEMARA, K. The motor cortex. Pyramidal System: Patterns of facilitation and inhibition on motoneurons innervating limb musculature of cat and baboon and their possible adaptive significance. In M.D. Yahr and D.P. Purpura (Eds.), Neurophysiological Basis of Normal and Abnormal Motor Activities, Raven Press, Hewlett, N.Y., 1967, pp. 61-72.

56 RAND, R.W. An anatomical and experimental study of the cerebellar nuclei and their efferent pathways in the monkey, J. Comp. Neurol., 101 (1954) 167-223.

57 RISPAL-PADEL, L., and MASSION, J. Relations between the ventrolateral nucleus and the motor cortex in the cat, Exp. Brain Res., 10 (1970) 331-339.

58 RISPAL-PADEL, L., LATREILLE, J., and VANUXEM, P. Repartition sur le cortex moteur des projections des differents noyaux cerebelleux chez le chat, C.R. Acad. Sc. Paris, 272 (1971) 451-454.

59 ROBERTS, T.S., and AKERT, K. Thalamo-cortical connections and cytoarchitecture of opercular and insular cortex in Macaca mulatta, Schw. Arch. Neurol. Neurochir. u. Psychiat., 92 (1963) 1-43.

60 RUSTIONI, A., KUYPERS, H.G.J.M., and HOLSTEGE, G. Propriospinal projections from the ventral and lateral funiculi to the motoneurons in the lumbosacral cord of the cat, Brain Research, 35 (1971) 255-275.

61 SCHEIBEL, M.E., and SCHEIBEL, A.B. Spinal motoneurones, interneurones and Renshaw cells. A Golgi study, Arch. ital. Biol., 104 (1966) 328-353.

62 SHAPOVOLOV, A.I., KURCHAVAYI, G.G., KARAMJAN, O.A., and REPINA, Z.A., Extrapyramidal pathways with monosynaptic effects upon primate αmotoneurons, Experientia, 27 (1971) 522-524.

63 SNIDER, R.S., and NIEMER, W.T. A stereotaxic atlas of the cat brain, The University of Chicago Press, Chicago, 1961.

64 STERLING, P., and KUYPERS, H.G.J.M. Anatomical organization of the brachial spinal cord of the cat. III. The propriospinal connections, Brain Research,

7, (1968) 419-443.
65 SZENTAGOTHAI, J. Propriospinal pathways and their synapses. In. J.C. Eccles and J.P. Schade (Eds.), Organization of the Spinal Cord, Progress in Brain Research, Vol. 11, Elsevier, Amsterdam, 1964, pp. 155-174.
66 TESTA, C. Functional implication of the morphology of spinal ventral horn neurones of the cat, J. Comp. Neurol., 123 (1964) 425-444.
67 THOMAS, D.M., KAUFMAN, R.P., SPRAGUE, J.M., and CHAMBERS, W.W. Experimental studies of the vermal cerebellar projections in the brain stem of the cat (Fastigiobulbar tract), J. Anat. London, 90 (1956) 371-385.
68 TORVIK, A. The ascending fibers from the main trigeminal sensory nucleus: An experimental study in the cat, Amer. J. Anat. 100 (1957) 1-15.
69 VOOGD, J. The cerebellum of the Cat. Structure and Fibre Connexions. Van Gorcum & Comp. N.V., Assen. 1964.
70 VOOGD, J. Comparative aspects of the structure and fibre connexions of the mammalian cerebellum. In C.A. Fox and R.S. Snider (Eds.), The Cerebellum, Progress in Brain Research, Vol. 25, Elsevier, Amsterdam, 1967, p. 353.
71 WAGMAN, I.H. Eye movements induced by electrical stimulation of cerebrum in monkeys and their relationship to bodily movements. In M.B. Bender (Ed.), The Oculomotor System, Harper & Row, New York, 1964, pp. 18-39.
72 WALBERG, F., and JANSEN, J. Cerebellar corticovestibular fibers in the cat, Exp. Neurol., 3 (1961) 32-52.
73 WALBERG, F., POMPEIANO, O., BRODAL, A., and JANSEN, J. The fastigio-vestibular projection in the cat. An experimental study with silver impregnation methods, J. Comp. Neurol., 118 (1962) 49-75.
74 WALKER, A.E. The Primate Thalamus, University of Chicago Press, Chicago, Ill., 1938, p. 305.
75 WILSON, V.J., and YOSHIDA, M. Comparison of effects of stimulation of Deiters' nucleus and medial longitudinal fasciculus on neck, forelimb and hind-limb motoneurons, J. Neurophysiol., 32 (1969) 743-758.
76 WOOLSEY, C.N., SETTLAGE, P.H., MEYER, D.R., SPENCER, W., HAMUY, T.P., and TRAVIS, A.M. Patterns of localization in precentral and "supple-mentary" motor areas and their relation to the concept of a premotor area, Res. Publ. Ass. nerv. ment. Dis., 30 (1950) 238-264.

DISCUSSION

COURVILLE:

I think that Dr. Kuyper's idea on the integration of the cerebellar efferents, the cortical efferents to the cord, as well as brain stem efferents to the spinal cord is very attractive. Concerning the projections of the fastigial nucleus to the thalamus, he has shown that in the monkey, the situation is very much similar to what has been observed in the cat. He has pointed out that the fastigial projections in the monkey reach the VM as well as the medial part of the VL nucleus. It seems to me that in Dr. Rinvik's figures, this is a portion of VL that is apparently devoid of terminal fibers from the cortex. In connection with these data, I would like to mention a few recent unpublished observations on cerebellar efferents in the monkey. As Dr. Kuypers has noted, the anterior part of the interpositus nucleus (that is the nucleus interpositus anterior) projects to the contralateral magnocellular part of the red nucleus. I can confirm this and add that the parvocellular part of the red nucleus receives its projection from the dentate nucleus. Concerning the posterior part of the interpositus nucleus, our studies in the cat have shown that it projects to the vestibular nuclei, mainly the descending and the medial nuclei, in addition to having scanty ascending projections.

KUYPERS:

I am quite grateful to Dr. Courville for his comments. I do think, however, that the findings of Dr. Rinvik (and those of Petras in the monkey, see elsewhere in this volume) are in keeping with our findings in that the medial part of the VL receives cortical projections e.g. from the gyrus proreus (Rinvik, Exp. Brain Res. 5, 129-152, 1968) in the cat and the premotor area in the monkey (Petras). In respect to Dr. Courville's comments on the efferents of the nucleus interpositus, his findings add further to the riddle of the organization of the cerebellar outflow. The existence of a pronounced projection from the N.I.P. to the vestibular nuclei would seem to be in line with findings of Voogd, which suggest that some of the projections from the N.I.P. are directed to cell groups of the medial bulbar reticular formation, which together with the vestibular complex project to the ventromedial part of the spinal intermediate zone, and would steer especially proximal movements (cf. also Shapovalov et al., Exp. 27: 522-524, 1971, in the monkey). The ascending projection from the N.I.P. to the thalamus, however, seems to behave differently since it influences mainly the caudal parts of the motor cortex which especially governs distal motor activity. In summary, the detailed organization of the cerebellar efferent is still very unclear to me.

HASSLER:

I would like to comment on this projection from the cerebellar nuclei to VL and VM. I must say we tried to get the degenerating fibers from the fastigial nucleus to the thalamus in the cat, but we avoided the dorsal approach to the fastigial nucleus. We made a ventral approach from the 4th ventricle, and were able, in two cases, to destroy the fastigial nucleus without any damage to the surrounding fibers. In both cases we did not see any degeneration in the ventrolateral or in the ventromedial nucleus of the thalamus. So I think that the experiments of Dr. Kuypers are clearing up the situation a little bit. The degeneration comes from crossing fibers that cross above the fastigial nucleus, and which are usually destroyed if one uses a dorsal approach to the fastigial nuclei. In such cases we can damage perhaps fibers originating in the interpositus nucleus and in other structures. So, mainly in the cat, I am very doubtful about this direct projection from the fastigial nucleus to VL; we could not find it in cases with restricted lesions.

KUYPERS:

To Dr. Hassler's question I would like to give the following comment. Thomas, et al. (J. Anat. (Lond.) 90: 371, 1956), Angaut and Bowsher (Brain Res. 24: 49, 1970) as well as Voogd (Thesis, Univ. Leyden, 1964) found ascending degenerating fibers to the thalamus following lesions of the fastigial nucleus. It might be possible that their lesions and electrode tracks partially involved fibers crossing in the cerebellum. However, according to Flood and Jansen (Acta Anat. 63: 137, 1966) transection of the superior cerebellar peduncle causes retrograde changes in neurons of the ipsilateral interpositus and lateral nucleus and in neurons of mainly the contralateral fastigial nucleus. These findings together led us to conclude that the ascending cerebellothalamic projections which we described are of fastigial origin. This is in agreement with the findings of Cohen et al. (J. Comp. Neurol., 109: 233, 1958), Voogd (Thesis, Univ. Leyden, 1964) and Angaut (Brain Res., 24: 49, 1970) who demonstrated that after small lesions of the interpositus nucleus degenerating fibers are present almost exclusively in the ipsilateral superior cerebellar peduncle. The fact that Dr. Hassler did not obtain degeneration in the VL and the VM nuclei of the thalamus after fastigial lesions might have been due to the location of the lesions since the fastigiothalamic fibers apparently are derived from specific portions of the nucleus.

JASPER:

I have some comments on Dr. Kuypers' paper. In discussing the fastigiothalamic pathway with Dr. Snider some time ago, he made the comment that these fibers did not seem to follow the course of the fibers in the brachium conjunctivum at the level of the red nucleus. But the fibers seem to be situated superior to the red nucleus and just lateral to the central gray, with some fibers actually penetrating the central gray. This pathway seemed to be intermingled with fibers in the old, so-called paleo-spino-thalamic system. I would like to ask Dr. Kuypers what he thinks about the projections of the fastigiothalamic pathway at this level of the red nucleus.

KUYPERS:

What Dr. Jasper has pointed out is absolutely correct. The ascending fastigial fibers as shown in our drawings travel dorsal to the red nucleus and—as other authors have shown also—terminate in part in the central gray matter and in the medial mesencephalic reticular formation. As a consequence the fastigial projections are not only related to the *descending* brain stem reticular and vestibular pathways to the spinal cord but also to the *ascending* brain stem reticular pathways. However, this does not mean that there is a controversy. Instead one could state in a somewhat popular fashion that the two groups of connections are in harmony in that the ascending reticular pathway keeps the cortex on its toes while the descending reticular and vestibular pathways keep the body on its toes.

ALBE-FESSARD:

I have two questions to ask. What are the bases for the recognition between VP and VL? Are the discrepancies made according to the different forms of the cells or to the sort of afferents going to these cells? I ask this question because electrophysiologically it is clear in the monkey that if cells lying posteriorly and inferiorly in VP receive afferents from the skin, the other cells that receive afferents only from the deep tissues are found at the limit between VP and VL. Are these cells to be put in VP or in VL? My other question deals with the effect of the injection into the nucleus ruber. Do you think that it can act differently in the large cells and in the small cells? And that some of the results may be due to the difficulty to find the termination of small cells with the technique used, as it is easier to see in this way the termination of the big cells?

KUYPERS:

In answer to Dr. Albe-Fessard's first question, we have come to the definite conclusion that fastigial and other ascending cerebellar fibers terminate in the VPLO of Olszewski, which is also called VIM nucleus of the thalamus. In respect to her second question; J. Dekker M.D. in our laboratory is also applying the autoradiographic technique to neuroanatomical questions. As far as I know there are no indications as yet that this technique demonstrates only the termination of one type of cells or the other. Further the findings of Dr. Edwards in respect to the rubrothalamic projections obtained with the autoradiographic technique have much in common with the findings of Dr. Lawrence and Dr. Hopkins in our department. They are studying the ascending rubral projections in the rhesus monkey, using, however, the Fink-Heimer silver impregnation technique. They first transected the brachia conjunctiva bilaterally. One year later, the degenerating cerebellar fibers in the thalamus could not be demonstrated any longer. After one year,therefore, they placed a second lesion in the rostral part of the red nucleus and studied the resulting degeneration after a survival period of seven days following the second lesion. Their findings so far suggest that in the monkey few, if any, rubral fibers ascend to the VL nucleus of the thalamus. This is also in keeping with the findings of Poirier and Bouvier (1966), which were obtained by means of the retrograde degeneration technique.

HASSLER:

May I answer to Dr. Albe-Fessard, that really the electrophysiological borderline you found in the human thalamus is between the nuclei with big cells and the nucleus VL or VoP, in the most rostral part of this big cell area, which should be called, after Crouch (1934), ventrointermedius nucleus. In this area are found the terminations of the Ia fibers laterally and vestibular afferents medially. So I think that all afferents coming from outside, from Ia fibers, from the skin, and so on, are going to thalamic nuclei with very big cells, the most rostral part of those is the ventrointermedius nucleus.

Corticothalamic Projections and Sensorimotor Activities
T. Frigyesi, E. Rinvik, and M.D. Yahr, editors. © 1972
Raven Press, New York.

Organization of Thalamic Projections to the Motor Cortex of the Cat

P. L. Strick, P. J. Hand, and A. R. Morrison

There have been many physiological studies investigating the connections between the ventrolateral nucleus of the thalamus (VL) and the motor cortex (1, 5, 24, 26). However, there is little anatomical information on the details of this pathway (20, 28). This study has been designed to answer two basic anatomical questions. First, to what region of the cortex does VL project and does this same cortical region also receive thalamocortical fibers from the ventrobasal complex (VB)? Second, how is the thalamocortical projection from VL organized? Studies of the cerebellum (10, 11) and motor cortex (23, 37) have suggested the existence of two systems which control different aspects of motor functioning: One system orients the animal in space by controlling posture and locomotion; a separate system controls more manipulative and skilled limb activities. Are both aspects of motor functioning also represented in VL? If so, is each represented in separate anatomical zones, as they are in the cerebellum (vermal-fastigial zone vs. paravermal-interpositus zone) and motor cortex (area 6 vs. area 4)?

The normal cyto- and myeloarchitecture of the ventrolateral nucleus reveals that it can be divided into a dorsal and a ventral zone. Figure 1 shows a low magnification view of the ventrolateral thalamus stained for myelinated fibers. The internal medullary lamina is the densely myelinated band at the top of the figure. Two regions of contrasting myelination can be seen: there is a dorsal zone (labelled A in the figure), which has few myelinated fibers and neighbors the internal medullary lamina; and a ventral zone (labelled B in the figure), which is more densely myelinated and neighbors the very densely myelinated VB (labelled C in the figure). Figure 2A, B, C show higher magnification views of the VL dorsal zone, ventral zone and VB respectively. Note the very sparse myelination in (A), the dorsal zone; the increase in fibers and bundles of myelin in (B), the ventral zone; and the great density of myelinated fiber bundles in VB (C).

The dorsal and ventral zones of VL also show distinct differences in cell type and cell distribution. The cells of the dorsal, myelin free zone (Fig. 3A) are moderately homogeneous in size (17 um x 26 um) and distribution. This contrasts with the more

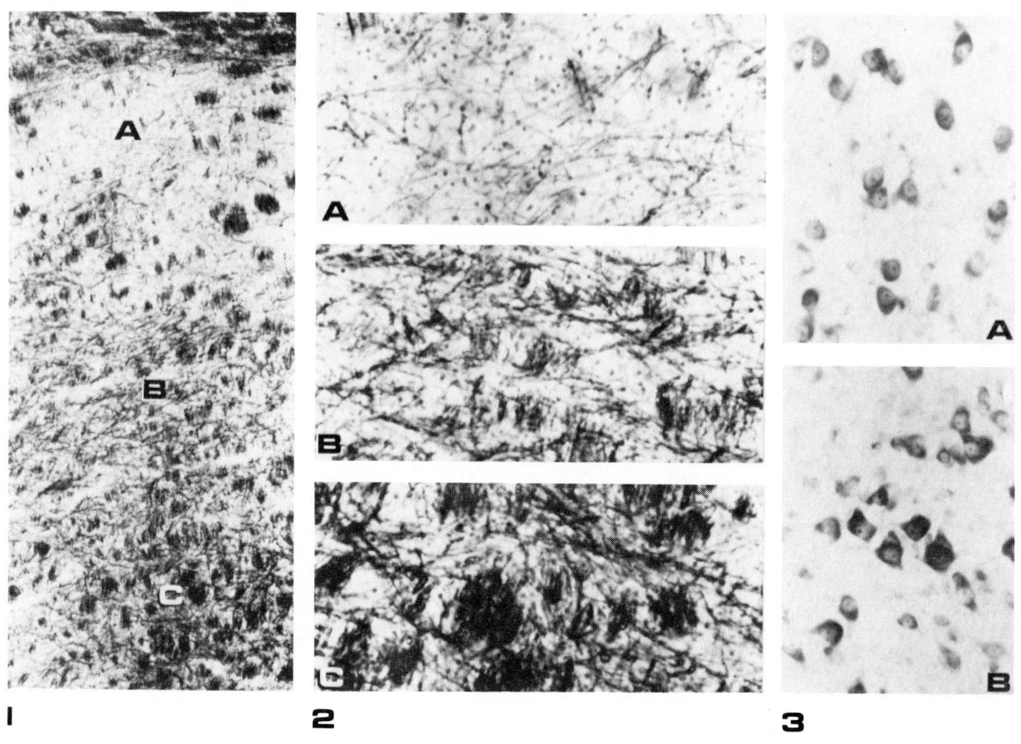

FIGURES 1, 2, 3. Normal cyto- and myeloarchitecture of ventrolateral thalamus. Fig. 1. Low magnification view of ventrolateral thalamus stained for myelinated fibers. The internal medullary lamina is the densely myelinated band at the top of the figure. A: dorsal zone of the ventrolateral nucleus (VL), B: ventral zone of VL, C: ventrobasal complex (VB) mag. 52x. Fig. 2. Higher magnification view of A: sparsely myelinated dorsal VL zone, B: densely myelinated ventral VL zone, C: very densely myelinated VB, mag. 208x. Fig. 3. Normal cell types in dorsal (A) and ventral (B) VL zones.

densely myelinated ventral zone (Fig. 3B) where large darkly stained cells (29um x 33um) appear in clusters of 2-4 cells, surrounded by smaller (15um x 19um) more lightly stained cells.

Our experimental approach has been to lower a bipolar electrode (consisting of two 150µm wires insulated except at their tips, separated by 0.5mm) into the thalamus of cats anesthetized with Nembutal (36mg/kg), and to electrically stimulate (0-60V, 50Hz, 0.05msec pulse duration) in order to cause contractions of somatic musculature. Only one penetration was made into each hemithalamus. After noting which muscles contract and which body part moves, a small electrolytic lesion is placed at the point of stimulation. Five to seven days after the lesion the animal was sacrificed under Nembutal anesthesia and the tissue processed according to Fink-Heimer staining methods (15, 16) in order to demonstrate degeneration occurring in the cerebral cortex as a result of the thalamic lesion. This procedure was performed in twelve cats, unilaterally or bilaterally. A total of twenty lesions form the basis of our results.

Utilizing these methods it has been possible to demonstrate that the two zones of VL project only to the motor cortex. Furthermore, the representation of trunk musculature and the thalamocortical projection to area 6 of the motor cortex originates from the dorsal myelin-free zone of VL, while the representation of limb musculature and the thalamocortical projection to area 4 originates from the ventral large-cell zone of VL.

Figure 4, animals I and II, illustrates these points, by demonstrating the results of stimulating and lesioning both the dorsal and ventral zones of VL. Since much of the cat's motor cortex is hidden from the surface, buried within the cruciate sulcus, (13, 14, 18) two views of the frontal cortex are illustrated, a rostral view on the left and a rostrodorsal view in which the cruciate sulcus has been schematically opened and the dorsal (D) and ventral (V) banks of the cortex placed side by side. The position and relative density of cortical degeneration caused by the thalamic lesion and the electrode penetration through cortex and thalamus is indicated by the stippling in the diagrams. According to control studies (17, 29, 30), the degeneration in cat I, located more caudally in the cortex around the ansate sulcus, and the very sparse degeneration on the ventral bank of the cruciate sulcus near the mesial wall of the hemisphere, is not a result of the VL lesion. This degeneration is caused by electrode penetration through caudal cortex, made in the process of thalamic stimulation and lesioning, and will therefore not be represented in the remaining figures. The figurines show the results of thalamic stimulation. The joint involved or surface above the contracting muscle is shaded.

In cat I, part of the dorsal zone of VL was electrically stimulated. This stimulation evoked flexion at the contralateral shoulder joint. The electrode was then lowered 1.5mm into the ventral zone of VL. Electrical stimulation at this new position evoked flexion at the contralateral elbow joint; the prime mover was the biceps. A small lesion was then made in the dorsal zone and a larger lesion in the ventral zone. These lesions caused degeneration in parts of area 6 and 4 previously shown to represent shoulder and elbow (4, 13, 14, 36). Prior investigations have shown that larger-sized VL lesions produce a greater density of thalamocortical degeneration than smaller

VL lesions (29, 30). There is a greater density of degeneration in cortical area 4γ than in cortical area 6aα in animal I. This is a result of the larger lesion in VL's ventral zone. Therefore, the region of the ventral zone of VL, where stimulation evokes elbow flexion, sends thalamocortical fibers to motor cortical area 4γ , while the region of the dorsal zone, where stimulation evokes shoulder movements, projects to area 6aα. Single lesions at this level of the thalamus, limited to either the dorsal or ventral zone, have also given this result. Cat II shows the results of stimulating and lesioning the ventral zone of VL only. Thalamic stimulation evoked a flexion withdrawal movement of the contralateral forelimb. The long head of the triceps (shoulder flexor) and the extensor carpi radialis (distal fixator and weak elbow flexor) muscles innervated by the radial nerve caused this movement. The lesion at this site caused degeneration in the region of area 4γ on the postcruciate gyrus and extended into the dorsal bank of the

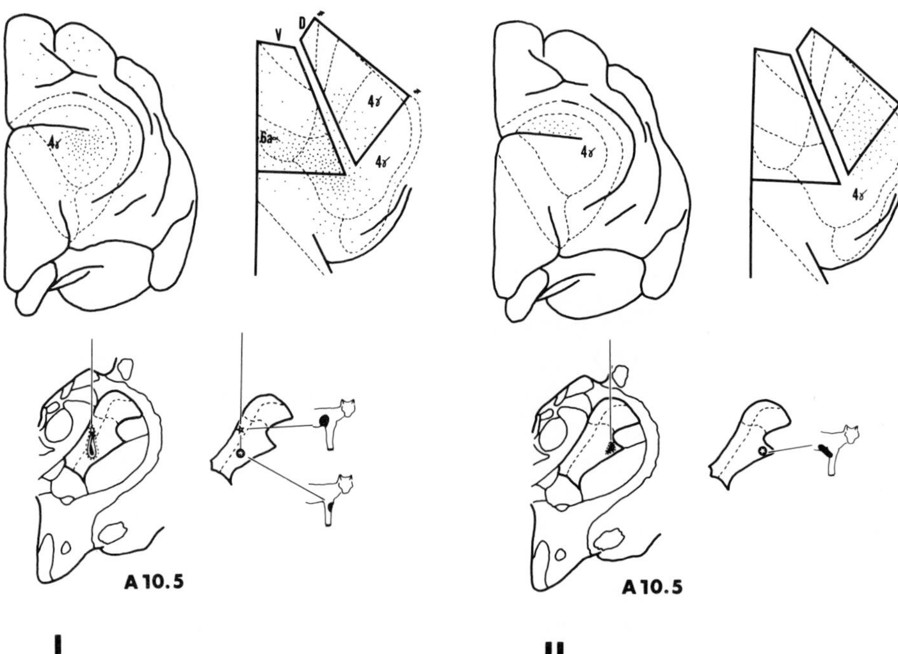

FIG. 4. Results of stimulating and lesioning dorsal and ventral VL zones. The top row of the figure shows two views of the frontal cortex for each animal: a rostral view on the left and a rostrodorsal view in which the cruciate sulcus has been schematically opened and the dorsal (D) and ventral (V) banks of the cortex placed side by side. The position and relative density of cortical degeneration caused by the thalamic lesion is indicated by the stippling in the diagrams. The bottom row of the figure shows the thalamic lesions plotted at one level of the thalamus (19). The figurines show the results of thalamic stimulation; the joint involved or the surface above the contracting muscle is shaded.

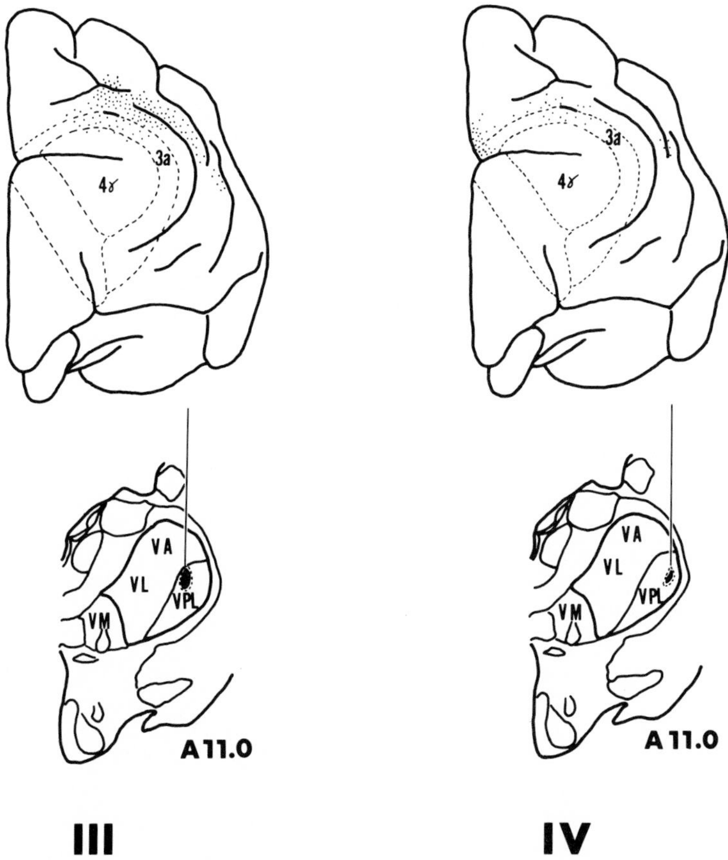

FIG. 5. Results of control lesions in VB. Animal III: forelimb VB lesion; animal IV: hindlimb VB lesion. See legend to Figure 4 for an explanation of the arrangement of the figure and the plotting of degeneration.

cruciate sulcus, which is normally hidden from the surface.

The findings in cats I and II clearly demonstrate that stimulating and lesioning the ventral zone of VL evokes contractions of distal somatic musculature and causes thalamocortical degeneration in area 4. Stimulating and lesioning the dorsal zone of VL evokes contractions of proximal somatic musculature and causes thalamocortical degeneration in area 6. Furthermore, neither the ventral nor dorsal zones of VL projected to cortical regions outside of the motor area (4 and 6). Figure 5 shows the results of control lesions in VB. In these experiments, neural activity in VB, evoked by natural stimulation of appropriate areas of the contralateral body surface, was monitored prior to lesioning, using previously described techniques (17). The lesion in cat III damaged part of VB where the forelimb is represented while the lesion in cat IV

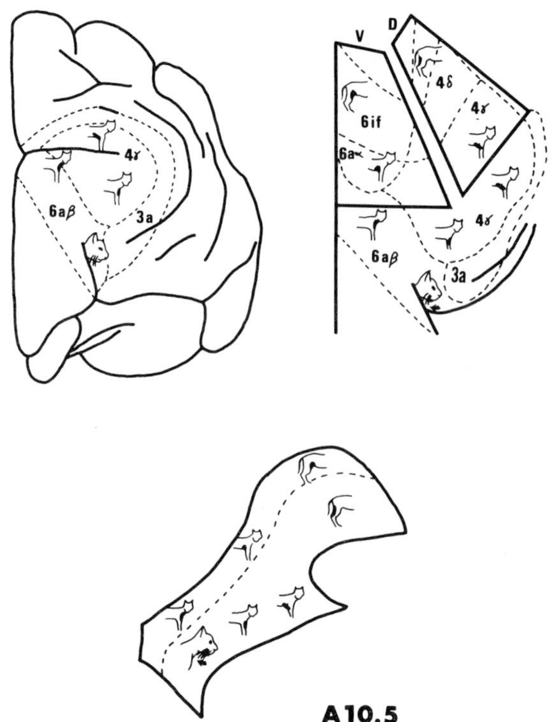

FIG. 6. Summary diagram illustrating the results of stimulating and lesioning in VL and part of the neighboring nucleus ventralis anterior (VA). The figurines in the thalamus show the points of thalamic electrical stimulation and lesioning in the various experiments. The shading over body parts indicates the muscle contractions evoked by the stimulation. The figurines on the two diagrams of the cortex show the region of the cortex where degeneration was produced by lesions at the thalamic site containing the same shaded figurine as that appearing on the cortical diagram.

damaged part of the VB hindlimb region. Both lesions caused thalamocortical degeneration totally within the somatic sensory cortical areas, including area 3a, the cortical zone adjacent to area 4. For example, the thalamic lesion in animal IV involved the rostral-dorsal pole of the ventroposterolateral nucleus. The thalamocortical degeneration in cat IV following this lesion was mainly situated on the most medial tip of the postcruciate gyrus and continued into the dorsal bank of the cruciate sulcus bordering the mesial wall of the hemisphere. This area of degeneration borders regions of area 4 on the postcruciate gyrus and dorsal bank of the cruciate sulcus. Recent studies of the VB thalamocortical projection, utilizing either small (17) or large lesions (21) and involving more caudal VB regions, also demonstrate VB projections only to somatic sensory cortical areas. These reports, combined with the present findings, support the notion that VL and VB project to separate cortical regions, with little or no overlap in these two thalamocortical systems.

Finally, Figure 6 is a summary diagram illustrating the results of stimulating and lesioning in VL and part of the neighboring nucleus ventralis anterior (VA).

The figurines in the thalamus show the position of electrical stimulation and lesioning. The shading over body parts indicates the muscular contractions evoked by the stimulation. The figurines on the two diagrams of the cortex show the region of the cortex where degeneration was located after lesions were placed at the thalamic site containing the same shaded figurine as that appearing in the cortical diagram.

For example, stimulation and lesions in the *medial* dorsal VL zone evoked contractions of neck musculature and caused degeneration in area 6aβ on the medial precruciate gyrus, extending into the ventral bank of the cruciate sulcus. *Lateral* dorsal zone VL stimulation and lesions caused contractions of shoulder musculature and degeneration buried in the cruciate sulcus, in area 6aα , rostrally on the ventral bank.

Note also that stimulation in the *medial* ventral zone of VL evoked retraction of the contralateral vibrissae and lesioning caused degeneration in the region of cortical area 6aβ bordering the presylvian sulcus, the only example of a ventral zone lesion that projects to area 6. However, the identification of this area as the motor region representing face musculature (4, 13, 14, 36) and the fact that this cortical zone borders area 3a, as do other regions of area 4 which control discrete aspects of movement, suggests that this region of area 6aβ is functionally different from the regions of area 6 related to postural musculature. Therefore there is no inconsistency in the ventral zone projection to this region of cortex.

An interesting finding is the separation of the two types of flexion withdrawal movements in the ventral zone of VL and their differential projections to cortical area 4. The most lateral VL region, where the extensor carpi radialis and the long head of the triceps predominantly control withdrawal movement by flexion of elbow and shoulder, projects to the postcruciate gyrus and rostral dorsal bank of the cruciate sulcus while the more medial ventral VL region, where elbow flexion is produced by predominant biceps activity, projects to the lateral precruciate gyrus and the ventral bank of the sulcus. Physiological studies have reported that the receptive field properties of neurons in the pre- and postcruciate cortex differ (6, 7, 9, 33, 34, 35). The anatomical findings now indicate that these cortical areas also receive input from different regions of the VL ventral zone.

During these experiments, stimulation of VL did not reveal a hindlimb region. However, in a neighboring region of caudal VA, stimulation evoked contractions of hindlimb musculature. Lesions at the point of stimulation caused degeneration in areas of motor cortex buried caudally in the cruciate sulcus on both its dorsal and ventral banks. Although the neurons in this region of VA are packed more densely than in VL, two VA zones morphologically similar to the VL zones could also be found. Stimulation in the dorsal VA zone evoked hip flexion,and lesions here caused degeneration in area 6if of the motor cortex situated in the caudal ventral bank of the cruciate sulcus. Stimulation in the ventral VA zone evoked knee flexion,and lesions caused degeneration in cortical area 4δ situated on the caudal dorsal bank of the cruciate sulcus. Control lesions in the rostral pole of VA showed that it did not project to the motor cortex and stimulation here did not evoke contractions of somatic musculature. These findings suggest that the boundary of VL (19) should be extended. The caudal portion of VA, from which hindlimb motor responses can be evoked and which projects to the hindlimb motor cortex (4, 13, 19, 30), should be considered anatomically and functionally as part of VL.

Physiological studies support this conclusion (1, 8, 27). They have shown that this caudal region of VA synaptically drives motor cortical neurons in a fashion identical to that of VL regions (1). Therefore, rather than suggest two separate thalamic inputs to the motor cortex, we prefer that this thalamic region be considered a unit; to be defined physiologically as that region of the thalamus from which stimulation can evoke contractions of somatic musculature, and anatomically, by its zonal cyto- and myeloarchitectural organization and projection to the motor cortex.

The identification of the dorsal and ventral VL zones and their differential projection to the motor cortex now provide an anatomical basis for interpreting inputs into this thalamocortical system. For example, recent studies of cerebellar nuclear projections to the thalamus(2, 3, 22) have shown that the fastigial nucleus sends efferents predominantly to the region of the dorsal VL zone, and the interpositus projects to the ventral VL zone. The present anatomy, in agreement with recent physiological observations (25), suggests that the fastigial nucleus influences area 6 predominantly and also the interpositus, area 4. Further anatomical study of cerebellar and pallidal systems, and of the inputs of other afferent fibers to the two VL zones, should provide information on the functional integration that proceeds in this thalamocortical system.

ACKNOWLEDGMENTS

This work was supported by U.S. Public Health Service Grants NS06716 and NS06376. P.L. Strick was supported in part by GM00281. We wish to thank Misses Graziella Mann and Anita Barsky for technical assistance.

REFERENCES

1 AMASSIAN, V.E. and WEINER, H. Monosynaptic and polysynaptic activation of pyramidal tract neurons by thalamic stimulation. In D.P. Purpura and M.D. Yahr (Eds.), The Thalamus, Columbia Univ. Press, New York, N.Y. 1966, p. 255-286.

2 ANGAUT, P. The ascending projections of the nucleus interpositus posterior of the cat cerebellum: An experimental anatomical study using silver impregnation methods. Brain Research, 24 (1970) 377-394.

3 ANGAUT, P. and BOWSHER, D. Ascending projections of the medial cerebellar (fastigial) nucleus: An experimental study in the cat. Brain Research 24, (1970) 49-68.

4 BORGE, A.F. The Motor Cortex of the Cat, Unpublished Master's Thesis, University of Wisconsin, 1950.

5 BROOKHART, J.M. and ZANCHETTI, A. The relationship between electrocortical waves and the responsiveness of the corticospinal system. Electroenceph. clin. Neurophysiol., 8 (1956) 427-444.
6 BROOKS, V.B., RUDOMIN, P. and SLAYMAN, C.L. Sensory activation of neurons in cat's cerebral cortex. J. Neurophysiol. 24, (1961) 286-301.
7 BROOKS, V.B., RUDOMIN, P. and SLAYMAN, C.L. Peripheral receptive fields of neurons in cat's cerebral cortex. J. Neurophysiol. 24, (1961) 302-325.
8 BUSER, P. Subcortical controls of pyramidal activity. In: D.P. Purpura and M.D. Yahr (Eds.), The Thalamus, Columbia Univ. Press, New York, N.Y., 1966, 323-347.
9 BUSER, P. and IMBERT, M. Sensory projections to the motor cortex in cats: a microelectrode study. In W.A. Rosenblith (Ed.), Sensory Communication, MIT Press, Cambridge, Mass. (1961), 607-626.
10 CHAMBERS, W.W. and SPRAGUE, J.M. Functional localization in the cerebellum. I. Organization in longitudinal corticonuclear zones and their contribution to the control of posture, both extrapyramidal and pyramidal. J. Comp. Neurol. 103 (1955) 105-129.
11 CHAMBERS, W.W. and SPRAGUE, J.M. Functional localization in the cerebellum. II. Somatotopic organization in cortex and nuclei. Arch. Neurol. Psychiat. 74, (1955) 653-680.
12 COHEN, D., CHAMBERS, W.W. and SPRAGUE, J.M. Experimental study of the efferent projections from the cerebellar nuclei to the brainstem of the cat. J. Comp. Neurol., 109 (1958) 233-260.
13 DELGADO, J.M.R. Hidden motor cortex of the cat. Amer. J. Physiol., 170 (1952) 673-681.
14 DELGADO, J.M.R. and LIVINGSTON, R. Motor representation in the frontal sulci of the cat, Yale J. Biol. Med. 28 (1955-56) 245-252.
15 EAGER, R.P. Selective staining of degenerating axons in the central nervous system by a simplified silver method: spinal cord projections to external cuneate and inferior olivary nuclei in the cat. Brain Research, 22 (1970) 137-141.
16 FINK, R.P. and HEIMER, L. Two methods for selective silver impregnation of degenerating axons and their synaptic endings in the central nervous system. Brain Research, 4 (1967) 369-374.
17 HAND, P.J. and MORRISON, A.R. Thalamocortical projections from the ventrobasal complex to somatic sensory areas I and II of the cat. Exp. Neurol., 26 (1970) 291-308.
18 HASSLER, R. and MUHS-CLEMENT, K. Architektonischer Aufbau des sensomotorischen und parietalen Cortex der Katze. J. Hirnforsch. 6 (1964) 377-420.
19 JASPER, H.H. and AJMONE MARSAN, C. A Stereotaxic Atlas of the Diencephalon of the Cat. National Research Council of Canada, Ottawa, 1954, 15pp.
20 JOHNSON, T.N. and CLEMENTE, C.D. An experimental study of the fiber connections between the putamen, globus pallidus, ventral thalamus and midbrain tegmentum in the cat. J. Comp. Neurol. 113 (1959) 83-102.

21 JONES, E.G. and POWELL, T.P.S. The cortical projection of the ventroposterior nucleus of the thalamus in the cat. Brain Research, 13 (1969) 298-318.

22 KIEVITT, J. and KUYPERS, H.G.J.M. Fastigial cerebellar projections to the VL nucleus of the thalamus in cat and Rhesus monkey. Anat. Rec., 169 (1971) 358.

23 KUYPERS, H.G.J.M. The descending pathways to the spinal cord, their anatomy and function: In J.C. Eccles and J.P. Schadé (Eds.), Organization of the spinal cord, Progress in Brain Research, Vol. II Elsevier, Amsterdam, 1964, 178-202.

24 PURPURA, D.P. and SHOFER, R.J. Cortical intracellular potentials during augmenting and recruiting responses. I. Effects of injected hyperpolarizing currents on evoked membrane potential changes. J. Neurophysiol., 27 (1964) 117-132.

25 RISPAL-PADEL, L., LATREILLE, J. et VANUXEM, P. Répartition sur le cortex moteur des projections des projections des différents noyaux cerebelleux chez le Chat. C.R. Acad. Sc. Paris, 272, (1971) 451-454.

26 RISPAL-PADEL, L. and MASSION, J. Relations between the ventrolateral nucleus and the motor cortex in the cat. Exp. Brain Res., 10 (1970) 331-339.

27 SASAKI, K., STAUNTON, H.P. and DIECKMAN, G. Characteristic features of augmenting and recruiting responses in the cerebral cortex. Exp. Neurol., 26 (1970) 369-392.

28 SMAHA, L.A., KAELBER, W.W. and MAHARRY, R.R. Efferent projections of the nucleus ventralis lateralis. An experimental study in the cat. J. Anat. (Lond.), 104 (1969) 33-40.

29 STRICK, P.L. Cortical projections of the feline thalamic nucleus ventralis lateralis. Brain Research, 20 (1970) 130-134.

30 STRICK, P.L. Experimental study of thalamocortical projections from the nuclei ventralis lateralis (VL) and ventralis anterior (VA). Anat. Rec., 166 (1970) 384.

31 STRICK, P.L. Functional zones in the cat ventrolateral thalamus. Proc. 1st Annual Mtg. Soc. for Neuroscience (1971) 122.

32 THOMAS, D.M., KAUFMAN, R.D., SPRAGUE, J.M. and CHAMBERS, W.W. Experimental studies of the vermal cerebellar projections in the brainstem of the cat (fastigio-bulbar tract). J. Anat. (Lond.), 90 (1956) 371-385.

33 TOWE, A.L., PATTON, H.D. and KENNEDY, T.T. Properties of the pyramidal system in the cat. Exp. Neurol. 8 (1963) 220-238.

34 TOWE, A.L., PATTON, H.D. and KENNEDY, T.T. Response properties of neurons in pericruciate cortex of cat following electrical stimulation of the appendages. Exp. Neurol., 10 (1964) 325-344.

35 TOWE, A.L., WHITEHORN, D. and NYQUIST, J.K. Differential activity among wide-field neurons of the cat postcruciate cerebral cortex. Exp. Neurol., 20 (1968) 497-521.

36 WARD, J.W. and CLARK, S.L. Specific responses elicitable from subdivisions of the motor cortex of the cat. J. Comp. Neurol., 63 (1935) 49-64.

37 WOOLSEY, C.N. Organization of somatic sensory and motor areas of the cerebral cortex. In H.E. Harlow and C.N. Woolsey (Eds.), Biological and Biochemical Bases of Behavior, Univ. Wisconsin Press, Madison, Wisc., 1958, 63-81.

Corticothalamic Projections and Sensorimotor Activities
T. Frigyesi, E. Rinvik, and M.D. Yahr, editors. © 1972
Raven Press, New York.

Does the Red Nucleus Project to VL and VA of the Thalamus? An Experimental Study of Rubral Efferents in the Cat Using a Protein Transport Tracing Method

Stephen B. Edwards

There are a number of reports in the literature describing projections from the red nucleus to various nuclei in the thalamus, including the VL-VA complex. The evidence for these projections derives largely from orthograde degeneration studies in which cerebellothalamic fibers were interrupted by rubral lesions (3, 7, 8), and studies of retrograde cellular changes in the red nucleus produced by diencephalic lesions too extensive to permit the determination of the course and terminal fields of the rubral efferents (6, 9, 12, 13). Bowsher and Angaut (2) attempted to avoid these experimental problems by tracing the fiber degeneration from red nucleus lesions made 15 months after ablating the cerebellum. Recently I have developed a technique by which the efferent projections of the red nucleus in the cat are traced by following with autoradiographic methods the transport of isotopically-labeled proteins from the cell bodies of red nucleus neurons to their terminals. Studies have shown that labeled amino acids injected locally in the brain are taken up and synthesized into transportable protein by neuron cell bodies only (10--review). Thus this technique permits one to trace the full extent of a pathway from identifiable cells of origin without contamination by fibers of passage.

Using a 10μl Hamilton fixed-needle syringe, a single injection of tritiated leucine was stereotaxically placed in the right red nucleus of adult cats. Each injection consisted of 1ul of normal saline containing 10 μC of L (4,5 ^{3}H) leucine (S.A.54C/mmole). The solution was injected continuously for a 5 to 15 minute period, and the syringe needle was then left in place 30 minutes before it was withdrawn. This procedure allows the leucine to be taken up by neuronal cell bodies and thus eliminates the spread of isotope along the needle track when the syringe is withdrawn. Eleven to eighteen days were allowed for the leucine to be incorporated into protein and the labeled protein to be transported down the axons to the terminals. The cats were sacrificed and perfused with saline and 10% formalin. Blocks of brain tissue were imbedded in paraffin, and 10μ serial transverse sections were cut from each block. Mounted dewaxed sections were dipped in Kodak NTB3 nuclear track emulsion and allowed to expose in light-tight boxes for 2 to 7 weeks. The slides were developed in concentrated

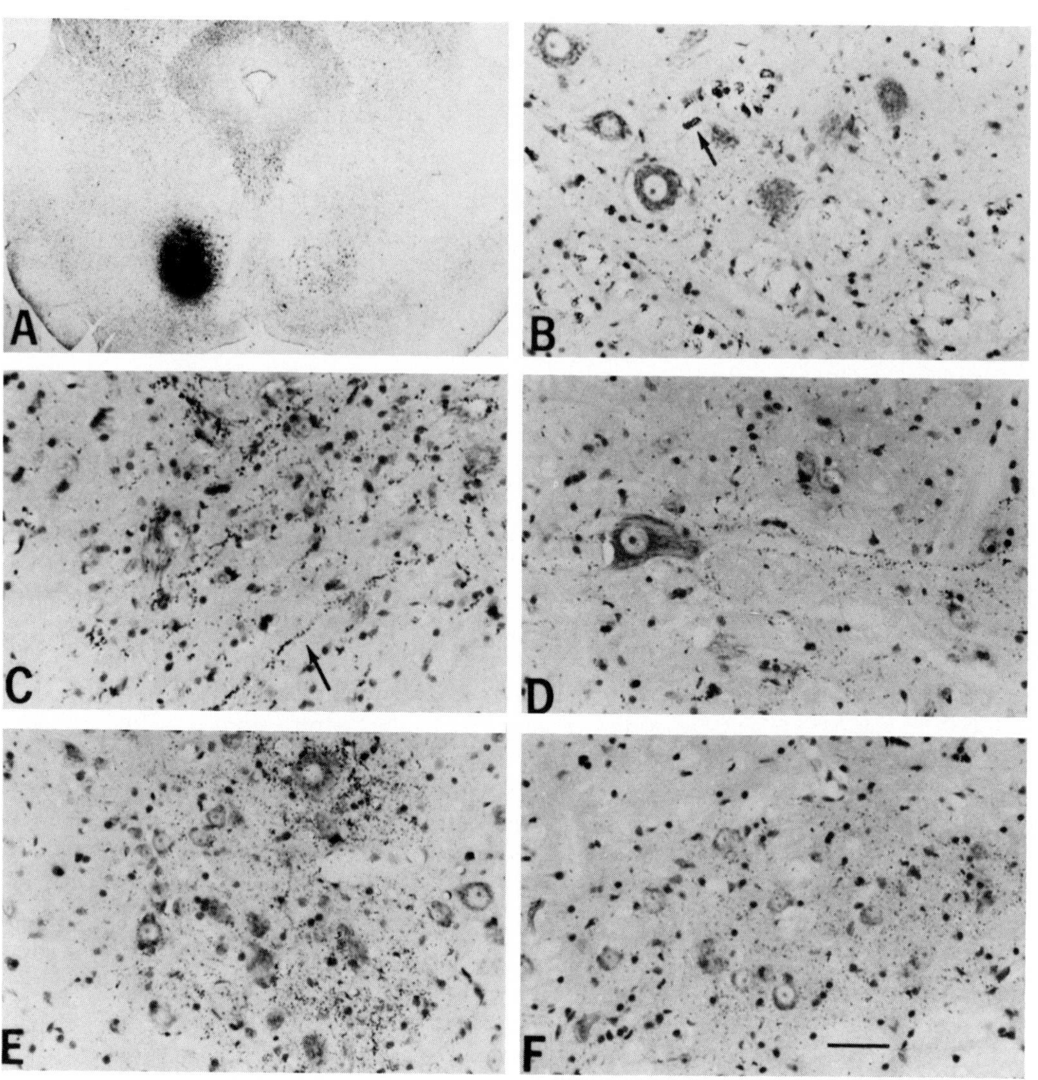

FIG. 1

Dekto1 for 2 minutes at 16°C, fixed, and stained with cresyl violet. The location of the radioactive label was determined by examining the pattern of reduced silver grains overlying the tissue. The density of grains constituting background was determined by examining "neutral" structures such as the optic tract, and in no experiment did it exceed 7 grains/1000u^2. A detailed discussion of this technique is in preparation.

Injections were placed in either rostral or caudal portions of the red nucleus and were restricted almost entirely to the nucleus itself (Fig. 1A). In both cases crossing fibers issuing from the ventromedial border of the nucleus were heavily labeled and could be traced throughout their course as they proceeded laterally and descended as a large but discrete collection of fascicles in the contralateral lateral funiculus of the brain stem and spinal cord. A contingent of these fibers could be observed ramifying in the transverse plane throughout the intermediate cell group of the facial nucleus (Fig. 1B) and to a much lesser extent in the dorsomedial and lateral cell groups, but not in the ventromedial cell group. Further caudally, large numbers of densely labeled fibers and terminal arborizations surrounded the cells of the lateral reticular nucleus, particularly its subtrigeminal portion. These observations agree in general with those of Courville (5) who traced these projections with fiber degeneration methods.

Several previously unreported projections in the cat were also found. As the descending rubral fibers turn ventrolaterally at the rostral pole of the superior olive, groups of labeled axons leave the tract, pierce the facial nerve, and terminate densely in restricted areas of pars ventralis and pars dorsalis of the superior sensory trigeminal nucleus (Fig. 1C). Labeled fibers could also be traced as they turned dorsally from the lateral funiculus to invade n. oralis of the spinal trigeminal nucleus (Fig. 1D). These fibers appeared to terminate in most regions of the nucleus, but terminal labeling was heaviest at the dorsal tip. A separate group of fibers descending in a position just dorsolateral to the spinal tract of V can be traced as they turn medially just ventral to the lateral cuneate nucleus and terminate profusely in the caudal pole of the descending vestibular nucleus (Fig. 1E). In confirmation of Walberg (14) and Hinman and Carpenter (7), a rubral projection to a restricted area of the dorsal lamella of the ipsilateral principal olive was found (Fig. 1F). The rubral projection to laminae V-VII

FIG. 1. A: Autoradiograms of the locus of injection in the red nucleus of cat 726RN and resultant sites of labeled terminal fields in the brain stem (B-F). B: Labeled fibers arborizing in the intermediate cell group of the contralateral facial nucleus. Pale grain-filled profiles (arrow) are cross sections of descending rubral fibers. C: Contralateral superior sensory trigeminal nucleus, pars dorsalis. Note heavily labeled fiber (arrow) in lower portion of micrograph. D: Contralateral n. oralis of the spinal trigeminal nucleus. Note rows of grains distributed along the dendritic tree of large cell. E: Dense terminal labeling in caudal pole of the contralateral descending vestibular nucleus. F: Site of termination of rubral fibers in a restricted portion of the dorsal lamella of the ipsilateral principal olive. Bar represents 30μ in micrographs B-F. The terminal field in the subtrigeminal portion of the lateral reticular nucleus is not shown.

of the spinal gray matter described by Nyberg-Hansen and Brodal (11) was also confirmed. Projections to the cerebellum were not studied.

Whether the injection was placed in the rostral or caudal portion of the red nucleus, the density of labeled fibers observed rostral to the nucleus was sparse compared to any one of the descending projections. Nevertheless, label could be detected ipsilaterally scattered throughout the zona incerta and fields of Forel. A few labeled fibers were also observed in the contralateral zona incerta. At more rostral levels it became increasingly difficult to distinguish any concentration of label from background levels, and at the level of VL-VA complex no unequivocal evidence of labeled fibers could be detected anywhere in the sections.

The largest outflow of the red nucleus in the cat, in terms of quantity of fibers, is that to the spinal cord and, in the present material,this projection appeared to be as massive as the direct corticospinal projection. Most of the remaining rubral efferents—direct rubro-cerebellar fibers, those to the contralateral lateral reticular nucleus and descending vestibular nucleus, and to the ipsilateral inferior olive—serve to link the red nucleus to various parts of the cerebellum. In addition, the red nucleus projects to two cranial nerve nuclei. The projections to the contralateral intermediate cell group of VII appear to be involved in activation of auricular and upper face musculature (4). Fibers to the superior sensory trigeminal nucleus and to n. oralis of the spinal trigeminal nucleus are probably involved in modulation of somato-sensory input from the face.

These preliminary observations indicate that the red nucleus does not participate in a path of transmission from the cerebellum to the VL-VA complex as has been suggested. This conclusion is supported by the physiological study of Anderson (1), who was able to drive red nucleus cells antidromically by stimulation of the spinal cord, medulla, and cerebellum, but was unable to do so when extensive regions of the VL and VA nuclei were stimulated.

A complete anatomical study of rubral efferent projections in the cat is under way.

REFERENCES

1 ANDERSON, M.E. Cerebellar and cerebral inputs to physiologically identified efferent cell groups in the red nucleus of the cat, Brain Res., 30 (1971) 49-66.

2 BOWSHER, D. and ANGAUT, P. Ascending projections of the red nucleus in the decerebellate cat, Experientia, 24 (1968) 262-263.

3 CARPENTER, M.B. A study of the red nucleus in the rhesus monkey. Anatomic degenerations and physiologic effects resulting from localized lesions of the red nucleus, J. comp. Neurol., 105 (1956) 195-249.

4 COURVILLE, J. The nucleus of the facial nerve; the relation between cellular groups and peripheral branches of the nerve, Brain Res., (1966) 338-354.

5 COURVILLE, J. Rubrobulbar fibers to the facial nucleus and the lateral reticular nucleus (nucleus of the lateral funiculus). An experimental study in the cat with silver impregnation methods, Brain Res., 1 (1966) 317-337.

6 GEREBETZOFF, M.A. Les bases anatomiques de la physiologie du cervelet, La Cellule, 49 (1941) 71-166.

7 HINMAN, A. and CARPENTER, M.B. Efferent projections of the red nucleus in the cat, J. comp. Neurol., 113 (1959) 61-82.

8 JOHNSON, T.N. and CLEMENTE, C.D. An experimental study of the fiber connections between the putamen, globus pallidus, ventral thalamus, and mid-brain tegmentum in cat, J. comp. Neurol., 113 (1959) 83-101.

9 KUYPERS, H.G.J.M. and LAWRENCE, D.G. Cortical projections to the red nucleus and the brain stem in the rhesus monkey, Brain Res., 4 (1967) 151-188.

10 LASEK, R.J. Protein transport in neurons, Int. Rev. Neurobiol., 13 (1970) 289-324.

11 NYBERG-HANSEN, R. and BRODAL, A. Site and mode of termination of rubro-spinal fibers in the cat. An experimental study with silver impregnation methods, J. Anat. (Lond.), 98 (1964) 235-253.

12 POMPEIANO, O. and BRODAL, A. Experimental demonstration of a somato-topical origin of rubro-spinal fibers in the cat, J. comp. Neurol., 108 (1957) 225-252.

13 PRESIG, H. Le noyau rouge et le pédoncle cérébelleux supérieur, J. Psychol. Neurol. (Leipzig), 3 (1904) 215-230.

14 WALBERG, F. Descending connections to the inferior olive. An experimental study in the cat, J. comp. Neurol., 104 (1956) 77-173.

Corticothalamic Projections and Sensorimotor Activities
T. Frigyesi, E. Rinvik, and M.D. Yahr, editors. © 1972
Raven Press, New York.

Some Substrates for Centrifugal Control over Thalamic Cell Ensembles

Madge E. Scheibel, Arnold B. Scheibel and Thomas H. Davis

> "...we believe that the essential organ of the optic thalamus is the centre of consciousness for certain elements of sensation......... the functions of this organ are influenced by the coincidental activity of the cortical centres, and this control is effected by means of paths from the cortex to the thalamus which probably end in its lateral nucleus."(H. Head and G. Holmes)

The aim of this communication is to reassess the substrate for centrifugal control over information processing mechanisms in somatosensory thalamus. In contrast to our earlier studies (26 – 30), we have been able to draw much of our data from Golgi-stained sections of neurally mature or adult animals. As a consequence, our consideration must include structures not previously seen in immature thalamus.

In the past few years, a number of electron microscopic studies of thalamic sensory nuclei have become available (4, 11, 16, 17, 21, 22, 23, 35, 37). These have served to stress the wealth of structural detail to be seen at this level of resolution and emphasize the richness of histological minutiae which remains beyond the scope of the light microscope. On the other hand, there are advantages inherent in the lower resolution and relative parsimony of detail of the Golgi image, especially insofar as the study of the neuropil field, the interrelationship of constituent elements and the patterns of synaptic linkage, are concerned.

The ensemble of neuronal end neuroglial elements which serve as receptive matrix for all thalamic afferent systems, ascending and descending, is among the most complex in the central nervous system. In many respects, the analysis of multilaminate cortical structures presents fewer problems than the thalamic ventral nuclear complex where patterns of organization are subtle and the nature of many profiles remain enigmatic. Study of a routine Nissl preparation of cerebral cortex is sufficient to give some idea of the nature and extent of horizontal lamination, distribution of cell types and, in a few cases, of vertical columnar organization providing discrete representations of the peripheral field (3, 13, 39). None of this is possible in the ventrobasal (VB) and ventrolateral (VL) nuclear fields even with the Golgi methods except through laborious reconstructions based on hundreds—or thousands—of sections. The result of this type of reconstruction is seen, in part, in figure 14. The modular organization of cortical fields to which we have called attention (7, 30) through analysis of Golgi preparations has no easily recognizable analogue in ventral thalamic nuclei, although study of firing patterns of populations of single units argues for their existence (2).

For these reasons, it seems useful to prefix our examination of descending elements exerting modulatory control over somatosensory thalamus with a brief review of those elements making up the ventrobasal field. This will also provide the opportunity to evaluate certain features of intrathalamic circuitry, a subject richer in physiological inference than in anatomical fact.

While questions of methodology have been discussed elsewhere, one point is worth emphasis. Adequate impregnations of adult tissue are possible with any one of a number of modifications of the rapid Golgi method, provided there is antecedent perfusion of the brain in situ. We have used perfusing solutions of 6 to 10% formalin, buffered and unbuffered, and formalin-glutaraldehyde mixtures in several ratios, all following an initial perfusion wash with cool isotonic saline or Ringers solution. So far, the normal variability of resulting Golgi impregnations has not allowed us to draw final conclusions as to the optimal perfusion fluid. Indeed, there may be none! On the other hand, where the Golgi technique is to be combined with electron microscopy, the somewhat more rigorous demands of the latter method may weight the selection of the initial perfusing fluid.

THE CELLULAR MATRIX

Thalamocortical relay cells. Figures 1, 2, and 3 illustrate a number of features which characterize thalamocortical neurons (T cells) throughout the specific projection nuclei of thalamus. Cell bodies are usually of moderate to large size, ranging from 20 to 35 u. The dendrites are arranged in sheaths or spreading bundles which develop out of 4 to 10 short primary dendrite stalks (24, 25, 26, 29, 36, 37) to generate a dendrite domain seldom more than 300 to 400 u in diameter. Although the dendrite surfaces are densely covered with hairy, pleomorphic 'pseudospines' in the perinatal preparation (32), the adult dendrite surface appears characteristically smooth and featureless except for tapering spike-like structures or appendages, individually or in clusters, usually on the outer half of most dendrite shafts (Figure 3 c'). We are in agreement with Tombol (37) that these structures probably represent presynaptic terminals rather than true dendritic structures. The dramatic loss of appendages from the dendritic surfaces of these cells during the maturative process matches a similar progression throughout the brain stem. On a significant proportion of T cells, we have also noted small tufted branches or rosettes similar to the larger ones characterizing adjacent local circuit cells. The possible significance of these will be considered below.

Although it has proven difficult to follow thalamocortical axons once the myelin sheaths develop approximately 100 to 150 u from the cell body, we traced a number of such fibers for appreciable distances (1000 to 2000 u) into thalamocortical bundles in

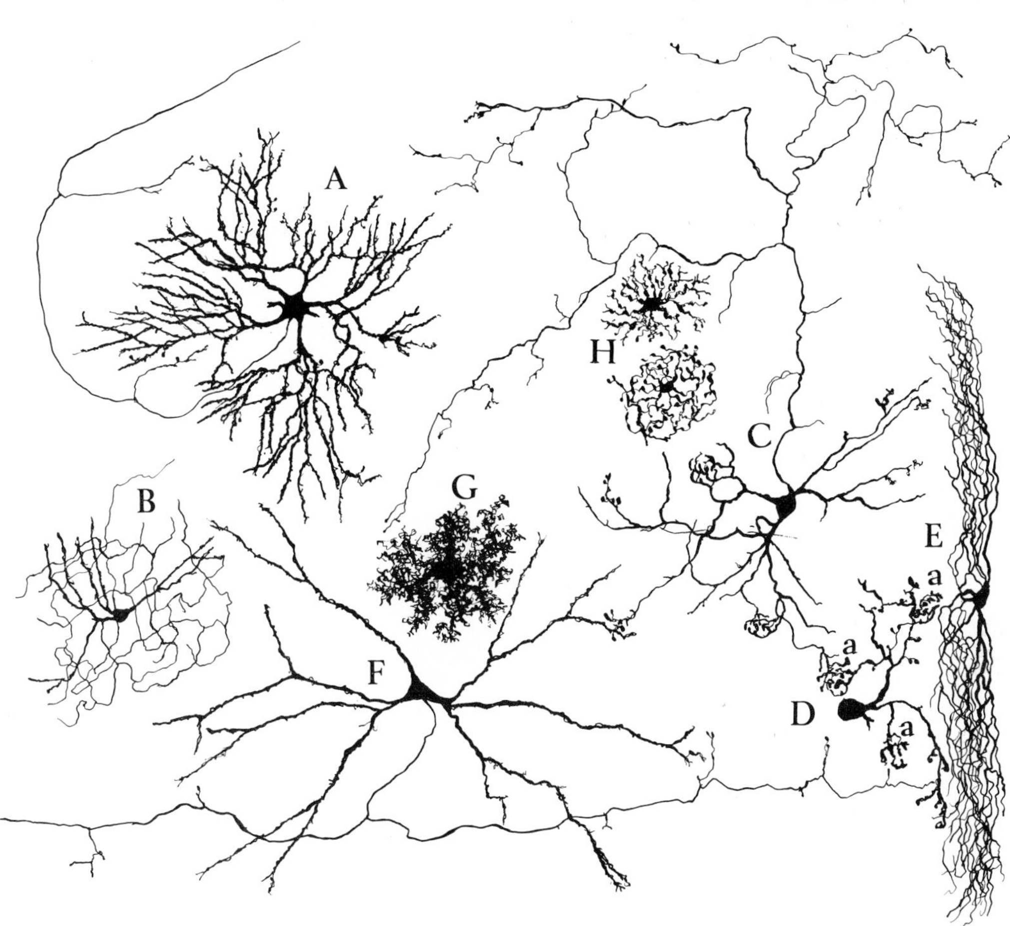

FIG. 1. Summary of cell types found in the ventrobasal complex of the thalamus. A. thalamocortical projections (T) cell. The axon is shown with 2 collaterals although this is unusual; B. local circuit (Golgi type II) or L cell with very restricted axonal path; C. L cell with more extensive axon system and claw or rosette-like terminals on some dendrites; D. similar L type cell but without demonstrable axon; E. local circuit cell with flattened axonal and dendritic domain; F. large reticular-like cell with bifurcating axon (integrator cell); G. protoplasmic astrocyte; H. oligodendrocyte variants with many swirled processes; a, mossy tuft-like structures on dendrite tips of some L cells. The very small axonless cells described in the text are not included in this illustration. Drawn from a number of sections of 20 to 70 day cat thalamus stained by Golgi variant. x 600.

10 day and 5 month cat material (Figure 2). Less than 15% (6 out of 51) of these axons bear collaterals (Figure 2 and 3, d), thereby appearing to offer little support for the recurrent collateral hypothesis of thalamic inhibition (1). This is in agreement with observations of Famiglietti made on geniculostriate neurons in the lateral geniculate nucleus (4).

Integrator Cells. Approximately 5% of VB cells are characterized by large somata (25 to 40 μ) and long, radiating, infrequently branched dendrites resembling the

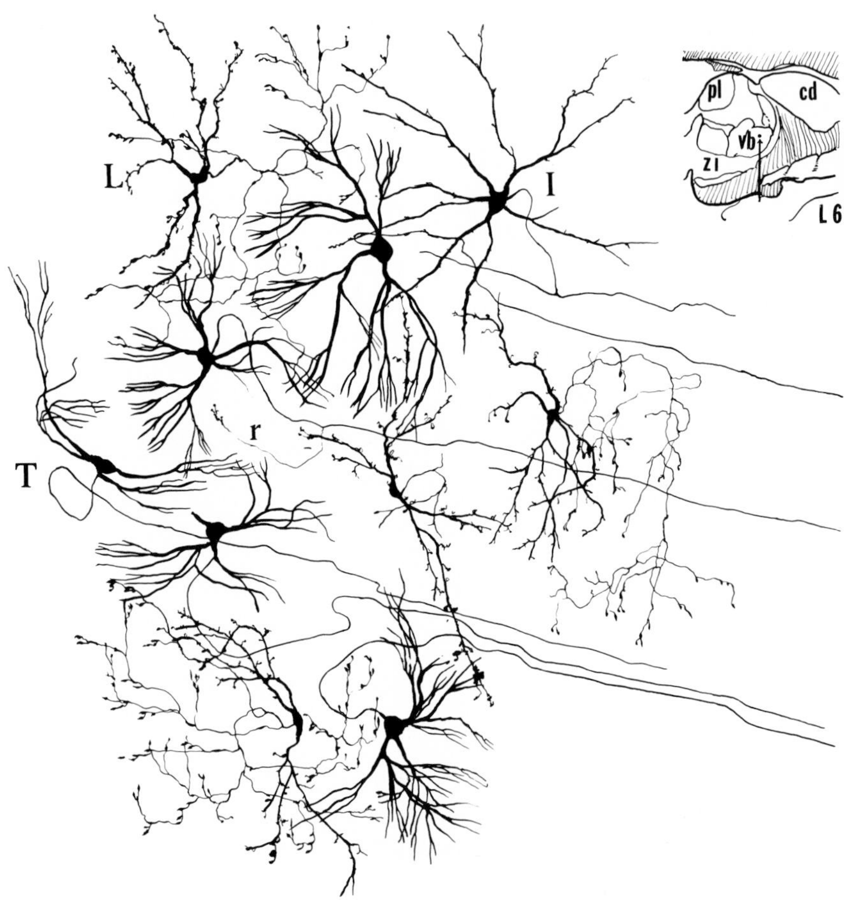

FIG. 2. Neuronal field in the ventrobasal complex (vb) showing several major cell types including T, thalamocortical projections cells; L, local circuit (Golgi type II) cells; I, integrator cells. Other abbreviations include r, recurrent collateral; pl, pulvinar; zi, zona incerta; cd, caudate. Section drawn from 6 month old cat stained with rapid Golgi variant. x 200.

generalized patterns of brain stem reticular cells (Figures 1, F and 2, I). Many of these neurons generate bifurcating axons which project both rostrally and caudally to unknown destinations. We have previously considered these elements as serving integrative functions (26) throughout the specific thalamic fields, possibly sampling activity patterns in thalamic cell clusters or modules, and passing this information on both rostrally and caudally to distant monitor systems. Recently Andersen and Andersson (1) have made use of this concept in constructing a model of sensory thalamic function. However, more extensive evaluation of their function is clearly indicated.

Local circuit interneurons. Golgi type II or L cells are infrequently stained in young rodent preparations, but in adult cats, they appear to represent at least one third of the total complement of VB cells. This figure is based on counts in Nissl and Kluver stained material and is comparable to estimates of Ralston (23) and of Tombol (37). Cell bodies range from 12 to 20 u in diameter and bear 2 to 6 lengthy dendrite shafts (Figures 2, L, 5, and 6). Their dendrite membrane surfaces bear many pleomorphic stalk-like structures, usually from 5 to 30 u in length, surmounted by one or more terminal enlargements or knobs (Figures 4, 5, and 6). Similar structures have been seen on local circuit neurons in various thalamic sensory nuclei (17, 22, 36, 37) and in the intralaminar system (31). There seems to be consensus that such structures are appreciably different from the smaller and more regularly arranged spines of cerebral cortex (8) (Figure 4, e). It is therefore considered appropriate that they receive a nonspecific name such as protrusion (35) or appendage (16).

Figure 1 indicates that there are a number of types of identifiable local circuit elements in the ventral complex of nuclei. Neuron 1, B is a classical Golgi type II variant of the L cell in that its axonal ramification is generated largely within the dendritic domain of the parent cell. The neuron illustrated at 1, C shows a frequent variant where the axon remains within the ventral complex and/or intralaminar pool while generating a number of branch patterns with a fairly extensive, if local, trajectory. Such cells may conceivably be responsible for the very short latency inhibition noted in nonspecific thalamic cells following stimulation in specific nuclei by Purpura (19).

In contrast, neuron 1, E is a highly specialized form whose axonal and dendritic fields are virtually coextensive. This type is usually found on the extreme edge of the ventral field complex such as the rostral and lateral borders of VA (28). The highly specialized, contour-moulded patterns of the demains appear to emphasize the powerful dynamic shaping factors operating at the interface between nuclear zones with different properties.

The element pictured at Figure 1, D represents an interesting problem in both the anatomy and physiology of the area. There are a certain number of cells (about 10%) which appear to be unequivocally neuronal in terms of cell body and dendrite patterns, but for which no axon can be demonstrated. This appears to be more than a problem of reliability of the Golgi impregnation. Ordinarily when a neuronal soma is stained, the axon hillock, at least, can be visualized even in the absence of axonal staining. In the case of these cells, no hillock has been visualized in the approximately 30 cases in which they have been identified. If these observations can be verified over a larger body of material, they raise the interesting problem of the role of axonless neurons.

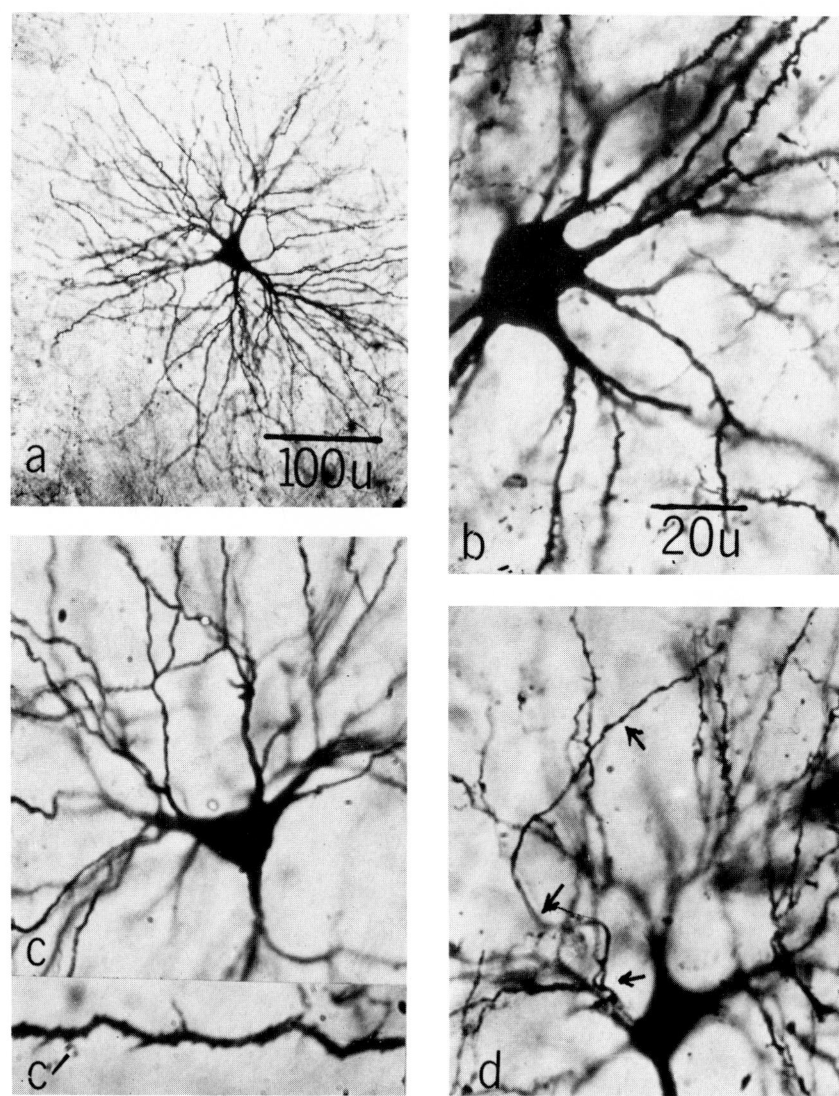

FIG. 3. Several thalamocortical (T) cells showing certain aspects of dendritic and axonal structure. a, dendritic domain developing from approximately 6 short primary dendrites; b and c, details of primary and secondary dendrite shafts showing essentially bare nature of dendrite surfaces; c', view of dendrite shaft at higher magnification to show tapering structures on dendrite surface believed to be presynaptic axonal terminals rather than dendrite structures. d, initial portion of axon of T cell. No collaterals could be identified. Photographs from 6 month old cat material stained with Golgi variant. x 100 and x 400. Inset photograph at c', x 880.

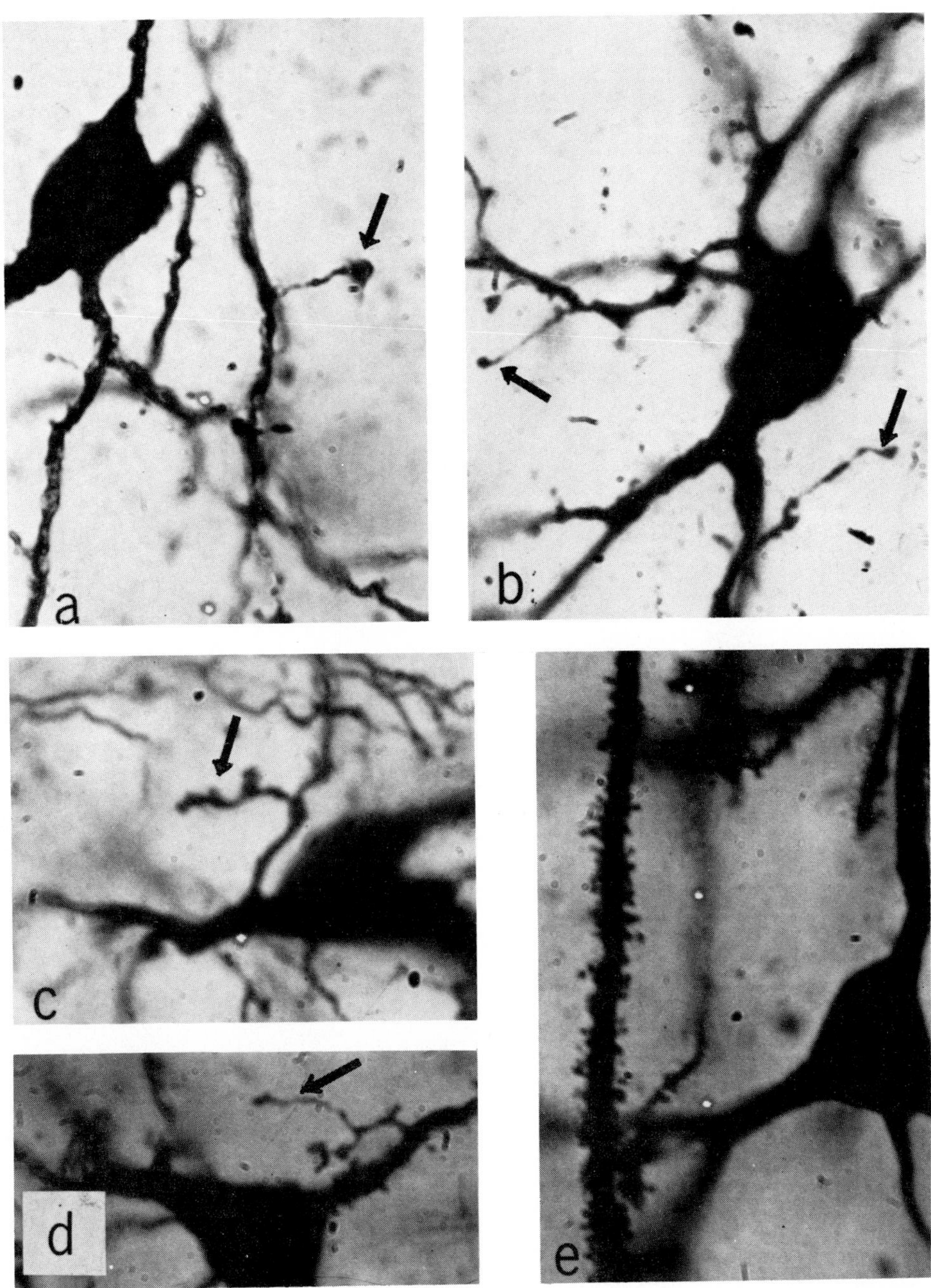

FIG. 4. Dendritic appendages or protusions on local circuit interneurons. a, b, c, and d; arrows mark typical structures. Some are as much as 20 to 30 μ in length. e, apical dendrite of cortical pyramid photographed at same magnification showing typical dendrite spines. Adult cat material stained with rapid Golgi variant. x 600.

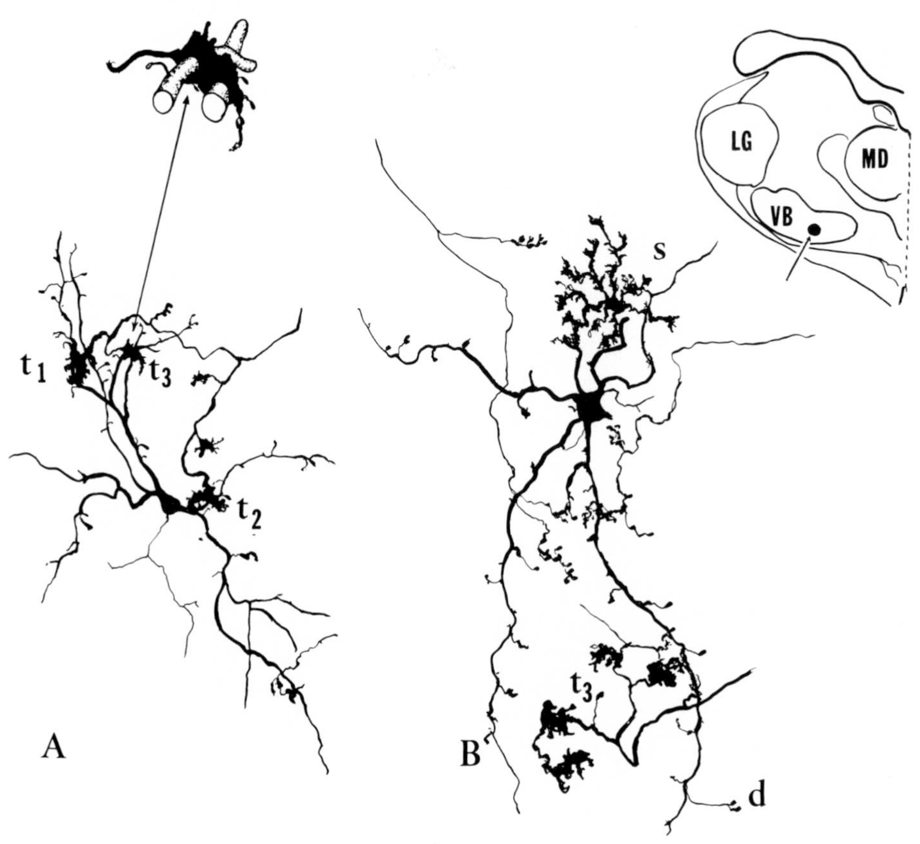

FIG. 5. Dendritic specializations on L cells and their interrelationships. In A, mossy tuft terminations t_1, t_2, t_3 on dendrite terminals belonging to other L cells make apparent synaptic contact with the pictured cell. The postsynaptic element is either the dendrite shaft itself as suggested in the inset diagram above A, or the dendrite appendages such as that pictured at d, in B. A small axonless cell is shown at s. Other abbreviations include VB, ventrobasal; LG, lateral geniculate; MD, dorsomedial nuclei. Drawn from adult cat material stained with rapid Golgi variants. x 200.

The best presently known example of this type is the amacrine cell of the retina, whose neuronal nature now seems well established (38). A necessary correlate of this type of neural activity is the capacity of dendrites to fulfill both presynaptic and postsynaptic functions. Adequate documentation already appears available for this type of dendritic role in a number of centers (4, 11, 17, 20, 21, 22, 23) including the VB complex, so the presence of functioning axonless neurons in ventral thalamic fields should provide no insoluble conceptual problems.

Another interesting feature of many of these cells is the presence of complex mossy tufts and clawlike rosettes on the terminals of a number of dendritic processes (Figures 1, C and 1, D, a; and Figures 5, 6, and 7). They have already been reported here and elsewhere (22, 36, 37) on the dendrites of short axon-bearing, local circuit (L) cells of this field, on some T cells, and in the intralaminar complex (31). They undoubtedly serve the same purpose for all of these elements, i.e., enabling participation at the pre- or postsynaptic level in synaptic complexes, nests, or glomeruli. The presence of these structures can only be inferred from Golgi studies but has been described in some detail by a number of electron microscopists (4, 11, 16, 21, 23, 35, 37).

Figures 6 and 7 illustrate the morphology of these tuft-like structures. Some of them appear to bear filamentous processes (Fig. 7, a) which terminate, in turn, in single knob-like enlargements or small clusters. Others appear fenestrated (Fig. 6, B and D) or show concave silhouettes suggesting close physical relationships with other structures which have not been stained. It is not possible to decide from Golgi data whether these tufts serve presynaptic or postsynaptic functions. However, certain deductions can be made about their role as will be shown below.

The simpler dendritic appendages found along dendrites of the L cells (Figs. 4, 6, and 11) appear appropriately sized and placed to form the central dendritic core of synaptic complexes or glomeruli described by Jones and Powell (11) and by Ralston (23). These are apparently postsynaptic to the remaining elements of the complex. The mossy tufts, on the other hand, would seem to correlate most convincingly with the rather enigmatic "large pale profiles" (11) shown to contribute to the glomerulus at the presynaptic level. If this interpretation were valid, it would suggest that the dendrite systems of L cells tend to operate presynaptically at their tips where most tufts are located and postsynaptically along the more proximal regions of the shafts where most of the appendages are found.

Granting that this possibility remains only an hypothesis at the moment, it suggests an interesting mode of interconnection among tuft and appendage-bearing neurons in the ventral nuclear complex. Terminal dendritic rosettes acting presynaptically effect synaptic contact with appendages generated along the shafts of similar L cells (Figs. 5 and 6, C). Each dendrite-to-dendrite articulation forms a potential glomerulus, to which a number of presynaptic axon terminals in varying combinations are added. This dendrite-to-dendrite linkage pattern extending throughout the nuclear fields is conceived as forming a 3 dimensional matrix with special properties for intranuclear spread of activity, resonant cycling, etc. The presence of similar tufted structures on many large thalamocortical cells suggests that some of these may participate

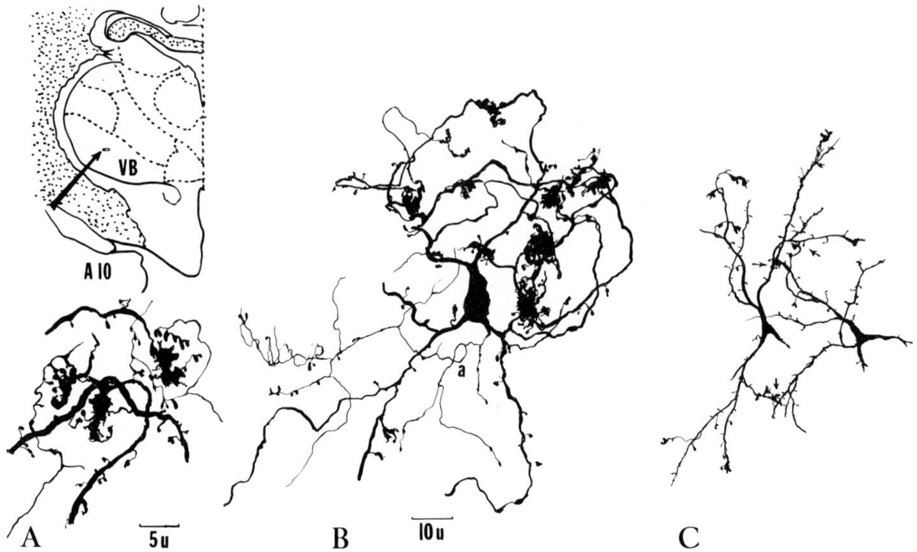

FIG. 6. Dendritic specializations (mossy tufts) on L cells. Mossy tuft terminals on L cell dendrites are shown at three levels of resolution. A gives some idea of the kind of structures which probably interrelate with the mossy tufts shown in B and C. Axonal terminal boutons and dendritic appendages may appear in very close relation and probably help to form the synaptic islands or glomeruli of electron microscopists. The arrows at C indicate probable points of tuft-appendage synaptic articulation significantly concerned in development of the dendro-dendritic matrix of interneurons (see text). Drawn from adult cat material stained with Golgi variants.

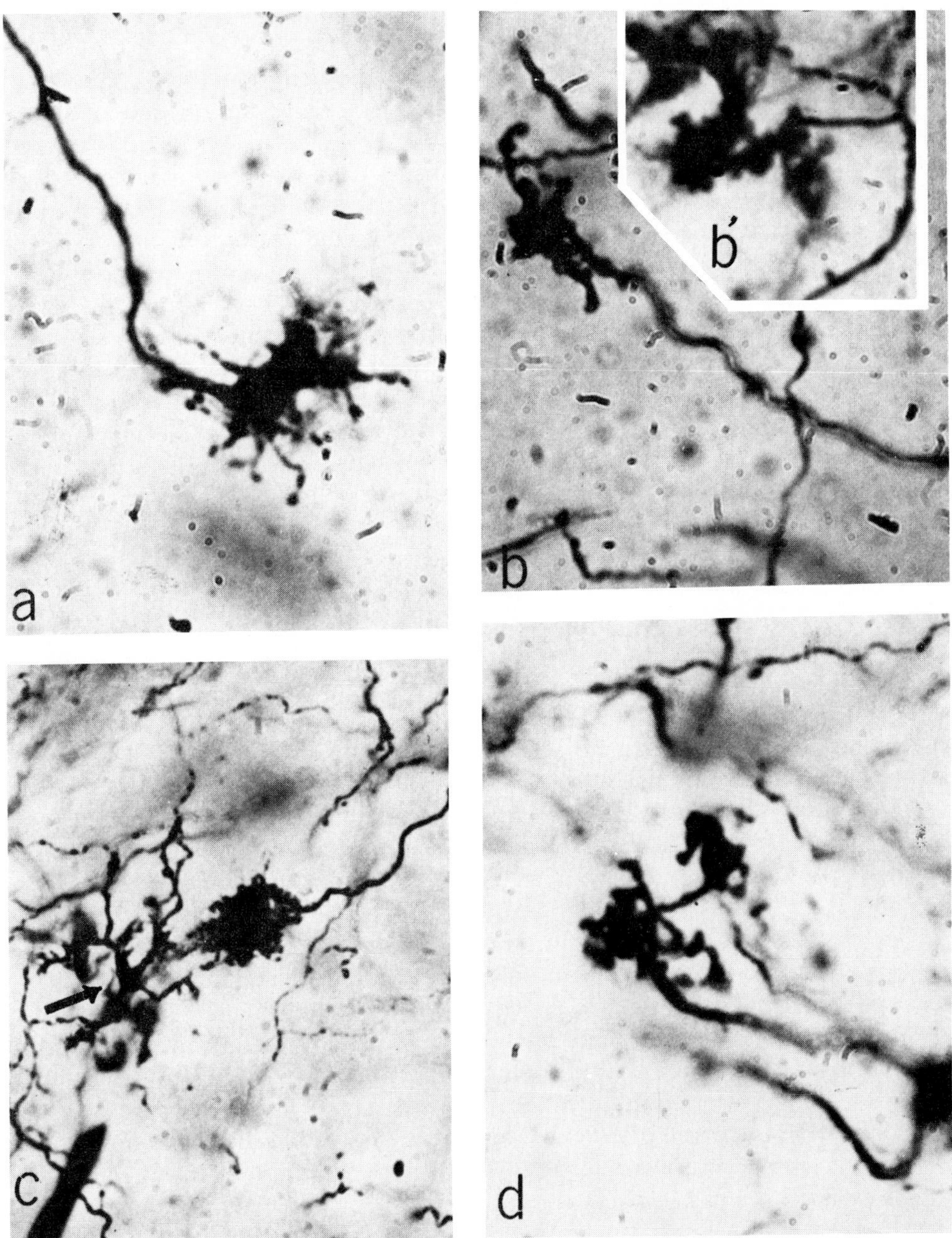

FIG. 7. Mossy tufts or rosettes on the terminals of L cells. Photographs a, b, b', and d, taken at the same magnification (x 800) show details of structure including terminal filaments, fenestration, concave profiles suggesting close contact with unstained structures, etc. Photograph c, taken at x 400 show a small axonless cell close to the tuft. In d, the cell body of origin can be seen out of focus at the lower right. Adult cat material stained with rapid Golgi variant.

to varying degrees in this type of dendritically spread activity.

The richly branched axons of the L cells undoubtedly provide a second mode of intercommunication among T and L cells within the nuclear field, modulating thalamic rhythms subserved by the dendrite-coupled chains. The axon-mediated connections might be concerned with short latency physiological phenomena, such as lateral inhibition and the rapid quenching of brachium-stimulated VL cells in the waking state as reported by Filion et al. (5).

Small axonless elements. While examining the problem of axonless cells, it seems appropriate to consider another population of cellular elements which are appreciably smaller in size than any local circuit neuron. These cells are pictured in Figs. 8, 9, and 10. They seem to be localized to the specific and intralaminar portions of dorsal thalamus with the possible exception of ventralis anterior and nucleus reticularis. The cell body is very small, seldom exceeding 3 to 5 u in diameter, and bears a variable number of short, sinuous dendrite-like processes with smooth or irregular surfaces. Each process bears upon its free end a tuft or partially formed claw or rosette. As a result, these elements bear some resemblance to cerebellar granules (Fig. 8, a), although the cell body is appreciably smaller and there is no demonstrable axon. Possible similarities to microglia and oligodendroglia are explored in Fig. 8, c and d, respectively. In each case, the morphological differences are notable, although it is obviously impossible to rule out the possibility that they represent some form of classical glial cell, specially adapted to the needs of the thalamic milieu. The tufts or rosettes which these small cells bear on the tips of their processes may ultimately provide some clue to their function. Among others, it seems reasonable to consider the possibility that these elements might participate through their terminal specializations in some type of synaptic complex, either as very small axonless neurons or as neuroglia.

From a purely speculative point of view, their ultimate identification as small neurons would add another intriguing note to an already complicated synaptic milieu. For without axons, they also would undoubtedly utilize their dendritic systems in both pre- and postsynaptic fashion. The small extent of their dendritic domains indicates functional roles limited to closely adjacent structures while, as already suggested, the invariable terminal rosettes could be interpreted as suggesting implication in glomerular structures. We accordingly propose as a working hypothesis that these small axonless cells, if neuronal in nature, may serve some type of transglomerular integrative function as indicated in Figure 11. This may include not only glomeruli based on adjacent local circuit neurons, but also glomeruli situated along the dendrite branches of a single neuron. The functional significance of such a unique arrangement, if indeed it exists, is not clear.

DESCENDING AXON SYSTEMS

Centrifugal axons entering the specific thalamic fields have been considered, at least for perinatal preparations, in several previous communications (24-27, 30, 31, 35-37). Reexamination of this problem with variants of the rapid Golgi methods in

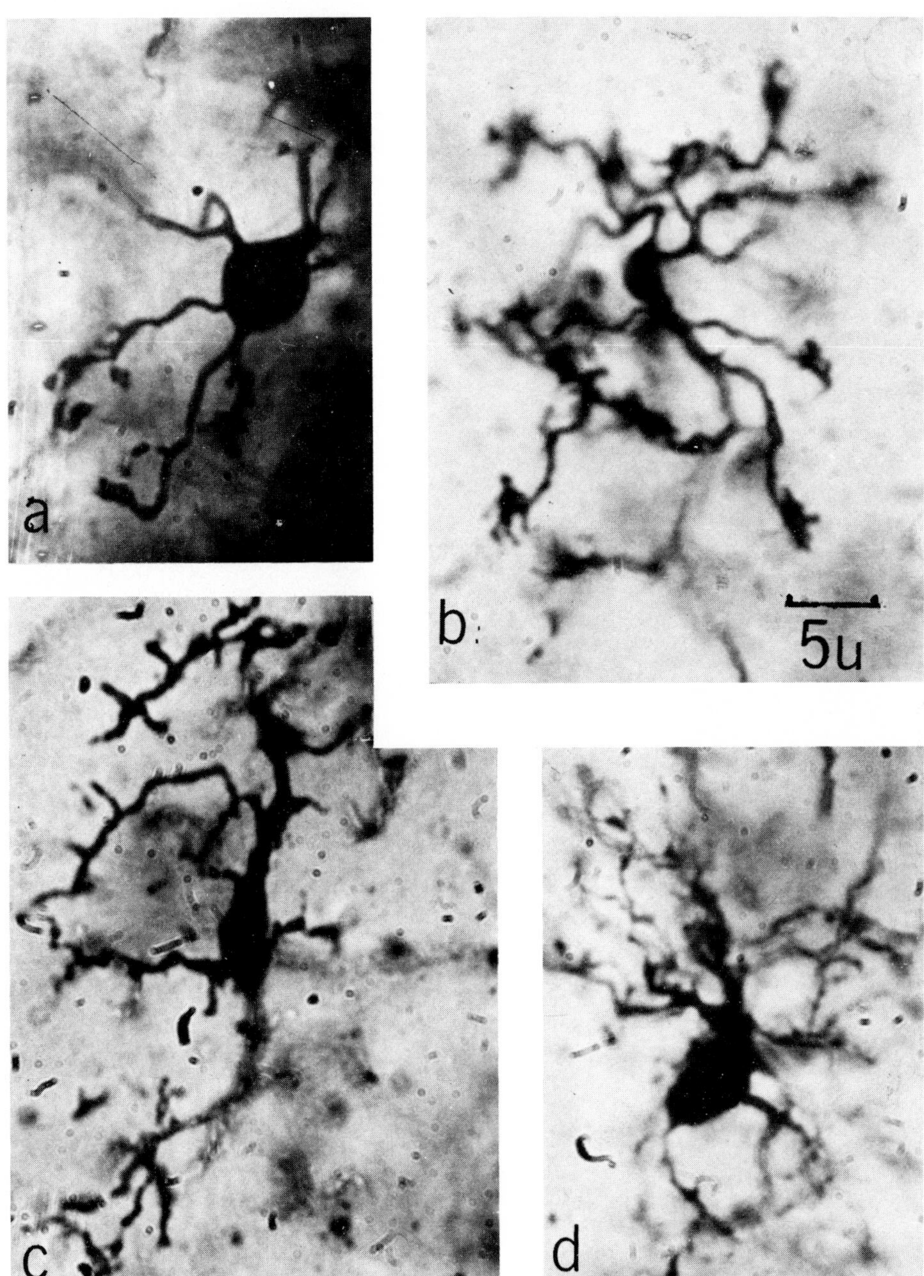

FIG. 8. Comparison of small axonless cell with other neural elements. These include a, cerebellar granule cell; c, microgliocyte; and d, oligodendrocyte. The size of the cell body, the pattern of the processes, and the presence of terminal rosettes tends to differentiate the small axonless cell, b, from the others. All photographed at 800 x. From sections of adult cat thalamus stained by rapid Golgi variants.

mature thalamus is fraught with difficulties. The sheer size and complexity of the adult carnivore or primate thalamus makes following axons for any distance at all a formidable problem. Even the mature rat and mouse, though simpler in thalamic organization, have proven difficult subject material for our work. Fortunately, most of the descending axonal pathways appear sketched in by the first or second week of life (24-27). Those parts of the system most likely to change would be the terminal patterns and modes of synaptic articulation. Thus far, we have not been able to examine sufficient numbers of well stained thalami to provide a complete picture. We must therefore continue to build on the data already culled from examination of perinatal

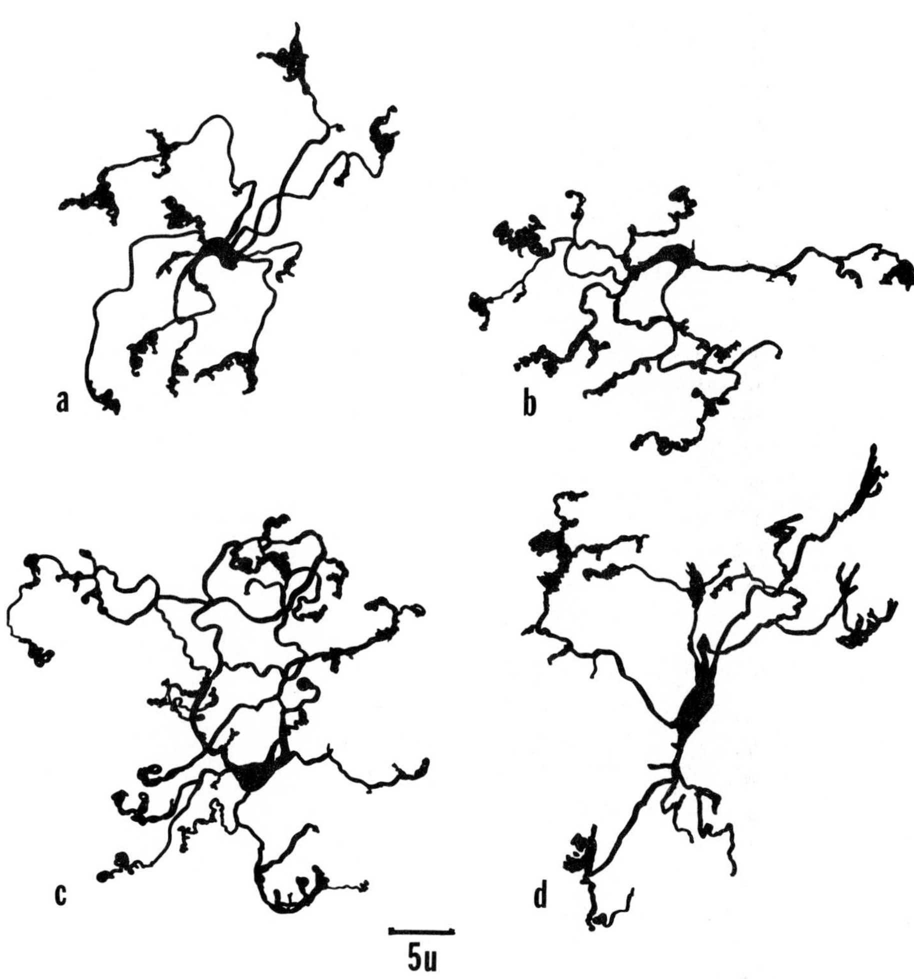

FIG. 9. Drawings of 4 different small axonless cells to show details of structure. Adult cat material stained with variant of rapid Golgi method.

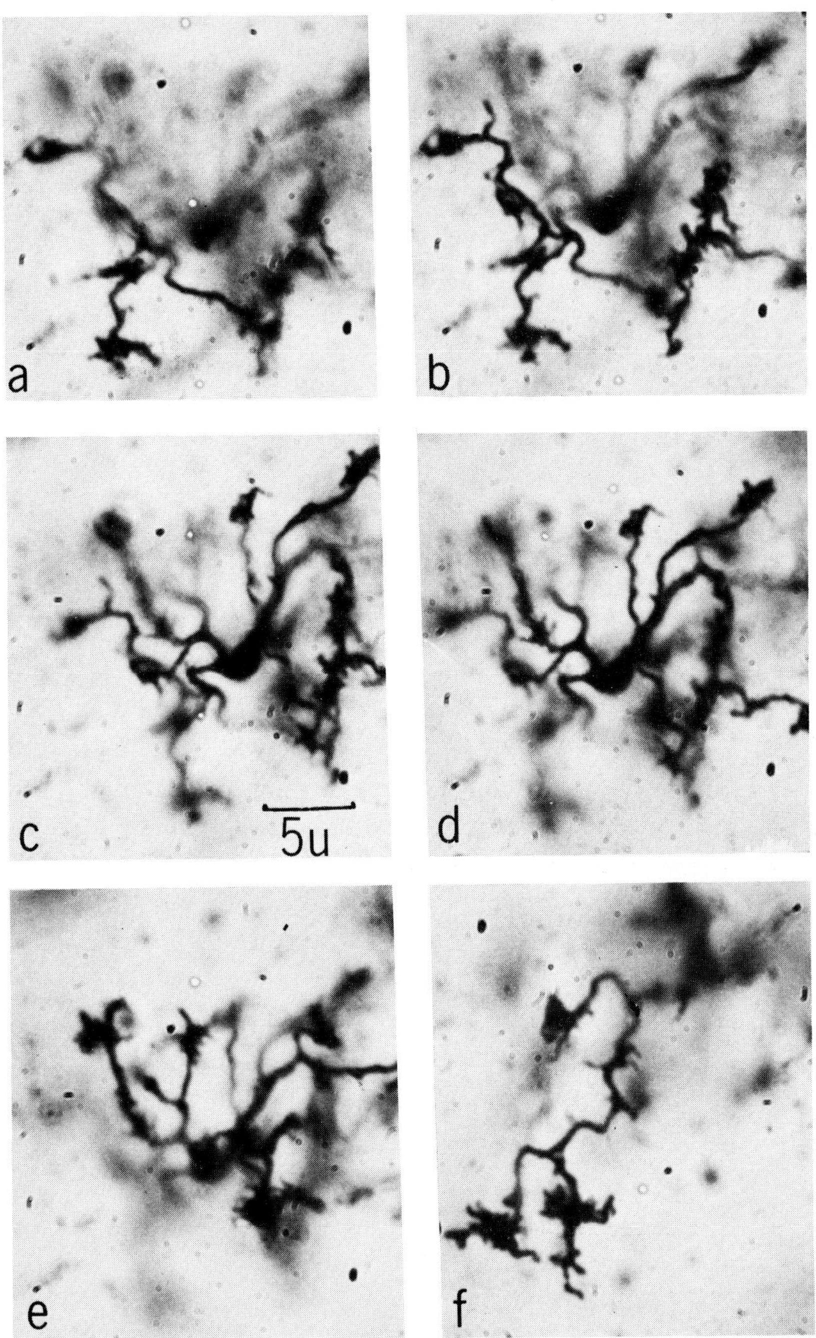

FIG. 10. Photographs a to f were taken of the same small axonless cell at different planes of focus to show all of the processes and terminal structures. Adult cat material stained with rapid Golgi variant. x 800.

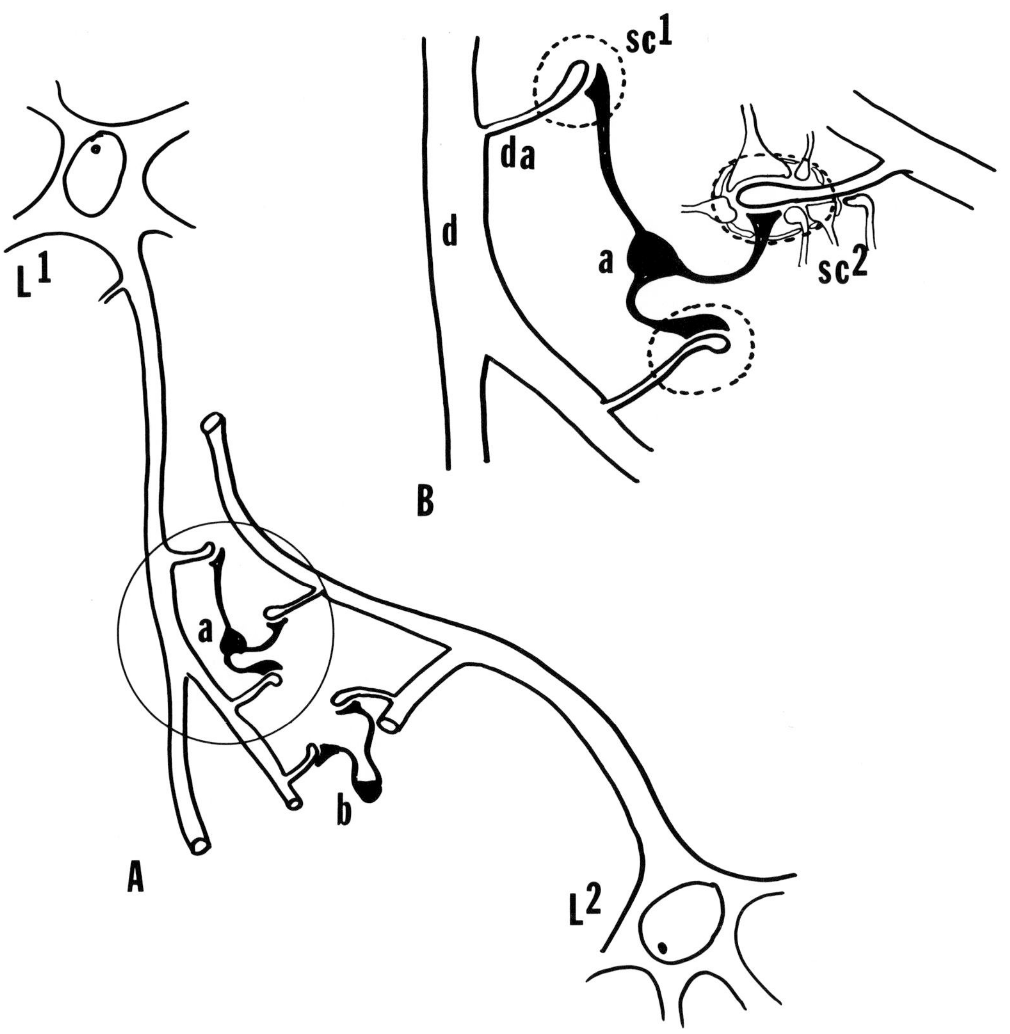

FIG. 11. Semischematic view of one possible type of relationship of small axonless cells with L cells. The small cells, a and b, make contact with dendritic protrusions such as da, by means of their tufted endings. These points of contact are probably the glomeruli or synaptic complexes, $sc^{1,2}$, described by electron microscopists. The role of these small axonless cells would appear to be some type of intercommunication between the various complexes on the dendrites, d, of the same cell L^1 or with adjoining L cells, L^2.

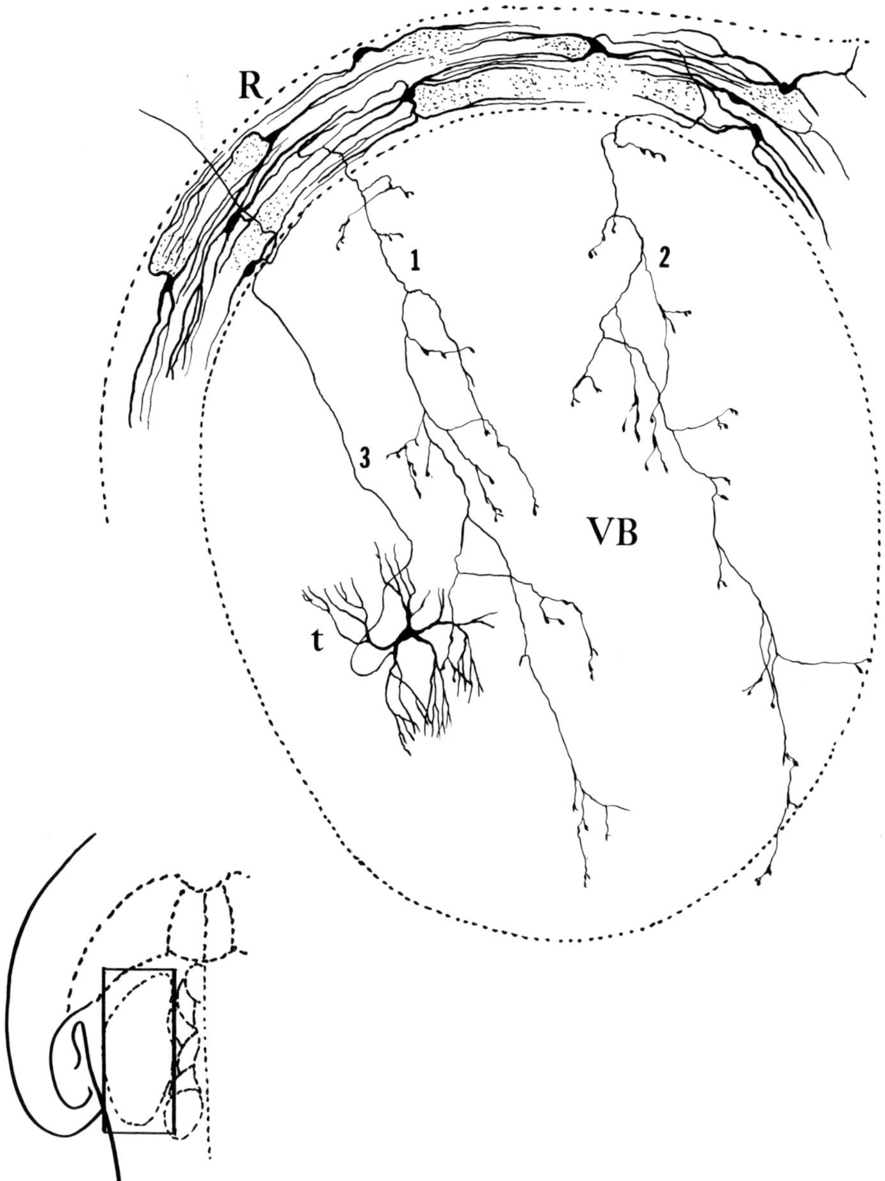

FIG. 12. The caudally directed projection of the nucleus reticularis thalami upon the ventrobasal complex (VB). Reticularis axons 1, and 2, generate a number of short collaterals with closely adjacent terminal structures to produce linear synaptic arrays along the rostro-caudal axis of the thalamus. Thalamocortical neuron, t, sends its unbranched axon, 3, rostrally through the nucleus reticularis toward cortex. Reconstruction from a number of sections of young rodent and kitten material stained with rapid Golgi variants.

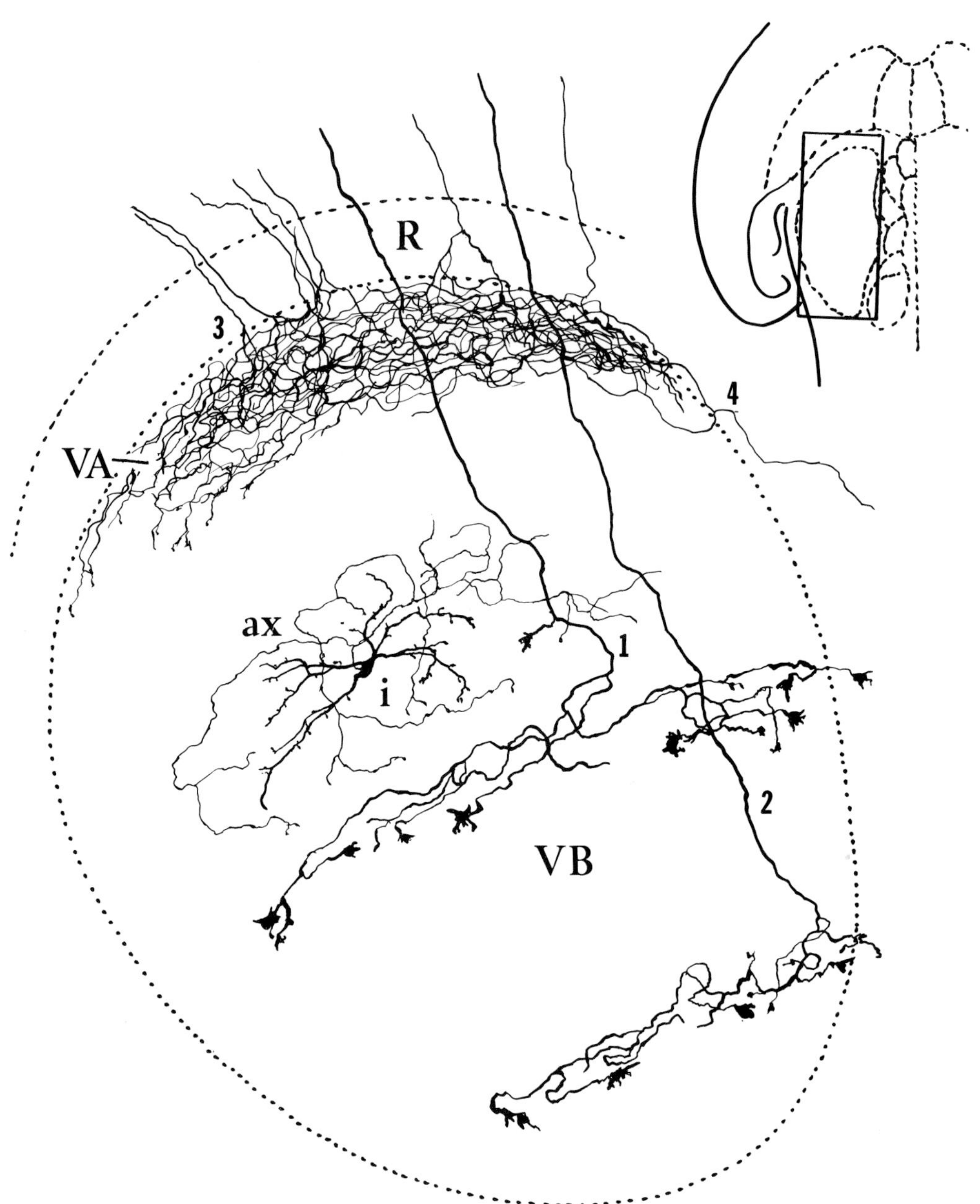

FIG. 13. One type of corticifugal projection upon the ventrobasal nuclear complex, VB. Fibers 1 and 2 penetrate the nucleus reticularis, R and the ventral anterior nucleus, VA to terminate in VB via transversely organized neuropil segments (see text). Synaptic contacts are thought to be made with the local circuit interneuron, i; the axon, a, of this cell is partly impregnated. Several axons, from cortex, 3, and from basal ganglia, 4, enter the VA nucleus. Reconstruction from a number of sections of young and adult rodents and cats stained with variants of the rapid Golgi methods.

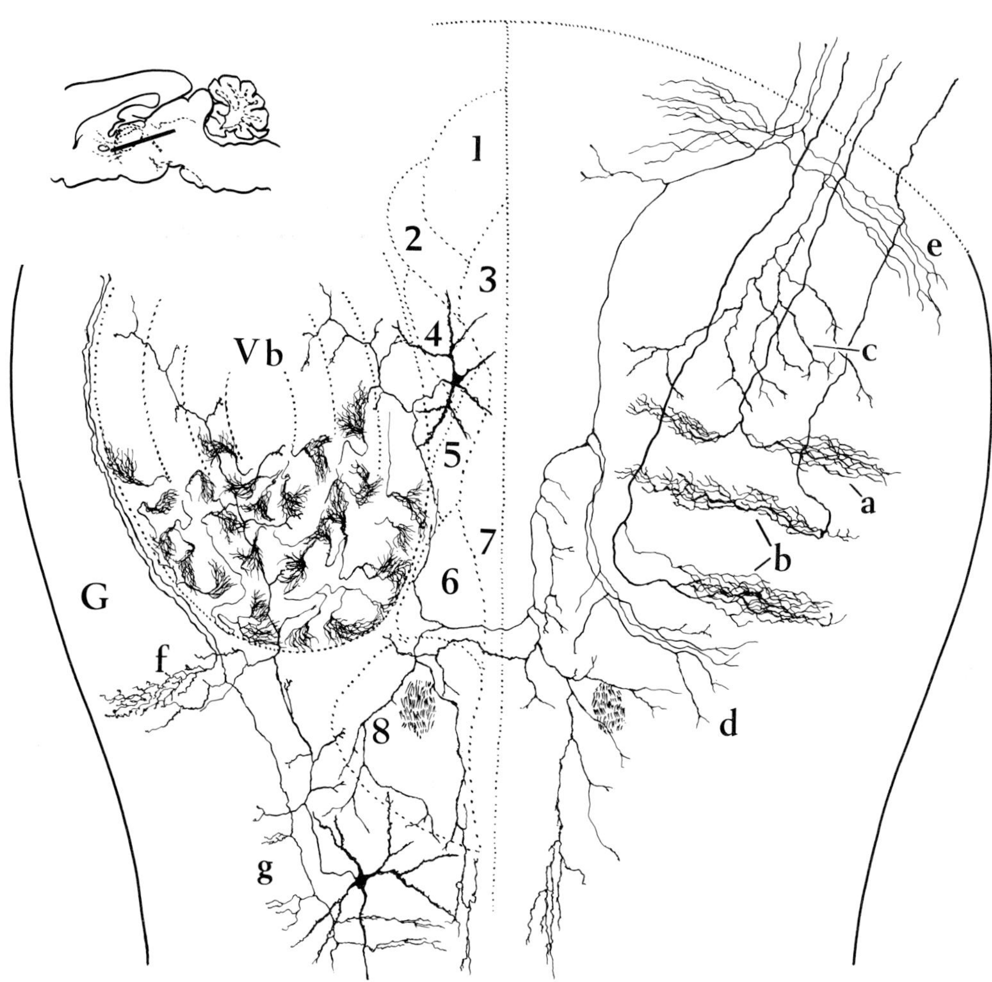

FIG. 14. Horizontal reconstruction showing neuropil patterns characteristic of thalamic fields. Vb, ventrobasal complex; G, lateral geniculate; a, corticothalamic discoid afferent terminal developing symmetrically from parent fiber; b, similar discoid afferents developing assymetrically from parent fiber; c, corticothalamic fiber generating broadly branching conical terminal pattern; d, part of the terminal system of a corticothalamic fiber to midline nonspecific system composed in part of 1, parataenial; 2, anterior ventral; 3, interanteromedial; 4, anterior medial; 5, central medial; 6, central lateral; 7, interventricular; 8, centre median-parafascicular nuclei, respectively. Also, e, part of plexus generated by centrifugal fibers in area of n. reticularsi thalami; f, afferent terminals in lateral geniculate nucleus; and g, in tegmentum. Drawn from several sections of 10 to 20 day old rat brain stem stained by rapid Golgi variant. From Scheibel and Scheibel (30). Reproduced by kind permission of publisher.

material, enriched by the insights derived from occasional vignettes of descending terminal circuitry in adult preparations. Degeneration studies employing both light and electron microscopy such as the one by Rinvik (Chapter in this volume) are, of course, invaluable in developing adequate ideas of the topography of such systems.

Axons of nucleus reticularis thalami cells provide a powerful system of descending afferents which appear to maintain a rather precise topographic relationship with adjacent specific thalamic fields (15). Following Cajal's observations that such axons appeared to run caudal rather than rostral (25), we were able to show that such fibers course backward through the length of specific and nonspecific thalamus, and in some few cases, overlap into upper mesencephalic tegmentum (27, 29). Although the precise mode of termination of this system has not been established, analysis of both Golgi (26) and degeneration material (15) point to the development of linear synaptic arrays (Fig. 12) arranged along each fiber in the rostro-caudal axis. We believe that synaptic contacts are established primarily with the thalamocortical relay cells, for the reasons mentioned below.

Axons of presumed cortical origin show several patterns of organization as they converge upon the thalamus from anterior and ventral lateral quadrants and penetrate deeply within specific and nonspecific thalamic fields. Of immediate concern are two major types of axon, both of which have already been described (26, 30). The heavier fibers characteristically generate a series of transversely oriented chip-like fields by virtue of their dense terminal neuropil generated across the long axis of the brain stem (Fig. 13). Careful examination suggests that many of these elements bear terminal structures somewhat like the mossy tufts already mentioned, though smaller and with larger filamentous secondary protrusions. Figures 13 and 14, a, and b, show how these neuropil complexes project across the specific thalamic field, fractionating neuronal ensembles in the vertical-transverse mode. In Figure 15, they are shown effecting synaptic contact entirely with local circuit cells. The evidence for this is still inferential, depending in part on the tuft-like axon terminals with their presumptive relationship to glomeruli found exclusively along L cells, and in part on the highly variable effects of cortical stimulation upon T cells (2, 10, 18, 33).

The second fiber type generates widely bifurcating axon branches which, in the rodent at least, may encompass one third to one half of the entire specific nucleus. Branch patterns of this fiber are very restrained (Fig. 14, c) and undoubtedly produce a low density type of synaptic engagement over a very large volume of tissue. We have likened the neuropil field generated by this axon to a cone, whose apex is rostral and whose base is caudal. Since a large number of such fibers descend upon the specific thalamic nuclei, generating the characteristic neuropil field at intervals, they can be compared to a stack of cones, completely investing the ventral complex of nuclei.

These two descending fiber systems when viewed jointly produce a terminal field system of interpenetrating chips and cones which must thoroughly fractionate the specific thalamic nuclei, undoubtedly providing multiple centrifugal innervation to each thalamic cell.

DISCUSSION

Remarkably little of a definitive nature can be said as yet about the mechanisms of cortical interaction with thalamus. From the anatomical point of view, the complex nature of centrifugal control is witnessed by the precision with which topographic relations are established (see Rinvik and Kuypers, chapters in this volume) and the highly specialized terminal patterns generated by these fibers (26, 30). Structural analyses are, in themselves, unlikely to tell us whether certain connections are facilitatory or inhibitory, but at a different level of complexity, they can provide clues as to the type of information processing operations which may be going on.

In Figure 15, a schematic view of the neuropil structure of the VB complex has been developed, partly from fact and partly from inference. While terminal patterns and specific receptive cell types have been indicated, a great deal more information will be needed at this level before a comprehensive picture of corticothalamic relations can be presented. Physiological studies such as those of Ogden (18), Iwama and Yamamoto (10), and Shimazu et al. (34) provide some evidence of the complex nature of cortical control over thalamic activity. Further support is added to such inferences by work reported elsewhere in this volume (see Petras, Albe-Fessard, Massion, Hollander, etc.) and by unpublished studies of our own (2). It is therefore hardly surprising that the structural substrate for these effects is also difficult to elucidate.

Figure 15 shows in highly schematic and oversimplified fashion, several features of the descending control system. Although there is convincing evidence that corticothalamic projections comprise several different fiber types, have a number of different cortical sources, and follow several different descending routes (26, 30, and Rinvik, Chapter in this volume), they are shown here as an essentially unitary system epitomized by those fibers leaving the pericruciate area, projecting caudally through the nucleus reticularis thalami, and terminating in successive compressed neuropil segments across the ventrobasal field. Synaptic links are pictured as being established exclusively with the L cells although there is no hard evidence that would preclude direct cortical links to T cells as well. However, as already indicated above, the presence of mossy rosettes on the terminals of many of these fibers suggests termination in some type of synaptic island or glomerulus and, in the thalamus, these appear to be localized to the L neurons. The range and variability of thalamic T cell response to cortical stimulation as reported by a number of workers (10, 18, 34) would also seem to argue for the existence of an intercalated neuron.

As we have indicated in discussing the interconnections of L cells, both axonal and dendritic paths may be available for transmission of cortically evoked effects beyond the receptive interneuron to T cells and to other L cells. In addition, there is another highly speculative possibility for transglomerular integrative activity in the presence of the tiny axonless cells already pictured in Figure 11 and labelled 'x' in Figure 15. The circuitry available even to this single paradigmatic corticothalamic line clearly offers many optional routes for the channeling and processing of information.

Since even fewer data are available on the exact mode and site of synaptic articulation of those fibers generating large conical fields (see above and Figure 14, c),

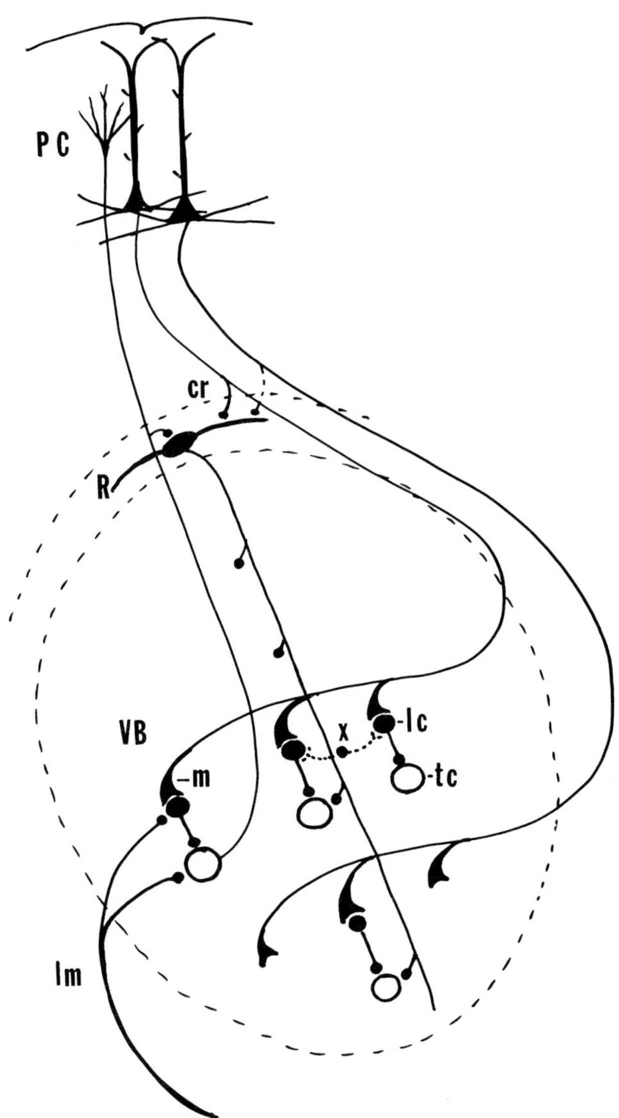

Fig. 15. Simplified schematic view of relations between sensory thalamus and centrifugal fiber systems. Medial lemniscus fibers, lm, terminate on both thalamocortical, tc and local circuit interneurons, lc in the ventrobasal complex, VB. Thalamocortical projection cells send axons through nucleus reticularis, R, giving off collaterals en route and reach pericruciate area of cortex, PC. Caudal projection of cortical pyramids, after sending collaterals to reticularis cells, terminate via their small mossy rosette-bearing endings on VB local circuit cells. These synapse in turn with thalamocortical cells and also may be synaptically linked to each other, in part, by small axonless cells, x. Descending projections from nucleus reticularis cells establish contacts with linear arrays of thalamocortical neurons.

it seems wise to delay further consideration of this corticifugal system until a later communication. Suffice it to say, we have suggested in a recent report (30) that, operating in concert, the tightly stacked terminal fields of these two corticifugal systems impose a three dimensional grid upon the matrix of VB neurons. Reasoning by analogy from the coincident current selection technique used in reading out individual cores from a computer memory array, such an arrangement could theoretically provide a cortical retrieval and readout capability over thalamic cell ensembles. Whether corticothalamic activity does actually include some type of information retrieval process cannot be decided with the physiological information presently available.

In Figure 15, the axonal projection running caudally from the nucleus reticularis thalami is seen to establish synaptic contact with linear arrays of thalamocortical cells arranged in rostro-caudal sequence. Once again there is insufficient evidence to document an exclusive synaptic relationship with T cells. On the other hand, the physiological data already in the literature (5, 12, 14, 33) suggest that a relatively constant inverse relationship exists between firing patterns of reticularis elements and neurons in the ventral complex of nuclei. Close coupling of this type implies, though does not necessarily demand, direct synaptic links without intervention of another neuron. Earlier suggestions that the nucleus reticularis thalami serves as a feedback control over thalamic firing patterns, providing phasic inhibition following evoked T cell discharge (26, 27, 29, 30) seem borne out by several physiological studies (5, 12, 14, 33). The rigorously arranged linear sequences (15, 27) along which this inhibitory control is exercised, introduces another impressive substrate for signal processing in an already complex field. The ultimate nature of this mechanism is still not clear, but we have suggested that the inhibitory sequencing of T cells by the nucleus reticularis may be causally related to rhythmic thalamocortical phenomena such as spindling and alpha activity.

While this schema emphasizes the importance of synaptic input from the ascending thalamocortical relay, the nucleus reticularis cells are unquestionably subject, also, to a number of other influences including inputs from cerebral cortex (Fig. 15, cr) and brain stem reticular core. Evidence of synaptic contributions from cortical systems has already been provided by the electron microscope studies of Rinvik (Chapter in this volume) while demonstrated variations in the functional relationship between nucleus reticularis and VL cells during waking, slow wave, and paradoxical sleep argue strongly for modulation by the reticular core. In this regard, it might be recalled that the nucleus reticularis represents a dorsal and rostral elaboration of the zona incerta, the projection pathway for the brain stem reticular core through posterior hypothalamus.

OVERVIEW

We conclude that the ventrobasal complex of the thalamus offers a complicated and still poorly understood matrix of interneurons under modulatory control of several centrifugal systems. The major neuronal subsystems with which these descending elements articulate are divisible into thalamocortical (T) cells and local circuit (L) cells. The latter, by virtue of specialized dendritic structures along their shafts (appendages) and at their tips (tufts or rosettes) are assumed capable of establishing interconnecting dendro-dendritic linkages to form a continuous three dimensional matrix with special properties for intranuclear spread (and inhibition) of neural activity, resonant cycling, etc. T cells are believed to be connected to this system of local circuit elements through tuft-mediated dendrite specializations of their own and through the axon systems of the local circuit cells. Some of the latter are thought to be without axons and accordingly perform their integrative functions exclusively through dendritic mechanisms, suggesting functional analogies with retinal amacrine cells. A very small axonless cell of unknown nature has also been described in the ventral thalamic nuclear complex of mature animals, and a putative transglomerular function has been assigned to it.

Two major corticothalamic fiber systems have been described on the basis of their terminal axonal patterns. At least one of these is conceived as operating upon the L cells rather than directly upon the T neurons. We have suggested that, operating in concert on somesthetic thalamus, the two fiber groups might provide a retrieval and readout capability for sensorimotor cortex.

The caudally-directed projection of nucleus reticularis may control T cell activity through direct synaptic linkage. Operating as a negative feedback, and in association with internuncial pools of L cells, nucleus reticularis neurons are probably instrumental in the sequencing of T cell excitability and thus, indirectly, in the development of rhythmic thalamocortical activities.

ACKNOWLEDGMENT

Supported by Grants NB 01063 and HD 00972, U.S. Public Health Service. Dr. Davies is a Postdoctoral Fellow, N.I.N.D.S.

REFERENCES

1 ANDERSEN, P. and ANDERSSON, S.A. (1968) Physiological Basis of the Alpha Rhythm. Appleton-Century-Crofts, New York.

2 DAVIES, T.L., SCHEIBEL, M.E. and SCHEIBEL, A.B. (In preparation.)

3 DROOGLEEVER FORTUYN, A.B. Cortical cell-laminations of the hemispheres of some rodents. Arch. Neurol. Psychiat. 6 (1914) 221-354.

4 FAMIGLIETTI, E.V. Dendro-dendritic synapses in the lateral geniculate nucleus of the cat. Brain Res. 20 (1970) 181-191.

5 FILION, M., LAMARRE, Y. and CORDEAU, J.P. Neuronal discharges of the ventrolateral nucleus of the thalamus during sleep and wakefulness in the cat. II. Evoked activity. Exp. Brain Res. 12 (1971) 499-508.

6 FRIGYESI, T.L. Organization of synaptic pathways linking the head of the caudate nucleus to the dorsolateral thalamus. Int. J. Neurol. (In press.)

7 GLOBUS, A. and SCHEIBEL, A.B. Pattern and field in cortical structure: The rabbit. J. comp. Neurol. 131 (1967) 155-172.

8 GRAY, E.G. Axo-somatic and axo-dendritic synapses of the cerebral cortex—an electron microscope study. J. Anat. (London) 93 (1959) 420-433.

9 HEAD, H. and HOLMES, G. Sensory disturbances from cerebral lesions. Brain

34 (1911) 102-254.
10 IWAMA, K. and YAMAMOTO, C. Impulse transmission of thalamic somatosensory relay nuclei as modified by electrical stimulation of the cerebral cortex. Jap. J. Physiol. 11 (1961) 169-182.
11 JONES, E.G. and POWELL, T.P.S. Electron microscopy of synaptic glomeruli in the thalamic relay nuclei of the cat. Proc. Roy. Soc. B172 (1969) 153-171.
12 LAMARRE, Y., FILION, M. and CORDEAU, J.P. Neuronal discharges of the ventrolateral nucleus of the thalamus during sleep and wakefulness in the cat. I. Spontaneous activity. Exp. Brain Res. 12 (1971) 480-498.
13 LORENTE de NO, R. La corteza cerebral del raton. Trab. Lab. Invest. biol. (Madrid) 20 (1922) 41-78.
14 MASSION, J. Etude d'une structure motrice thalamique, le noyau ventrolateral et de sa regulation par les afferences sensorielles. These de doctorat d'Etat es sciences naturelles. Faculte des Sciences de Paris. (1968)
15 MINDERHOUD, J.M. An anatomical study of the efferent connections of the thalamic reticular nucleus. Exp. Brain Res. 12 (1971) 435-446.
16 MOREST, D.K. The neuronal architecture of the medial geniculate body of the cat. J. Anat. (London) 98 (1964) 611-630.
17 MOREST, D.K. Dendodendritic synapses of cells that have axons: The fine structure of the Golgi type II cell in the medial geniculate body of the cat. Z. Anat. Entwick.-Gesch. 133 (1971) 216-246.
18 OGDEN, T.E. Cortical control of thalamic somato-sensory relay nuclei. Electroenceph. clin. Neurophysiol. 12 (1960) 621-634.
19 PURPURA, D.P. Operations and processes in thalamic and synaptically related neural systems. In The Neurosciences, Second Study Program (Ed., F.O. Schmitt), Rockefeller Univ. Press (1970) pp. 458-470
20 RALL, W., SHEPHERD, G.M., REESE, T.S. and BRIGHTMAN, M.W. Dendodendritic synaptic pathway for inhibition in the olfactory bulb. Exp. Neurol. 14 (1966) 44-56.
21 RALSTON, H.J. The synaptic organization in the dorsal horn of the spinal cord and in the ventrobasal thalamus in the cat. In Oral-Facial Sensory and Motor Mechanisms (Eds., R. Dubner and Y. Kawamura), Appleton-Century, Crofts, N.Y. (1971) 229-250.
22 RALSTON, H.J. Evidence for presynaptic dendrites and a proposal for their mechanism of action. Nature 230 (1971) 585-587.
23 RALSTON, III, H.J. and HERMAN, M.M. The fine structure of neurons and synapses in the ventrobasal thalamus of the cat. Brain Res. 14 (1969) 77-97.
24 RAMON y CAJAL, S. Contribucion al estudio de la vie sensitiva central y de la estructura del talamo optico. Rev. trim. Microgr. 5 (1900) 185-198.
25 RAMON y CAJAL, S. Histologie du Systeme Nerveux de l'Homme et des Vertebres. A. Maloine, Paris, 1911, 2 vols.
26 SCHEIBEL, M.E. and SCHEIBEL, A.B. Patterns of organization in specific and nonspecific thalamic fields. In The Thalamus (Eds., D.P. Purpura and M.D. Yahr), Columbia Univ. Press, N.Y. 1966, pp. 13-46.
27 SCHEIBEL, M.E. and SCHEIBEL, A.B. The organization of the nucleus reticularis

thalami: a Golgi study. Brain Res. 1 (1966) 43-62.
28 SCHEIBEL, M.E. and SCHEIBEL, A.B. The organization of the ventral anterior nucleus of the thalamus: a Golgi study. Brain Res. 1 (1966) 250-268.
29 SCHEIBEL, M.E. and SCHEIBEL, A.B. Structural organization of nonspecific thalamic nuclei and their projection toward cortex. Brain Res. 6 (1967)60-94.
30 SCHEIBEL, M.E. and SCHEIBEL, A.B. Elementary processes in selected thalamic and cortical subsystems—The structural substrates. In The Neurosciences, Second Study Program (Ed., F. Schmitt), Rockefeller Univ. Press, N.Y., pp. 443-457.
31 SCHEIBEL, M.E. and SCHEIBEL, A.B. Input-output relations of the thalamic nonspecific system. (In press.)
32 SCHEIBEL, M.E., DAVIES, T.L. and SCHEIBEL, A.B. Unpublished data, and in press.
33 SCHLAG, J. and WASZAK, M. Characteristics of unit responses in nucleus reticularis thalami. Brain Res. 21 (1970) 286-288.
34 SHIMAZU, H., YANAGISAWA, N. and GAROUTTE, B. Cortico-pyramidal influences on thalamic somatosensory transmission in the cat. Jap. J. Physiol. 15 (1965) 101-124.
35 SZENTAGOTHAI, J. The structure of the synapse in the lateral geniculate body. Acta. anat. (Basel) 55 (1963) 166-185.
36 SZENTAGOTHAI, J. Models of specific neuron arrays in thalamic relay nuclei. Acta morphol. Acad. Sci. Hung. 15 (1967) 113-124.
37 TOMBOL, T. Short neurons and their synaptic relations in the specific thalamic nuclei. Brain Res. 3 (1966) 307-326.
38 WERBLIN, F.S. and DOWLING, J.E. Organization of the retina of the mudpuppy, Necturus maculosus. II. Intracellular recording. J. Neurophysiol. 32 (1969) 339-355.
39 WOOLSEY, T.A. and VAN DER LOOS, H. The structural organization of layer IV in the somatosensory region (SI) of mouse cerebral cortex. Brain Res. 17 (1970) 205-242.

DISCUSSION

CARPENTER:

Although the thalamus is a relatively small part of the central nervous system, it has long been regarded as the key to understanding the organization and function of the central nervous system. Thalamic inputs are derived from virtually all sensory systems, from the reticular formation, from the cerebellum and from the basal ganglia. Thalamic output constitutes the major source of impulses projecting to the cerebral cortex and is an important source of impulses passing to parts of the basal ganglia. While it has been customary to regard thalamic subdivisions as simple relay nuclei, it is obvious that thalamic neurons, impinged upon by multiple afferent systems, perform many integrative functions, not all of which are known. Attempts to elucidate the integrative functions of thalamic neurons and related neuronal subsystems have utilized mainly intracellular recording techniques, which indicate that these structural elements play important roles in high-fidelity, modality specific impulse transmission, in input selection, in output tuning, in synchronization, in desynchronization, and in parallel processing. While the functional properties and interrelations of certain neuronal subdivisions of the thalamus are clear, many functional relationships remain obscure, because it has not been possible to define their morphological basis. The internuclear synaptic pathways which link different neuronal subdivisions of the thalamus probably are among the most profuse and complex of all internuncial systems. This situation appears further complicated by the fact that the neuronal populations of recognized thalamic subdivisions are not homogeneous and possess intrinsic synaptic mechanisms that control the functional properties of that unit and the impulses it transmits to the cortex and other sites.

The Scheibels, in using the Golgi method, probably have selected the only method which at our current level of understanding can be expected to yield information concerning the morphological substrates that regulate the functional properties of populations of thalamic neurons. This approach seems certain to form the foundation for later studies at the ultrastructural level and for better insight into the interpretation of microelectrode studies.

The present study of the ventrobasal (VB) complex addresses itself to two points: (1) cells of the postsynaptic matrix, and (2) descending presynaptic terminals. Cells of the ventrobasal complex include at least three types of neurons: (1) the thalamocortical relay neuron, (2) the Golgi type II neuron, and (3) a small pleomorphic neuron, which has no apparent axon.

Thalamocortical relay neurons (20-30) in adult animals appear to differ from those found in immature animals. In the immature animal multiple dendritic shafts leave the cell body directly and break up into tufted or bushy arbors that greatly enlarge the postsynaptic surface and are thought to contribute to the high synaptic security which characterizes impulses conveyed by this lemniscal system. In the adult animal, dendrites of these cells differ in that they are arranged in bundles, are relatively smooth and only occasionally show a shaggy pseudospine system. A finding of considerable importance is that less than 15% of the axons of these cells appear to have collaterals in their proximal segments. This observation does not lend support to the recurrent collateral hypothesis of thalamic inhibition.

While studies in immature animals revealed very few Golgi type II neurons in the VB complex, data from mature cats indicate that such cells are relatively numerous, constituting about one-third the number of relay neurons. This new observation indicates that axons of these cells not only remain in the vicinity of the parent cell, but also project several millimeters in various planes. Such short-axoned cells could be involved not only in producing local or surround inhibition, but might be implicated in the short latency inhibition by certain specific thalamic nuclei upon nonspecific systems. It is thus apparent that these short-axoned cells, not previously recognized, may play a role in synchronization of thalamic activities.

A small proportion of cells in the ventrobasal complex (approximately 5%) resemble neurons of the brain stem reticular formation in that they have long, infrequently branched dendrites and bifurcating axons which project both rostrally and caudally. The extent and regions of terminations of these cells are unknown, but it is postulated that these cells serve as "integrator" elements for ensembles of VB cells.

A cellular element not previously identified in the thalamus is a small neuron (3 to 5) with variable numbers of shaggy or hairy dendrites and no apparent axon. Dendritic terminals of these cells are described as not unlike those of granule cells in the cerebellar cortex. These dendritic terminals appear to bear close relationships with terminals of corticothalamic fibers. It is not known if these dendrites enter a glomerular formation, but glomeruli have been described in the lateral geniculate body (2) and in the ventrobasal complex (1). The observation that these cells are without axons suggests that they may function like the amacrine cells of the inner plexiform layer of the retina. The retinal amacrine cell, linked to both the bipolar and ganglion cells, appears to exert inhibitory influences upon ganglion cells which result in surround inhibition.

Finally, the authors have described the descending presynaptic terminals which probably originate in the cerebral cortex. These fibers are massive and sweep into broad regions of the thalamus. These terminals are arranged in discoid arrays. Other fibers of cortical origin terminate in cone-shaped formation.

The frequent association of the tufted terminals in the discoid arrays with the dendrites of the amacrine-like small cells in the VB complex suggests that these corticothalamic fibers, acting via interneurons, may exert inhibitory effects upon relay cells of the VB complex.

1 Jones, E.G., and Powell, T.P.S. An electron microscopic study of the mode of termination of corticothalamic fibres within the sensory relay nuclei of the thalamus. Proc. Roy. Soc. (Lond.) Series B. 172 (1969) 173-185.

2 Szentagothai, J. Glomerular synapses, complex synaptic arrangements and their operational significance. The Neurosciences, Second Study Program. Ed. by F.O. Schmitt. Rockefeller University Press, 1970, pp. 427-443.

FOX:

I have not much to say for I have not studied the thalamus as the Scheibels have. Looking at Golgi impregnations of the adult monkey thalamus, I have the impression that the large relay cells have large cell bodies with short dendritic trunks that divide very rapidly, like a brush. This pattern is found throughout the thalamus; also it is found in the lateral geniculate nucleus. On the other hand, the small cells are short axon cells and they have extremely long dendrites. This is their appearance in the lateral geniculate nucleus and in VL. (I can't see much difference between VL and VB but then I have not studied them intensively.) The terminal portions of the long dendrites give rise to complicated beaded branches which form claws or nests. These processes may be much better developed in the monkey than in the cat. They are dendritic processes but I have often thought, "What beautiful axons they would make."

In Golgi impregnations of the thalamus it is often difficult to tell which nucleus one is looking at. In Nissl preparations nuclear boundaries are much better outlined. But when a few cells are impregnated it is often difficult to decide whether a particular cell is on the boundary of one nucleus or the other. I am certain of the identification of one nucleus I have looked at recently; it is the parafascicular nucleus and the finding here may also be true of the other intralaminar nuclei. The cells are completely different; they are not like those in the typical thalamic nuclei. The neurons of the parafascicular nucleus have many body spines and extremely long dendrites; They resemble somewhat the large cells in the reticular formation.

I have not seen the small granular cells that the Scheibels show. When I first saw them on the screen I though they looked somewhat like oligos. But the Scheibels demonstrate their neuronal character by showing their contact with mossy rosette-like terminals. In the striatum Ramon y Cajal described "dwarf" or "neurogliaform" nerve cells which he illustrated in his figure 325, D and E (1911). We are convinced now that one of these cells (E) is an oligo because in fortunate impregnations of the striatum we have seen similar cells with their processes in continuity with myelinated fibers.

PURPURA:

Perhaps Dr. Fox can respond to a question of a general nature. A number of years ago the question of recurrent inhibition in the thalamus was brought into focus in discussion about whether there were sufficient Golgi cells and axon-collaterals of relay cells. The Scheibels were also quite concerned about the morphological basis of recurrent inhibition in the spinal cord. Now we know that Renshaw cells are indeed present in the ventromedial region of the ventral horm but they do not have short axons. Rather they possess long axons that may extend for several segments. Golgi cells have now been seen by the Scheibels in the thalamus but this still raises the question of the extent to which specific relay cells such as in ventrobasal thalamus possess axon-collaterals?

FOX:

I would like to see the Scheibels' preparations. In the adult monkey we have not succeeded in impregnating the axons of the large neurons. We have been able to impregnate only the initial segment of these axons and we assume that at this point the axon acquires a myelin sheath. This is not to say that myelinated fibers cannot be impregnated by the Golgi technique. Maybe it's a matter of luck. The axons of Purkinje cells are medullated and we have found them in our adult preparations but we have not found the axons of the relay thalamic cells impregnated.

PURPURA:

But collaterals?

FOX:

You see, if you don't get the axons impregnated, you're not going to get the collaterals. (Laughter.)

Corticothalamic Projections and Sensorimotor Activities
T. Frigyesi, E. Rinvik, and M.D. Yahr, editors. © 1972
Raven Press, New York.

Cortical Control of Thalamic Sensorimotor Relay Activities in the Cat and the Squirrel Monkey

Tamas L. Frigyesi and Robert Schwartz

The concept that corticofugal control operates on corticopetal inflow at various levels of the neuraxis has gained prominence in current understanding of neural function (3, 8, 14, 26, 37). This phenomenon has been extensively studied with respect to various sensory systems (1, 2, 7, 28, 34, 36, 61, 65). However, only meager consideration has been given to the issue of the control which the motor cortex exerts over proprioceptive activities. It has long been recognized that operations of thalamic nuclei are dependent on the integrity of those cortical fields upon which they project; that is, thalamic nuclei connected to the cerebellum function properly only when they are also linked to an intact motor cortex (27). The present study focuses attention on the centrifugal control in the dorsal thalamus over activities of proprioceptive origin which supply prominent inputs to corticospinal neurons; it also attempts to expound on the mechanisms which are involved in the corticofugal gaiting of corticopetal activities in the dorsal thalamus.

It has been demonstrated in previous studies that the specific cerebellar outflow system, the brachium conjunctivum (BC), provides a major input to corticospinal neurons (17, 21). Proprioceptive impulses arising in the muscle spindle, joint, tendon, skin and end-organs of the vestibular, visual and auditory systems converge in cerebellar subsystems which, in turn, project onto the motor cortex by relaying through various nuclei of the dorsal thalamus (17, 21, 22). Nucleus ventralis lateralis (VL) is the principal relay nucleus in the dorsal thalamus involved in establishing functional contact between the motor cortex and deep cerebellar nuclei. BC axons radiate profusely into VL but also impinge on neurons in many other nuclei of the rostral half of the dorsal thalamus (22). VL neurons are engaged not only by BC axons but also by fibers which originate in dorsal thalamus, basal ganglia (BG), substantia nigra (SN) or reticular formation (RF) (19—21, 23, 46—50). On the other hand, virtually complete disappearance of VL neurons was observed following extirpation of the motor cortex (MC).(40). These diverse inputs and the virtually unimodal output of this nucleus indicate that VL is not only a relay station serving merely to direct the transmission of impulses between the cerebellum and motor cortex, but is also a region where signals of proprioceptive origin are processed prior to reaching neurons in the motor cortex. Intra-VL transactions effected by medial and midline thalamic nuclei, various components of BG, SN and brain-stem RF have previously been subjected to scrutiny (15-17, 19-25, 44-52). It was demonstrated that activities generated in these structures gain access, via synaptic pathways, to VL neurons where they transform patterns of activities in the cerebellothalamic projections to different patterns of activities in the thalamocortical radiation. The purpose of this paper is to define mechanisms and operational characteristics of those corticothalamic projection activities which effect intra-VL transactions and transform patterns of prethalamic impulses to different patterns of postthalamic discharges within the cerebellocortical projections system.

The experiments were performed on encéphale isolé or gas (Penthrane) anesthetized cats and squirrel monkeys (Saimiri sciureus) in a manner described previously (19, 24).

FIG. 1. Characteristics of rostral internal capsule (IC, at open triangles) evoked intracellularly recorded activities from VL neurons in the cat. Upper traces in this and in all subsequent figures are surface recordings from the motor cortex (MC): negativity is signalled by an upward deflection. Lower traces are intracellular recordings from VL neurons; negativity is signalled by a downward deflection. Voltage calibrations in all figures refer to the intracellular recordings. A and B illustrate identification of a relay neuron. A, brachium conjunctivum (BC, at upward arrow) stimulus elicits a monosynaptic EPSP of 0.9 msec latency, a superimposed spike discharge and a succeeding IPSP in this VL neuron, and a relayed potential in the MC. B, IC stimulus elicits an antidromic spike in the VL neuron. Capsular stimulation also elicits a small EPSP following the antidromic spike and a succeeding prolonged IPSP in this unit. Concomitantly, complex multiphasic potentials are demonstrable in MC. C-E, recordings from another VL neuron are shown on superimposed traces. C, IC stimuli elicited antidromic potentials and succeeding EPSP-IPSP sequences are shown. Capsular stimuli elicit complex potentials in MC. D, recordings from the VL neuron at two levels of polarization. IC stimuli now fail to elicit antidromic potentials, but generate monosynaptic EPSPs which trigger single spike discharges. An IC evoked monosynaptic EPSP is seen in isolation in the hyperpolarized trace. The IC evoked polysynaptic EPSPs and prolonged IPSPs exhibit similar temporal properties on both traces. E, IC stimuli elicit, in one trace, an antidromic, in the second trace, an orthodromic (monosynaptic) spike discharge. The evoked polysynaptic excitatory and inhibitory potentials exhibit identical electrographic properties in both traces. F-H demonstrate recordings from a third VL neuron. F, the IC stimulus elicits a monosynaptic EPSP which triggers a spike discharge and succeeding complex polysynaptic excitatory and inhibitory potentials. G, concomitant with the capsular stimulus, a spontaneous spike occurs which prevents the IC evoked monosynaptic EPSP from triggering a spike discharge. The latency of the late spike discharge, G, coincides with that of the polysynaptic EPSP, seen in isolation during hyperpolarization, H.

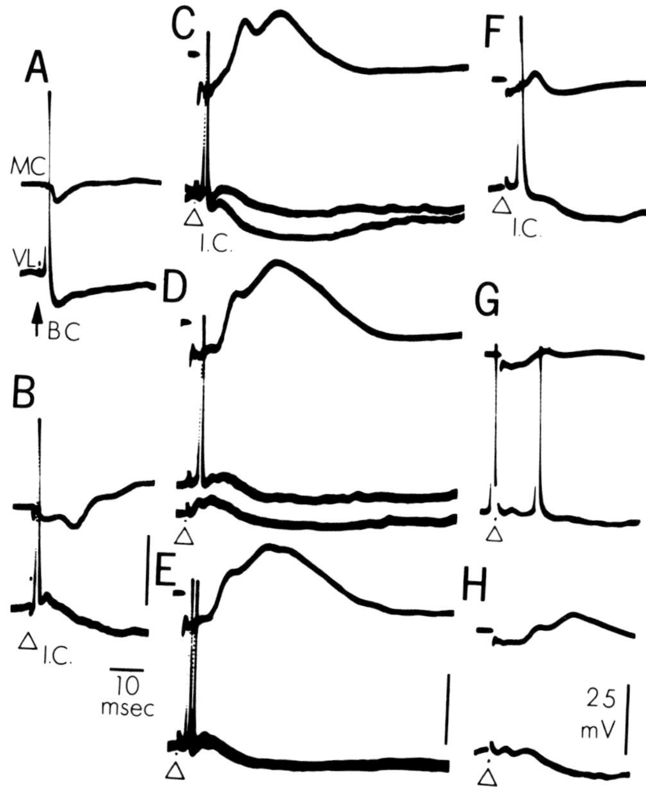

FIG. 1.

Operational Characteristics of the Reciprocal Projections Between the Motor Cortex and VL.

VL* neurons have conveniently been divided into two groups by electrophysiologists: 1. relay, and 2. non-relay neurons (19, 42, 57, 62, 63). This dichotomy is

----

*The difficulties involved in delineating the VA-VL boundary in the cat based only on cytoarchitecture have been well documented (39, 54). There are also inherent difficulties in determining the exact thalamic locations from which intracellular recordings are obtained even when the tapered shaft of the recording glass micropipette is identified histologically, but intracellular staining had not been employed. Therefore, the identification of neurons here was based on combined histological and electrophysiological methods. Consequently, the thalamic area designated here as VL includes caudal parts of VA and excludes the most dorsal layer of VL where neurons are uninfluenced by cerebellofugal activities. The differences in species introduce additional difficulties in identifying the primate homologues of those feline neurons whose electrophysiological properties were extensively studied in the cat (vide infra).

based on the observed presence or absence of MC evoked antidromic invasion of those VL neurons which exhibit orthodromic responsiveness to cerebellar nuclear or BC stimulation. The group of non-relay VL neurons has been further subdivided according to their mono- or polysynaptic responsiveness to cerebellofugal activities (19, 20). Fig. 1 A and B depict characteristics of intracellular recordings from a VL relay neuron. Figure 1, C-E, illustrates another VL neuron whose axon radiates to the motor cortex, as indicated by the antidromic invasion of its soma during low-frequency (8/sec) stimulation of the internal capsule (IC); but failure of antidromic invasion by capsular stimulation was frequently encountered in this neuron (Fig. 1, D and E). In view of the high incidence of similar observations in VL, it cannot be stated that neurons such as illustrated in Fig. 1 F-H are non-relay neurons because antidromic spike generation was not observed during the entire period of capsular stimulation. Most investigators who have studied VL neurons during IC or MC stimulation have uniformly reported that only 15-40% of VL neurons exhibited antidromic spikes under these conditions (19, 55, 57, 62, 63). These findings, however, do not imply that only a similar percentage of VL neurons project onto the motor cortex. Although antidromic stimulation generally is an effective technique for identification of neurons, its frequent failure to invade the soma of thalamic neurons restricts its usefulness as a guiding criterion for the dichotomy of VL neurons. The prominent limitations of this technique in this respect are obviated, however, by those anatomical studies (vide supra) which reveal that virtually all neurons in VL degenerate after extensive destruction of the motor cortex. Consequently, the dichotomy of VL neurons among relay and non-relay elements based on electrophysiological criteria stands on tenuous grounds and is in conflict with anatomical observations.

FIG. 2. Long-latency excitation of VL neurons by corticofugal and cerebellofugal projection activities. A-C, D-F, and G-I, intracellular recordings from 3 VL neurons. A-C, responsiveness of this VL neuron to IC stimulation is similar to that described in Fig. 1 B and C. In this neuron, however, IC stimuli induced late EPSPs arising from the IC evoked IPSPs are also demonstrable. D-F, responsiveness of this neuron to BC stimulation is similar to that described in Fig. 1A. In this neuron, however, BC stimuli induced late EPSPs arising from the BC evoked IPSPs are also demonstrable. Note the relatively small variations of latencies of these late depolarizations. In E, the BC evoked late EPSP triggers a spike discharge. F, after prolonged impalement, the neuron has deteriorated and the BC evoked monosynaptic and late EPSPs are seen uncomplicated by spike discharges. G, BC evoked monosynaptic EPSP triggers a spike discharge. Late depolarization is seen arising from the BC evoked IPSP. H, IC evoked polysynaptic EPSP triggers a spike discharge and is succeeded by a prolonged IPSP. Late depolarization is seen arising from the IC evoked IPSP. I, IC evoked monosynaptic EPSP and late depolarization arising from the IC evoked IPSP are seen. H-I, latencies of the IC evoked late depolarizations are longer than those elicited by BC stimulation.

Less uncertainty exists with respect to the orthodromic responses in VL neurons generated via corticothalamic projections during MC or IC stimulation. Low-frequency (8/sec) stimulation of corticothalamic projections elicited short and long-latency excitatory and inhibitory postsynaptic potentials (EPSPs and IPSPs) in VL neurons. The short (less than 8 msec) latency orthodromic responses were 1. monosynaptic EPSPs, 2. polysynaptic EPSPs and 3. IPSPs (Fig. 1). Development of evoked EPSPs and succeeding IPSPs were not dependent upon prior antidromic invasion of the soma of VL neurons (Fig. 1). Moreover, IC evoked excitatory-inhibitory sequences in these neurons exhibited similar electrographic properties irrespective of the presence or absence of an

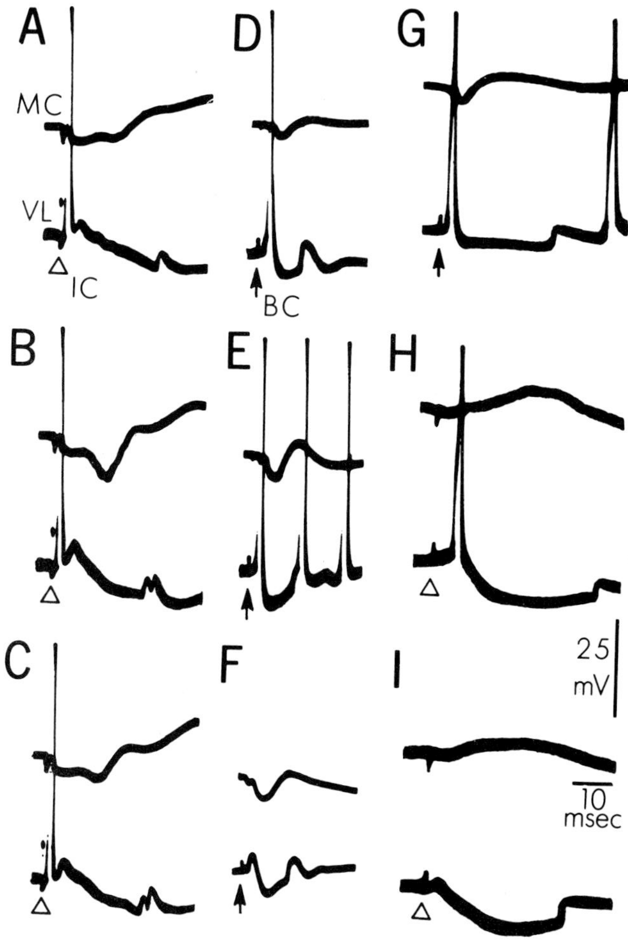

FIG. 2

initial antidromic spike in these elements (Fig. 1 E). The existence of recurrent collaterals in ventrolateral and medial thalamus has been a controversial issue, whereas abundant cortico-VL fibers have been convincingly demonstrated in anatomical studies (53). It follows therefore, that the virtual omnipresence of orthodromic postsynaptic potentials (PSPs) in VL neurons during electrical stimulation of MC or IC indicates the operation of an extensive corticothalamic projection system.

In this study, electrical stimulations which elicited anti- and orthodromic potentials in a VL neuron were frequently confined to discrete areas in the corona radiata (CR) immediately below the motor cortex. In contrast to IC stimulation, which elicited PSPs in the vast majority of VL neurons, CR stimulation, with a single pair of electrodes, was frequently ineffective in generating PSPs in these units. However, a search along pairs of electrode arrays inserted to CR generally resulted in the location of a restricted area wherefrom antidromic potentials and subsequent PSPs in the same VL neurons could be induced. We can state therefore that restricted areas in the motor cortex are orthodromically linked to the regions within VL which project upon them. These findings indicate that the motor cortex and the dorsal thalamus are reciprocally linked to one another in a highly topographical manner. It is to be emphasized, however, that evidence for reverberating activities (11) within this corticothalamic circuit was not obtained.

During MC and IC stimulation, the antidromic and evoked short-latency orthodromic PSPs were frequently followed by long-latency (15-50 msec), small EPSPs in many VL neurons (Fig. 2 A-C, H and I). During BC stimulation, long-latency (8-30 msec) EPSPs were encountered in many of these elements which also exhibited monosynaptic EPSPs with a superimposed spike discharge and a succeeding IPSP (Fig. 2 D-F and G).

The latencies of these IC and BC evoked late EPSPs varied extensively in the sample (8-50 msec) but in each neuron they varied only over a narrow range. Since the prominent background activity of VL neurons hindered the identification and measurement of latencies of these small, late EPSPs, the latency histograms were derived from only those late depolarizing waves which arose from a level of prominent hyperpolarization when the background activities were virtually abolished. Thus these late EPSPs were seen in isolation, and their latencies were precisely measured. The latency histogram shown in Fig. 3 indicates that these late EPSPs in VL neurons were not random occurrences following MC, CR or IC and BC stimulation. The distribution of latencies indicates that 1. late EPSPs exhibiting the shortest latencies (8-14 msec) were driven by only BC stimuli; 2. those exhibiting intermediate latencies (15-30 msec) were driven by both MC and BC stimuli; and 3. those exhibiting the longest latencies (35-50 msec) were driven by only MC stimuli (see also Steriade, Chapter in this volume). Since these late EPSPs were elicited by axonal stimulation of corticofugal and cerebellofugal projections, and since both of these projections are comprised of relatively large axons (Rinvik, Chapter in this volume), the long latencies of these EPSPs can be accounted for by conduction through intrathalamic (intra-VL?) polysynaptic chains. The diagram in Figure 3 illustrates three arrangements of intrathalamic synaptic organizations which may account for the generation of these late EPSPs in VL neurons. The diagrams are justified on the grounds of parsimony and not by excluding alternative hypotheses. (In view of Rinvik's observations, Chapter in this volume, and Jones and Powell's findings (31) conduction through complex intra-VL dendrodendritic chains is very likely.) The data suggest the operation of at least three types of intrathalamic (VL) polysynaptic excitatory chains which are: 1. available only to cerebellofugal but unavailable to corticofugal activities; 2. available to cortico-VL but unavailable to cerebellofugal activities; and 3. available to both

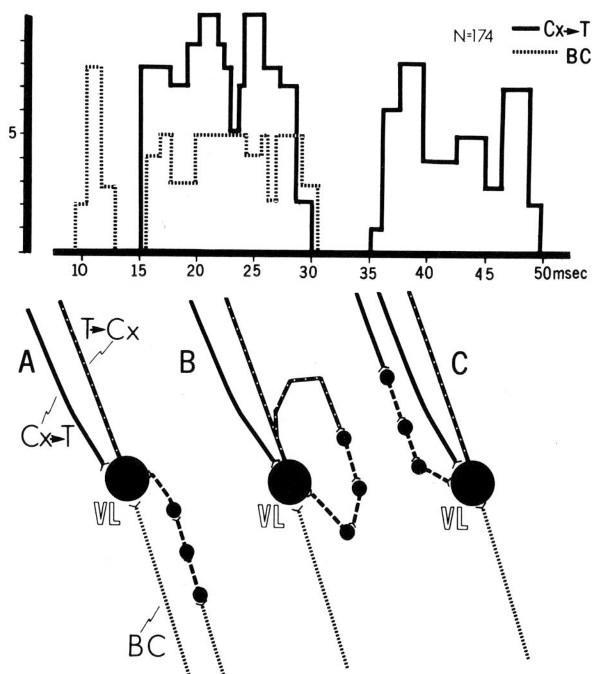

FIG. 3. Frequency distribution of the late EPSPs in VL neurons during stimulation of corticothalamic and cerebellothalamic projections. Ordinates denote the number, abscissae indicate the latencies (in msec) of late EPSPs. Abbreviations: BC, brachium conjunctivum; VL, n. ventralis lateralis; Cx → T, corticothalamic projections; T → Cx, thalamocortical projections. A illustrates an intrathalamic polysynaptic chain which is engaged only by BC fibers. B illustrates an intrathalamic polysynaptic chain which is available to both cortico- and cerebellothalamic projection activities via a recurrent collateral. C illustrates an intrathalamic polysynaptic chain which is engaged only by corticothalamic fibers. In view of Rinvik's observations regarding the abundance of dendrodendritic synapses in VL (Chapter in this volume), these polysynaptic chains may reflect dendrodendritic synapses arranged in series. Further description in text.

corticofugal and cerebellofugal activities. Since the latencies were measured in a highly selected sample (vide supra), the histogram showing their distribution does not reflect the actual proportion of these three types of synaptic organizations in VL; it merely indicates that they are constituents of intra-VL synaptic systems. However, these functional data are not being used here as evidence of the existence of anatomic structures not yet or only provisionally demonstrated (41). The intrathalamic polysynaptic chains illustrated in Figure 3 are considered as solely functional entities. A powerful argument may be raised against the foregoing interpretation of the data: all long fiber systems entering the thalamus exhibit reduction of diameter of the constituent axons when compared to their prethalamic sizes (30, 31, 53). Moreover, some corticothalamic fibers follow a tortuous route. These facts make it virtually impossible to determine the conduction velocities of corticothalamic fibers with any degree of certainty when only stimulating-recording site distances and latencies of evoked EPSPs are available for this purpose. It may also be noted that inasmuch as the line of inquiry is solely dependent upon intracellular recordings or other electrophysiological techniques, the question of what kind of VL cells (relay, non-relay, or "interneuron") are engaged by corticothalamic axons, cannot be answered with certainty (41).

These studies, utilizing intracellular recording techniques to obtain information about the functional properties of VL neurons, restricted the scope of inquiry. These studies have indicated that: 1. VL neurons are connected serially as well as reciprocally with the motor cortex in a topographical manner; 2. single stimuli to corticofugal projections elicit complex effects in VL neurons; and 3. a variety of synaptic pathways impinge on VL neurons which generate prominent ongoing activities and constant interactions in these elements. These observations are in consonance with numerous anatomical (27, 30-32) and electrophysiological studies (17, 19, 20, 23, 25, 29, 44, 45). Nevertheless, these observations also indicate that intracellular recordings from VL neurons provide ambiguous information regarding the mechanisms and operations of these elements as separate entities. Individual characteristics of VL neurons are virtually embedded in the operation of the MC-VL-MC circuit which is powerfully affected by complex interactions in the thalamus (vide infra). While the studies described above have highlighted the elaborately interrelated operation of single VL neurons, they alone have little obvious relevance to the role of VL units in the intact MC-VL-MC circuit. Therefore it was deemed necessary to extend the scope of inquiry to the study of whole-circuit properties of the reciprocal VL-MC relationship. Since effective isolation of VL neurons is unfeasible, it was conjectured that the analysis of averaged effects taking place simultaneously in populations of VL neurons would yield a more complete picture of the contribution of thalamic neurons to the operation of the MC-VL-MC circuit.

The highly topographical arrangement of the reciprocal thalamocortical projections (vide supra) permits the concomitant anti- and orthodromic activation of VL neurons by simultaneously stimulating both fiber systems (corticothalamic and thalamocortical) which link discrete areas in MC to respective discrete areas in VL, provided that localized stimuli are applied to discrete areas within CR. Under these conditions, focal potentials (population responses) (21) in the electrothalamogram indicate the generation of both antidromic and succeeding orthodromic potentials in VL (Fig. 4A).

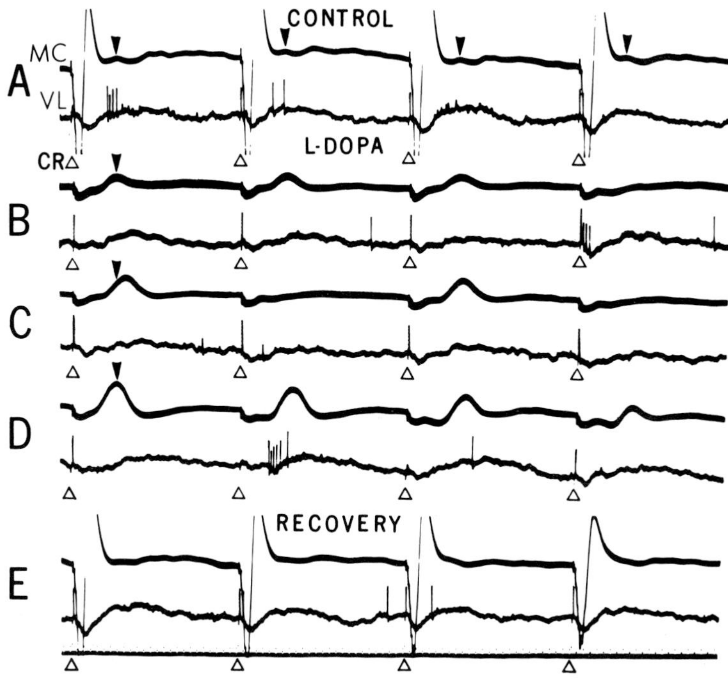

FIG. 4. Effects of L-DOPA on evoked potentials in VL and MC elicited by low-frequency (8/sec) stimulation of corona radiata (CR, at open triangles) in the squirrel monkey. B, 8 minutes; C, 15 minutes; and D, 20 minutes after i.p. administration of 200 mg L-DOPA in combination with a decarboxilase inhibitor, 32 mg MK-486 (alpha-methyl dopa hydrazine). A, control responses evoked by stimulation of CR. In VL, antidromic potentials and succeeding orthodromically evoked negative-positive waves are demonstrable. In MC, complex waves are seen reflecting anti- and orthodromic activation of fibers of the reciprocal thalamocortical circuit. Downward arrow heads are equidistant from the stimulus artifacts, and point to small surface negative deflections. B-D, following administration of L-DOPA: In VL, CR evoked antidromic potentials continue to be demonstrable, but the orthodromic potentials are severely attenuated. In MC, CR evoked prominent early responses are virtually abolished. Under these conditions, CR evoked negativities, which were barely detectable in the control record (at arrow heads), B, become prominent, and C, exhibit alternating, incrementing and, D, decrementing characteristics. E, recorded 40 minutes after administration of L-DOPA. These recovery records are essentially similar to those of the control, A. Time marker: 5 msec.

These orthodromic potentials were diphasic (negative-positive), reflecting extracellularly the EPSP-IPSP sequences simultaneously generated in a relatively large number of VL neurons (46). Surface activities, recorded concomitantly from the MC, also revealed short-latency anti- and orthodromic potentials (Fig. 4 A). Thus, low-frequency (8/sec) stimulation of restricted areas within CR brought the thalamocortical circuit into action.

The trajectories of the major components of this VL-MC-VL circuit have been demonstrated in anatomical (40, 43, 53) and characterized in electrophysiological (4, 19, 20, 57, 63, 66) studies. However, the contributions of the individual elements of this subsystem were obscured by the whole-circuit operation. It appeared that partial decomposition of this complex subsystem of thalamocortical circuits would provide an understanding of its internal organization. L-DOPA and strychnine, administered systematically, were used in attempts to reduce this complex circuit into its constituents. Both of these drugs were equally effective and induced similar effects in simplifying the CR evoked effects in VL and MC. The effects of L-DOPA on the operation of this thalamocortical circuit are shown in Fig. 4 B-D. In VL, CR evoked antidromic potentials were unaffected but the orthodromic potentials (excitatory-inhibitory sequences) were severely attenuated following administration of L-DOPA. In MC, components of the CR evoked early complex potentials were either abolished or severely reduced in amplitude. Under these conditions, CR stimulation elicited prominent negative waves which exhibited 20-30 msec latencies, and incrementing, alternating and decrementing characteristics during prolonged 8/sec stimulation. The control record in Fig. 4 indicates that 8/sec CR stimulation, prior to the administration of L-DOPA, elicited only barely detectable negativities of comparable latencies in MC. Surface negative waves in the MC exhibiting similar properties were commonly observed during 8-12/sec stimulation of medial and midline thalamic nuclei. (Reasons for the use of this terminology, instead of "nonspecific" or "diffuse" projection systems, were discussed previously (19)). These data are consonant with the notion that 8/sec CR stimulation, following administration of L-DOPA, orthodromically activates MT and MeT nuclei as effectively as localized thalamic stimulation does. Inasmuch as anatomical studies (Rinvik, Chapter in this volume) have revealed that discrete loci in MC project to both VL and MeT nuclei, stimulation of restricted areas in CR obviously activates MC-VL and MC-MeT (33) projections. But since in the untreated animal the MC-MeT projections elicited only rudimentary late negative potentials in MC characteristic of low-frequency activation of MeT structures, it is suggested that CR stimulation evoked excitatory effects elsewhere (in the thalamus) and activated mechanisms which, in turn, exerted inhibitory effects on neurons in MeT.

Motor Cortical Effects on Medial Thalamic Neurons.

Figure 5 shows that corticofugal synaptic pathways indeed engage neurons in MeT and generate prolonged inhibitory effects in these units (25). Low-frequency stimulation of CR elicited PSPs in the vast majority of MeT neurons. In virtually all instances the initial CR evoked synaptic effect was an EPSP which exhibited a latency of 2–3 msec. Two types of early EPSPs were encountered: 1. those of long duration and compounded of several components; and 2. those of short duration. Both types of EPSPs were succeeded by evoked, prolonged (50–100 msec) IPSPs. Although the data do not reveal the exact latencies for the CR evoked apparently long-latency IPSPs in MeT neurons, those depicted in Fig. 5 A–D show latencies of less than 5 msec. Inasmuch as the shortest latencies exhibited by CR evoked EPSPs in ventrolateral and

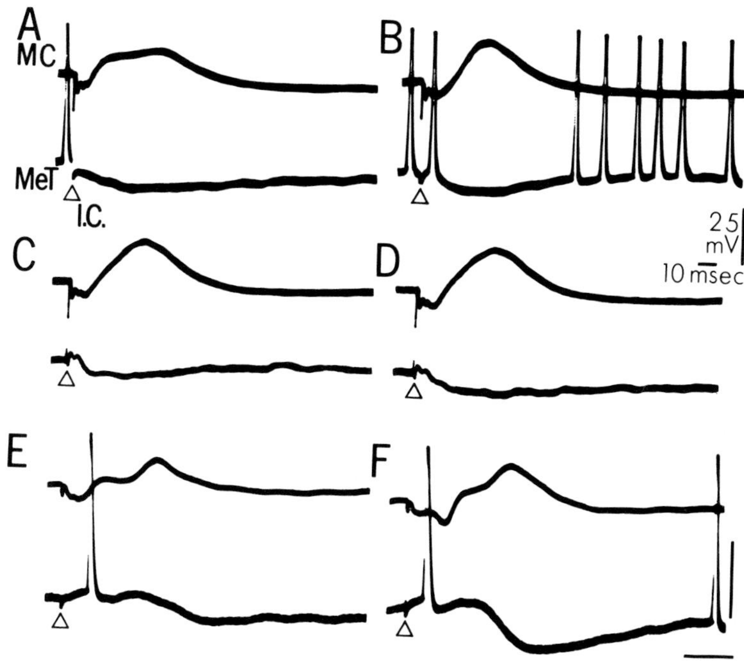

FIG. 5. Corticofugal projection activities evoked PSPs in medial thalamic (MeT) neurons in the cat. Stimuli to the rostral internal capsule (IC) delivered at 8/sec. A, IC stimulus coincides with the declining phase of a spontaneous spike discharge in a MeT neuron. The IC evoked IPSP exhibits the shortest latency under this condition. B, same cell, IC evoked IPSP is preceded by a short-latency EPSP with a superimposed spike discharge. C–D, another cell. IC stimulation elicits short latency (less than 3 msec) EPSPs and succeeding prolonged (30–70 msec) IPSPs. Small field potentials are seen anterior to the evoked EPSP. E–F, a third neuron. IC stimulation elicits prolonged EPSPs which are compounded of several components indicative of polysynaptic excitation of this neuron. In E, abrupt development of a second major component of the EPSP is seen 10 msec following the shock to IC. In F, prominent late component of the IC evoked IPSP is seen. E–F, IC evoked EPSPs are succeeded by prolonged (50–80 msec) IPSPs. A–F, IC stimuli evoked typical anti- and orthodromic responses are demonstrable in MC.

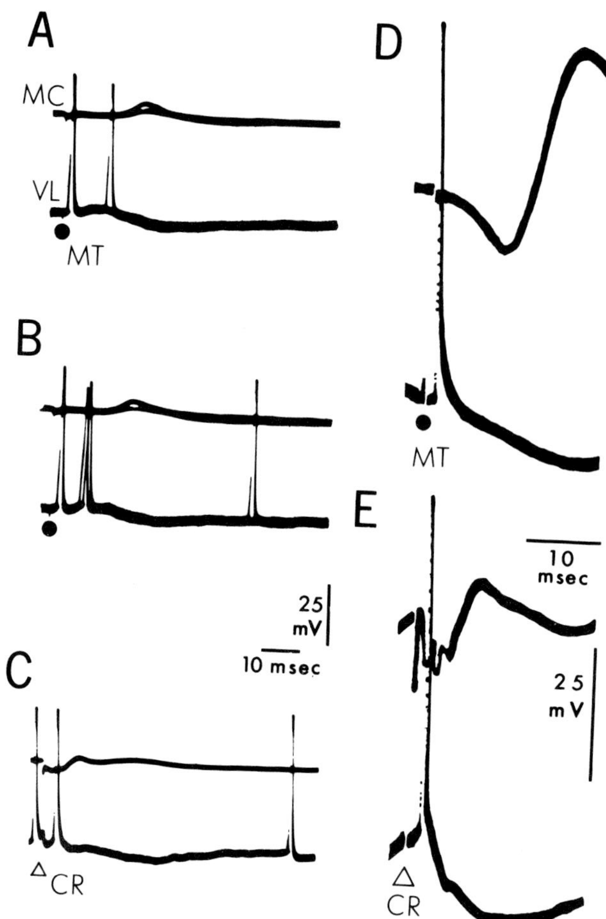

FIG. 6. Antidromic potentials in VL neurons during low-frequency (8/sec) midline thalamic (MT) stimulation, A–C, in the cat and, D–E in the monkey. A–C, same neuron. A–B, superimposed traces, which illustrate recruitment of surface negative waves in the motor cortex, and the stability of latencies of the shortest latency spike discharges in the ventrolateral neuron during MT stimulation (at dots). MT stimuli also elicited prolonged EPSPs in this neuron. Spike discharges are demonstrable at various phases of development of MT evoked EPSPs in this unit. Prolonged IPSPs are seen succeeding the MT evoked EPSPs. C, CR stimuli elicit monosynaptic EPSPs and associated spike discharges in this unit. D–E, same neuron. D, an antidromic spike discharge in the VL neuron, and a recruiting wave in the motor cortex are demonstrable following a stimulus of an 8/sec train to MT. E, a monosynaptic EPSP, in the VL neuron, and a multiphasic potential in the motor cortex are demonstrable following the CR stimulus.

medial thalamic neurons were 1.5-3 msec, temporal properties of the CR evoked short latency IPSPs indicate that they were generated via relatively simple synaptic pathways. These findings also reveal that medial thalamic neurons, similar to VL neurons, are reciprocally linked to the motor cortex.

The great heuristic importance of the problem of motor cortical inhibition in medial thalamus necessitates further discussion of the trajectories involved in the generation of MC evoked IPSPs in MeT neurons. In principle, MC evoked short-latency IPSPs could be generated via 1. recurrent collaterals, impinging on inhibitory neurons with MeT projections, activated antidromically by stimulation of MeT-MC pathways; 2. a monosynaptic pathway from MC to MeT; or 3. an oligosynaptic pathway from MC to MeT with an interposed relay. The first possibility is confronted with strong experimental evidence to the contrary (5, 44). The second possibility may, in fact, be a probability (Albe-Fessard, Chapter in this volume). Experimental data, however, compel one to consider and scrutinize the third possibility. It has recently been reported that electrical stimulation of VL elicits prolonged IPSPs, which exhibit latencies as short as 1.5 msec, in MeT neurons (13). In our study we demonstrated antidromic potentials in VL neurons (Fig. 6) which exhibited 1 msec latencies during MT stimulation. These last two reports indicate the operation of a monosynaptic pathway from VL to MeT. Whether this VL-MeT pathway is inhibitory or it excites inhibitory neurons within MeT cannot be determined from the data at hand. However, consideration of latencies of MC evoked EPSPs in VL and IPSPs in MeT neurons, as well as the latencies of VL evoked IPSPs in MeT neurons (13) indicates that the shortest latency IPSPs in MeT neurons during MC or CR stimulation could have been generated disynaptically by relaying through VL (25). This mechanism readily accounts for observations showing disinhibition of medial thalamic neurons following ablation of the motor cortex (Hassler, Chapter in this volume). Our data further indicate that this MC-VL-MeT projection system is sensitive to metabolites of L-DOPA (Fig. 4). Disinhibition of MeT neurons is induced because MC evoked excitation of VL neurons is abolished following administration of L-DOPA (vide supra).

These findings highlight the structural context and orientation of the parallel circuits which link discrete areas in MC to VL and MeT neurons. Activities arising in MC monosynaptically excite VL neurons (Fig. 1) which, in turn, generate prolonged inhibitory effects in MeT neurons. These MC evoked relayed inhibitory effects on MeT neurons render the MC evoked excitatory effects, other than monosynaptic, ineffective in triggering spike discharges in these elements. The MC evoked monosynaptic excitation in MeT neurons may trigger spike discharges because these synaptic effects develop prior to the MC evoked disynaptic inhibition in these elements. It has long been established that activities arising in MeT generate polysynaptic, prolonged inhibitory effects in VL neurons (46). It was recently shown that such MeT evoked IPSPs could, in part, be the function of neurons in the reticular nucleus (16). Thus the MC-MeT-thalamic reticular nucleus-VL projections represent a feedforward inhibitory system of MC-VL excitatory activities. Discrete points in MC, thus, reciprocally innervate VL and MeT subsystems. This flip-flop arrangement of VL and MeT neurons with respect to effects of MC stimulation (which dictate the operation of reciprocally acting inhibitory pathways) is distinctly different from effects of low-frequency, localized electrical stimulation of VL or MeT structures which are commonly associated with generation of augmenting or recruiting responses, respectively, in the MC. The most interesting new observation here is that pharmacological inactivation of an intrathalamic inhibitory system operating on MeT neurons permits the orthodromic (from MC) activation of the medial thalamic recruiting system (Fig. 6). These processes are germane to the synchronization of activities in the thalamocortical radiations, such as in the VL-MC pathway which receives tonic input from deep cerebellar nuclei (17). The data further corroborate the theorem (44-46) that synchronization of thalamocortical activities depends primarily upon modulatory influences, in this case from the MC, which operate upon thalamic neurons rather than on the pacemaker or autorhythmic properties of thalamic neurons (5-7, 64).

The Mesencephalic Route of Corticothalamic Fibers.

Three trajectories for corticothalamic fibers have been described in anatomical studies: two enter the thalamus from the internal capsule, whereas the third descends to the cerebral peduncle (10, 30, 35, 53, 59) where it turns dorsally and, after funneling through the substantia nigra, radiates into the dorsal thalamus (Fig. 7 K). Particular attention is paid here to those corticothalamic fibers which follow this latter, tortuous route because of their intimate spatial relations to SN. These anatomical observations have prompted an inquiry into the feasibility of studying SN evoked thalamic potentials in isolation, uncomplicated by spurious effects elicited by the concomitant, inadvertent and unavoidable activation of corticothalamic fibers during electrical stimulation of SN. A comparison of Fig. 7I and J shows that the negative waves of the focal VL potentials elicited by IC stimulation were altered by a retrothalamic, prenigral transsection (at the level and direction indicated by arrow, J, in Fig. 7 K), whereas simultaneously recorded surface potentials from the motor cortex appeared to be unaffected. Similar observations were made in cats acutely denigrated by 6-OH Dopamine injected to the ipsilateral substantia nigra (18). These indicate that axons descending into areas caudal to the thalamus are also involved in the generation of thalamic potentials during rostral IC stimulation. Examination of synaptic potentials in VL neurons elicited by IC and *rostral* SN stimulation disclosed that latencies and durations of the IC and rostral SN evoked monosynaptic EPSPs in these elements were virtually identical. However, in contrast to IC stimulation, rostral SN stimulation failed to generate prolonged IPSPs in VL neurons. That is, *rostral* SN stimulation reproduced some of the synaptic events induced by motor-corticofugal activities in VL neurons. Taken together, these data indicate that 1. monosynaptic EPSPs in VL neurons during *rostral* SN or IC stimulation could have been generated via the same pathway, through corticothalamic fibers following the mesencephalic route; and 2. the descending loop of corticothalamic fibers is primarily involved in the generation of excitatory effects in VL neurons. Consequently, activities arising in MC which exert prolonged inhibitory effects in VL neurons by extensive involvement of neurons in the thalamic reticular nucleus (vide infra) traverse primarily along those corticofugal pathways which enter the thalamus from the internal capsule. These findings also indicate that evaluation of evoked effects in thalamic neurons during stimulation of

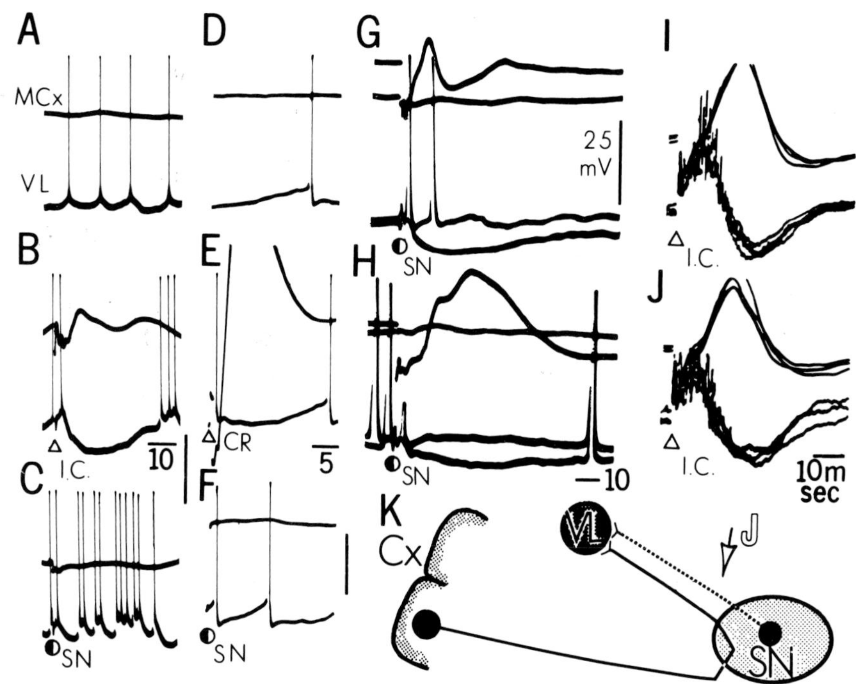

FIG. 7. Activities mediated via the descending loop of corticothalamic fibers. Spatial characteristics of this fiber system is diagrammatically illustrated in K. A–C, intracellular recordings from a VL neuron in the cat. A, background discharges of the neuron. B, rostral internal capsule (IC) evoked monosynaptic EPSP and a succeeding IPSP are seen. C, central substantia nigra (SN) evoked monosynaptic EPSP and the subsequent activities in this neuron are fundamentally different from those seen in B. D–F, intracellular recordings from a VL neuron in the monkey. E, corona radiata (CR) evoked antidromic spike discharge succeeded by small depolarizations arising from an IPSP are demonstrable prior to development of a slow-rising EPSP which is terminated by a spike discharge in much the same way as in the control record, D. F, central SN evoked monosynaptic EPSP. G and H, different VL cells (cat). Two recordings from each neuron are superimposed: one trace was obtained during rostral capsular, the other during rostral nigral stimulation. Note the differences in motor cortex recordings. The shock artifacts of the SN and IC stimuli were aligned and indicated by a symbol, labeled SN. In both cells the monosynaptic EPSPs elicited by both modes of stimulation exhibit similar electrographic properties, whereas the ensuing synaptic events are different. I, capsular stimulation evoked focal potentials in VL and complex surface responses in the motor cortex. J, following retrothalamic, prenigral transsection (at the level indicated by the arrow in the diagram) the capsular evoked surface activities and the focal positivity in VL remained essentially unchanged whereas the focal negativity was reduced in amplitude. Further description in text.

rostral SN demands extreme caution. On the other hand, evoked PSPs in VL neurons during IC or CR and central SN stimulation exhibited prominent differences (Fig. 7 A-F), which indicate that they were generated through different pathways. An inference, of more than heuristic importance, may be drawn from these findings: the descending loop of corticothalamic fibers traverses predominantly the rostral pole and not the central regions of SN. This inference is in accord with the recently reported anatomical study of Carpenter and Peter (10) who observed that appreciable numbers of corticothalamic fibers which project profusely to the CM-Pf complex and paracentral nucleus traverse even caudal parts of SN. But in our electrophysiological study VL neurons were explored in order to gain an understanding of the functional relationship between the descending loop of corticothalamic fibers and nigrothalamic projections. Our observations are also consonant with those of Rinvik (53) showing that only a minority of corticofugal fibers to VL descend to the mesencephalon and pierce only the rostral pole of substantia nigra.

Cortical regulation of transmission in the thalamic relays of the cerebello-corticospinal projection system.

The basic operational characteristics of the specific cerebellofugal projection system and its relationship to the sensorimotor organization in higher mammals has been discussed in detail elsewhere (17). It is pertinent to recall here that, when electrical stimulation is applied only to the specific cerebellofugal projection system (deep cerebellar nuclei or brachium conjunctivum (BC)) of the encéphale isolé or gas (Penthrane) anesthetized, succinylcholine paralized cat, each action potential in the BC axons induces an action potential in the thalamocortical radiation, which, in turn, elicits an action potential in the corticospinal tract (21). That is, one-to-one synaptic relationships and high synaptic security are prominent characteristics of the cerebello-corticospinal projection system.

It has also been established that high-frequency (up to 100/sec) BC stimulation evokes trains of discharges in the cerebellothalamic pathway, which are converted to phasic activities in the thalamocortical radiation and in the corticospinal tract during low-frequency (8/sec) stimulation of MeT nuclei, head of the caudate nucleus, or internal pallidal segment as well as following systemic administration of atropine, or barbiturates and during slow-sleep (17-23, 44-53). Under these conditions, evoked EPSP-IPSP sequences are observed in the thalamic relay neurons of the cerebellocortical projection system; BC discharges reaching the thalamic relay neurons during the evoked EPSPs elicit mono- or oligosynaptic excitation in these elements and trigger spike discharges which through the thalamocortical pathway provide a powerful input to neurons in the MC. BC discharges reaching the thalamic relay neurons during the evoked IPSPs elicit mono- or oligosynaptic excitation in these elements which fail to trigger spike discharges. Fig. 8 illustrates that when BC stimuli are timed to occur during corticothalamic projection evoked IPSPs, BC stimuli evoked monosynaptic EPSPs fail to trigger spike discharges in the VL neurons. Thus, corticothalamic projection activities may elicit periodically recurring functional discontinuity in VL and other thalamic relays of the cerebellocortical projection system. Since the

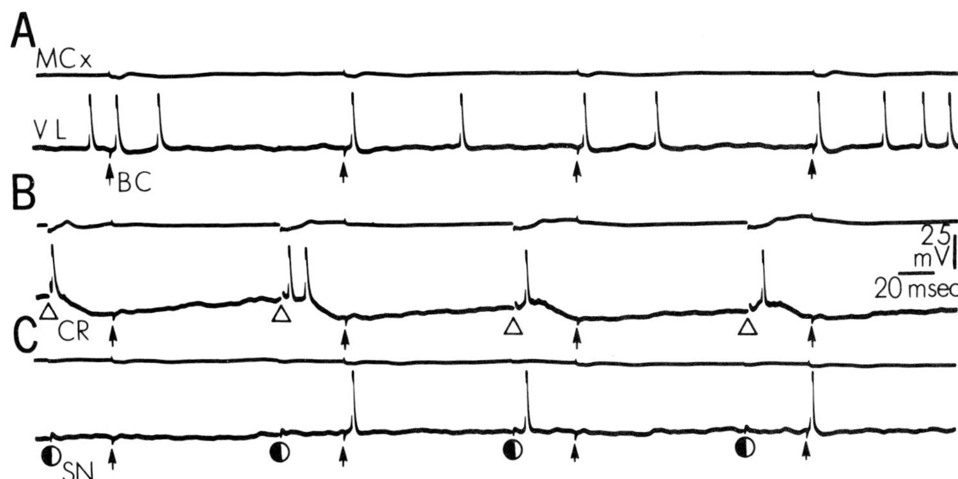

FIG. 8. Patterns of inhibition of VL cell discharges initiated by 8/sec stimulation of brachium conjunctivum (BC, at upward arrows) conditioned by 8/sec stimulation of corona radiata and substantia nigra in the cat. B, CR, and C, SN, stimuli lead the BC stimuli by 35 msec during interactions. A, BC stimuli elicit short-latency spike potentials and succeeding IPSPs in the VL neuron. B, CR stimuli elicit prolonged IPSPs posterior to the evoked EPSPs in this unit. BC evoked discharges and succeeding IPSPs are inhibited and the underlying BC evoked small EPSPs are revealed. C, central SN stimulation. Only alternate BC stimuli trigger cell discharges.

specific cerebellofugal activities form a major input to neurons in the MC, the MC is capable of regulating its own input through this mechanism.

Analyses of probability of firing of BC evoked oligosynaptic EPSPs in the thalamic relay neurons of the cerebellocortical projection pathway in the cat have revealed that corticofugal projection activities induce several patterns of phasic discharges in the thalamocortical radiation concomitant with tonic activation of the BC pathway. During activation of corticothalamic projections, these patterns of transformation of long trains of prethalamic impulses to bursts of postthalamic discharges depend on the mode of development, latencies and durations of evoked IPSPs in neurons in the thalamus between the cerebellum and MC. Four examples of the most commonly observed patterns of IPSP development in VL neurons in the cat during IC stimulation are shown in Fig. 9. These data indicate that the gamut of MC evoked functional discontinuity in the cerebellocortical projection system ranges from a persistent one, through 1:4, 1:5 transformation, to none at all, depending upon development of 1. sustained hyperpolarization due to IPSP summation, 2. EPSPs of 15-25 msec and IPSPs of 60-100 msec duration, and 3. no or barely detectable IPSPs, respectively, during corticothalamic projection activities in the cat.

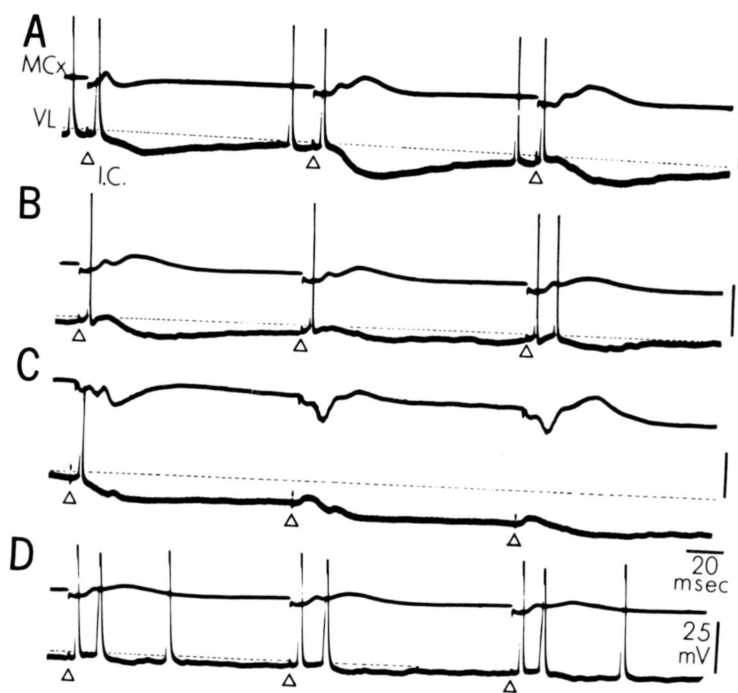

FIG. 9. Examples of characteristics of evoked IPSPs in four different VL neurons during 8/sec internal capsule (IC) stimulation in the cat. Dotted lines are drawn through base of spikes to show relationship between the assumed firing level and synaptically induced membrane potential oscillations. A, IC stimulation elicits EPSP-IPSP sequences. The repetitive stimuli induce gradual prolongation of the evoked EPSPs with resultant curtailment of the evoked IPSPs. B, evoked IPSPs exhibit maximal amplitude following the first capsular stimulus, and attenuate gradually during continued stimulation. C, a prolonged IPSP is seen following the first stimulus which carries the membrane potential below the firing level of the EPSP evoked by the second stimulus. The IPSP evoked by the second stimulus summates with that of the first. Summation of evoked IPSPs during continued stimulation results in a sustained hyperpolarization of the neuron which prevents the capsular evoked EPSPs from triggering cell discharges. D, barely detectable evoked hyperpolarization and a recurrent sequence of spike initiation following each capsular stimulus in an 8/sec train.

Although the basic characteristics of regulation of transmission in the thalamic relay neurons of the specific cerebellofugal projection system in the squirrel monkey are essentially similar to those in the cat (21), certain interaction patterns were commonly encountered in the primate which were only occasionally observed in the

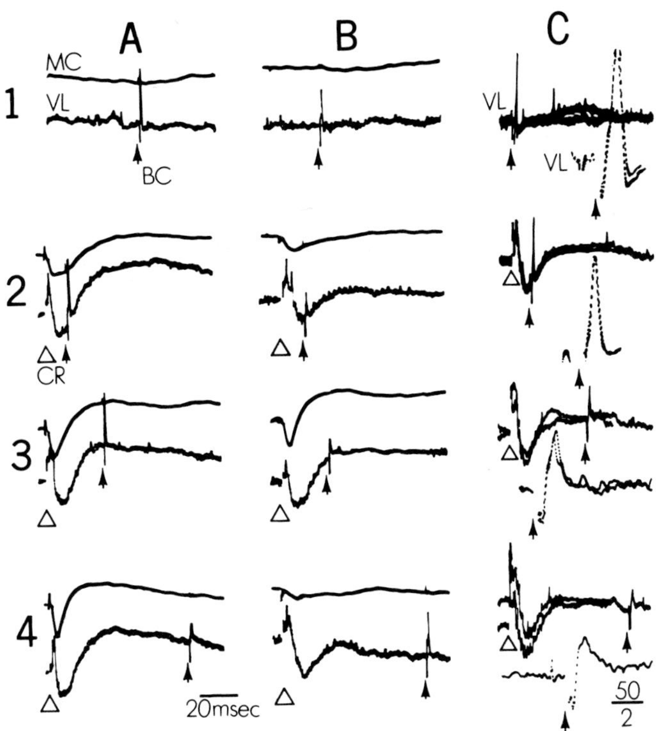

FIG. 10. Inhibition of BC evoked focal potentials in VL by 8/sec stimulation of corona radiata (CR) in the monkey. Surface recordings from the motor cortex are illustrated only in A and B. Unconditioned BC evoked focal potentials are shown in A1, B1 and C1. In C, BC evoked focal VL potentials are illustrated on two time bases; the faster one is at higher amplification. A–C, 2–4, conditioning CR stimuli elicit excitatory-inhibitory (negative-positive) sequences in VL. The duration of these diphasic waves is much shorter in the monkey (30 msec) than in the cat (80–120 msec). B, inhibition of the postsynaptic components of BC evoked focal VL potentials coinciding with the CR evoked focal positivity in VL. A and C, BC evoked focal potentials exhibit amplitudes comparable to those in the control recordings during CR evoked focal positivities in VL; they are severely attenuated or abolished at 40 to 100 msec following each CR stimulus when CR evoked focal activities are no longer demonstrable in VL.

feline thalamus (cf. Hassler, Chapter in this volume). Figure 10 B shows that the most commonly demonstrable interaction pattern between corticofugal and cerebellofugal projection activities in VL in the cat is also demonstrable in the primate. However, Figure 10 A and C illustrate the most commonly encountered patterns of cortical in-

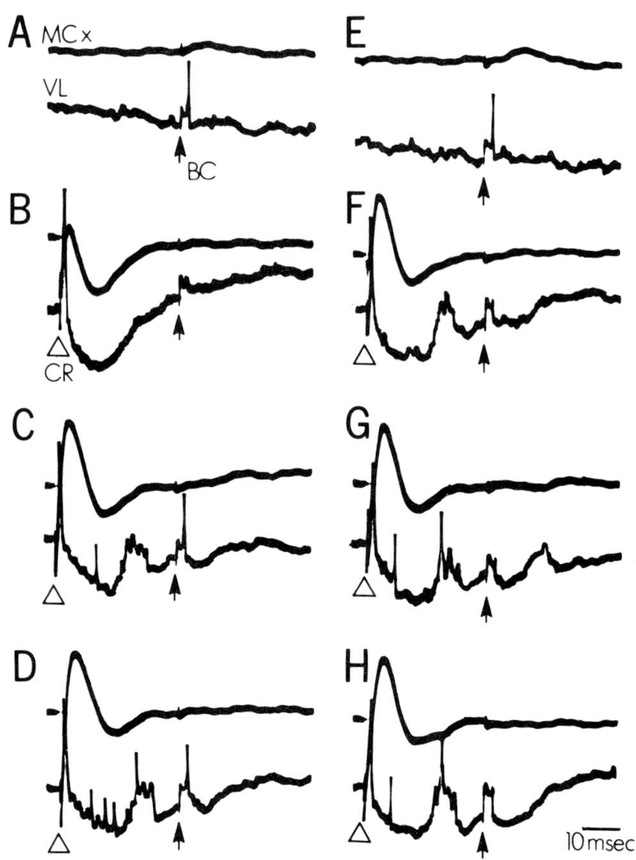

FIG. 11. Characteristic patterns of focal potentials in the primate VL elicited by corticothalamic projection activities. A–D, and E–H, recordings from two intra-VL sites, about 2 mm apart, during the descent of a microelectrode. A and E, 8/sec BC stimuli elicit similar focal potentials at both sites. B–D, and F–H, 8/sec stimulation of corona radiata (CR) elicits short-latency spike discharges and subsequent prominent positive waves. During repetitive stimulation, gradual development of unitary firing and a negative wave are generated by the 8/sec CR stimulation. This negativity arises from the CR evoked prominent positive wave in VL. B shows the inhibitory effects of CR stimuli on BC evoked focal potentials (at 35 msec conditioning-testing intervals). C and D, the CR evoked inhibitory effects are abolished when the negative waves develop despite the prolongation of the CR evoked positivities. F–H, under similar conditions, CR evoked inhibitory effects are sustained at the other recording site.

hibition of cerebellar evoked activities in the primate VL; these patterns were rarely seen in the cat.

Examination of dorsal thalamic areas in the squirrel monkey in which neurons are oligosynaptically driven by cerebellofugal projection activities revealed that corticothalamic projections elicit focal potentials in these regions which exhibit properties unlike those in corresponding regions in the cat. Figure 11 illustrates two recording sites (A-D and E-H), about 2 mm apart, in the monkey thalamus where BC stimulation generated oligosynaptic focal potentials (Fig. 11 A and E). In these regions, CR stimulation evoked short-latency spike discharges and succeeding prominent (20-30 msec duration) positive waves (Fig. 11 B). These potentials are considered to be extracellular reflections of antidromic, mono- and oligosynaptic spikes and succeeding IPSPs demonstrated in intracellular studies (Fig. 7 E), and generated simultaneously in a large population of VL neurons (22). Continued 8/sec stimulation of CR was commonly associated with prolongation (up to 100 msec) of the CR evoked positive waves in the thalamus (Fig. 11, C, D, G and H). Evoked prominent negative waves and spike discharges arose from these prolonged positive waves. These indicate that in the population of neurons in the propinquity of the recording electrode, the constituent neurons had selective and heterogeneous inputs arriving in labelled lines characterized by minimal cross-modality dispersion (45). CR stimulation generated short-latency inhibitory effects in some of these elements while long-latency excitatory effects in others. When BC stimuli were timed to occur coincident with the CR evoked focal positivity in the thalamus (Fig. 11 B), inhibitory interactions were demonstrable. However, during continued stimulation, concomitant with the development of the late excitatory effects in some elements of this neuronal population, CR-BC stimulation at the same conditioning-testing intervals elicited either excitatory (Fig. 11 C, D) or inhibitory (Fig. 11 F-H) interactions. These observations indicate a highly topographical arrangement of corticofugal and cerebellofugal converging pathways on thalamic neuronal organizations in the monkey. This clustering of excitatory and inhibitory intrathalamic systems engaged by corticofugal projections is in apparent contrast with the orderly columnar arrangement (20) of the corresponding pathways converging on thalamic neurons in the cat.

Figure 12 depicts a further elaboration of the complexities of these primate VL neuronal clusters, as opposed to the feline orderly columns, whose constituents receive selective inputs from extra- and intrathalamic sources. The data show that low frequency (8/sec) BC stimuli elicited a multiphasic focal potential in VL, and two short (less than 4 msec) latency positive deflections in the MC (Fig. 12 A). Every alternate BC stimulus triggered a discharge of 2.8-3.1 msec latencies in one of the units of this neuronal cluster in VL and a diphasic evoked potential in the motor cortex. Conditioning CR stimuli severely attenuated the focal potentials but failed to affect the alternating unit discharges in VL, and virtually abolished the relayed potentials in the MC elicited by the testing BC stimuli (Fig. 12 B). On the other hand, conditioning MT stimuli, at the same conditioning-testing intervals, suppressed the BC evoked alternating spike discharges of this unit, but failed to alter the BC evoked focal potentials generated in this VL neuronal cluster, and also increased the probability of development of BC evoked relayed potentials in the MC (Fig. 12 C). Simi-

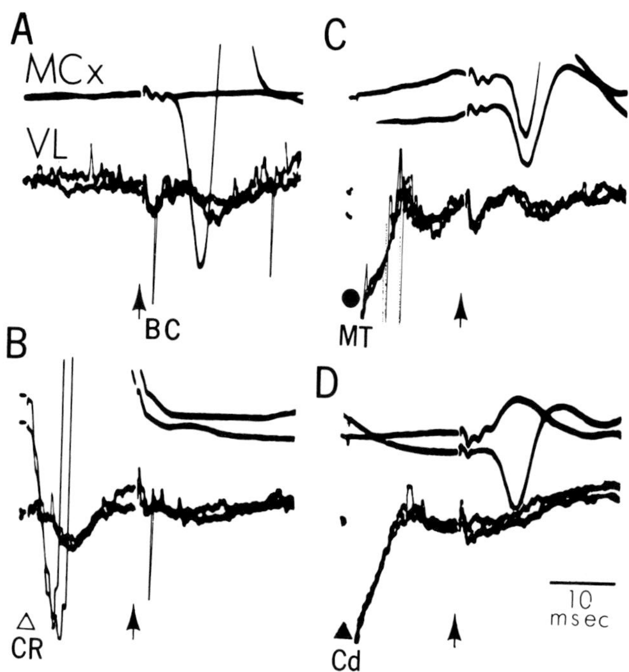

FIG. 12. Characteristics of effects mediated by four intra- and extrathalamic converging pathways on a neuronal population in VL in the monkey. A-D, two traces are superimposed. All stimulations at 8/sec. A, each BC stimulus elicits a multiphasic focal potential in VL and two small positive deflections in the motor cortex. Every alternate BC stimulus elicits a unit discharge in VL and a prominent diphasic (positive-negative) relayed potential in MC. Conditioning stimulation of CR, in B, of midline thalamus (MT), in C, and caudate (Cd), in D, precede the BC stimuli by 20 msec. B, CR stimuli virtually abolish all components of the BC evoked focal VL and relayed cortical potentials but leave the alternating unit discharges unaffected. C, MT stimuli generate short latency (5 msec) negative focal potentials associated with discharges of another VL unit. MT stimuli fail to affect the evoked focal potential, but suppress the alternating unit discharges in VL and facilitate the development of the relayed potential in the cortex following BC stimuli. D, Cd stimuli abolish virtually all BC evoked effects in VL. In the cortex, they abolish the second small positive deflection in one trace, and induce a third small positive deflection as well as inversion of the relayed potential in the other trace following the BC stimuli.

larly timed conditioning Cd stimuli abolished both the BC evoked focal potential and alternating unit discharges in VL but failed to affect the probability of the development of BC evoked relayed potentials in the MC (Fig. 12 D). These data indicate that this neuronal cluster was engaged by cerebellofugal, corticofugal, medial thalamic and caudatofugal synaptic pathways. However, the individual elements within this cluster with different convergence characteristics were not arranged in a plane as in the feline thalamus (20). These data also indicate that the intrathalamic synaptic networks attached to BC axons in the squirrel monkey exhibit complexities which were not observed in studies of the intrathalamic parallel pathways linking the cerebellum to the MC in the cat (19-23). Corticofugal, medial thalamic, basal ganglia and substantia nigra projection activities, in general, lose their modality specificities upon entering the intrathalamic interneuronal machinery in the cat. Polysynaptic responses in medial and ventrolateral thalamic neurons elicited by these projections are remarkably similar, and exhibit notable differences only in their latencies. Accordingly, the interaction patterns between cerebellofugal and MC, MeT, BG or SN projection activities are virtually identical in the feline thalamic neurons. In the squirrel monkey, however, MC, MeT, BG or SN pathways engage intrathalamic synaptic networks with largely different internal organizational characteristics. Each of these intrathalamic polysynaptic systems projects in a distinct manner upon thalamic neurons with cerebellar input. Individual characteristics of MC, MeT, BG or SN projection activities are obliterated within these intrathalamic synaptic machineries to a lesser degree in the squirrel monkey than in the cat. Accordingly, the interaction patterns between MC, MeT, BG or SN and cerebellar projection activities are prominently dissimilar in the primate thalamic neurons.

The Thalamic Reticular Nucleus and Motor Cortex Evoked Inhibition in VL.

The foregoing data have indicated that corticothalamic projections elicit excitatory-inhibitory sequences in thalamic neurons in the cerebellocortical projection system in both the cat and squirrel monkey. The data also show that the inhibitory components of these MC evoked rhythmic activities in the thalamus induce periodic functional discontinuities in the cerebellocortical projection system. Several patterns of phasic activities in thalamocortical radiation have been described in this study as dependent upon modes of development, durations and latencies of IPSPs in the thalamic neurons induced by corticothalamic projection activities. The mechanisms involved in the generation of these IPSPs, which effectively gait cerebellofugal activities in thalamic neurons, have aroused considerable interest and several theories have been advanced to account for them (5-7, 44-46, 64).

It has been previously proposed, on the basis of structural data, that neurons in the thalamic reticular nucleus (nR) may initiate episodic suppressive activity (59) in the principal thalamic nuclei upon which they project (12, 58). Electrophysiological data from several laboratories have indicated that reciprocal relationships exist between extracellularly recorded unitary firings in VL (38, 46, 60) and several other thalamic nuclei (64) and in rostral nR. Figure 13 A and B show intracellular recordings from a neuron in the dorsolateral nR, and from another neuron in the adjacent VL during 8/sec stimulation of corticothalamic projections. The major effect of low-frequency CR or IC stimulation on dorsolateral nR neurons is the development of

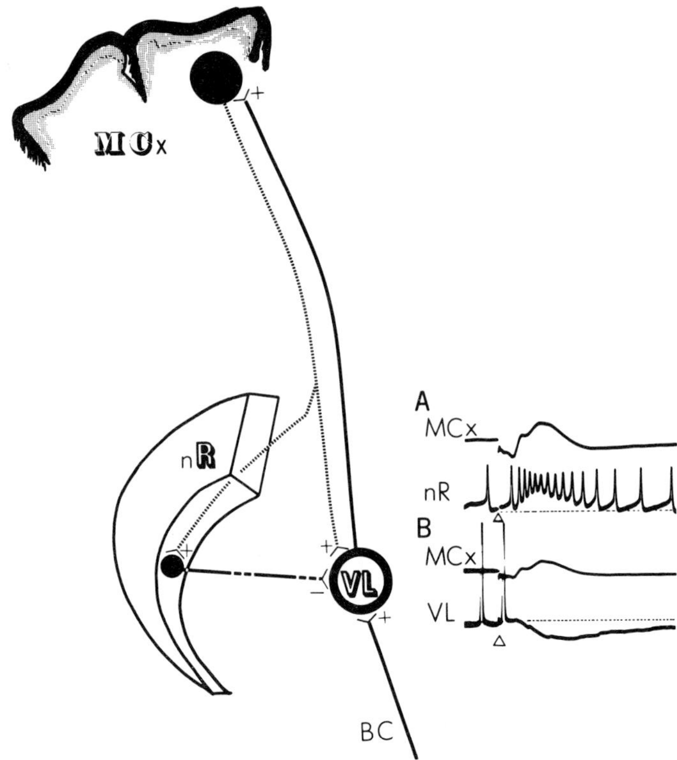

FIG. 13. The functional relationship between neurons in the dorsolateral thalamic reticular nucleus (nR) and the reciprocal corticothalamic circuit. The diagram illustrates that the neuron in VL engages a neuron in the motor cortex (MCx), which, in turn, projects back to the same VL neuron. The cortico-VL axon sends off an axon collateral to nR, and an nR neuron radiates back to the VL neuron, which is also engaged by a cerebellothalamic (BC) axon. A, B: lower traces, intracellular recordings from an nR neuron, A, and an adjacent VL neuron, B, following stimuli to the reciprocal thalamocortical circuit (at triangles); upper traces are surface recordings from the motor cortex. In the nR neuron a prolonged burst, and in the VL neuron a prolonged IPSP are seen following the stimulus to the corona radiata. B, the same CR stimulus also elicits an antidromic spike potential and an EPSP anterior to the IPSP in the VL neuron. The broken horizontal lines are drawn through the level of resting potentials of neurons to emphasize the similar temporal properties of the CR evoked burst in the nR and the CR evoked IPSP in the VL neuron. Further description in text. Cortically evoked monosynaptic EPSPs in dorsolateral nR neurons were not seen in this study. However, it is to be noted that Steriade, and also Massion (this volume) report on motor cortex evoked and extracellularly recorded monosynaptic excitatory effects from nR. (Modified from Frigyesi, Brain Res. 1972, in press.)

prolonged (up to 100 msec) burst discharges. In the same animal, latencies, durations and buildup patterns of evoked burst discharges in nR neurons and IPSPs in VL and MeT neurons exhibit remarkable similarities during stimulation of the same area of the corticothalamic projections using similar parameters for stimulation (Fig. 14). Moreover, the late, prominent negative waves on the surface recordings from the MC exhibit close time relations to the bursts in nR neurons and they increment or decrement pari passu with the buildup and attenuation of nR bursts during IC or CR stimulation (Fig. 13 A). Thus, the same stimulus which induces the prolonged, gaiting IPSPs in

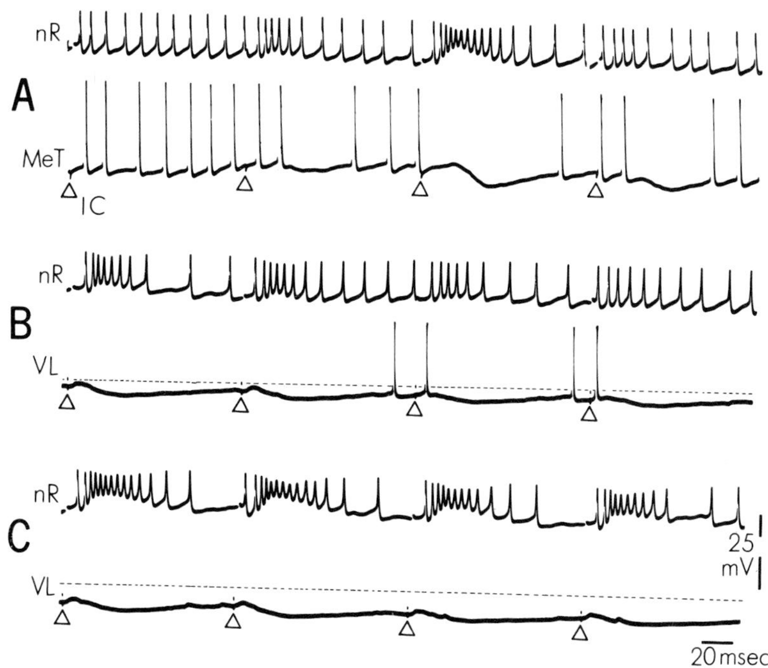

FIG. 14. Similarities of patterns of development of burst discharges in neurons in the dorsolateral thalamic reticular nucleus (nR) and IPSPs in neurons in the dorsal thalamus during low-frequency (8/sec) stimulation of the internal capsule (IC) (at open triangles). Upper traces, intracellular recordings from nR neurons and lower traces, a medial thalamic neuron, A, and two VL neurons, B and C. A, gradual buildup and alternation of burst discharges are seen in the nR neuron during repetitive IC stimulation. Pari passu, gradual buildup and alternation of IPSPs are seen in the MeT neuron. B, gradual attenuation of capsular evoked burst discharges are seen in the nR neuron. Parallel attenuation of capsular evoked IPSPs are seen in the VL neuron. The assumed firing level of the neuron is indicated by the broken horizontal line. C, sustained burst discharges in the nR neuron and IPSP summation in the VL neuron during repetitive stimulation of IC.

VL neurons also generates burst discharges of similar temporal characteristics in neurons in the dorsolateral nR. These observations suggest that the burst discharges in dorsolateral nR neurons and the IPSPs in VL neurons are causally related (16, 17). It is tempting to speculate that the corticofugal projection evoked burst discharges in dorsolateral nR neurons are associated with the persistent release of an inhibitory transmitter in VL which causes the development of the prolonged IPSPs. Furthermore, although the anatomical studies have yielded conflicting reports (Hassler, Chapter in this volume, and 9, 40, 56, 58) regarding the existence of nR-MC axons or axon collaterals, the close temporal relations between the evoked bursts in nR and the same stimulus evoked incrementing-decrementing negativities in MC could be most parsimoniously explained by the assumption of the operation of such an axon collateral of an nR neuron whose main axon projects back upon VL (29, and Mettler, Chapter in this volume).

Essentially similar relationships were observed between evoked burst discharges in dorsolateral nR neurons and evoked IPSPs in VL neurons during 8/sec stimulation of MeT, and Cd (16, 17). However, dorsolateral nR neurons so far explored have failed to show convergence between these projections. This contrasts starkly with observations made about neurons in the rostral pole of nR, where convergence between these projections was commonly encountered (cf. the Scheibels, Chapter in this volume). It is also noteworthy that similar burst discharges in dorsolateral nR were not observed during stimulation of cerebellofugal projections.

SUMMARY

Effects of stimulation of pathways arising in the motor cortex (MC) on responses in neurons in ventrolateral (VL) and medial (MeT) thalamus were studied to delineate further the properties of corticothalamic projection activities. Intracellular recordings from thalamic neurons revealed that reflux from discrete areas in MC operates upon those regions in VL which project upon them. Furthermore, discrete areas in MC radiate dual projections in a topographical manner to both VL and MeT. The data also revealed that some of the corticothalamic fibers descend to the mesencephalon and, anterior to radiating back to the dorsal thalamus, traverse the rostral pole but not the central and caudal regions of the substantia nigra. Alternating, relatively short EPSPs and prolonged IPSPs are the major synaptic events in neurons in VL and MeT, as are prolonged burst discharges in neurons in dorsolateral n. reticularis thalami (nR) during low-frequency (8/sec) stimulation of the corticothalamic projections. Close similarities were observed between durations, latencies and buildup patterns of MC evoked burst discharges in nR neurons and IPSPs in VL and MeT neurons. These observations, together with anatomical findings which show that nR neurons project back upon the principal nuclei of the dorsal thalamus, indicate that nR neurons may be involved in the generation of MC evoked IPSPs in VL and MeT neurons. Additional data, however, indicate that MC evoked IPSPs in MeT neurons could also be generated by involvement of those neurons in VL which project medially. The results indicate that transmission of activity in the cerebello-cortico-corticospinal projection system is dramatically influenced in thalamic neurons by IPSPs induced by corticothalamic projection activities.

The primary inference here is that the MC and the dorsal thalamus are reciprocally linked in a topographical manner. Pathways interconnecting these structures carry two-way traffic and engage in a diversity of mutually complementary or alternative subsystems. Consequently, activities in the MC may be profoundly affected by diencephalic influences and diencephalic neuronal transactions may be profoundly affected by corticothalamic projection activities.

ACKNOWLEDGMENTS

This work was supported by grants from the National Institute of Neurological Diseases and Stroke, NINDS #NS-09898-01 and #NS-09898-02.

REFERENCES

1 ADKINS, R.J., MORSE, R.W. and TOWE, A.L. Control of somatosensory input by cerebral cortex. Science 153 (1966) 1020-1022.

2 ADEY, W.R., SEGUNDO, J.P. and LIVINGSTON, R.B. Corticofugal influences on intrinsic brainstem conduction in cat and monkey. J. Neurophysiol. 20 (1957) 1-16.

3 AJMONE MARSAN, C. The Thalamus. Data on its functional anatomy and on some aspects of thalamo—cortical integration. Arch. ital. Biol. 103 (1965) 847-882.

4 AMASSIAN, V.E. and WEINER, H. Monosynaptic and polysynaptic activation of pyramidal tract neurons by thalamic stimulation. In: The Thalamus. Eds. D.P. Purpura and M. Yahr, Columbia U. Press, N.Y. 1966 pp: 255-286.

5 ANDERSEN, P. and ANDERSSON, S.A. Physiological basis of the alpha-rhythm. Appleton-Century-Crofts, New York, 1968.

6 ANDERSSON, S.A. and MANSON, J.R. Rhythmic activity in the thalamus of the unanesthetized decorticate cat. Electroenc. clin. Neurophysiol. 31 (1971) 21-34.

7 ANDERSEN, P., ECCLES, J.C., and SEARS, T.A. Cortically evoked depolarization of primary afferent fibers in the spinal cord. J. Neurophysiol. 27 (1964) 63-77.

8 CAJAL, RAMON y S. Las fibras nerviosas de origen cerebral del tuberculo cuadrigemino anterior y talamo optico. Trab. Lab. Invest. biol. Univ. Madr. 2 (1903) 5-21.

9 CARMAN, J.B., COWAN, W.M. and POWELL, T.P.S. Cortical connexions of the thalamic reticular nucleus. J. Anat. (London) 98 (1964) 578-598.

10 CARPENTER, M.B. and PETER, P. Nigrostriatal and nigrothalamic fibers in the rhesus monkey. J. comp. Neurol. 144 (1972) 93-116.

11 CHANG, H.-T. The repetitive discharges of corticothalamic reverberating circuit. J. Neurophysiol. 13 (1950) 235-257.

12 CHOW, K.L. Regional degeneration of the thalamic reticular nucleus following cortical ablations in the monkey. J. comp. Neurol. 97 (1952) 37-59.

13 DESIRAJU, T. and PURPURA, D.P. Organization of specific-nonspecific thalamic internuclear synaptic pathways. Brain Res. 21 (1970) 169-181.

14 DUSSER de BARENNE, J.G. and McCULLOCH, W.S. Sensorimotor cortex, nucleus caudatus and thalamus opticus. J. Neurophysiol. 1 (1938) 364-377.
15 FELDMAN, M.H. and PURPURA, D.P. Prolonged conductance increase in thalamic neurons during synchronizing inhibition. Brain Res. 24 (1970) 329-332.
16 FRIGYESI, T.L. Intracellular studies of neurons in the thalamic reticular nucleus. Fed. Proc. 30 (1971).
17 FRIGYESI, T.L. Organization of synaptic pathways linking the head of the caudate nucleus to the dorsal thalamus. Int. J. Neurol. 8 (1972) In press.
18 FRIGYESI, T.L., IGE, A., IULO, A. and SCHWARTZ, R. Denigration and sensorimotor disability induced by ventral tegmental injection of 6-hydroxy-dopamine. Exptl. Neurol. 33 (1971) 78-87.
19 FRIGYESI, T.L. and MACHEK, J. Basal ganglia-diencephalon synaptic relations in the cat. I. An intracellular study of dorsal thalamic neurons during capsular and basal ganglia stimulation. Brain Res. 20 (1970) 201-217.
20 FRIGYESI, T.L. and MACHEK, J. Basal ganglia-diencephalon synaptic relations in the cat. II. Intracellular recordings from dorsal thalamic neurons during low frequency stimulation of the caudatothalamic projection systems and the nigrothalamic pathway. Brain Res. 27 (1971) 59-78.
21 FRIGYESI, T.L. and PURPURA, D.P. Functional properties of synaptic pathways influencing transmission in the specific cerebello-thalamocortical projection system. Exptl. Neurol. 10 (1964) 305-324.
22 FRIGYESI, T.L. and PURPURA, D.P. Acetylcholine sensitivity of thalamic synaptic organizations activated by brachium conjunctivum stimulation. Arch. int. Pharmacodyn. 164 (1966) 110-132.
23 FRIGYESI, T.L. and RABIN, A. Basal ganglia-diencephalon synaptic relations in the cat. III. An intracellular study of ansa lenticularis, lenticular fasciculus and pallidosubthalamic projection activities. Brain Res. 35 (1971) 67-78.
24 FRIGYESI, T.L. and PURPURA, D.P. Electrophysiological analysis of reciprocal caudato-nigral relations. Brain Res. 6 (1967) 440-456.
25 FRIGYESI, T.L. and SCHWARTZ, R. Reciprocal inhibition of ventrolateral and medial thalamic neurons by corticothalamic projections. Fed. Proc. 31 (1972).
26 GRANIT, R. Receptors and sensory perception. Yale U. Press, New Haven, 1955 pp. 369.
27 HASSLER, R. Über die Rinden- und Stammhirnanteile des menschlichen Thalamus. Psychiat., Neurol., Med. Psychol. 1 (1949) 181-187.
28 HEAD, H. and HOLMES, G. Sensory disturbances from cerebral lesions. Brain, 34 (1911) 102-254.
29 JASPER, H.H. Diffuse projection systems: the integrative action of the thalamic reticular system. EEG. clin. Neurophysiol. 1 (1949) 405-421.
30 JONES, E.G. and POWELL, T.P.S. The projections of the somatic sensory cortex upon the thalamus in the cat. Brain Res. 10 (1968) 369-391.
31 JONES, E.G. and POWELL, T.P.S. Electron microscopy of synaptic glomeruli in the thalamic relay nuclei of the cat. Proc. Roy. Soc. B. 172 (1969) 153-171.
32 JONES, E.G. and POWELL, T.P.S. An electron microscopic study of the mode

of termination of cortico-thalamic fibres within the sensory relay nuclei of the thalamus. Proc. Roy. Soc. B. 172 (1969) 173-185.

33 KEMP, J.M. and POWELL, T.P.S. The connexions of the striatum and globus pallidus: synthesis and speculation. Phil. Trans. R. Soc. Lond. B. 262(1971) 441-457.

34 KRAUTHAMER, G. and ALBE-FESSARD, D. Inhibition of non-specific sensory activities following striopallidal and capsular stimulation. J. Neurophysiol. 28 (1965) 100-124.

35 KUYPERS, H.G.J.M., and LAWRENCE, D.G. Cortical projections to the red nucleus and the brainstem in the rhesus monkey. Brain Res. 4: 151-188, 1967.

36 LEVITT, M., CARRERAS, M., LIU, C.N., and CHAMBERS, W.W. Pyramidal and extrapyramidal modulation of somatosensory activity in gracile and cuneate nuclei. Arch. ital. Biol. 102 (1964) 197-229.

37 LIVINGSTON, R.B. Central control of afferent activity. In: H.H. Jasper, et al. Reticular formation of the Brain. Little, Brown and Co. Boston. 1958, pp. 177-185.

38 MASSION, J. Étude d'une structure motrice thalamique, le noyau ventrolateral, et de sa régulation par les afferences sensorielles, These de Doctorat. Paris 1968.

39 METTLER, F.A. Neuroanatomy. Mosby, 1948. 536 pp.

40 METTLER, F.A. Extensive unilateral cerebral removals in the primate: physiologic effects and resultant degeneration. J. comp. Neurol. 79: 185-246, 1943.

41 METTLER, F.A. Anatomic structures and physiologic systems. Psychiat. Quart. 38 (1964) 1-45.

42 NAKAMURA, Y. and SCHLAG, J. Cortically induced rhythmic activities in the thalamic ventrolateral nucleus of the cat. Exp. Neurol. 22 (1968) 209-221.

43 PETRAS, J.M. Some fiber connections of the precentral and postcentral cortex with basal ganglia, thalamus and subthalamus. Trans. Amer. Neurol. Ass. 91 (1965) 274-275.

44 PURPURA, D.P. Interneuronal mechanisms in thalamically induced synchronizing and desynchronizing activities. In: The Interneuron. M.A.B. Brazier, Ed. U. Calif. Press (1969) Berkeley. pp. 467-496.

45 PURPURA, D.P. Operations and processes in thalamic and synaptically related neural subsystems. In: The Neurosciences. Second Study Program. Eds. G.C. Quarton, T. Melnechuk and G. Adelman. Rockefeller U. Press. New York, 1970 pp 458-470.

46 PURPURA, D.P. and COHEN, B. Intracellular recording from thalamic neurons during recruiting responses. J. Neurophysiol. 25 (1962) 621-635.

47 PURPURA, D.P., DESIRAJU, T., PRELEVIC, S. and SANTINI, M. Excitability changes in dendrites of thalamic neurons during prolonged synaptic activation. Brain Res. 10 (1968) 457-459.

48 PURPURA, D.P., FRIGYESI, T.L., McMURTRY, J.G. and SCARFF, T. Synaptic mechanisms in thalamic regulation of cerebello-cortical projection activity. In: The Thalamus, Ed. D.P. Purpura and M.D. Yahr. Columbia U. Press. New York 1966. pp. 153.172.

49 PURPURA, D.P., FRIGYESI, T.L. and MALLIANI, A. Intrinsic synaptic organization and relations of the corpus striatum. In: Neurophysiological basis of normal and abnormal motor activities. Ed. M.D. Yahr and D.P. Purpura, Raven Press, Hewlett, N.Y. 1967. pp. 177-214.

50 PURPURA, D.P., McMURTRY, J.G. and MAEKAWA, K. Synaptic events in ventrolateral thalamic neurons during suppression of recruiting responses by brain stem reticular stimulation. Brain Res. 1 (1966) 63-76.

51 PURPURA, D.P., SCARFF, T. and McMURTRY, J.G. Intracellular study of internuclear inhibition in ventrolateral thalamic neurons. J. Neuroph. 28: 487-496, 1965.

52 PURPURA, D.P., SHOFER, R.J. and MUSGRAVE, S.F. Cortical intracellular potentials during augmenting and recruiting responses. II.Patterns of synaptic activities in pyramidal and nonpyramidal tract neurons. J. Neurophysiol. 27: (1964) 133-151.

53 RINVIK, E. The corticothalamic projection from the pericruciate and coronal gyri in the cat. Brain Res. 10 (1968) 79-119.

54 RINVIK, E. A re-evaluation of the cytoarchitecture of the ventral nuclear complex of the cat's thalamus on the basis of corticothalamic connections. Brain Res. 8 (1968) 237-254.

55 RISPAL-PADEL, L. and MASSION, J. Relations between the ventrolateral nucleus and the motor cortex in the cat. Exp. Brain Res. 10 (1970) 331-339.

56 ROSE, J.E. and WOOLSEY, C.N. Organization of the mammalian thalamus and its relationship to the cerebral cortex. Electroenc. clin. Neurophysiol. 1 (1949) 391-404.

57 SAKATA, H., ISHIJIMA, T. and TOYODA, Y. Single unit studies on ventrolateral nucleus of the thalamus in cat: its relation to the cerebellum, motor cortex and basal ganglia. Jap. J. Physiol. 16 (1966) 42-60.

58 SCHEIBEL, M.E. and SCHEIBEL, A.B. The organization of the nucleus reticularis thalami: a Golgi study. Brain Res. 1 (1966) 43-62.

59 SCHEIBEL, M.E. and SCHEIBEL, A.B. Structural organization of nonspecific thalamic nuclei and their projection toward cortex. Brain Res. 6 (1967) 60-94.

60 SCHLAG, J. and WASZAK, M. Characteristics of unit responses in nucleus reticularis thalami. Brain Res. 21 (1970) 286-288.

61 SHIMAZU, H., YANAGISAWA, N. and GAROUTTE, B. Cortico-pyramidal influences on thalamic somatosensory transmission in the cat. Jap. J. Physiol. 15 (1965) 101-124.

62 STERIADE, M., APOSTOL, V. and OAKSON, G. Control of unitary activities in cerebellothalamic pathway during wakefulness and synchronized sleep. J. Neurophysiol. 34 (1971) 389-413.

63 UNO, M., YOSHIDA, M. and HIROTA, I. The mode of cerebello-thalamic relay transmission investigated with intracellular recording from cells of the ventrolateral nucleus of the cat's thalamus. Exp. Brain Res. 10 (1970) 121-139.

64 VERZEANO, M. Pacemakers, Synchronization and Epilepsy. In: Synchronization of EEG activities in epilepsies. H. Petche and M.A.B. Brazier, Eds. Springer Verlag, Vienna, In press.

65 WALBERG, F. Corticofugal fibers to nuclei of the dorsal columns. Brain, 80 (1957) 273-287.

66 YOSHIDA, M. YAJIMA, K. and UNO, M. Different activation of the two types of the pyramidal tract neurones through the cerebello-thalamocortical pathway. Experientia, 22 (1966) 331-332.

DISCUSSION

SAX:

I'd like to ask Dr. Frigyesi what the activity of the cortical neurons were when he used lower doses of L-DOPA. At the range of 200 mg. per kilo plus the use of the alphamethyldopa-hydrazine, you are really using massive doses of this drug. Therapeutically, you can get your effects with only 75-100 mg. of L-DOPA. My comment is that at this range, in a clinical situation, you can produce paradoxical effects: hypotonia and an extreme sleep state.

PURPURA:

Purpura, Einstein. What I wanted to ask Dr. Frigyesi—the issue that really is going to be joined here, and I think we probably ought to put it on the table because it has been suggested already by the earlier Scheibels' data—is whether we're going to really put into the nucleus reticularis all the inhibitory elements that are going to generate IPSPs all over the thalamus. That's essentially what we're getting to. I personally don't like the idea although I can't see any reason why some elements of the rostral pole of reticularis can't function this way since they have the kinds of multiple inputs that one is looking for. But I think we're going to run into trouble because the characteristics of these PSPs, the IPSPs in particular, are quite different in different nuclear groups. I doubt whether the kinds of neuronal synchronization observed in some of them could be effected largely through the reticularis input, because in addition to the very phasic kinds of IPSPs, one sees rather prolonged IPSPs also. So we're going to have to include interneurons rather diffusely distributed in the thalamus. Then why only focus on the IPSPs which are seen everywhere in the thalamus? For example, when you stimulate the medial thalamus, you've got, preceding these IPSPs, EPSPs which also tend to synchronize throughout the thalamic regions. I may be as guilty as anyone for emphasizing the IPSPs, but there are the EPSPs. Why can't they also be generated by bursting elements of the reticularis? I think it's an interesting suggestion. One will have to see how it fares over the course of time. Might I ask another question though: why must the effect of the dopa be to block the inhibition between VL and the medial thalamus when, in fact, there is as much excitation generated in these elements by stimulating the medial thalamic and the VA-VL areas, as there is inhibition. So I think it would be nice, Tamas, if we had records in the medial thalamic regions during the effects of dopa to see what's happening in the subcortical relays which are presumably controlling the tonic input, that is generating that late negative wave in the cortex.

STERIADE:

Concerning the problem: "Are the reticularis neurons responsible for the inhibitory effects seen in the VL?", as suggested by the elegant study of Frigyesi, showing that IPSPs in VL cells are time-locked with long spike barrages in the reticularis nucleus, I would like to anticipate some data which will be included in my presentation of the afternoon session. The VL synchronizing process is very efficiently set in motion by orthodromic volleys arising in the precruciate motor cortex. Corticofugal fibers may engage monosynaptically both reticularis neurons and VL interneurons as recognized by their high-frequency spike barrages. But the powerful sequences of rhythmic inhibition elicited in VL principal cells by precruciate stimuli, comprising long-lasting firing suppression, rhythmic spike clusters and associated 8-12/sec spindle waves, have not been found to be related to the events recorded from the cells encountered in the rostral pole of the reticularis nucleus. Neither the spontaneous firing of reticularis cells, nor their cortically evoked pattern of discharge could possibly account for the stereotyped rhythmic activity found in VL relay cells. This relation was, however, evident with VL intrinsic interneurons which proved to be the best candidates for sculpturing the cortically evoked rhythmic excitatory-inhibitory sequences of VL relay cells (see Fig. 21 of my chapter in this Symposium).

FRIGYESI:

With respect to Dr. Sax's question: we also applied lower doses of L-DOPA and L-DOPA without a MAO inhibitor; the results were essentially similar to those reported here. The advantage of the high dose of L-DOPA in combination with MK-486 is that the phenomena could be obtained much faster than without MK-486. With respect to Dr. Purpura's question whether all IPSPs are generated by the involvement of thalamic reticular neurons, the answer is a probable no. The data which I presented, and the data of others, suggest that neurons in the thalamic reticular nucleus are very likely involved in the generation of *some* of the IPSPs seen in VL during capsular stimulation. Of course, this data, by no means, exclude that there are other mechanisms operating within the thalamus which are also capable of inducing prolonged IPSPs in VL neurons. Why the dorsolateral part of the thalamic reticular nucleus and not the rostral part? In our experience, neurons in the dorsolateral part of the thalamic reticularis nucleus behaved entirely differently from those in the rostral pole during capsular, midline thalamic, caudate and BC stimulation. For example, in the dorsolateral part of the thalamic reticularis nucleus, we have not observed convergence between corticofugal, midline thalamic, substantia nigra and entopeduncular projections. We didn't observe any cell in this particular area of nR which was driven by BC stimulation. This is in sharp contrast from what we have observed in the rostral pole of nR; there we observed not only convergence between the preceding projection systems, but we also found neurons which were driven by cerebellofugal projection activities. How about the EPSPs? We do not have data as to how the evoked EPSPs in VL neurons are generated; whether there are neurons in the thalamic reticularis nucleus which are also capable of contributing to the generation of these evoked EPSPs in VL neurons, we cannot say at present. Finally, your point is very well taken that we have to extend our studies and investigate medial thalamic neurons following the administration of L-DOPA.

JASPER:

Just two questions to Dr. Frigyesi. First, I enjoyed very much your beautiful colored diagrams, more impressive by their color. But I'm sure that you present them rather tentatively. The interneurons you've shown in these diagrams and the axon collaterals, of course especially the latter, are brought into some question by previous anatomical reports in this meeting: Do you still believe the diagrams will hold with the present lack of solid anatomical information to support them. The second question is concerning the nature of the fiber spectrum in some of these pathways. For example, your BC-VL system, what is the fiber spectrum in this group of fibers, to make you assume that these longer latency EPSPs are truly due to a multisynaptic interneuronal system? Are there a group of very fine fibers that might contribute to this long latency?

FRIGYESI:

The first question of Dr. Jasper relates to the intra-VL interneuronal chains, and I presume that you made particular reference to the recurrent collaterals which I had illustrated. The recurrent collateral system which I described generates excitatory effects on VL neurons; the data neither implied nor supported the proposition that recurrent collaterals would contribute to the generation of prolonged inhibition in VL neurons. The issue is controversial whether there are any recurrent collaterals in the thalamus; Tömböl and the Scheibels have reported recurrent collaterals of presumed relay cells. I would also like to point out that the histogram was prepared from a highly selected sample of intracellular recordings, therefore the data do not reveal the actual distribution of the recurrent collaterals; they merely show that they do operate in VL. In view of Rinvik's presentation today, which showed an abundance of dendro-dendritic synapses in VL, the diagram may indeed need a revision; the various types of intra-VL synaptic chains may be effected, to a presently unknown extent, by transmission through serially arranged dendro-dendritic, rather than axo-dendritic, contacts. Dr. Jasper's second question raises the issue that could the delayed EPSPs be accounted for by conduction through small fiber systems? The spectrum of diameter for myelinated BC fibers is 3-10μ, and for cortico-VL fibers is 0.5-2.5μ. The diameter generally diminishes after these fibers enter the thalamus. The pivotal issue, however, is that the proven monosynaptic responses in both systems exhibited high synaptic security and negligible variation in latencies. The contrary was observed for the late EPSPs. Therefore, it appears reasonable to assume that the delayed EPSPs were generated via polysynaptic chains.

HASSLER:

I want to return to this question of the reticular nucleus of the thalamus because you pointed out that in the dorsolateral part of the reticularis nucleus you observed evoked effects different from those in the most rostral pole. That should be so because the reticular nucleus of the thalamus is not a unit, but that there are at least 15 subnuclei of this reticular complex; this is not only an architectonic joke, but it really exists. Each subnucleus has special afferent pathways. Every ventral nucleus has a special reticular nucleus related to it; they both receive the same afferent pathways and have the same cortical relations; this was now demonstrated again by Minderhoud. Only the rostral pole of the thalamus has a related big reticular nucleus. In fact, it has the bigest reticular nucleus, with a large number of cells; this rostral pole relates to the VA nucleus; fibers here have longer extensions than in other parts of the reticular nucleus. But, perhaps, I agree a little bit with Purpura; we should not overestimate this reticular nucleus. Every morphologist is now so happy that we have, for the last two years, from the Scheibels and Minderhoud, a new concept for this nucleus which was completely enigmatic for us so long. I think that in the thalamic nuclei the small cells, which are described in every thalamic nucleus except in the ganglion habenulae, are quite important, and I don't believe that they are really axonless. I am so afraid that these small cells will swallow all EPSPs and IPSPs; and then they must digest them—where, I don't know. I think that we should believe in Dr. Fox's comments, which were very cautious, that perhaps these small cells also have axons but they are very difficult to demonstrate in the Golgi material.

METTLER:

Exercising my prerogative as a Chairman, may I return to a question with regard to the Scheibel discussion. Unfortunately, the Scheibels weren't here to defend themselves against the possibility that these small cells might be neuroglia. There is one body of evidence that might be called upon in this connection, that is the electron microscope. What do you think about this Rinvik?

RINVIK:

I was very excited by the paper of the Scheibels; in particular, by their finding of these small neurons, with an apparent lack of axons, from several hundred consecutive sections in the nucleus ventralis lateralis of the thalamus. I had seen parts of dendritic branchlets which, in serial reconstructions, would give an appearance of claw-like sinuous structures that the Scheibels have now described in the VB complex. They do not actually say specifically the VB complex, they say "ventralis lateralis and parts of the midline nuclei," so I think that this certainly should be taken into consideration. I would also like to add to the comment to Professor Hassler about the heterogeneity of the nucleus reticularis. I completely agree with him. I am presently making an electron microscopical study of the normal nucleus reticularis. It is very clear, though the results are preliminary, that the synaptological organization of the nucleus reticularis differs at the various levels throughout the whole thalamus; the organization in the rostral cap is different from that seen in reticularis bordering on lateralis posterior, and is different from that seen in reticularis bordering on VL or on the VB complex. So I think this is a very important point.

Corticothalamic Projections and Sensorimotor Activities
T. Frigyesi, E. Rinvik, and M.D. Yahr, editors. © 1972
Raven Press, New York.

Chairman's Summary

Fred A. Mettler

The purposes of symposia being various it is advisable to identify the intentions of the present activity. If I understand these correctly they are to express what we know about those connections of the cerebral cortex which proceed to the thalamus, with a view to ascertaining how these mediate what we ultimately call sensory and motor activity. By the use of the term thalamus here, the dorsal thalamus (including the metathalamus) is understood. This is an ambitious goal which we shall do well if we approach without attaining. Obviously it will be necessary, in view of the limited time available, to make the assumption that those who are here, and those who read the proceedings later, already know a good deal about these matters and are more concerned with the illumination of controversial or obscure details, than with a systematic presentation of the subject as a whole. With this *caveat* in mind we have before us four principal presentations, together with a not inconsiderable body of discussion.

Thus far, morphologic data on the corticothalamic projections of only one cortical region have been presented but it is probably the most important one, from the point of view of the general purpose of this symposium. It is the frontoparietal area in which the endings of the afferent pathways from touch and proprioception, and the cells of origin of the corticospinal efflux lie in close proximity. Rinvik has employed silver staining and electron microscopic techniques in order to examine the corticifugal fibers which pass from this territory into the thalamus. We learn that, in addition to the well-known recurrents which connect this cortex back to those thalamic nuclear masses which project upon it, there are also projections to other thalamic nuclei the primary corticipetal projection of which is to somewhat different regions. One very interesting projection is that from the medial cortex to bilateral thalamic foci. As I have previously mentioned, there is a considerable body of literature which supports the view that the corpus callosum contains corticifugal projection fibers which descend on the opposite side of the neuraxis. According to the literature (references will be found on page 1468 of Kappers, Huber and Crosby's Comparative Anatomy of the Nervous System) these include elements long enough to even get into the spinal cord. It is only fair to point out, however, that the literature on this subject is very inconclusive and that the course taken by the fibers described by Rinvik is through the anterior commissure and not corpus callosum.

Our attention has also been drawn to the circuitous route which some of the homolaterally distributed corticothalamic fibers follow. It has long been known that pathways which are relatively straight and direct, in the embryonic stages of lower forms, tend to become diverted from such a direct course as the brain matures and evolves, being caught up, as it were, in masses of fibers which pass through or alongside of them. In recent years we have an example of practical importance of this principle in the rostral rolling of the caudate nucleus, and in the manner in which nigrostriatal fibers are carried far forward into the anterior limb of the internal capsule. Now Rinvik calls our attention to the way in which corticothalamic fibers are carried caudally for a considerable distance before they are able to attain the caudal part of the dorsal thalamus.

An interesting aspect of Rinvik's paper is an excursion into the examination of the possible existence of dendrodendritic synapses which he points out may be of importance in determining what type of cell is the target of the corticothalamic fibers.

Kuypers and Kievit present a summary of the descending pathways of the cord and, with a discussion of cerebellar, rather than cortical, afferents, open the subject of the physiologic role of the ventrolateral nucleus—which is probably the focal point of most current work on the thalamus. Such an investigation broadens our concept of the deep somatic afferent input beyond that of the conventionally considered, more direct, proprioceptive input.

The Scheibels' presentation is based upon Golgi preparations made from mature animals. In these a more complex pattern is discernible than was revealed in their earlier immature material. One of the principal differences is the large number of small elements which the Scheibels call local circuit cells, to be distinguished from their previously noted, integrator cells which are much larger and compose only 5% of the ventrobasal population. The local circuit cell is evidently interposed between the corticothalamic fiber and principal thalamic neurons. This material opens the way to an interpretation of the manner in which the corticothalamic projection may operate and the Scheibels have presented a theoretical diagram to explain this. Such a theoretical conclusion also appears in the next presentation. Frigyesi and Schwartz offer a considerable body of factual electrophysiologic material and inferences drawn therefrom which requires very close attention to digest. It is in such concentrated presentations as this one, especially when they conclude on the note of theory, that the summarizer's role acquires something more than perfunctory significance. However, it also exposes him to the risk of misinterpreting what the speakers have intended to convey. If I understand Frigyesi and Schwartz correctly, and I assume they will immediately let me know if I do not understand them correctly, they have made eight objective points and drawn some inferences from each of these as they have gone along and have then wound up with a general theoretical interpretation of the whole. It appears that these points, the inferences and general conclusions are somewhat as follows:

1. Electrical stimulation of the motor cortex elicits antidromic potentials and succeeding mono- and polysynaptic responses in VL neurons which are also orthodromically linked to the cerebellum. From this the authors conclude that VL is the site of extensive information processing as well as a relay in the unidirectional transmission of information.

2. VL neurons exhibit antidromic and monosynaptic excitatory potentials upon

localized neocortical stimulation. From this they infer the existence of a topographically arranged system of reciprocal connections between VL and the motor cortex.

3. Latency histograms have been presented to indicate that evoked late EPSPs, in the brachium conjunctivum and internal capsule, cluster in three groups: a. polysynaptic EPSPs exhibiting 9-12 msec latencies, temporally related to brachium conjunctivum stimulation alone; b. 15-30 msec latencies, driven by stimuli in both the brachium conjunctivum and internal capsule; and c. 35-50 msec latencies were only driven by internal capsular stimulation. Frigyesi and Schwartz feel that these relationships indicate the operation of three types of intrathalamic interneuronal organizations: one activated by recurrent collaterals, another which is available to brachium conjunctivum fibers only, and a third type which is only activated by corticofugal neurons.

4. Directing their attention to Rinvik's morphologic studies which have demonstrated that some corticothalamic axons descend as far as the mesencephalon and traverse the rostral pole of the substantia nigra before attaining the dorsal thalamus, these investigators have stimulated the nigra generally and recorded from VL and found that rostral nigral stimulation reproduces some of the synaptic events in VL neurons which are elicited by motor cortex stimulation. However, localized stimulation of the central part of the substantia nigra elicited synaptic events in VL neurons which were fundamentally different from those observed during motor cortex stimulation. It is believed that the data indicate that stimulation or destruction of the rostral substantia nigra generally involves the corticothalamic fibers which follow the route described by Rinvik.

5. Stimulation of the internal capsule elicits complex motor cortex potentials and an antidromic-orthodromic excitatory sequence, and succeeding inhibition, in large populations of VL neurons. Intraperitoneally administered L-DOPA abolished all components of such evoked motor cortical potentials and also the capsular evoked orthodromic responses in VL. It is inferred that the medial thalamic nuclear group is inhibited by activities arising in VL neurons which are orthodromically activated by projections from the motor cortex. It is also inferred that L-DOPA selectively inhibits motor cortex projections impinging on VL neurons, and that frontal corticifugal fibers to the medial nuclear group are L-DOPA insensitive.

6. When brachium conjunctivum stimulation occurs during cortical evoked EPSPs in VL neurons, brachium conjunctivum-evoked EPSPs, and superimposed spike discharges continue. When brachium conjunctivum stimulation is timed to occur during cortical evoked IPSPs in VL neurons, brachium conjunctivum-evoked monosynaptic EPSPs usually fail to induce spike discharges in VL. It is believed that these data suggest that corticothalamic projections produce a functional discontinuity in the cerebello-thalamo-cortical projection system and also that the role of cortical inhibition does not reproduce the pattern of inhibition of nonspecific thalamic origin, on the parallel projections through the thalamus linking the cerebellum to the motor cortex, but has characteristics of its own.

7. The probability of firing particular units in the thalamus by stimulating the brachium conjunctivum, has been analyzed into 5 patterns. Most particularly, maximal IPSP development follows the first stimulus and then gradual IPSP attenuation

occurs during repetitive stimulation, or gradual buildup of IPSPs occurs during repetitive stimulation, or IPSP summation results in sustained hyperpolarization, or only orthodromic excitation and no detectable IPSPs occur.

8. Eight/sec motor cortex stimulation elicits intracellular burst discharges in the nucleus reticularis. Latencies, durations and buildup patterns of such evoked bursts corresponded with latencies, durations and development patterns of motor cortex-evoked IPSPs in neighboring VL neurons. It is proposed that cortically evoked activity in the nucleus reticularis results in the development of IPSPs in VL neurons already activated from the motor cortex.

The general theory evolved from these eight points and inferences would seem to be that the corticifugal and intrathalamic arrangements involve

A. Topographically organized reciprocal motor cortex-VL linkages.

B. Independent and interrelated topographical organization of cortico-VL and cerebello-VL projections.

C. Reciprocal inhibition of specific and nonspecific thalamic nuclei by corticofugal projections.

D. Operation of intrathalamic interneuronal organizations attached to corticofugal projections; and,

E. Cortico-VL projections give off axon collaterals to neurons of the nucleus reticularis which, in turn, radiate into VL. Corticofugal excitation of these reticular nucleus neurons results in persistent release of an inhibitory transmitter generating prolonged inhibition in VL neurons during activation of corticofugal projections.

Corticothalamic Projections and Sensorimotor Activities
T. Frigyesi, E. Rinvik, and M.D. Yahr, editors. © 1972
Raven Press, New York.

Corticostriate and Corticothalamic Connections in the Chimpanzee

J. M. Petras

Studies of the primate thalamus have concentrated heavily on the architectonics of the region and on the origin of thalamocortical projections (13, 14, 17, 18, 23, 24, 26, 27, 54, 58, 60, 62, 64,65). Analysis of the terminal connections of the primate spinothalamic, trigeminothalamic and medial lemniscus fibers has been disappointingly limited(e.g.,8,15,64). Similarly the number of studies describing the corticothalamic projections of the precentral gyrus have provided very limited information (34, 41, 61); this is due in large measure to the fact that the Marchi method fails to stain adequately areas of terminal degeneration.

With the introduction in 1951 of the Nauta technique for anterograde fiber degeneration (43), and its subsequent modifications (12, 44, 46), together with the recent development of the Fink and Heimer methods in 1967 (21), it has been possible to re-investigate in greater detail the organization of the afferent systems of the primate thalamus. In the same period Olszewski (1952) (47) published his architectonic evaluation of the rhesus monkey thalamus, and Nauta method studies of the spinothalamic (39), the medial leminiscal (6), cerebellothalamic (38, 40), and pallidothalamic (45), projections in the monkey followed. In 1964 we demonstrated the existence of corticothalamic connections arising in Brodmann's area 4 that projected chiefly to the nucleus ventralis lateralis and the nucleus centrum medianum (48). We subsequently have found that ablations of area 4 in the chimpanzee also result in abundant degeneration to selected subdivisions of the nucleus ventralis lateralis and to the nucleus centrum medianum. The present communication will present, in abridged form, some observations on the corticothalamic projection of the "motor" cortex in the chimpanzee as it compares with our previous findings in the monkey.

MATERIALS AND METHODS

This report is based on observations made on the brains of five chimpanzees. Three animals had surgical ablations of the precentral gyrus while the brains of the two other animals were utilized to study the normal architectonics of the forebrain.

Despite all precautions to limit the lesions to the cortical mantle, some involvement of the adjacent white matter of the cortex appeared inevitable. A large dorsoventral lesion was placed in the precentral gyrus in the first case and, in an attempt to extend the lesion more ventrally, damage was inflicted to the inferior quarter of the postcentral gyrus. Cytoarchitectonically the lesion in the precentral gyrus was limited to area gigantopyramidalis of Brodmann (1925) (area FA of Bailey, von Bonin and McCulloch, 1950). Injury to the postcentral gyrus appeared in area PC of Bailey, von Bonin and McCulloch (1950). The lesions in our two other chimpanzees were more limited, however. In the second case the dorsal-third of the precentral convolution was ablated along the convexity and the defect was extended medially to involve area gigantopyramidalis of the paracentral lobule as far as the cingulate sulcus. The cortex along the middle-third of the central sulcus was removed in the third case. In the latter two cases the lesions were limited to Brodmann's area gigantopyramidalis (FA of Bailey, von Bonin and McCulloch, 1950). These animals survived for 16, 12 and 10 postoperative days, respectively.

The animals were anesthetized and injected intravenously with heparin, then perfused transcardially with physiological saline and 10% formalin solutions. The brains and spinal cords were dissected free and thereafter kept in formalin. The brains were cut on the freezing microtome at 26μ and 52μ and the sections collected in serial order. Serial sections were impregnated for degenerated fibers using the Nauta uranyl nitrate modification (Nauta, unpublished) of the Nauta and Gygax (43, 44) techniques, and in two chimpanzees the Fink and Heimer (21) method (procedure I) was also applied. The method of Albrecht-Fernstrom (1) was applied in one case. Alternate sets of adjacent serial sections were stained with cresylechtviolett and others with the Weil method to provide additional cytoarchitectural and myeloarchitectural controls for the course and termination of degenerated fibers observed in the silver preparations. Additional material available for the study of the normal anatomy included two additional chimpanzee brains, one cut frozen at 208μ thickness and stained with cresylechtviolett, and the other celloidin embedded and cut at 36μ thickness with adjacent serial sections alternately stained with cresylechtviolett and the Loyez technique. The terminal distribution of fine fibers as identified microscopically was recorded on projection drawings of selected sections.

RESULTS AND DISCUSSION

This preliminary report is limited to a general consideration of the connections of the corticostriate and corticothalamic projections from the "leg" region of the precentral cortex in a single animal. Further observations on this case and other animals will be published later. An architectonic analysis of the lateral nuclear mass of the chimpanzee thalamus has paralleled our experimental work, but detailed consideration of these data also will be reported elsewhere. The latter studies of the chimpanzee diencephalon have revealed a striking number of cytoarchitectonic and myeloarchitectonic similarities with nuclei of the thalamus of the rhesus monkey as described by Olszewski (47), and for this reason the nomenclature used here follows that of Olszewski.

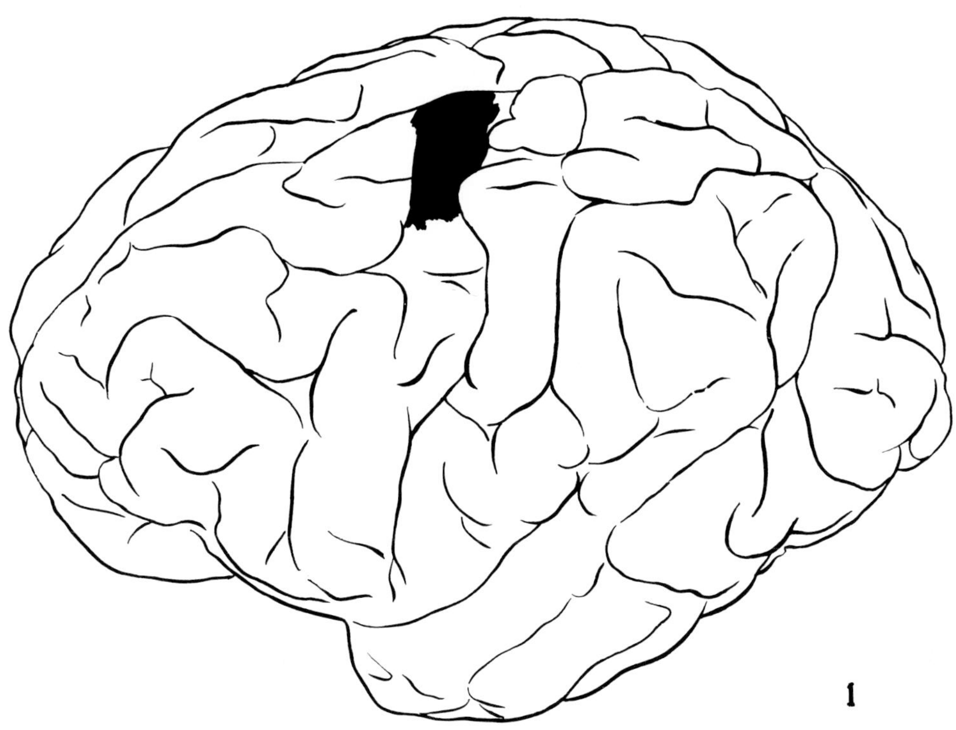

FIG. 1. Drawing of the left cerebral hemisphere of a chimpanzee. The lesion, represented in solid-black, was placed in the dorsal two-thirds of the precentral gyrus. The medial portion of area 4 was also destroyed, but is not represented in this figure.

The Corpus Striatum and Globus Pallidus

Corticofugal fibers leave the lesion area in the precentral gyrus (Fig. 1) and enter the extreme, external and internal capsules and the corpus callosum. Fine caliber, corticostriate fibers form a dense terminal field in the dorsolateral two-thirds of the ipsilateral putamen (Figs. 2-4). This field occupies a large dorsal sector of the nucleus and tapers to a narrow lateral zone in a more ventral part of the nucleus. The projection extends caudally to a level just anterior to the disappearance of the medial segment of the globus pallidus, and in the rostral direction to the putaminal part of the caudo-putamen at the level of the genu of the corpus callosum. At precommissural levels of the putamen the quantity of fiber degeneration diminshes abruptly. Some terminal degeneration also is present in the body and head of the caudate nucleus ipsilaterally, the fibers being distributed along the lateral-third of the nucleus adjacent to the internal capsule. Some of the cellular bridges between the head of the caudate nucleus and putamen also contain degenerated fibers. Fibers utilizing the extreme and external capsules furnish sparse numbers of fibers to the claustrum. Fiber degeneration in the claustrum parallels rostrocaudally the terminal field of distribution in the adjacent putamen and, like the putamen, degeneration is limited to the dorsal two-thirds of the nucleus. There were no degenerating fibers in the medial or lateral segments of the globus pallidus.

Similar corticocaudate and corticoputaminal fibers from the precentral gyrus have been identified in the rhesus monkey by Petras (48, 49, 52) and Kemp and Powell (25). There is a wide overlapping of corticostriate connections originating along different points in the precentral gyrus (49, 50, 52). The corticostriate projection of the postcentral gyrus in the rhesus monkey also overlaps approximately the same dorsolateral area of the putamen as covered by fibers from the precentral convolution (25, 49, 52).

Corticothalamic Connections

1. The nucleus ventralis lateralis pars oralis and nucleus reticularis thalami. In the present study, fiber degeneration coursing in the posterior limb of the internal capsule enters the dorsolateral aspect of the nucleus ventralis lateralis pars oralis (VLo) after supplying connections to the immediately adjacent cells of the nucleus reticularis thalami (R) (Fig. 4). Fine-caliber fibers weave among the cellular island of VLo and form still finer terminal tendrils. More medial areas of the lateral thalamic mass do not contain fiber degeneration; these nuclei, areas corresponding to the nucleus ventralis anterior (VA) and nucleus ventralis anterior pars magnocellularis (VAmc) of Olszewski (47), lie outside the field of distribution of the corticothalamic projections.

The nucleus ventralis lateralis pars oralis (VLo). The region of termination, and some adjacent areas, in the rostral part of the lateral nuclear mass of the thalamus of the chimpanzee shows sufficient cytoarchitectural similiarities to the nucleus ventralis lateralis pars oralis (VLo) in the rhesus monkey to justify labeling it VLo in the chimpanzee. The nucleus is characterized by darkly stained, large angular cells distributed in irregular groups, in the form of cell islands. In the chimpanzee these islands are developed best along the lateral-third of the lateral nuclear mass and extend ventralward to the lateral portion of nucleus ventralis lateralis pars medialis (VLm). The precentral corticothalamic fibers to VLo appear not to furnish additional fibers to the adjacent VLm.

Neither in the rhesus monkey nor the chimpanzee have we found fiber degeneration in VLm following lesions of the precentral gyrus, but we have not yet studied the fiber projections of other areas of the chimpanzee's frontal lobe. The subcortical afferent connections of VLm and VAmc are somewhat more controversial. In the present study neither VAmc nor VLm receive precentral corticothalamic connections. Anterograde fiber degeneration studies (10, 16) have described nigrothalamic fiber connections with VLm and VAmc. In the rhesus monkey Mettler (42) did not find retrograde changes in the substantia nigra following thalamic lesions of VLm or VAmc. He suggests that the nigrofugal projection goes principally to the striatum and globus pallidus

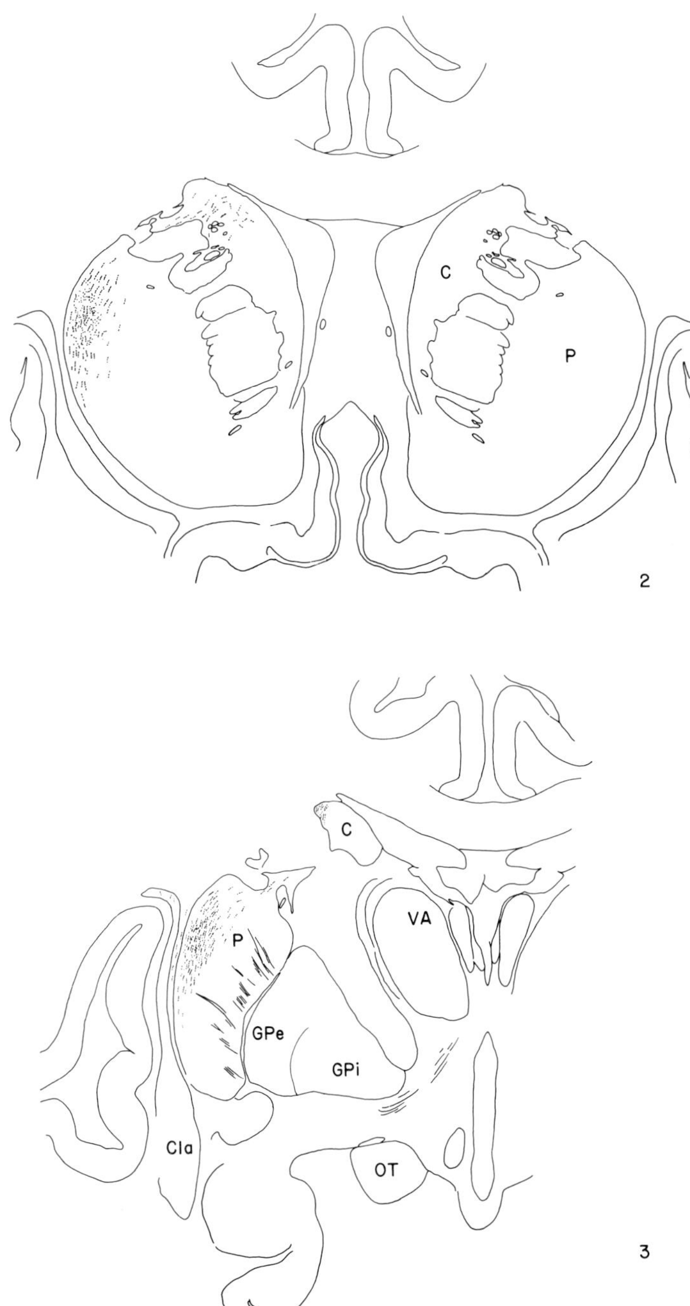

FIGS. 2 & 3. Fiber degeneration observed in a chimpanzee with a lesion of the "hind-limb area" of the precentral gyrus (see Fig. 1). In these and subsequent drawings, coarse dots indicate fibers of passage, fine stipple terminal degeneration. Abbreviations: see p. 212.

while the nigrothalamic elements are perhaps formed by small collaterals of the main trajectory.

Cerebellothalamic fibers are more widely distributed in the nucleus ventralis lateralis and nucleus ventralis anterior of the thalamus. Mehler (38) reports terminal connections of ascending cerebellofugal fibers with the pars caudalis (VLc), pars oralis (VLo), and pars medialis (VLm), of the nucleus ventralis lateralis, and both the pars principalis (VA), and pars magnocellularis (VAmc) of nucleus ventralis anterior in the rhesus monkey.

2. The nucleus ventralis lateralis pars caudalis (VLc). At more caudal thalamic levels the dorsal portion of VLo is replaced by a more densely cellular region, the nucleus ventralis lateralis pars caudalis (VLc). In the case under discussion an exceedingly dense terminal arbor of fine degenerating fibers is distributed within VLc and occupies a dorsolateral sector of the nucleus. At more caudal thalamic levels this degeneration continues in a ventrolateral direction into an area medial to the external medullary lamina and dorsal to the ventral posterior nuclear complex (VPLo and VPLc). This segment of the nucleus ventralis lateralis is topographically reminiscent of the nucleus ventralis lateralis pars postrema (VLps) in the rhesus monkey (47).

The massive corticothalamic connections established with VLc in the rhesus monkey (49, 52) are supplemented by a dense cerebellothalamic pathway (38; Petras, unpublished observations) in the same species. Pallidothalamic fibers, however, do not establish connections with this component of the nucleus ventralis lateralis according to Nauta and Mehler (45). Nigrothalamic connections with this nucleus have not been reported (10, 16).

3. The intralaminar nuclei of the thalamus. Degenerated fibers sweep medially and ventrally through the thalamus destined for distribution in selected intralaminar nuclei. Small numbers of fibers continue further medially, penetrate the internal medullary lamina and terminate in the paralaminar part of the nucleus medialis dorsalis (MD) designated as pars multiformis (MDmf) by Olszewski (47). Among the intralaminar nuclei, some connections are present in nucleus centralis lateralis (Cl), but the nucleus centrum medianum (CM) is perhaps the main intralaminar terminus. A rather large and dense terminal field is most prominent in the dorsomedial half of the nucleus centrum medianum (Fig. 5). Sporadic fiber degeneration also is seen medial to the nucleus centrum medianum among the small flattened neurons embedded in the internal leaf of the internal medullary lamina which separates the centrum medianum-parafascicular nuclear complex from the nucleus medialis dorsalis. Terminations of a fiber contingent present in the nucleus medialis dorsalis region are restricted to a few small-celled fields, in the lateral and ventrolateral paralaminar portion of MD similar to Olszewski's (47) MDmf of the rhesus monkey, a region which Mehler (36) includes in the "ill-defined" caudal limits of Cl.

At rostral thalamic levels in this case and in previously published monkey cases, evidence could not be found for fiber degeneration in the nucleus paracentralis and the nucleus medialis dorsalis pars parvocellularis (MDpc of Olszewski) (47), or the midline thalamic nuclei.

Thalamo-striate connections. The thalamo-striate projections were

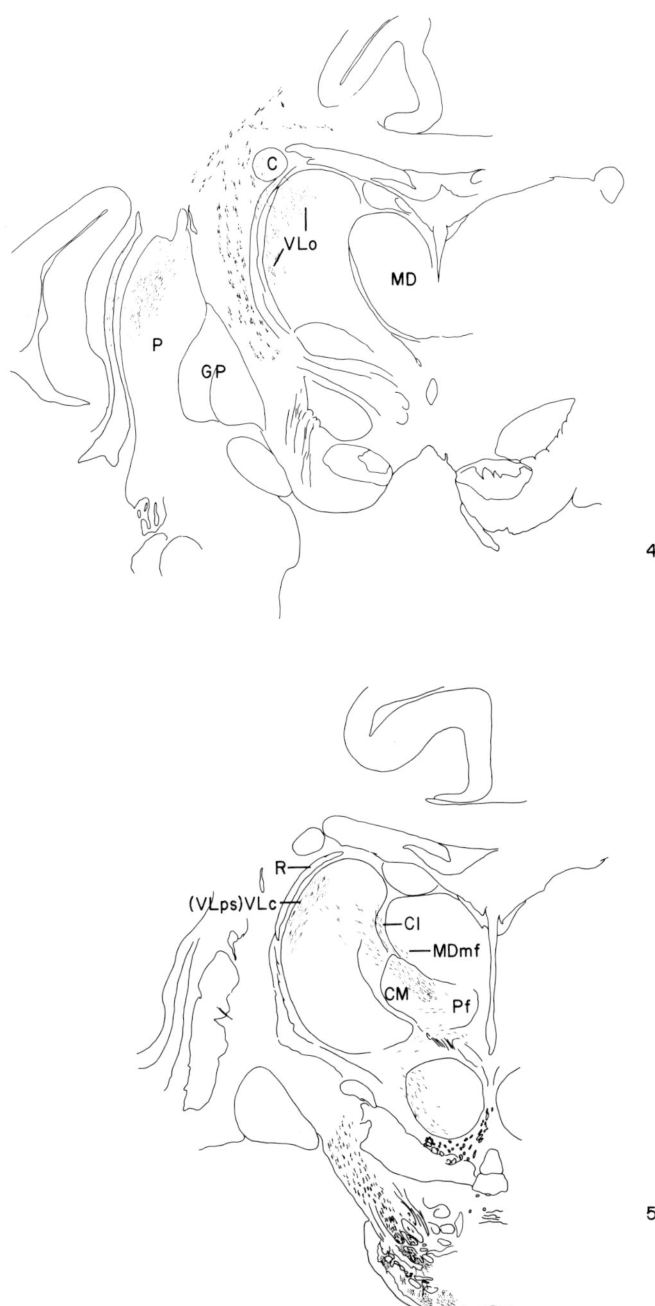

FIGS. 4 & 5. The fiber degeneration occurring in the rostral and caudal thalamus is described in the text. Figure 5 also shows fiber degeneration in the nucleus ruber and around cells in the griseum pontis.

investigated in human autopsy cases with hemispheric lesions involving the striatum (22, 55, 63) and despite the interpretative limits imposed by the extensive destruction of superficial as well as deep structures in the hemispheres, these studies amply demonstrate a thalamo-striate connection for the nucleus centrum medianum. The value of these early data are confirmed by Powell and Cowan's (56) experimental study in the rhesus monkey. Following more selective lesions of the striatum these workers concluded that the head of the caudate nucleus receives fibers from the nuclei centralis medialis, centralis lateralis (Cl) and paracentralis (Pcn), while the putamen receives fibers mainly from the nucleus centrum medianum (CM) and nucleus parafascicularis (Pf). Evidence further confirming the projection of the centrum medianum to the striatum was provided by Mehler (36) in a rhesus monkey case with a discrete lesion of the nucleus centrum medianum. Anterograde fiber degeneration was traced ipsilaterally to the striatum and ended chiefly in the putamen.

The nucleus centrum medianum. Lesions involving the centrum medianum and closely adjacent intralaminar nuclei fail to abolish or ameliorate the dyskinesia produced by primary destruction of the subthalamic nucleus of Luys in the rhesus monkey (11). The effects of thalamic lesions in VLo and CM on experimentally produced cerebellar dyskinesia have also been studied. Carpenter and Hanna (9) found in a case with a CM lesion, accompanied by destruction of the adjacent areas of VPM and VPLc, that tremor at rest was abolished while ataxic tremor was reduced. In a second rhesus monkey with a lesion in CM and the adjacent VPLo and VPLc nuclei, simple tremor (tremor at rest) and ataxic tremor were abolished for a four week period. Occasional short periods of tremor returned, however, and at six weeks both simple tremor and ataxic tremor recurred; the severity of these abnormal movements was never as pronounced as that which was first encountered following cerebellar injury. Other forms of dyskinesia such as generalized ataxia and dysmetria, and the generalized motor hypokinesis of these monkeys, was unaffected by CM lesions.

While the functional properties of the CM have eluded precise neurological analysis, the recently identified afferent connections from the globus pallidus and precentral gyri strongly implicate the CM as an important thalamic component in the "control" of movement; a rather interesting fact in view of the large size of the CM in some cebid monkey genera, in cercopethecid monkeys, and in the anthropoid apes and man. A substantial corticothalamic connection with CM exists in the rhesus monkey (48)

FIG. 6. This is a photomicrograph of a cresylechtviolett-stained frozen section through the caudal thalamus. The architectonic divisions of the thalamus may be easily appreciated here and particularly noteworthy is the distinction between VLc and VLps. The VLc cell group lies more medially and appears to be comprised of a denser cellular population. The VLps cell group is "broken-up" by many large bundles of myelinated fibers (pale areas) oriented dorsolaterally to ventromedially in the nucleus. In the case under consideration a dense terminal arbor is seen in the VLps. The asterisk indicates terminal areas of fiber degeneration in this case, the two locations appear to correspond to the paralaminar parts of MDmf in the rhesus monkey.

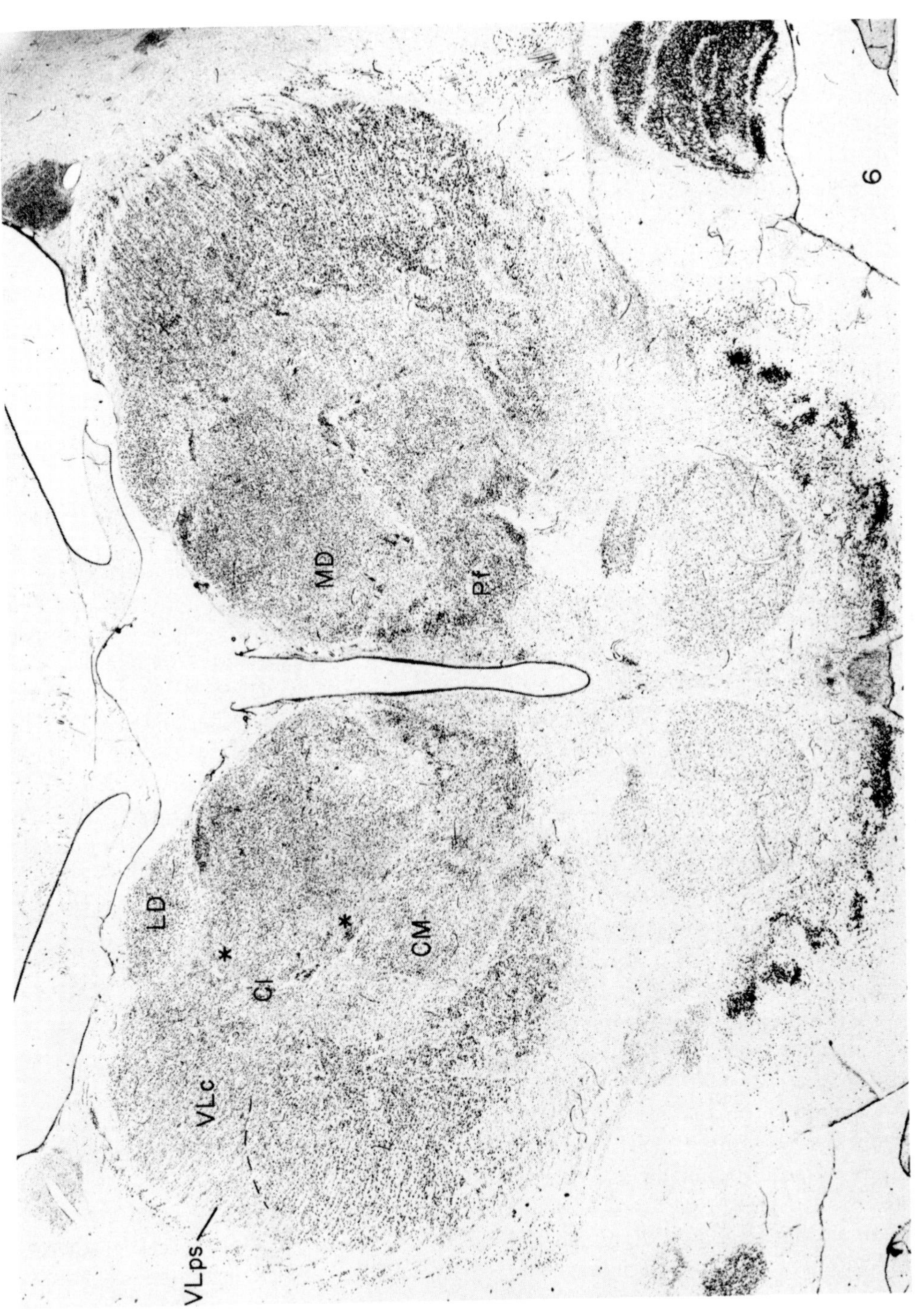
MD
Pf
LD
Cl
CM
VLc
VLps
9

and is also present in the chimpanzee (49, 50). Kuypers (see 36) has identified similar connections following ablations of the precentral gyri of the same species. Ablations of the precentral gyri in several genera of New World and Old World primates (52) confirmed a topographically organized distribution of precentral fibers to the nucleus centrum medianum (CM). In the rhesus monkey, the large corticothalamic connection from the precentral gyrus to the CM is supplemented by an important efferent projection from the internal segment of the globus pallidus (45).

Divergent opinions exist regarding the sources of ascending afferent connections to the CM. A substantial spinothalamic connection can be demonstrated with Cl, but a comparable terminal connection with the CM has not been identified in the rhesus monkey (37, 39); or the chimpanzee (37). A cerebellothalamic projection to the CM-Pf nuclear complex was reported for the cat by Thomas et al. (59), however, Mehler (36, 38) was unable to confirm such a projection in the rhesus monkey. Current observations (Petras, unpublished) with the cerebellothalamic connections in the rhesus monkey indicates that a rich stream of fibers passes through CM-Pf, but evidence clearly demonstrating terminal connections with neurons of either of these two cell groups cannot be found.

The nucleus centralis lateralis. Unlike the afferent relationships of the nucleus centrum medianum (CM) the afferent connections of the nucleus centralis lateralis (Cl) appear to originate from widely different regions of the central nervous system: the isocortex of the hemispheres, cerebellum, spinal trigeminal nucleus (Mehler, personal communication), and the spinal cord. Cortical projections from the precentral gyrus of the rhesus monkey have been reported (48-50, 52) and cortico-intralaminar connections with this nucleus have been identified following ablations of frontal cortical areas 6 (48, 49) and 8 (3, 4) of the rhesus monkey. Evidence has not been found for Cl intralaminar afferent connections originating in parietal somesthetic or parietal association cortex, that is, from the postcentral gyri, or the superior and inferior parietal lobules (50, 52, 53). Although a significant pallidal fiber component, originating in the internal segment of the globus pallidus, furnishes terminal fibers to the cells of the nucleus centrum medianum (CM) of the rhesus monkey (45), a pallidothalamic projection to the intralaminar and paralaminar components of the Cl have not been reported.

Ascending afferent connections to Cl are numerous. Mehler, Feferman and Nauta (1960) traced a component of the spinothalamic tract through the brain stem reticular formation and into the internal medullary lamina of the thalamus where fibers were distributed throughout Cl. Mehler (1969) subsequently found in the chimpanzee spinothalamic connections with Cl neurons. Comparison of our data on corticothalamic connections in the chimpanzee and of the distribution of spinothalamic fibers in the chimpanzee (37; Mehler, personal communication) reveals a consistent overlapping of connections in the Cl and paralaminar regions of the nucleus medialis dorsalis, namely, those sectors of MD corresponding to Olszewski's (47) MDmf in the rhesus monkey.

A review of recent literature suggests the following picture of the afferent and efferent connections of the striatum, globus pallidus and thalamic nuclei (2, 3, 10, 16, 19, 25, 36-39, 42, 45, 49, 52, 56). The caudate nucleus and putamen receive a strong corticostriate projection from the precentral gyrus and this connection appears to overlap in part with a corticostriate projection originating in the postcentral gyrus. Evidence for corticopallidal fibers, however, have not been found in either the rhesus monkey or the chimpanzee. An important fine-fibered, nigrostriatal projection has been demonstrated and nigropallidal connections also have been reported for the rhesus monkey. The simian nucleus ventralis anterior (VA) of the thalamus receives afferent fibers from the globus pallidus and the cerebellum. The nucleus ventralis anterior pars magnocellularis (VAmc) receives afferent fibers from the substantia nigra and cerebellum. Area X (47) of the nucleus ventralis lateralis receives fibers from the cerebellum but not from the striatum, globus pallidus, substantia nigra or precentral gyrus. Pallidothalamic, corticothalamic, and cerebellothalamic connections converge in the nucleus ventralis lateralis pars oralis (VLo) while the pars caudalis (VLc) receives projections only from the precentral gyrus and cerebellum. While the exact cortical area of origin of fibers to the nucleus ventralis lateralis pars medialis (VLm) has not been established, projections from the globus pallidus and substantia nigra have been reported. The nucleus ventralis lateralis pars postrema (VLps) of the rhesus monkey, and its probable equivalent in the chimpanzee, receive an important projection from the area gigantopyramidalis of the precentral gyrus, and also from convergent afferent fibers from the cerebellum (see Fig. 14 in (53)). Thus, considerable anatomical data have become available regarding afferent connections of the ventral lateral nuclear complex of the thalamus. These data suggest that significant functional differences exist among the various cytoarchitectural subdivisions of the nucleus ventralis lateralis.

The intralaminar nuclei differ dramatically from other thalamic nuclei, their efferent fibers establishing connections chiefly with the corpus striatum rather than the cerebral cortex. Killackey and Ebner, however, recently have found anterograde fiber degeneration in the opossum and hedgehog, suggesting that certain intralaminar nuclei have cortical connections. Current anatomical consensus still holds that the intralaminar nuclei and the CM-Pf complex are non-cortical dependents. The nucleus centrum medianum projects mainly to the putamen and parafascicularis. The nucleus centrum medianum receives connections from the pallidothalamic fasciculus arising from the internal segment of the globus pallidus and is overlapped by a prominent cortical projection from the precentral gyrus. The dorsal paralaminar portion of Cl receives some overlapping connections from the "premotor" cortex (field 6 or area frontalis granularis of Brodmann; or FB of von Bonin and Bailey),but this cortical field of the frontal lobe cortex appears to project more selectively to the nucleus parafascicularis (48, 49). The nucleus centralis lateralis (Cl) is provided with numerous afferent connections from divergent sources, and it in turn projects to the corpus striatum, chiefly the caudate nucleus. Its cells may be excited by multimodal signals "originating" in the cerebral cortex, cerebellum, spinal cord, and perhaps the reticular formation, before it may in turn signal information to the corpus striatum.

Although I have, in this brief survey, restricted both the observations and remarks to anatomical observations on the nucleus ventralis lateralis and intralaminar nuclei and their inter-connections, it must be kept in mind that the efferent connections of the precentral gyri converge upon important cell groups at all levels of the neuraxis: subthalamic regions, midbrain tegementum, griseum pontis, reticular formation and spinal cord. Studies of these connections in the rhesus monkey, chimpanzee and man may be found in the accounts of Kuypers (28–30), Kuypers, Fleming and Farinholt (32), Liu and Chambers (35), Schoen (57), Kuypers and Lawrence (33), and Petras (51,52).

SUMMARY

The fiber degenerations resulting from lesions of the precentral gyrus (Brodmann's field 4 or area gigantopyramidalis; FA of Bailey, von Bonin and McCulloch) were studied in the chimpanzee by the aid of various Nauta method variations. Identification of the areas of terminal degeneration was aided by supplemental material from two normal chimpanzee brains stained with a cresylechtviolett technique and the Loyez method. The following observations were made:

(1) Corticostriate connections from the precentral gyrus converge ipsilaterally upon the dorsolateral two-thirds of the putamen at precommissural levels of the nucleus and the "body" of the putamen as far caudally as the "middle" thalamus. Cortical projections to the head of the caudate nucleus appear limited to the dorsolateral aspect of this cell group and to a comparable lateral area in the body of the caudate.

(2) A sparse cortical projection to the dorsal region of the claustrum is present. This connection appears approximately coextensive rostrocaudally with the corticoputaminal field.

(3) Corticopallidal fibers to the internal and external segments of the globus pallidus were not seen.

(4) Corticothalamic fibers utilizing the posterior limb of the internal capsule are distributed ipsilaterally to the nucleus reticularis thalami (R) adjacent to VLo, the nucleus ventralis lateralis pars oralis (VLo), pars caudalis (VLc), and pars postrema (VLps). Evidence of fiber degeneration in the nucleus ventralis lateralis pars medialis (VLm) could not be found in our case with restricted precentral gyrus ablation.

ABBREVIATIONS FOR ALL FIGURES

C	Caudate nucleus
Cl	Nucleus centralis lateralis
Cla	Claustrum
CM	Nucleus centrum medianum
GPe	Globus pallidus, external segment
GPi	Globus pallidus, internal segment
MD	Nucleus medialis dorsalis
MDmf	Nucleus medialis dorsalis pars multiformis
OT	Optic tract
P	Putamen
Pf	Nucleus parafascicularis
VA	Nucleus ventralis anterior
VLc	Nucleus ventralis lateralis pars caudalis
VLo	Nucleus ventralis lateralis pars oralis
VLps	Nucleus ventralis lateralis pars postrema

REFERENCES

1 ALBRECHT, M.H. and FERNSTROM, R.C. A modified Nauta-Gygax method for human brain and spinal cord. Stain Technol., 34 (1959) 91-94.

2 ARANSON, L.R. and PAPEZ, J.W. The thalamic nuclei of Pithecus (Macacus) Rhesus. II. Dorsal Thalamus. Arch. Neurol. Psychiat., Chicago, 32 (1934) 27-44.

3 ASTRUC, J. Cortico-fugal fiber degeneration following lesions of area 8 (frontal eye field) in Macaca mulatta. Anat. Rec., 148 (1964) 256.

4 ASTRUC, J. Corticofugal connections of area 8 (frontal eye field) in Macaca mulatta. Brain Research, 33 (1971) 241-256.

5 BAILEY, P., von BONIN, G. and McCULLOCH, W.S. The isocortex of the chimpanzee. The University of Illinois Press, Urbana (1950).

6 BOWSHER, D. Projection of the gracile and cuneate nuclei in Macaca mulatta: An experimental degeneration study. J. Comp. Neurol., 110 (1958) 135-155.

7 BRODMANN, K. Vergleichende Lokalisations lehre der Grosshirnrinde, 2. Auflage., J.A. Barth, Leipzig, (1925).

8 CARPENTER, M.B. The dorsal trigeminal tract in the rhesus monkey. J. Anat., Lond., 91 (1957) 82-90.

9 CARPENTER, M.B. and HANNA, G.R. Effects of thalamic lesions upon cerebellar dyskinesia in the rhesus monkey. J. Comp. Neurol., 119 (1962) 127-148.

10 CARPENTER, M.B. and PETER, P. Nigrostriatal and nigrothalamic fibers in the rhesus monkey. J. Comp. Neurol., 144 (1972) 93-116.

11 CARPENTER, M.B., STROMINGER, N.L. and WEISS, A.H. Effects of lesions in the intralaminar thalamic nuclei upon subthalamic dyskinesia. A study in the rhesus monkey. Arch. Neurol., Chicago, 13 (1965) 113-125.

12 CHAMBERS, W.W., LIU, C.Y. and LIU, C.N. A modification of the Nauta technique for staining of degenerating axons in the central nervous system. An Rec., 124 (1956) 391-392.

13 CHOW, K.L. and PRIBRAM, K.H. Cortical projection of the thalamic ventrolateral nuclear group in monkeys. J. Comp. Neurol., 104 (1956) 57-75.

14 CLARK, W.E. LeGROS. The structure and connections of the thalamus. Brain, 55 (1932) 406-470.

15 CLARK, W.E. LeGROS. The termination of ascending tracts in the thalamus of the macaque monkey. J. Anat., Lond., 71 (1936) 7-40.

16 COLE, M., NAUTA, W.J.H. and MEHLER, W.R. The ascending efferent projections of the substantia nigra. Trans. Amer. Neurol. Assoc., 89 (1964) 74.

17 CROUCH, R.L. The nuclear configuration of the thalamus of Macacus rhesus. J. Comp. Neurol., 59 (1934) 451-485.

18 CROUCH, R.L. and THOMPSON, J.K. The efferent fibers of the thalamus of Macacus rhesus. J. Comp. Neurol., 69 (1938) 255-271.

19 DeVITO, J.L. Projections from the cerebral cortex to intralaminar nuclei in monkey. J. Comp. Neurol., 136 (1969) 193-202.

20 KILLACKEY, H. and EBNER, F.F. Two different types of thalamocortical projections to a single cortical area in mammals. Brain, Behav. Evol. (in press).

21 FINK, R.P. and HEIMER, L. Two methods for selective silver impregnation of degenerating axons and their synaptic endings in the central nervous system. Brain Research, 4 (1967) 369-374.

22 FREEMAN, W. and WATTS, J.W. Retrograde degeneration of the thalamus following prefrontal lobotomy. J. Comp. Neurol., 86 (1947) 65-93.

23 FRIEDEMANN, M. Die Cytoarchitektonick des Zwischenhirns der Cercopitheken mit besonderer Berucksichtigung des Thalamus opticus. J. Psychol. Neurol., 18 (1911) 309-378.

24 HEINER, J.R. A reconstruction of the diencephalic nuclei of the chimpanzee. J. Comp. Neurol., 144 (1960) 217-238.

25 KEMP, J.M. and POWELL, T.P.S. The cortico-striate projection in the monkey. Brain, 93 (1970) 525-546.

26 KRIEG, W.J.S. A reconstruction of the diencephalic nuclei of Macacus rhesus. J. Comp. Neurol., 88 (1948) 1-52.

27 KRUGER, L. and PORTER, P. A behavioral study of the functions of the Rolandic cortex in the monkey. J. Comp. Neurol., 109 (1958) 439-469.

28 KUYPERS, H.G.J.M. Corticobulbar connections to the pons and lower brainstem in man. An anatomical study. Brain, 81 (1958a) 364-388.

29 KUYPERS, H.G.J.M. Cortico-bulbar connections from the pericentral cortex to the pons and lower brain stem in monkey and chimpanzee. J. Comp. Neurol. 110 (1958b) 221-256.

30 KUYPERS, H.G.J.M. Central cortical projection to motor and somato-sensory cell groups. Brain, 83 (1960) 161-184.

31 KUYPERS, H.G.J.M. (See discussion of 36)

32 KUYPERS, H.G.J.M., FLEMING, W.R. and FARINHOLT, J.W. Subcorticospinal projections in the Rhesus monkey. J. Comp. Neurol., 118 (1962) 107-137.

33 KUYPERS, H.G.J.M. and LAWRENCE, D.G. Cortical projections to the red nucleus and brain stem in the rhesus monkey. Brain Research 4 (1967) 151-188.

34 LEVIN, P.M. The efferent fibers of the frontal lobe of the monkey, Macaca mulatta. J. Comp. Neurol., 63 (1936) 369-419.

35 LIU, C.N. and CHAMBERS, W.W. An experimental study of the cortico-spinal system in the monkey (Macaca mulatta). The spinal pathways and preterminal distribution of degenerating fibers following discrete lesions of the pre- and postcentral gyri and bulbar pyramid. J. Comp. Neurol., 123 (1964) 257-284.

36 MEHLER, W.R. Further notes on the center median nucleus of Luys. In: The Thalamus, D.P. Purpura and M.D. Yahr, Eds., New York: Columbia Univ. Press. 1966, pp. 109-122.

37 MEHLER, W.R. Some neurological species differences—A posteriori. Ann. N. Y. Acad. Sci., 167 (1969) 424-468.

38 MEHLER, W.R. Idea of a new anatomy of the thalamus. J. Psychiat. Res., 8 (1971) 203-217.

39 MEHLER, W.R., FEFERMAN, M.E. and NAUTA, W.J.H. Ascending axon degeneration following anterolateral cordotomy: An experimental study in the monkey. Brain, 83 (1960) 718-750.

40 MEHLER, W.R., VERNIER, V.G. and NAUTA, W.J.H. Efferent projections from dentate and interpositus nuclei in primates. Anat. Rec., 130 (1958)430-431.
41 METTLER, F.A. Corticifugal fiber connections of the cortex of Macaca mulatta. The frontal region. J. Comp. Neurol., 61 (1935) 509-542.
42 METTLER, F.A. Nigrofugal connections in the primate brain. J. Comp. Neurol., 138 (1970) 291-319.
43 NAUTA, W.J.H. and GYGAX, P.A. Silver impregnation of degenerating axon terminals in the central nervous system: (1) Technic (2) Chemical notes. Stain Technol., 26 (1951) 5-11.
44 NAUTA, W.J.H. and GYGAX, P.A. Silver impregnation of degenerating axons in the central nervous system: a modified technique. Stain Technol., 29 (1954) 91-94.
45 NAUTA, W.J.H. and MEHLER, W.R. Projections of the lentiform nucleus in the monkey. Brain Research, 1 (1966) 3-42.
46 NAUTA, W.J.H. and RYAN, L.F. Selective silver impregnation of degenerating axons in the central nervous system. Stain Technol., 27 (1952) 175-179.
47 OLSZEWSKI, J. The thalamus of the Macaca mulatta. An atlas for use with the stereotaxic instrument. S. Karger, Basel, 1952.
48 PETRAS, J.M. Some fiber connections of the precentral cortex (areas 4 and 6) with the diencephalon in the monkey (Macaca mulatta). Anat. Rec., 148 (1964) 322.
49 PETRAS, J.M. Fiber degeneration in the basal ganglia and diencephalon following lesions in the precentral and postcentral cortex of the monkey (Macaca mulatta); with additional observations in the chimpanzee. Eighth Internat'l. Anat. Congr., Wiesbaden,Germany, 1965, p. 95.
50 PETRAS, J.M. Some fiber connections of the precentral and postcentral cortex with the basal ganglia, thalamus and subthalamus. Trans. Amer. Neurol. Assoc., 90 (1965) 274-275.
51 PETRAS, J.M. Corticospinal fibers in New World and Old World simians. Brain Research, 8 (1968) 206-208.
52 PETRAS, J.M. Some efferent connections of the motor and somatosensory cortex of simian primates and felid, canid and procyonid carnivores. Ann. N.Y. Acad. Sci., 167 (1969) 469-505.
53 PETRAS, J.M. Connections of the parietal lobe. J. Psychiat. Research, 8 (1971) 189-201.
54 PINES, J.L. Zur Architektonik des Thalamus opticus beim Halbaffen (Lemur catta). J. Psychol. Neurol., 33 (1927) 31-72.
55 POWELL, T.P.S. Residual neurons in the human thalamus following hemidecortication. Brain, 75 (1952) 571-584.
56 POWELL, T.P.S. and COWAN, W.M. A study of thalamo-striate relations in the monkey. Brain, 79 (1956) 364-390.
57 SCHOEN, J.H.R. Comparative aspects of the descending fiber systems in the spinal cord. In: Organization of the spinal cord, Progress in Brain Research, Vol. 11, J.C. Eccles and J.P. Schadé, Eds., Elsevier Publ. Co., Amsterdam, 1964, pp. 203-222.

58 SHIPS, J.G. The nuclear configuration and cortical connections of the human thalamus. J. Comp. Neurol., 83 (1945) 1-56.

59 THOMAS, D.M., KAUFMAN, R.P., SPRAGUE, J.M. and CHAMBERS, W.W. Experimental studies of the vermal cerebellar projections in the brain stem of the cat (fastigiobulbar tract). J. Anat., Lond., 90 (1956) 371-385.

60 TONCRAY, J.E. and KRIEG, W.J.S. The nuclei of the human thalamus: A comparative approach. J. Comp. Neurol., 85 (1946) 421-460.

61 VERHAART, W.J.C. and KENNARD, M.A. Corticofugal degeneration following thermocoagulation of areas 4, 6 and 4-s in Macaca mulatta. J. Anat., Lond., 74 (1940) 239-254.

62 VOGT, C. La myéloarchitecture du thalamus du cercopithèque. J. Psychol. Neurol., 12 (1909) 285-324.

63 VOGT, C. and VOGT, O. Thalamuss studien I-III. I. Zur Einführung. II Homogenitat und Grenzgestaltung der Grisea des Thalamus. III. Das Griseum centrale (centrum medianum Luys). J. Psychol. Neurol., Leipzig, 50 (1941) 31-154.

64 WALKER, A.E. The thalamus of the chimpanzee I. Terminations of the somatic afferent systems. Confin. Neurol., 1 (1935) 99-127.

65 WALKER, A.E. The primate thalamus. The University of Chicago Press, Chicago (1938).

66 WALKER, A.E. The thalamus of the chimpanzee. II. Its nuclear structure, normal and following hemidecortication. J. Comp. Neurol., 69 (1938) 487-507.

DISCUSSION

YAKOVLEV:

I would like to ask Dr. Petras how he envisages the distribution of terminal branches of each of these corticofugal fibers in various structures on their way downstream. Do they run without branching until they reach to some particular subcortical region where they branch? After all, each fiber must have specific cells of termination. Or is it that each fiber sends collaterals distributed at many levels along the way down, the axon terminals of some of these fibers reaching to the cells in the brainstem and spinal cord?

PETRAS:

I do not have any data on the points that you raise, therefore, my comments must be considered speculative. My lesions are large, and considered from the neurocytological point of view, it is impossible in these experiments to deal with the problem of the morphology of corticofugal axons and their terminal and collateral branches. The large portions of a single gyrus that are ablated in our experiments result in the destruction of all cell laminae in the cortex. It is generally believed that the infragranular layers of the cortex contain neurons with axons that project subcortically. If pressed to speculate on the points you raise, I would be inclined to the view that the parent axon of each cell is a complex process of the cell with major collateral branches arborizing in many subcortical nuclei; the striatum, thalamus and other subcortical structures in the brain stem and spinal cord. Scheibel and Scheibel have described the large isodendritic type cells (Ramon-Moliner) of the reticular formation. These cells possess very long axons with numerous collaterals to nuclei of the brain stem and with intrathalamic terminals. Perhaps there are cortical neurons with similarly complex axonal arbors, although this does not rule out the possibility of other neuronal types with long axons projecting to one or just a few subcortical sites.

JASPER:

For those of us who are not so familiar with the technique, how far can you go with the modified Nauta in determining or getting the answer to this question, as to whether you are dealing with fine collaterals or real terminals? Is it always distinct?

PETRAS:

The silver methods stain degenerated axons and their terminal fields. It is possible to make qualitative estimates of fiber-caliber, but it is not possible to routinely distinguish the parent axons from fine collateral arbors. I would like to distinguish between the terms *terminal connections* and *synaptic complexes*, the latter being visible under the electron microscope. Experience with the silver methods enables us to determine fibers of passage from areas of terminal degeneration. We constantly compare the areas of ipsilateral terminal degeneration with adjacent nuclei and with contralateral nuclear groups. We look for areas of dense fiber degeneration where pericellular or peridendritic arbors may be present. Finding dense fiber degeneration, we call these nuclear areas *terminal fields*. The presence of a few degenerated fibers can be very problematical, unless the fibers occur in discrete bundles and suggest passing elements only. To recapitulate, the silver methods enable us to trace fiber tracts over long distances and to locate their areas of *terminal connections*. With the methods of electron microscopy we can take a forward step in describing the morphology of neural circuits, namely, we can visualize the actual structure of *synaptic complexes* themselves and attempt to describe where each synaptic type is ending be it on dendrites, cell body or the axon hillock.

YAKOVLEV:

I would like to point out that, generally speaking, there are three patterns of connectivity: at random, seriatim, and in-parallel. The connectivity in-parallel assumes the prevalent role with the development of the neocortex of mammals. The corticofugal fibers, such as the pyramidal tracts,are an example of connectivity in parallel. All levels are connected to the motor cortex in-parallel. It would be of interest to know how far this principle of connectivity might apply to the axons of the individual Betz pyramid of the kinesthetic analyzer.

HASSLER:

I must congratulate you for this really unique material you demonstrated for us, and for the very nice evaluation in the thalamus. May I ask two questions: One question is: Did you see this cluster-like appearances only in the anterior part of VL, VLo. of Olszewski, Vo.a. of my nomenclature, or also in other places? The other question is: Did you also perform lesions anterior to the precentral gyrus? I am astonished that there is no degeneration from the cortex to the pallidum, and in your sections I sometimes had the impression that you also have some stippling in the most anterior part of the substantia nigra; or did I have the wrong impression?

PETRAS:

The clustering of cells occurs in the rostral part of VL. The regions between these cellular islands are occupied by fiber bundles and are thus "neuron poor" or "neuron-free" areas. I have labeled this region VLo.

I have chimpanzee cases with lesions rostral to the motor cortex, however, this data is only now being stained.

Despite repeated efforts in the rhesus monkey, gibbon and chimpanzee I have not found evidence for the presence of fiber degeneration in the globus pallidus. So far as I can determine, the putamen is the chief terminal target for the corticofugal projection of the precentral and postcentral gyri, and of the superior and inferior parietal lobules in the case of the rhesus monkey.

The degenerating fibers you noticed in the substantia nigra were intended to symbolize fibers of passage which descend along the ventral margin of the nigra or through the substance of the pars reticulata of this nucleus. The other fibers which I represented on the drawings, in both the gibbon and chimpanzee, are also fibers of passage. The latter fibers are not descending elements but are "collateral fibers" eminating from the fiber tract in the cerebral peduncle. These "collaterals" traverse the pars reticulata and pars compacta of the nigra before eventual distribution to the nucleus ruber. I have never found evidence in monkeys or apes for the presence of terminal degeneration in the nigra following lesions of the precentral or postcentral gyri.

KUYPERS:

About lesions rostral to the precentral gyrus, we have tried to do the same thing as you did, and we were not so successful in staining the thalamus so beautifully, but we got degenerating fibers in the medial thalamus close to the intralaminar nuclei following lesions rostral to the precentral gyrus. Does that fit with your observations?

PETRAS:

Yes, in the case of the rhesus monkey.

KUYPERS:

When you see the thalamic distribution of the cortical fibers, they all seem to avoid the most ventral part of the VL.

PETRAS:

Yes, there is an important and anatomically distinct ventral area in VL which does not appear to contain fiber degeneration. I did not mention this in my presentation, because I did not think I would have time to cover the subject. This ventral area in the chimpanzee is reminiscent of the same region in the rhesus monkey thalamus which is called VLm by Olszewski. In the present chimpanzee cases I found no evidence of fiber degeneration in this nucleus.

HASSLER:

Did you try to differentiate between areas 4 and 6?

PETRAS:

Yes, I have tried to do this, especially in rhesus monkey experiments. I prefer to leave this question open, however, as the studies are still in progress and I have no comparable data in the chimpanzee.

YAKOVLEV:

I would like to ask about the collateralization of the corticofugal systems. I wonder whether it follows the intracortical collateralization of the axons.

PETRAS:

I cannot answer your question.

Corticothalamic Projections and Sensorimotor Activities
T. Frigyesi, E. Rinvik, and M.D. Yahr, editors. © 1972
Raven Press, New York.

Corticofugal Projections Governing Rhythmic Thalamic Activity

M. Steriade, P. Wyzinski* and V. Apostol**

This chapter essentially deals with corticothalamic projections revealed by electrophysiological recordings and the cortically elicited thalamic events underlying the spindle waves of the electroencephalogram. It is usually thought that such EEG activity is an intrathalamic affair. Some of the data reported below will merely add new evidence for the idea that a paramount role is played by the internuclear thalamic relationship in the maintenance and development of 8-12/sec spindles and related neuronal clustered firing. But the chief objective of our study was to enlarge the picture of intrathalamic circuitry governing EEG synchronization by analyzing the possible supplementary role of corticothalamic projections in the determination of the spindle activity.

This is not an unprecedented idea. In a series of papers more than three decades old, Dusser de Barenne and McCulloch (20) stated that, after a lesion in the monkey's sensory thalamus, the corresponding subdivision of the sensory cortex shows a diminution of its electrical activity; in addition, abnormal activity (contrasting with well-developed oscillatory rhythms from intact thalamus) appears in the thalamus which had been separated from the cortex by undercutting; they therefore concluded that the mutual connections are essential for the normal spontaneous electrical activity. However, only the dependence of cortical spindle rhythm upon the appropriate thalamic specific nucleus was later firmly emphasized (2). On the other hand, removal of cortical matter led to contradictory conclusions; some reported lack (39, 86), others the presence (2, 9, 47) or even increase (88) of spindles in the thalamus of decorticate preparations. This deceiving picture is the likely result of differences between topical and large ablations of the cortical mantle which comprises areas with different

----

*Holder of a Centennial Scholarship from the National Research Council of Canada.
**Visiting investigator, on leave of absence from the Institute of Neurology, Bucharest (Rumania).

or even opposite influences on thalamic spindles*, between the acute, semichronic and chronic experimental conditions, and of the different nature of the investigated spindling, occurring spontaneously or induced by large amounts of barbiturate. In any case, there is general agreement that thalamic spindle activity gives rise to the appearance of similar rhythmic waves in the cortex, while it is largely independent of the control of corticofugal mechanisms.

Why hark back to this topic? The main reason is that the ability of the thalamus to exhibit spindles in the absence of the cerebral cortex does not necessarily imply that in intact animals cortical areas have no role in modulating, enhancing or even triggering the basic mechanisms of spindling, which are certainly held in the thalamic neuronal network. This mechanism might be operating through the precise topographical arrangements of corticothalamic projection disclosed by morphological studies (60). If this were so, the control could be revealed by artificially setting in motion an orthodromic volley in corticofugal pathways and recording rhythmic neuronal activities in critical thalamic zones more efficiently than by studying the thalamic residuum following a cortical ablation. In the latter effort, the difficulty of interpreting both acute (irritative phenomena) and chronic (compensation or even overreaction) conditions cannot be emphasized enough. Consequently, a methodological question arises concerning the reliability of such procedures. The choice of electrical stimulation (and recording the evoked spindle waves enveloping the related unitary events) is dictated by the necessity of a *stringently controlled* factor which may act *reversibly* during EEG fluctuations indicating different levels of vigilance. These effects can be easily *compared* with periods of preceding and subsequent background activity; moreover, the use of testing corticofugal volleys can *reveal the synaptic pathways* and disclose the best neuronal candidates underlying the elicited rhythmic activity among the thalamic target populations.

Stimulation creates a caricature which is perhaps as far from reality as that induced by the ablation technique. But actively provoking a structure has some advantages in discovering its hidden properties, and simulation of a pattern of activity by electrical stimulation may provide clues to the understanding of mechanisms, despite the fact that "natural" events are always more nuanced and less predictable than "artificial" ones. The diversity of types of spontaneous spindles, as recently recognized in various thalamic areas (9), was certainly not exhausted through the stereotyped recruiting waves evoked by low-rate electrical pulses to the so-called "nonspecific" thalamic system, but such analyses, as presented in the pioneering works of Morison and Dempsey (48), Dempsey and Morison (15) and Jasper (37), and in the subsequent intracellular studies of Purpura and his group (52-54, 56), did give major answers to the problem of EEG synchronization.

The question now is whether other projection systems contribute to the genesis of

----

*Even the authors who found an increased thalamic spindling after decortication, when discussing contradictory results in the literature, admit that in some cases the cortical lesioning may involve areas which enhance spindles (88).

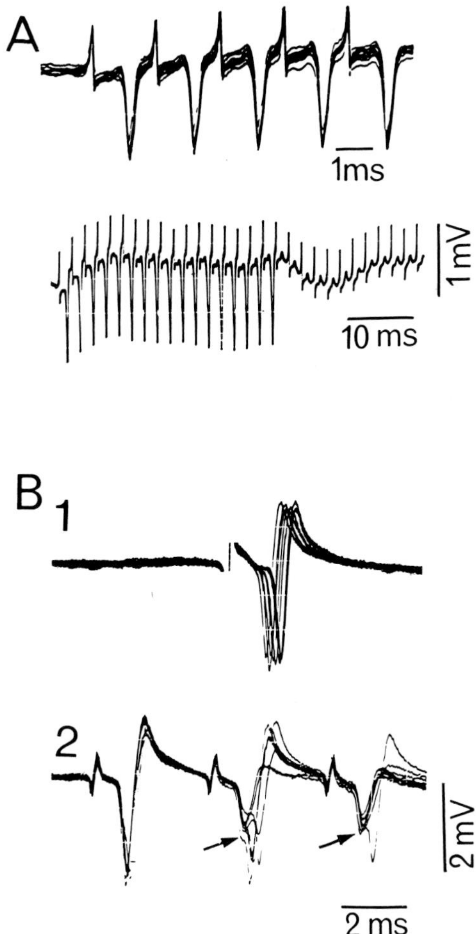

FIG. 1. Identification of a neuron in the dentate cerebellar nucleus projecting monosynaptically to the VL thalamic nucleus (A) and of a VL relay neuron (B). A: antidromic spikes following VL shocks. Note ability to follow fast stimuli (about 550/sec) without failure, at constant (1 msec) latencies; inhibition occurred only after 32 msec, likely due to a pathway involving the cerebellar cortex, simultaneous with the appearance of a slow positive shift. B: VL relay cell activated monosynaptically (note variations in latency; shortest value at 1 msec) following shocks to the cerebellothalamic pathway at the level of the red nucleus (1), and antidromically invaded (at around 0.85 msec latency) following a train of three shocks to the precruciate cortical area (2; arrows indicate IS-SD break). In this and following figures, negativity upwards. From Steriade, Apostol and Oakson (72).

thalamic rhythmic activity, defined as waxing and waning 8-12/sec oscillatory waves and related neuronal spike clusters interspersed with periods of silence, characteristic of decreased vigilance of the brain. The unaltered pattern of neuronal firing characteristic of EEG spindling in the thalamic motor relay following an extensive lesion of deep cerebellar nuclei, and the persistence of abortive spindle elements following a lesion destroying practically all the medial thalamus (73) (see also Figs. 13-14, in this chapter), contrasting with the disappearance of spindling in the respective cortical projection area after an elective lesion of the specific thalamic relay (2, 74), suggests that the specific—nonspecific intrathalamic pathways (16, 17) are complemented by other projection systems involving the complex organization of neuronal aggregates in specific thalamic nuclei for the control of EEG synchronization. The corticothalamic pathways, which have been revealed in the motor system by anatomical (10, 40, 59, 60) and electrophysiological (18, 27, 50, 61, 63, 73, 85) studies, are powerful projections which may directly contact the *interneuronal* apparatus in the ventrolateral (VL) thalamus and, thus, share the origin of the localized EEG spindling in this specific thalamocortical system. This is the core of our work.

The results derived from experiments reported below, on locally anesthetized *encephale isole* cats, will show that motor cortex stimulation induces 8-12/sec rhythmic waves in the VL nucleus, which exhibit a striking similarity in configuration, intraburst frequency and corresponding unitary events to both the EEG spindles occurring during spontaneous "sleepiness" and those induced by a very small amount of a short-acting barbiturate. When the EEG shows a low-voltage, fast activity, the elicited rhythmic VL sequence, transferred back to the motor cortical area, is confined to the period immediately following the testing cortical shock-train, but when there is an EEG background showing a decreased vigilance, it can take the pattern of the continuous spindling. Several data will champion the idea that, at least for the VL of the non-barbiturized cat, the orthodromic corticothalamic projections are mainly involved in the genesis of this cortically elicited activity, rather than the previously suggested (1, 4) inhibitory mechanism activated by the recurrent collaterals of specific thalamocortical axons. It will be also shown that, within the frame of the complex corticothalamic synaptic pathways, both the cells in the thalamic reticularis nucleus and the intrinsic VL interneurons can be driven monosynaptically by corticofugal volleys. The rhythmic elements are, however, the VL interneurons. Some findings are presented and the suggestion is made that the rich and rhythmic spike clusters of some interneurons, elicited by cortical stimuli in the spindle frequency range, may exert a powerful excitatory impingement on VL relay cells when they recover from the long-lasting inhibitory period, and thus contribute to the rebound activity.

RECIPROCAL SYNAPTIC PATHWAYS BETWEEN THE VENTROLATERAL THALAMUS AND THE MOTOR CORTEX

A. *The VL relay function* applies to the transfer of cerebellar (and striatal) messages towards the motor cortex. This can be demonstrated electrophysiologically by the evidence of neurons in the contralateral interpositus and dentate cerebellar nuclei projecting monosynaptically to the VL, and by recording this relayed ac-

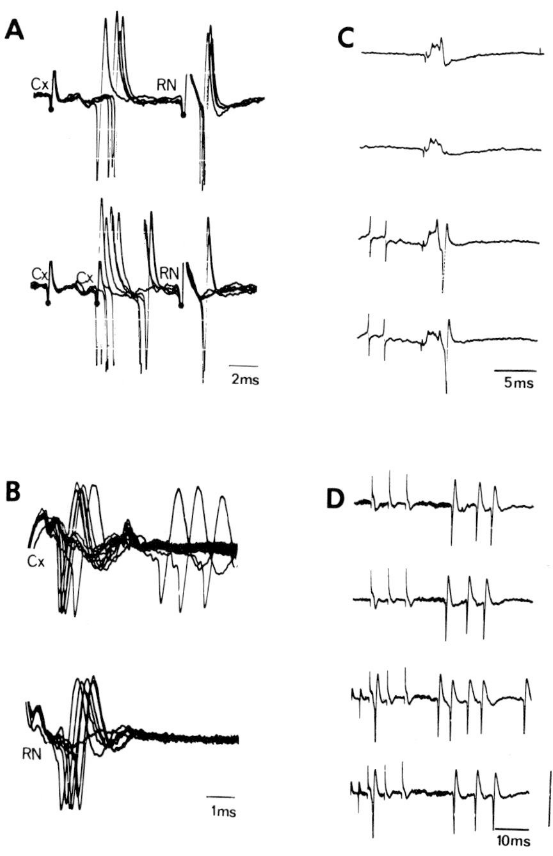

FIG. 2. Cerebellar and cerebral cortical converging inputs on single VL neurons. A-D, four different neurons. Testing stimuli applied to the cerebellothalamic pathway at the level of the red nucleus (RN) and to the lateral part of the precruciate gyrus (Cx); Dots indicate stimulus artifacts in A; in B, the sweeps were triggered by the stimuli; in C and D, the first two traces indicate the effect of the RN stimulation (one shock in C, a train of three shocks in D), and the last two traces show the same testing volleys preceded by two cortical shocks. Vertical bar: 1 mV. Full explanation in text.

tivity in VL cells, which can be also identified by their direct projection to the motor cortical area. Antidromic invasion in deep cerebellar nuclei following VL shocks* occurred at latencies from 1.0 to 1.8 msec in different units (Fig. 1A), indicating that the conduction velocity in the cerebellothalamic pathway (calculated for a distance of about 17 mm between the VL and the cerebellum) ranges roughly between 10 and 17 m/sec. This is somewhat slower than the 20 m/sec conduction velocity reported in the cerebello-rubral pathway (33). Monosynaptic excitation following shocks applied to the cerebellothalamic pathway could be obtained in VL cells (Fig. 1, B_1) which were also antidromically invaded by stimulating the depth in the lateral part of the precruciate gyrus (Fig. 1, B_2), an area where mass potentials were evoked with maximal amplitudes by brachium conjunctivum (63) and VL (68) stimulation. The latencies of cortically elicited antidromic spikes in VL, from 0.5 to 4.0 msec (50, 61, 63, 73, 85), reflected (on a basis of an approximated distance of 20 mm between the VL and the precruciate gyrus) a wide range of conduction time (between 5 and 40 m/sec) in this pathway.

A comparison of patterns of successive antidromic spikes in dentate and interposital cells with those in VL neurons indicates the ability of the former to follow 500-600/sec shocks for periods as long as 35-60 msec (Fig. 1A; see also Fig. 6 in ref. 73) which contrasted with the fragmentation between the initial segment (IS) and somadendritic (SD) spikes or complete inhibition usually seen in the latter only a few msec after the initial sign of invasion (Fig. 1, B_2). This suggests, from the very beginning of this story, the ability of cortical stimulation to set in motion the powerful equipment of inhibitory Golgi II type cells lying in the VL (82, 83) and it casts doubt on the existence of such short axon inhibitory cells in deep cerebellar nuclei (36).

B. The feed-back cortical control on VL principal cells parallels, in a descending way, the ascending transmission, relayed in the VL, of cerebellar and striatal information. Transsynaptic activation has been reported in association with antidromic spikes in the same VL unit following cortical (61, 63, 85) or capsular (27) stimulation. The existence of a thalamo-cortico-thalamic loop, and its subtle modalities of influencing the VL relay neurons, had to be proved by recording

----

*Monosynaptic activation (at around 2 msec) in the cerebellar dentate nucleus following VL stimuli, as previously reported from this laboratory (73), might be explained by recurrent cerebellar intranuclear collaterals (57). Another challenging inference, in spite of the fact that a thalamocerebellar pathway has not been yet described by anatomists, is that there is a feed-back information from the thalamic motor relay to the deep cerebellar nuclei. In fact, rubrocerebellar projections have already been disclosed in both anatomical (13) and electrophysiological (8, 24) studies, and orthodromic spikes follow VL stimuli in red nuclear cells (8) (the latter have been, however, ascribed in other experiments to an axon reflex in brachium conjunctivum fibers (84)).

unitary activities at the two extremities of the chain, to check the possibility of monosynaptic convergences of cerebellar and cortical inputs onto the same VL cell, to disclose different (direct and circuitous) pathways involved in the cortical control of single VL principal neurons, to obtain evidence on the cortical source of the descending fibers, and to reveal the nature of this influence. These data are presented.

1. It has been found that short-latency, excitatory corticothalamic linkages are convergent with cerebellothalamic fibers onto the same VL cells. Such a unit (Fig. 2A) was synaptically driven with one impulse discharge at 1.3-1.5 msec latency by a shock to the red nucleus*, and at 3-4 msec latency by stimulating the depth of the lateral part in the precruciate gyrus. It might be argued that the longer latency of a cortically evoked response and its dispersed spikes in this case do not necessarily imply plurisynaptic excitation, since it was recently reported that the conduction velocity of the cortico-VL fibers is significantly slower (4-14 m/sec) than that of cerebellothalamic axons, and that the cortically evoked EPSPs in VL cells have a much slower time-course than those elicited by cerebellothalamic stimulation (85). The existence of a slow negative field potential after the cortical shock and before the appearance of the evoked spikes (even more pronounced in Fig. 6A) may, however, suggest that another VL population was synaptically driven by the corticofugal volley at a shorter latency. This was actually shown for the cell depicted in Fig. 2B, which undoubtedly exhibits monosynaptic convergence of cerebellothalamic and corticothalamic pathways. This neuron discharged almost identically to both precruciate and red nuclear stimulation, with one impulse discharge to one single shock, at around 1.0 msec latency, thus indicating (if 0.3-0.5 msec is subtracted for the synaptic delay) that some corticothalamic fibers may have a conduction velocity as fast as 30-40 m/sec.

At short (3-6 msec) intervals, cortical stimulation proved to exert a facilitatory influence on the probability of monosynaptic VL firing in response to a subsequent cerebellothalamic testing shock, even when the precruciate conditioning volley did not by itself discharge the unit under observation (Fig. 2, C-D). This facilitatory effect exerted by the corticofugal projections upon VL responsiveness supports our previous data on depression of both spontaneous background activity and red nuclear evoked VL mass responses following an acute or chronic ablation of the pericruciate area (70).

----

*The stimulation of the cerebellothalamic fibers was performed in the present experiments at the red nuclear level (F 4-5). A synaptic relay at this level of the ascending pathway, however, is difficult to conceive in either felines or primates, if one takes into consideration the anatomical findings stating that both magno- and parvocellular parts of the red nucleus discharge exclusively downwards in the monkey (51), and recent electrophysiological data showing that cat's rubral cells may be antidromically excited from the contralateral spinal cord, ipsilateral medulla and contralateral brachium conjunctivum, but not from the thalamus, although the electrode placements in this series of experiments included extensive areas from L 3 to L 6 of ventralis anterior (VA) and VL (8).

It can be also related to some results from experiments done on the somatosensory thalamocortical system, showing depression of spontaneous firing in the ventrobasal (VB) complex after KCl application or cooling of the somesthetic cortical area (89), as well as cortically induced improvement of synaptic transmission in the VB expressed by the decreased latency of peripherally elicited discharges (6).

Reduced amplitude of the monosynaptically relayed wave evoked in the VL by cerebellothalamic stimulation, occurring at longer (10–100 msec) intervals after motor cortex stimulation (29, 50, 75) and associated with silenced firing in multiunit recordings of VL neurons (70), has to be ascribed to IPSPs always following the orthodromic spikes (27, 28, 50, 85).*

2. Cortical cells giving rise to descending, thalamopetal axons have been recognized in the pericruciate area by their antidromic invasion following VL shocks. In most cases, stimulating the pyramidal tract (PT) in the medulla or pes pedunculi could not also backfire these neurons, even if the stimulus strength was increased and the current spread to neighbouring structures, as can be seen from the different components of the cortical field response without or with lemniscal contamination (32, 35). However, a few motor cortical cells have been antidromically invaded in the precruciate gyrus and just behind the cruciate sulcus both from the VL (Fig. 3A) and PT (Fig. 3D), with corresponding latencies but with identical patterns of IS-SD break at successive shocks, and transsynaptically excited when the stimulating electrode was moved deeper in the VL (Fig. 3B). Such units were found in each of the two groups of fast and slow (the antidromic spikes in Fig. 3D have 4.7 msec latency when stimulating the medulla) PT cells. The physical spread of current from the VL to the internal capsule may be precluded since stimulation of other thalamic points, in the lateral part of the VB complex, closer to the internal capsule than the VL, did not elicit antidromic spikes in these cases even at higher intensities (Fig. 3C).

Neurons such as depicted in Fig. 3 are to be regarded as relaying messages from the VL (in B) to the PT (in D), and sending axon collaterals back to their main source of afferences (in A). This confirms previous evidence, by means of the evoked potential technique, of a collateral pathway from the PT to the thalamus (12), in spite of subsequent negative results reporting the lack of mass postsynaptic activity in the VL following PT stimulation (19). The failure to evoke mass responses may be ascribed to the rather scanty projections of PT axon collaterals to the VL, as found in the present unitary study. It should be recalled in this respect that the synaptic excitation of VB neurons by recurrent collaterals of PT axons has also been found to occur in less than 30% of the tested cells (66).

The motor feed-back regulation may also be assisted by the contralateral pre-

----

*Cortically elicited inhibition in VL cells without preceding spikes might be ascribed to cell depolarization, as seen in the large amplitude of the hyperpolarization in Fig. 4 (18); see also the evolution from IPSP preceded by spike discharge to IPSP in isolation with progressive depolarization of the membrane potential in the neuron depicted in Fig. 4A in another work (50).

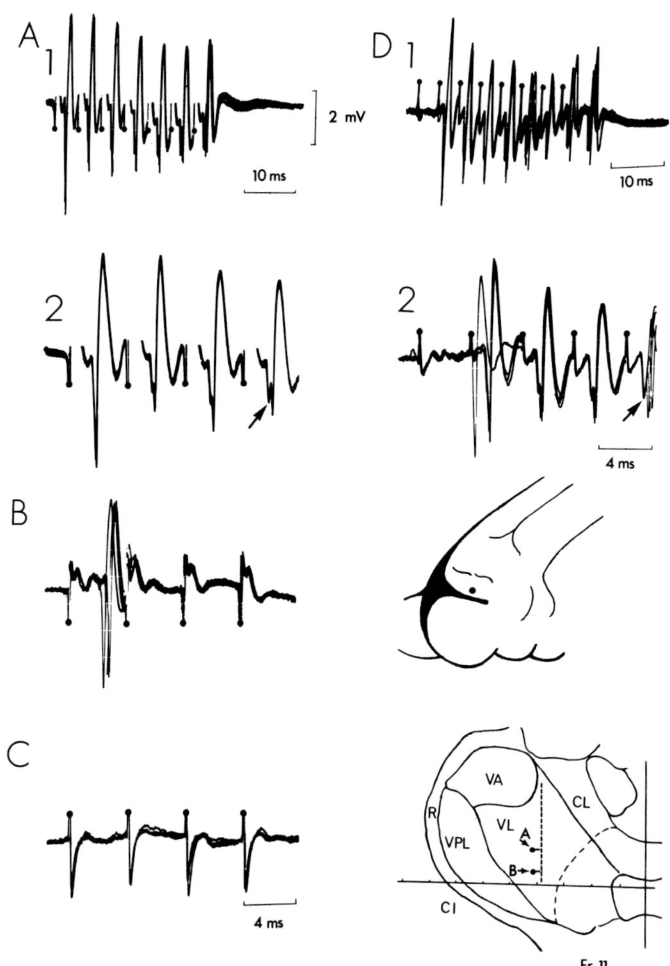

FIG. 3. Suggestion of a thalamo-cortico-thalamic loop through pyramidal tract axon collaterals. Recording of a motor cortical cell in the postcruciate gyrus at the point indicated in the brain drawing. In A, VL stimulation (at the point marked on the thalamic track) elicited antidromic spikes at 1.85 msec latency; note IS-SD break (arrow) at successive shocks. In B, the stimulating VL electrode was moved deeper; the same cell became activated synaptically (spike diminished in amplitude); note variations in latency and unresponsiveness to subsequent stimuli. In C, no response to VB stimulation at F9, L6, D1, closer to the internal capsule than the VL stimuli in A. This cell was identified as a slow PT neuron, as invaded antidromically (at 4.7 msec latency) from the medulla (D), with a pattern of IS-SD break similar to that elicited by VL stimuli (compare A_2 to D_2). Recordings made in the depicted order: A to D. Further comments in text.

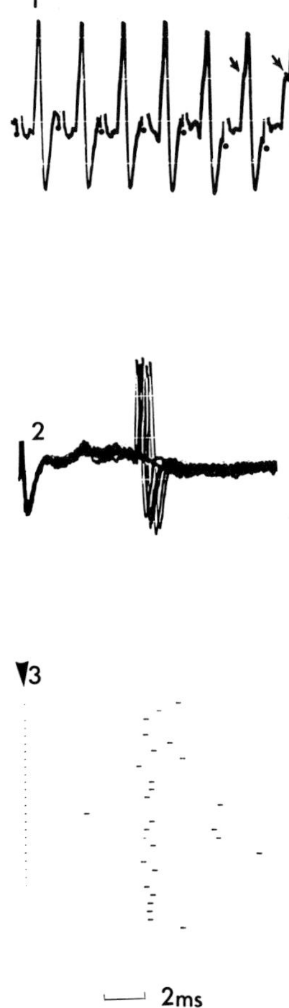

FIG. 4. Contralateral cortical control on thalamic VL nucleus through callosal pathways. Chronically implanted, behaving Macaca mulatta. Recording in the arm area of the left precentral cortical gyrus. Stimulation of the left VL nucleus (in 1) elicited antidromic spikes (at 0.8 msec latency) with IS-SD break (arrows). Stimulation of the homotopic contralateral (right) cortical points evoked synaptic discharges (original spikes superimposed in 2, dotgram in 3). Unpublished data by Steriade and Halle.

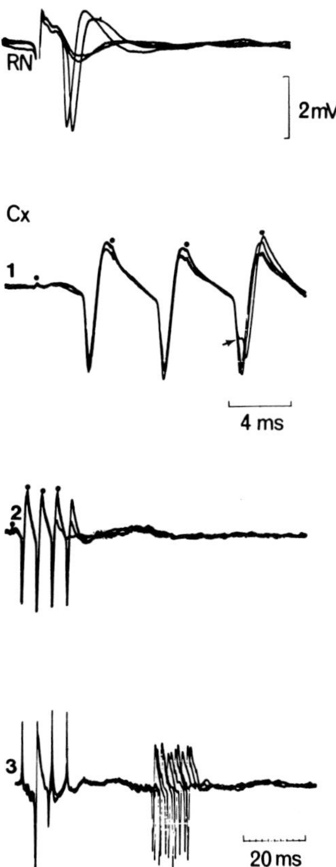

FIG. 5. Cortically elicited long – latency discharges in a VL relay cell, identified by red nuclear (RN) evoked synaptic discharges and antidromic spikes following pre-cruciate cortical (Cx) stimulation. 1 and 2: antidromic invasion of the cell, depicted at fast and slow speed. In 3: increasing intensity of Cx stimulation led to inhibition of antidromic responses following the first full spike and appearance of long-latency (25-40 msec) synaptic discharges.

cruciate cortex. The synaptic excitation of identified VL relays cells by shocks to the opposite motor cortical area (reported in detail elsewhere (80)) usually required temporal summation and the latency of the response fluctuated markedly, with the shortest spike latency between 6 and 15 msec. Consequently, the following inhibition and postinhibitory rebounds, in the form of spike clusters, were less pronounced than with ipsilateral cortical stimuli, although essentially the same features were exhibited in both cases (compare Fig. 16 and Fig. 19). The contralateral cortical control is presumably exerted by the callosal pathways. This seems to be a function common to felines and primates, since in another series of experiments (77) we recorded single units in the precentral arm area of the chronically implanted, behaving Macaca mulatta, antidromically invaded by ipsilateral VL stimulation and synaptically driven at short latencies (4-6 msec) by stimulating the homotopic points in the contralateral motor area (Fig. 4).

3. Long-latency (25-40 msec) bursts of 6-10 repetitive (200-300/sec) spikes in VL neurons following precruciate stimulation were seen in previous experiments from this laboratory (73). Such bursts of high-frequency discharges were not related to the late (150-300 msec latency) postinhibitory rebound in the same cell, as was shown by their independent changes with increasing intensities of testing cortical stimuli, and their different behavior during slow sleep: the former were abolished even during minimal and transient signs of EEG synchronization, which contrasted with preservation, in the same functional state, of the late, postinhibitory spike clusters (see Fig. 14 in ref. 73; see also these differential effects in our Fig. 6). The bursts occurring at 25-40 msec latency reflect a powerful excitatory corticofugal drive, probably exerted through a complex chain of internuncial thalamic (VL?) neurons. When evoked in an identified VL relay cell or in association with short-latency spikes indicating more direct cortico-VL linkages, these bursts always require temporal summation by repetitive shocks, appearing only after the end of the testing train (see Fig. 6). But once set in motion, they may occur even during the inhibitory period following the first antidromic spike of the same neuron, inhibition which is evidenced by the failure of the IS spike to invade the SD membrane (at the second shock) or by complete inhibition of backfiring to successive stimuli (Fig. 5). These data are supported by intracellular recordings (see Frigyesi and Schwartz, Chapter in this volume) showing late (at comparable, 35-45 msec, latencies) EPSPs in VL neurons, elicited by capsular stimulation, occurring during period of prominent hyperpolarization of these cells (Fig. 2, H-I, in their paper). It has to be emphasized that such cortically evoked spike barrages in VL relay neurons, as identified by their monosynaptic spikes to red nuclear stimulation and antidromic invasion following precruciate shocks (Fig. 5), were never elicited at latencies shorter than 25-30 msec. This is stressed to infer an interposed chain of excitatory interneurons driven by corticofugal fibers and acting on VL relay cells, and to differentiate the principal cells from the VL interneurons engaged directly by corticofugal fibers (vide infra, Fig. 7).

As mentioned above, cortical stimulation could result in short-latency (4-5 msec) single spikes and long-latency (25-40 msec) repetitive discharges in the same neuron (Fig. 6), which suggest two different, oligo- and multisynaptic corticothalamic linkages acting on VL cells. When recording also the slow focal waves, the repetitive discharges were constantly superimposed on a negative (N) field potential, indicating depolarization in a pool of neighbouring neurons; only then, the positive (P) wave, regarded as reflecting neuronal inhibition, developed and was followed by a spike cluster in the single unit or, contingently, in most or all of the simultaneously recorded cells, possibly triggering another cycle of similar events. The repetitive discharges superimposed on the N wave were abolished following administration of Surital, in an amount as small as 1 mg/Kg (occasionally the amplitude of the related slow wave was also reduced), while the late spike cluster was left intact (Fig. 6, compare C with D).

This sequence apparently resembles that described in VB neurons by Andersen and

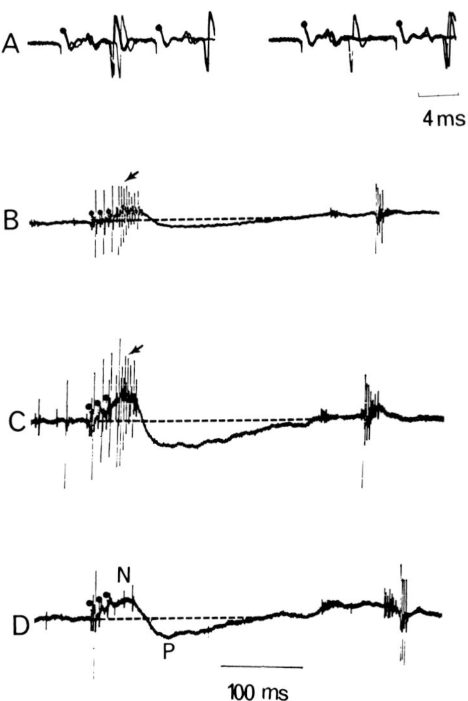

FIG. 6. Oligo- and plurisynaptic cortico-VL linkages. The same VL unit was recorded in A-D, without (A) and with focal slow waves (B-D); in C-D the gain was in creased 2.5 times, because of the diminution in spike amplitude. Note the smaller spikes recorded (especially in C-D) simultaneously with the large positive-negative discharge. Short-latency (4-5 msec) discharges (in A), and both short- and long-latency (arrow) discharges (in B). 1 mg/Kg i.v. Surital was administered between C and D. See further explanation in text.

his colleagues (1, 3). Several difficulties in reconciling their hypothesis with the interpretation of our findings will be discussed in the last section, when different features of EEG spindling and related unitary events induced by cortical stimulation will be presented. For now it is sufficient to mention some factual dissimilarities. The N-P sequence was seen in the VB following an a s c e n d i n g volley arising along the lemniscal axons, while essentially only the P wave was produced following cortical stimulation (see Fig. 1 in ref. 3); accordingly, they ascribed the N wave to postsynaptic excitation evoked in VB relay cells by the afferent lemniscal stimulation, while the P component was exclusively ascribed to the mechanism of recurrent collaterals of thalamocortical axons exciting local inhibitory interneurons. In our experiments, too, the P wave might occasionally occur in the VL without a preceding depolarizing component (see Fig. 17C), but, as a rule, it followed a powerful excitatory corticothalamic

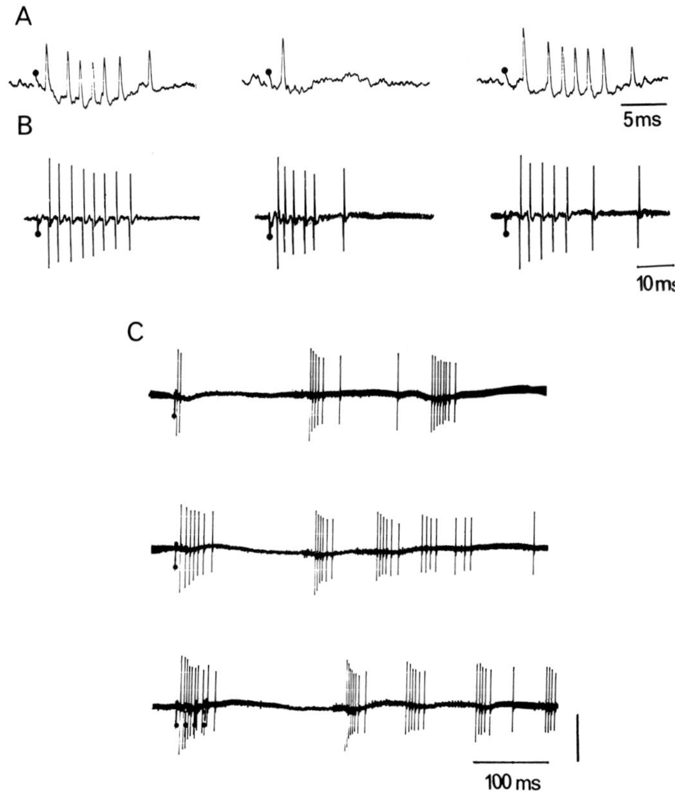

FIG. 7. High-frequency barrage discharges elicited by precruciate cortical shocks in presumed interneurons recorded within the VL anatomical limits. Three different cells (A–C). Vertical bar: 0.5 mV in A, 1 mV in B–C. Full description of latencies and intraburst frequencies in text. Note in C, the relation of the richness and rhythmicity in the late clusters with different degrees of the early excitation; one (first and second trace during periods of EEG desynchronization and synchronization, respectively) and four testing shocks (last trace); compare the discharge modality of this cell with the very similar pattern of cortically evoked discharge in the interneuron depicted in Fig. 20C.

drive. When a fully developed N wave with superimposed synaptic unit discharges were seen following the cortical shock train, the initiation of the P wave could be delayed and reached latencies as long as 60–70 msec (Fig. 6). The lack or the presence of the cortically elicited N component suggests that the synaptic discharges elicited by corticofugal volleys can be seen in precise VL districts by checking the adequate point for stimulating the motor cortex, as expected from a consideration of the fine topographical and somatotopical arrangements of cortico-VL projections (60). Finally, let us anticipate that the N-P sequence followed by a postinhibitory rebound and a similar series of cyclic events were seen in the VL of the encephale isole cat by cortical, but not by cerebellothalamic, stimulation (vide infra, Fig. 17D).

C. The VL Golgi 2nd type neurons or "cellules à cylindre-axe court," as termed by Ramon y Cajal (57) in the VB region, may be recognized from their high-frequency (up to 600/sec) spike barrages, recalling Renshaw (58) cells in the spinal cord and interneurons within the cerebellar cortex (21). It has been demonstrated in this study that such cells, recorded within the VL anatomical limits,* may be synaptically engaged by direct fibers arising in the motor cortical area. Some of these units showed monosynaptic excitation following precruciate stimulation (latency of the first evoked spike at 1.1 msec), with a high-frequency (500-600/sec) burst of up to seven or eight discharges, the changes in latency of the first spike displacing correspondingly the entire group (Fig. 7A). The frequency of the spike barrage in other cells was lower (300/sec in Fig. 7B; 150-200/sec in Fig. 7C) and the latency of the first cortically elicited discharge in the burst ranged between 1.5 and 2.5 msec. This pattern of evoked discharges cannot be ascribed to cell injury, since it was observed in neurons exhibiting small negative, healthy spikes, which suggests a certain distance from the recording microelectrode (Fig. 7A), and because of the unchanged spike amplitude and configuration throughout the long period of recording required for studying the spontaneous firing and the evoked discharges during different periods of synchronizing and desynchronizing EEG patterns (see Fig. 20). None of the cells showing such a pattern of discharge could be invaded antidromically by exploring all cortical foci in the pericruciate area. Synaptic activation of an interneuron by recurrent collaterals of specific thalamocortical axons cannot be definitely ruled out in these cases. However, since none of these cells could be driven, and since such a pattern of discharge was not elicited by cerebellothalamic stimulation giving rise to action potentials in the thalamocortical radiation, the possibility of direct linkages of corticofugal fibers with the VL interneuronal apparatus seems more likely.

It should be noted parenthetically that such a direct and high-security cortical descending pathway was also disclosed by recording synaptic discharges at 0.9-1.2 msec latency (which were able to follow all the shocks in a train at 100/sec) evoked by precruciate stimulation in cells lying in the rostral pole of the thalamic reticular complex (see Fig. 21), which could also be recognized by their long, high-frequency spike barrages during EEG synchronization, as recently described by Schlag and Waszak (65). The behavior of cortically evoked discharges in reticularis cells during EEG patterns of waking and slow sleep paralleled the changes undergone during the same functional states by cortically evoked discharges in VL interneurons (Fig. 21), and both these changes were opposite in sign to the fluctuations in responsiveness of VL relay

----

*Their ratio to the VL principal neurons appeared to be roughly 1:5 which is within the limits (1:3-1:6) reported in anatomical studies (45, 82) and electrophysiological recordings of VB cells (5), but the difficulty of recording such neurons makes any inference concerning their true ratios hypothetical.

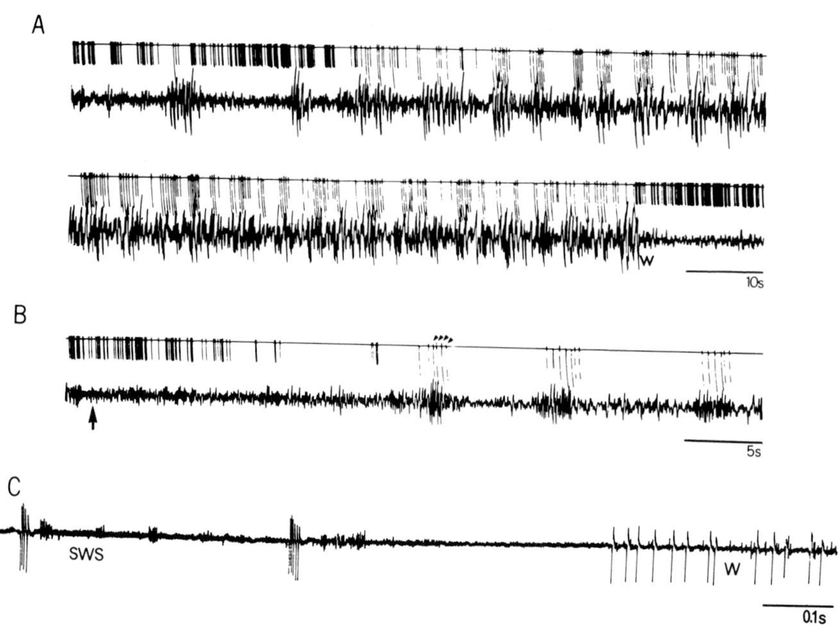

FIG. 8. Fluctuations in the spontaneous firing of VL cells during EEG patterns of waking (W) and synchronized sleep (SWS). In A-B of this figure (as well as in other similar recordings of subsequent figures), EEG was recorded from the ipsilateral pericruciate cortical area and VL unit spikes displayed on the oscilloscope were used to deflect one pen of the ink-writing machine; each deflection exceeding the common level (in A, or marked by small arrows in B) represents a group of 3 to 7 high-frequency spikes, as depicted with original discharges in C. Spontaneously occurring SWS in A and C; EEG synchronization induced by 1 mg/Kg i.v. Surital at the arrow in B. Note: sudden, long-lasting depression of spontaneous firing at the very onset of EEG synchronization (B); rhythmic (3-4/sec) spike clusters in close time-relation with groups of EEG spindles during both natural (A) and barbiturate-induced (B) synchronization; regularization and increased mean-rate of discharges on spontaneous arousal (W, in A and C); bursts of spikes at different rhythmicities in two simultaneously recorded spikes in C, during SWS. Modified from Steriade, Apostol and Oakson (73).

cells. Several anatomists (46, 64) reported that reticularis cells do not project axons to the cerebral cortex; therefore, their synaptic activation following cortical stimuli is not attributable to recurrent collateral excitation by antidromic invasion. The present disclosure of monosynaptic corticoreticular linkages is an electrophysiological correlate of corticoreticular fibers revealed by morphological studies (60)(see also other references in the discussion of ref. 46 and 60). Similarly, intracellular (Frigyesi and

Schwartz) and extracellular (Massion and Rispal-Padel) data are reported in this volume; the longer latencies seen in those records (at least 2.5 msec) probably imply indirect, oligosynaptic, corticoreticular linkages.

The early cortically evoked excitation of the presumed VL interneurons was followed by long-lasting (100-200 msec) silence and, thereafter, by rhythmic spike clusters in the frequency range of 8-12/sec. The latency and prominence of these late events were generally related to the frequency and number of spikes in the early group of evoked discharges (Fig. 7C). The richness in spikes, and the number and rhythmicity of late clusters, were always much more pronounced in such presumed VL interneurons than similar events recorded from the VL relay cells.

Since, to the best of our knowledge, the present and a previous work by Marco *et al.*(43) are the only available reports on interneuronal barrage discharges in the VL region (the failure to record such cells in other experiments is ascribed by some authors (65) to different characteristics of the microelectrodes), it seems worthwhile to compare the features of response in these two studies. The spontaneous firing of such interneurons cannot be related with data resulting from their recordings in deeply barbiturized preparations, where the presumed interneurons, as opposed to the principal cells, did not usually fire except in response to shocks. In our experiments, longer intervals at the beginning of a *spontaneous* interneuronal barrage with progressively increasing spike frequency to the middle of the burst (see Fig. 20A) contrasted with the spike organization in the spontaneous spike clusters occurring during synchronized sleep in VL relay cells, which exhibited the shortest interval at the beginning and successively increasing intervals towards the end of the burst (see Fig. 8C; see also Fig. 4 in ref. 73). Such a pattern, with a longer interval between the first two than between the second and third spikes, was also seen in some of the *evoked* barrages (Fig. 7A), and it was also described for 65% of the cells in the study of Marco *et al.* (43) (see their Fig. 6). Because these authors stimulated the VL intranuclearly, the identity of the input was reasonably qualified as "unknown" in their interneurons discharging transsynaptically at 2-20 msec. It can be supposed that the interneurons excited in the present work at significantly shorter latencies (1.1-1.5 msec) by precruciate stimuli, belong to a specific, cortically driven neuronal population, and that their testing shocks mostly affected medial thalamic, reticular thalamic and other as yet unknown projection systems implicated in the extraordinary complexity of the thalamic interneuronal networks (52), which makes any tentative scheme provisional and oversimplified. We have no data about the nature of such interneurons, which they believe to be inhibitory (Renshaw-like), in view of the good time relation between a hyperpolarizing potential and a spike barrage recorded from the vicinity, but we think that an excitatory nature can be attributed to at least some of these cells, as we will later infer.

CONTROL OF ACTIVITIES IN PRINCIPAL CELLS OF THE VENTROLATERAL THALAMUS DURING WAKING AND SYNCHRONIZED SLEEP

A. *The spontaneous discharges* of more than 90% of the VL cells showing fluctuations in their background firing during EEG patterns of waking and slow sleep were regularized and they increased the mean-rate of discharges on spontaneous and reticular or sensory elicited arousal (Fig. 8A) (41, 72-74). The increase of the overall amount of spikes during wakefulness (mean-discharge rates of 7-40/sec, compared to 1-5/sec during slow sleep) was generally more dramatic during the first few seconds of arousal than during the subsequent steady state of waking (73). Mono- and plurisynaptic EPSPs induced in VL neurons by stimulating the brain stem tegmentum are probably the basis of tonic impingement from the waking reticular system onto the thalamic motor relay (55).

The sudden decrease or even complete silence of the spontaneous unit activity at the very onset of slow sleep, which was valid for both the naturally occurring synchronization and the EEG changes induced by a very small (1-2 mg/Kg) amount of Surital (Fig. 8B), could result from abrupt withdrawal of tonic excitatory reticulo-VL impulses. The clustered firing appeared when 8-12/sec EEG spindles developed within the frame of synchronizing patterns. The spike clusters lasted 10-15 msec and consisted of 3-7 spikes at about 300-500/sec (Fig. 8C). This high intraburst frequency was reflected by an early, major modal interval at 2-3 msec, whereas such extremely short intervals are absent during wakefulness when the intervals are dispersed between 20 and 75 msec (see Fig. 13), as during waking, they are usually lacking at the extremities of this neuronal chain, in cerebellar (72, 73) and motor cortical (22, 77) cells. The rhythmicity of spike clusters was seen by a late, minor interval mode around 200 msec, reflecting the more or less regular periods of about 200-500 msec between the bursts of spikes (41, 72, 73).

The close time-relation between the VL spike clusters and the motor cortex spindle waves was always observed when the EEG synchronization was induced by barbiturates (7, 41), even in a very small (1 mg/Kg i.v.) dose (Fig. 8B) (73). When spontaneous cortical spindling is considered, this relation is a matter of controversy: it was ascertained (73) or denied (41). Moreover, in the latter case, no clear relationship was found even between a local thalamic spindle sequence (recorded with the same microelectrode) and the bursts of unitary discharges (41). There are several aspects to be discussed in this respect, clearly dissociating (1) the problem of time-relation between VL spike clusters and *local* spindles, from (2) that of relation with *cortical* spindles.

(1) After a re-analysis of this problem, there is no doubt in our opinion that VL spike clusters, occurring spontaneously during the EEG synchronization in the non-barbiturized *encephale isole* cat, are closely related with spindles and that they are superimposed on negative slow waves, belonging to local spindle sequences at around 10/sec; such focal negative components likely reflect depolarization in a large pool of elements. Certainly, when a single unit is recorded, the frequency of its spike clusters is generally lower than that of 8-12/sec in the spindle waves, but with multiunit recordings frequently spontaneous local negative waves envelop a superimposed burst of spikes of *one* or *another* of the cells under observation; occasionally, almost *all* the units from the recorded population discharge on the negative slow shift (Fig. 17B). This is similar to what happens during natural drowsiness and light sleep in the VB complex of the chronically implanted, behaving cat, where

multiunit recordings also proved that rhythmic bursts of discharges are superimposed on negative waves of the local spindles, with similar frequencies (31). As with all biological, "spontaneously" occurring phenomena, their less predictable whims (due, in fact, to interference with still active desynchronizing mechanisms, much more affected with barbiturate anesthesia) may put the spike cluster on the crest of the negative wave, occasionally on the declining phase or, exceptionally, even during the slow positivity (Fig. 17A), which simply implies that this unit discharged in spite of the

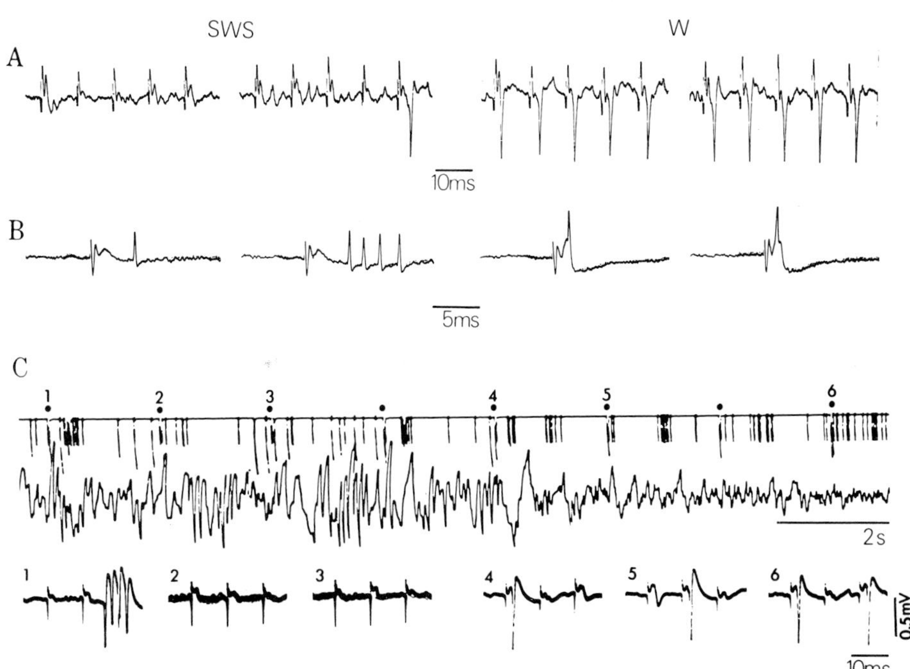

FIG. 9. Synaptic excitation of VL neurons elicited by red nuclear stimulation during wakefulness (W) and spontaneously occurring slow wave sleep (SWS). Three different cells (A–C). Note: short-latency discharges (B) and ability to follow without failure a train of shocks (A) during W; increase in latency, sometimes with repetitive firing (B) or near disappearance of evoked spikes (A) during SWS. In A and B, two testing stimulations (single shock in B and a train of five pulses in A) are depicted during both W and SWS. C, another cell: simultaneously analyzed background firing (first trace, as in the preceding figure), EEG activity (second trace), and, at the bottom, oscilloscopic records corresponding to figures at the top trace and showing the discharges evoked by a train of three shocks during different patterns of EEG rhythms. Note: during SWS (1–3) lack of short-latency evoked discharges (a spontaneous burst of 450–500/sec spikes in relation with the beginning of a EEG spindle appeared in 1); during EEG arousal (6) and even preceding it by a few seconds (4–5), monosynaptic discharges to one or two of the testing shocks. From Steriade, Apostol and Oakson (73).

fact that most of its neighbours were inhibited. But, generally, a consistent relation could be found between the spike clusters of different neurons and each negative slow component of the local spindle (Fig. 17B). The variable correspondence actually depends on the level of the synchronization; the slow waves of slightly-, fully-, or hypersynchronized states are time-related with some, many or almost all simultaneously recorded neurons, as also shown by Verzeano et al. (87) in the monkey's thalamus.

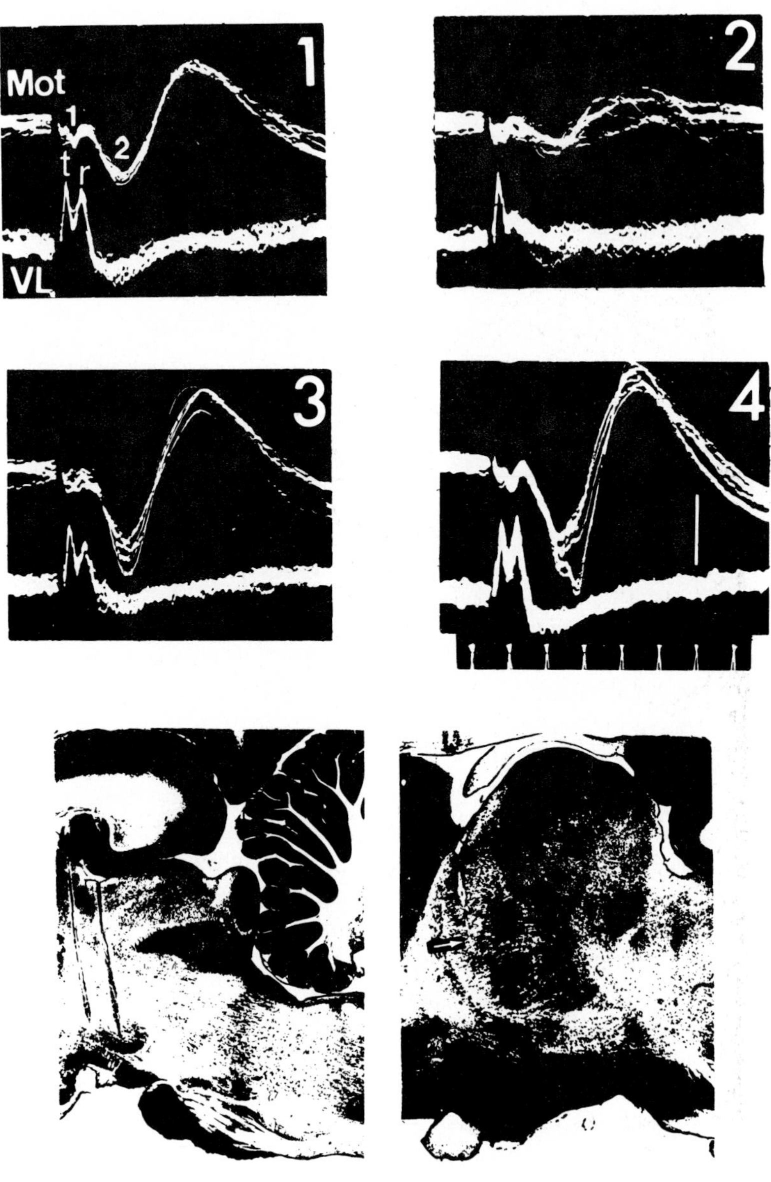

FIG. 10

(2) The relation between the VL spike clusters and a group of spindle waves recorded from the motor cortex was also more evident when the EEG synchronization was induced by a very small amount of barbiturate (Fig. 8B) than with naturally occurring spindles, but in the latter case too, the two events were well time-locked, as can be observed in Figs. 8A, 11B and 12A $_2$. Some failures in detecting this correspondence (as seen, f.i., in Fig. 9C, where a group of cortical spindles occurred between two groups of VL spike clusters) might be due to the position of the recording cortical electrode, which must be at the very point of projection of the observed VL relay neuron when the relation is checked. Actually, more or less accurate synchrony between thalamic rhythmic activity and cortical spindle waves was obtained by moving the cortical electrode by only 0.75 mm (7). This correspondence is not entirely due (even if it is rendered more evident) to the artificial condition created by the barbiturate anesthesia, since a good time relation was also seen between VB rhythmic unitary discharges and spindles of the electrocorticogram during behavioral light sleep in the chronically implanted cat (31). Certainly, such a correspondence between thalamic and cortical events is easier to detect in acute than in chronic experiments with unchangeable locations of the cemented wires or silver balls. As already emphasized (73), the gross temporal relation between a group of EEG spindle waves and a series of thalamic bursts of spikes did not imply the same frequency in both phenomena. The frequency in the former ranged invariably between 8 and 12 or 14/sec, while in the latter it was usually 2-5/sec, but occasionally at 10-12/sec (see these differences in the two spikes depicted in Figs. 8C and 12A$_3$), and the same unit might display both

---

FIG. 10. Modifications undergone by simultaneously recorded mass responses elicited by red nuclear stimulation in the VL nucleus and motor cortical area during wakefulness (1), drowsiness with EEG spindles (2), slow wave sleep (3) and paradoxical sleep (4) in a chronically implanted, behaving cat. Time marker: 2 msec. Vertical bar: 0.3 mV. At the bottom, location of stimulating and recording deep electrodes used in these experiments; left: two stimulating electrodes inserted in the middle and in front of the red nucleus; right: the electrode was located in the anterior part of the VL (arrow), used for recording rubrally evoked potentials (this figure) or for evoking mass responses in the motor cortex and the pyramidal tract. In 1, t indicates the presynaptic, and r the monosynaptically generated component of VL response; the first positive deflection (1) of the cortical response is closely related to the r VL component and could still be recorded in acute experiments from the white matter following cortical ablation; the second positive component (2) is cortically generated, as shown (78) by its selective disappearance following topical ablation of the motor area. Note: striking reduction of the VL postsynaptic (r) component during drowsiness (in 2) and its enhancement during waking (in 1) and paradoxical sleep (in 4), without concomitant alterations of the presynaptic (t) component; increase of cortically elaborated component (2) during slow wave sleep (in 3), in spite of the reduction in the output from the VL, evidenced by decrease of the VL relayed (r) component and early (1) cortical deflection. Modified from Steriade, Iosif and Apostol (78).

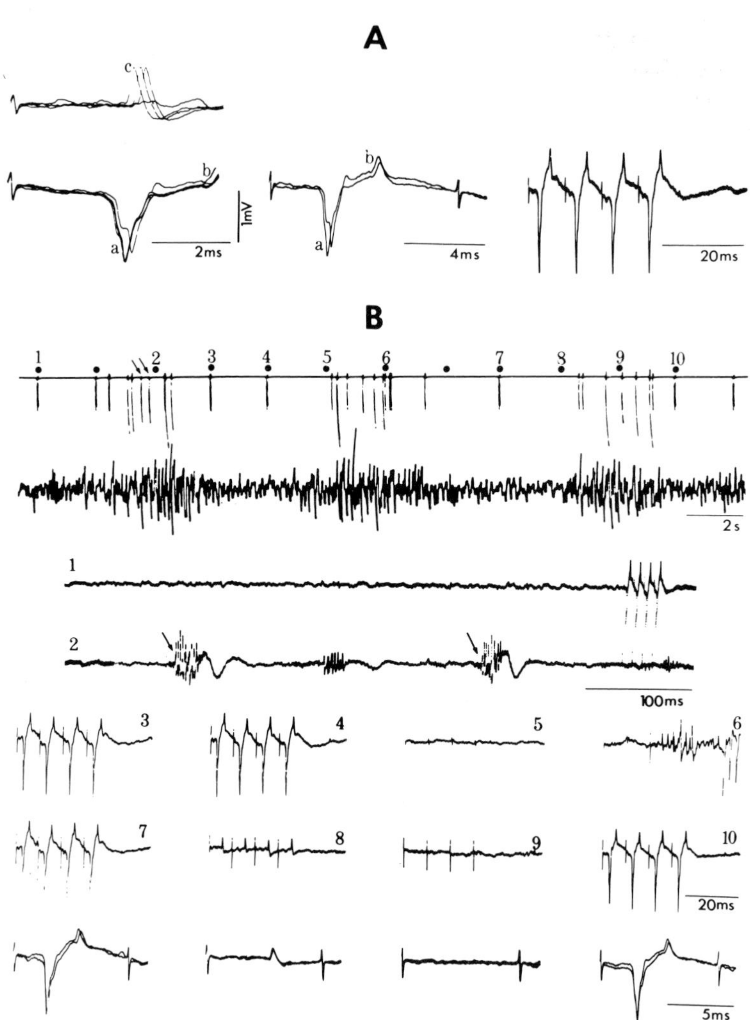

FIG. 11. Suppression of antidromic invasion induced in VL cells by cortical precruciate stimulation during EEG spindles. Three neurons (a: large positive-negative spike, b: small negative spike, and c: larger negative spike) were simultaneously recorded and identified by stimulating in the depth of the lateral part of the precruciate motor cortex. Neuron c was synaptically excited (note variations in latency) with the shortest latency at 2.8 msec (A, at the top); by increasing the voltage from 7V to 9V (the shock triggered the sweep), cells a and b became antidromically invaded at 2.45 msec and 4.8 msec latencies, respectively, as shown by ability to follow fast stimuli without fail-

basic frequencies during EEG spindles. The cortical spindle waves may be partially ascribed to the spike discharges within the clusters of VL relay neurons, transferred to the appropriate point in the pericruciate area. This view is supported by the close time-relation between a burst of spikes in VL cells and the surface-positive (41) or depth-negative (73) phases (reflecting neuronal excitation of cortical cells receiving VL messages) of spindle-like activity appearing in the motor cortex under different experimental conditions. But the mechanism of cortical spindles exceeds that of a simple reflection of the thalamic spindling; the complexity can be ascribed to interference of the latter with intrinsic synchronized alternating excitatory and inhibitory postsynaptic potentials of motor cortical neurons (38). This is probably the reason behind the reduced, but still obvious, correspondence of VL spike clusters with cortical than with local thalamic spindle waves.

B. The evoked discharges of the relay type of VL neurons were inhibited during EEG synchronization and especially when spindle waves were associated with clustered firing in the background neuronal activity. Synaptic discharges elicited by cerebellothalamic stimulation practically disappeared for many cells (Fig. 9A); occasionally they presented a high-frequency repetitive burst at a longer latency than that observed for single evoked spikes during waking (Fig. 9B) (26, 73, 74). Reappearance of the evoked monosynaptic discharges could precede the EEG signs of arousal by a few seconds (Fig. 9C). This confirms earlier results from macroelectrode recordings of reticular induced enhancement of the VL field potentials evoked by brachium con-

---

ure at fixed latencies, and the cell c was prevented to discharge; superimposed sweeps triggered by each of the four shocks in a train at around 100/sec is shown at left (note IS-SD break), the first and the third sweeps are superimposed in the middle, and all the testing shocks are depicted at right at lower speed; the long latency of spike b was unusual for antidromic activation of VL cells, however the reality of this spike (superimposed on the negative hump of spike a) became evident by testing its all-or none character and especially when it was evoked in absence of spike a (see 8, at bottom). In B, the traces of the ink-written records show the spontaneous firing of cell c and the EEG rhythms with spontaneously occurring spindles. Figures on the EEG record indicate application of the testing train inducing antidromic invasion of cells a and b, and corresponding to those depicting the evoked discharges on the oscilloscope (1-2: moving film, 3-10 single sweeps; at the bottom: 7-10 again, at faster speed). Note groups of spike clusters of neuron c in good time relation with spindle sequences; all the three neurons showed quite identical clustered firing during spindling, as shown by the spontaneous clusters of these neurons in 6; two spike clusters of the neuron c (arrows in 2) correspond to the deflections indicated by arrows on the ink-written record. Note that during EEG spindle bursts (2, 5, 6, 9) antidromic invasion of both neurons was suppressed. Note also that in 8 the a spike disappeared 500 msec prior to the appearance of the EEG spindle, when the spike b was still responding. Modified from Steriade, Apostol and Oakson (73).

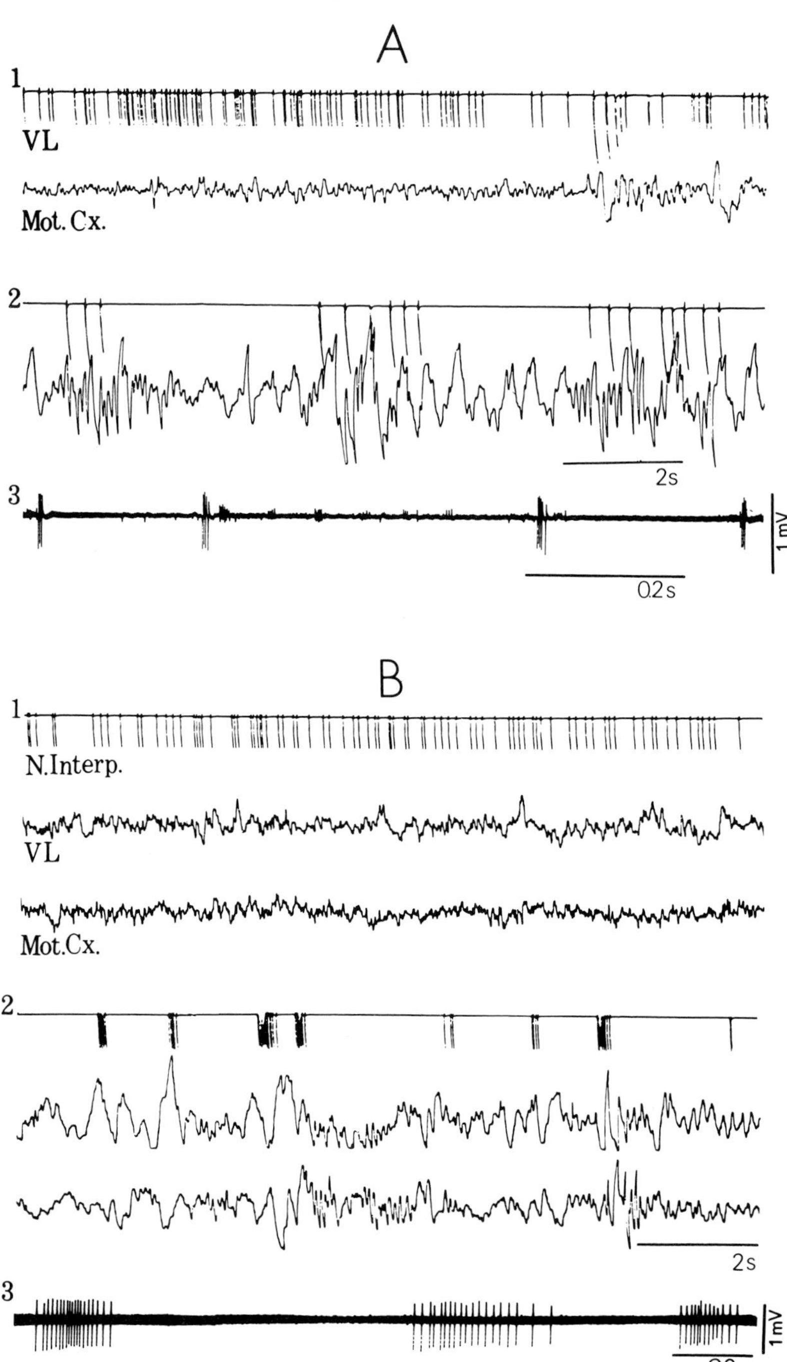

FIG. 12

junctivum (29) or red nuclear (68) stimulation, responses which were inhibited during periods of EEG synchronization. These data are explained by intracellular studies of Purpura and his collaborators showing prolonged IPSPs generated during EEG synchronization in VL neurons through pathways linking the medial thalamus with the lateral nuclei (56), and blockade, during high-frequency reticular stimulation, of IPSPs evoked in the VL nucleus by low-frequency midline thalamic stimulation (55).

It may be argued that all the above reported fluctuations in VL responsiveness, resulting from experiments on paralyzed animals, can not be translated in terms of the events occurring during the behavioral sleep-wakefulness continuum, and that they constitute only an amusing neurophysiological game, played under rather artificial conditions. That these findings can actually be extrapolated to the phenomenology of natural sleep was shown by identical changes undergone by the monosynaptic VL mass response to a cerebellothalamic stimulus during waking and various stages of sleep in the chronically implanted, behaving cat (Fig. 10) (78). Striking depression or virtual disappearance of the thalamic relayed wave (r component) was seen especially at the onset of sleep, during drowsiness with EEG spindles, which deprived the motor cortex of the input required for elaborating the intrinsic cortical component (wave 2). With partial recovery of the VL output during slow wave sleep, the intrinsic cortical wave may develop and become even greater than during wakefulness. This latter, unexpected event is due to the decreased responsiveness during waking of motor cortex neurons relaying VL messages, in spite of the increased input from the VL; it was seen by recording mass (68, 71, 78) and unit (77) VL-evoked activities in both paralyzed animals and freely moving cats and monkeys. Finally, the enhancement of the VL relayed wave during the deepest phase of sleep, with EEG fast activity, may reach values over those recorded during waking. Let us emphasize that the obliteration, during

---

FIG. 12. Comparative patterns of unit firing during EEG patterns of wakefulness and slow sleep in thalamic VL and cerebellar interpositus nuclei. VL cell driven monosynaptically by red nuclear stimulation (A) and interposital neuron antidromically invaded by VL stimuli (B). In both cases, unit spikes were depicted on the EEG machine (1-2) as in the preceding figures, and typical patterns of original spikes during slow sleep are depicted in 3. EEG spontaneous rhythms recorded from the motor precruciate cortex (Mot. Cx.) and VL nucleus. Note: regular discharges during waking (A_1 and B_1) in both VL (10/sec) and interpositus (7-8/sec) nuclei; short and rhythmic bursts of high-frequency spikes in the VL neuron during slow sleep; the bursts of spikes appeared in VL associated with the first signs of EEG spindles (A_1) and they were seen later in close time relation with cortical high-voltage sequences of spindles but not with pure slow waves (A_2); each deflection exceeding the common level represents a cluster of 3-5 spikes, as depicted in the oscilloscopic record (large spike in A_3). On the other hand, the bursts of spikes appearing during slow sleep in the interposital neuron (B_{2-3}) were of much longer duration and lower frequency; they were sometimes related with VL slow waves, but not with thalamic or cortical spindles. From Steriade, Apostol and Oakson (72).

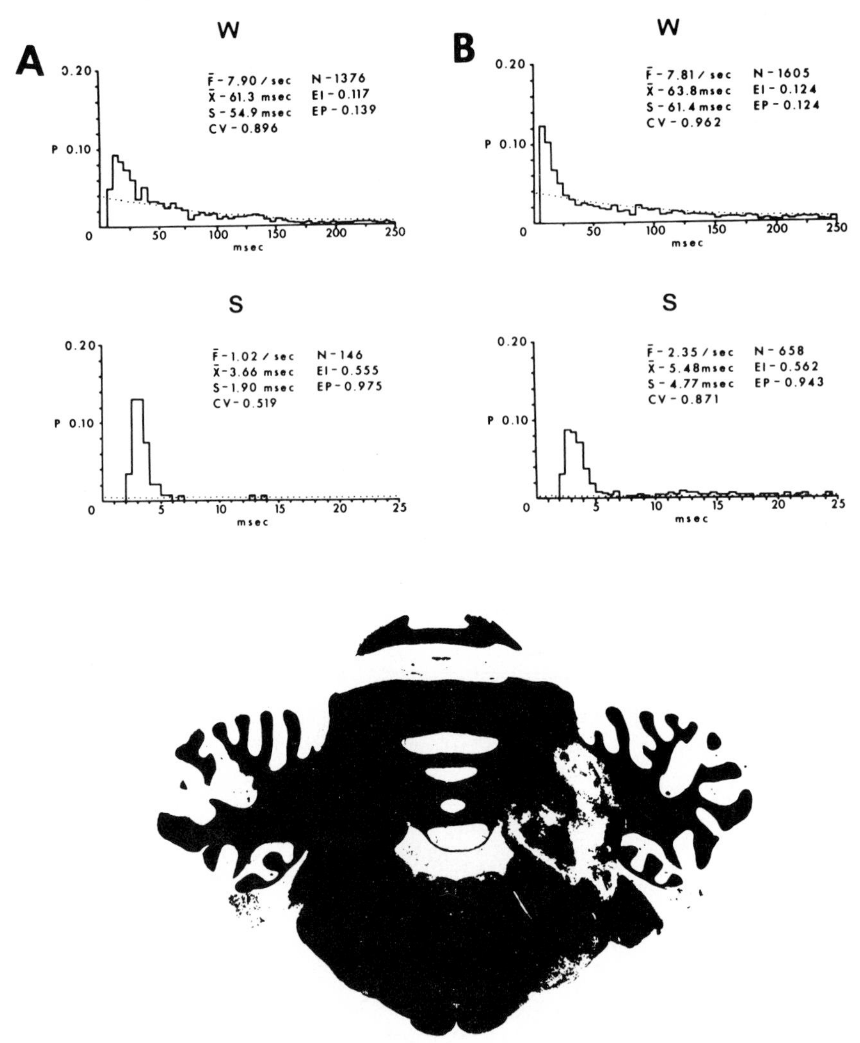

FIG. 13. Interspike interval histograms (solid curves) and computed Poisson interval histograms (dotted curves) of a VL relay cell during EEG patterns of wakefulness (W) and slow sleep (S), before (A) and following (B) an extensive lesion of the contralateral interpositus and dentate cerebellar nuclei (see the extent of this lesion at the bottom). Note lack of significant differences after the cerebellar lesion. Symbols: $\overline{F}$ = mean firing rate; $\overline{X}$ = mean interval; $\overline{S}$ = standard deviation; CV = coefficient of variation; N = number of intervals analyzed; EI = fraction of measured intervals falling outside depicted time range; EP = fraction of computed Poisson intervals falling outside depicted time range. Modified from Steriade, Apostol and Oakson (73-74).

drowsiness and slow sleep, of the VL monosynaptic wave occurred without any alteration in the presynaptic (tract, t) component (Fig. 10), thus indicating that the depression of the synaptic transmission through the VL nucleus during these stages of sleep does not require postulation of presynaptic inhibitory mechanisms. These results, concerning both the postsynaptic changes and unaltered presynaptic events during natural sleep and wakefulness, have been recently confirmed (25).

Inhibition of the evoked discharges in VL relay cells during EEG spindles was seen not only during transsynaptic excitation, but also during antidromic invasion following precruciate stimuli (73). EEG synchrony profoundly affected the ability of VL projection cells to fire as a result of stimulation of their axons, but the depressing effect on the tested antidromic spikes was not exerted to the same extent on all neurons. This was shown by recording simultaneously two antidromically invaded cells (Fig. 11A). The evoked backfiring was abolished in both neurons during EEG spindles; however, the biphasic, initially positive spike a disappeared 400-500 msec prior to the development of the EEG spindle sequence, when the spike b was still responding (Fig. 11, B_8), which indicates that they were unequally affected by the EEG synchronization. Inhibition of discharges blocked both the IS and SD spikes (see the IS-SD break in the spike a, the last of the four shocks in the train, Fig. 11A); all spindle wave sequences were associated with complete failure to invade the cell. It may be inferred that the blockage affected not only the SD membrane, but also the low-threshold IS region. Blocking of both IS and SD spikes by recurrent inhibition in pyramidal tract neurons suggested that inhibitory synapses may be located on or near the axon hillock (67). These data on decreased probability of antidromic invasion in VL cells during EEG synchronization (73) are corroborated by the reduced amplitude, during behavioral light sleep, of mass potentials reflecting the antidromic response upon stimulation of the corresponding radiation, as found in sensory (lateral geniculate and VB) thalamic nuclei (14).

Summing up, all the evidence indicates that behavioral light sleep or EEG synchronizing patterns in paralyzed animals, and especially periods of spindle waves with related clustered firing, are associated with a powerful inhibition of synaptic transmission through the VL relay. The following step was undertaken to determine the mechanisms controlling the VL clustered firing and the accompanying EEG phenomena.

C. The independence of the VL rhythmic activity from the major specific input was concluded by studying the thalamic effects following the destruction of deep cerebellar nuclei. Fluctuations, during EEG patterns of waking and synchronized sleep, in the spontaneous firing of cerebello-VL projecting cells (as identified by their antidromic spikes elicited by thalamic stimuli, see Fig. 1A) revealed that clustered firing during EEG synchronization is not an exclusive feature of thalamic and cortical neurons, but that it also occurs in the dentate and interposital cerebellar nuclei. Regular cerebellar discharges during waking (Fig. 12, B_1) developed into irregular (0.2-2/sec) and relatively long (150-250 msec) bursts of 80-220/sec spikes during spontaneously occurring synchronization of the encephale isole cat, sometimes in fairly close time-relation with high-amplitude VL slow waves, but not with thalamic or cortical spindles (Fig. 12, B_2). Such clusters, unaltered by ablation of the sensorimotor cortex, were unlike those recorded from the VL principal cells during the same functional state (Fig. 12, compare A_3 to B_3), having a lower frequency (major interval mode during slow sleep between 5 and 10 msec), a longer duration (accounting for the increased mean-rate of discharge during slow sleep compared to waking), and a marked irregularity, all in contrast with those of VL bursts of spikes (72, 73). In spite of these differences in configuration and significance (see discussion in refs. 73 and 77), the independence of the VL patterns of discharge upon the cerebellum had to be further checked by interrupting cerebellothalamic projections. The temporal patterns of discharge in VL relay neurons remained unaltered following extensive lesions of the contralateral dentate and interposital nuclei. Some VL neurons, which were studied before and after such lesions, presented no significant changes in the interval interspike histograms during waking and slow sleep (Fig. 13) (73, 74).

D. The influence of the midline and intralaminar thalamic nuclei on VL rhythmic activity, as might be suggested by EPSP-IPSP sequences set in motion in the thalamic motor relay by stimulating the medial thalamus (56), was checked by studying the effect of lesions placed between frontal planes 7.5 and 12.5, between lateral planes 0.0 and 2.5-3.0, at a depth between +4.5 and 0.0 or -1.0, which destroyed the rostral pole of the centro-median nucleus, the nuclei centralis medialis, paracentralis, reuniens, ventralis medialis, medialis dorsalis, the parts of the centralis lateralis and VA located medially to the lateral plane 3.0, and the very medial part of the VL, but spared the great lateral part of the VL and all the VB complex. These lesions (Fig. 14) left untouched the VL cells relaying cerebellofugal messages, as shown by rubrally elicited monosynaptic spikes recorded lateral to the plane 3.0 and by a normal cortical mass response (73). Following this destruction, slow (2-5/sec) waves were not altered, but the amplitude of 8-12/sec EEG spindles was clearly decreased. Spindle waves preserved the same frequency as before

---

FIG. 14. Effect of an acute unilateral (left) thalamic lesion (3 medial mm) on ipsilateral EEG spindles, induced by 2 mg/Kg Surital i.v. (A, C_1 at the arrow), an additional dose of 8 mg/Kg Surital (C_2) or occuring spontaneously (B), and on related clustered firing in the ipsilateral VL nucleus. Unit activity recorded on the EEG machine (top traces); EEG activity from the left and right motor cortex recorded on the second and third traces (B and C, as A). Three different cells; A and C: monosynaptically driven by cerebellothalamic stimulation; B: inhibited by precruciate shocks (dots) with subsequent rebound (arrows). Note reduction in amplitude of spindles in the ipsilateral motor cortex (A-C) in spite of no reduction in pure slow waves (B); rhythmic sequences of spike clusters, as occurring during EEG spindles in intact brain animals, were absent (C_1) or reduced to inconstant, single clusters (arrows in A); with higher doses of Surital, VL spike clusters became rich and rhythmic (C_2); postinhibitory rebounds following cortical shocks were still present (B, arrows). Modified from Steriade, Apostol and Oakson (73).

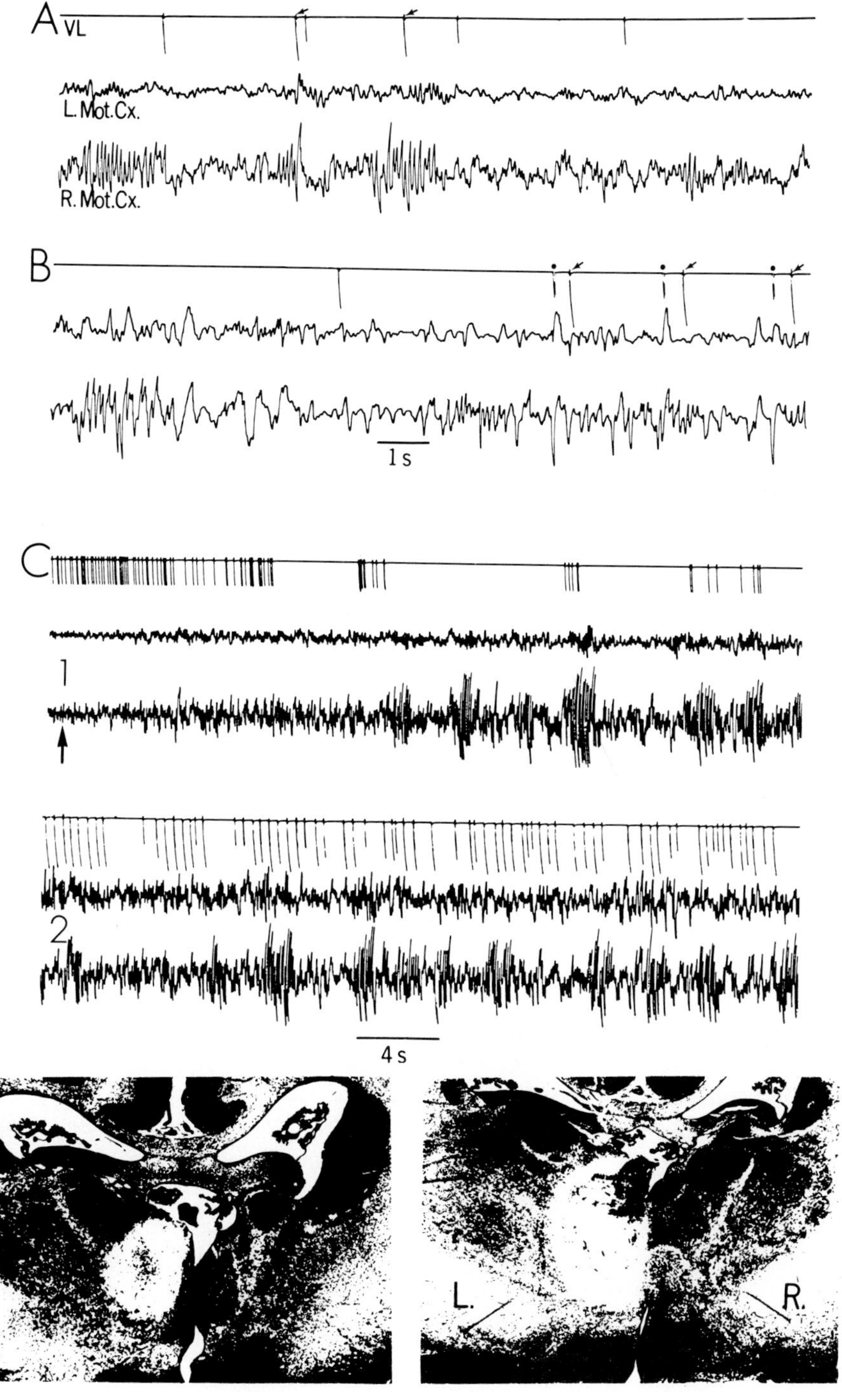

FIG. 14

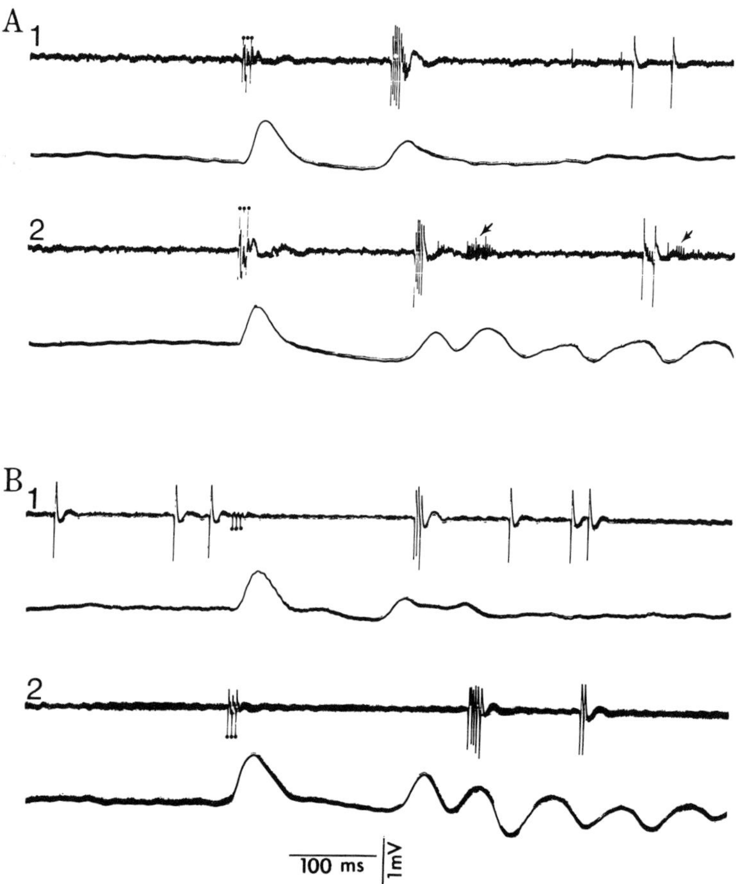

FIG. 15. Cortically elicited VL spike clusters and EEG spindle-like afterdischarge. A and B: two different neurons (in A simultaneous recording of another, small spike indicated by arrows). Trains of three shocks applied to the depth of the precruciate area with different voltages (6 V, 0.1 msec in 1; 15 V, 0.1 msec in 2). First trace: the VL neuronal activity; second trace: EEG recorded by a macroelectrode in the depth of the precruciate gyrus, close to the stimulating electrode. Note increases in latencies, and in frequencies and number of spikes, of the clusters following cortical stimulation, related to increased amplitude of the EEG spindle-like afterdischarge, by increasing voltages of stimulation. Note also in A_{1-2} the correspondence between the first EEG waves belonging to the afterdischarges evoked by different stimulation intensities and the similar variations in latencies of the preceding VL spike clusters; the second EEG wave in A_2 is time-related with a cluster of the small spike (at arrow). B is from Steriade, Apostol and Oakson (73).

the lesion, but remained at a stage of abortive elements, without their normal waxing in a burst, thus contrasting with the EEG recorded from the homotopic points of the contralateral sensorimotor cortex. Correlatively, the rhythmic VL spike clusters were replaced in most cells by single, isolated clusters, occurring much less frequently. This was valid especially for spontaneously occurring EEG synchronization (Fig. 14B), and also for spindling induced by a very small amount (2 mg/Kg i.v.) of a short acting barbiturate (Fig. 14, A and C_1). With higher doses of Surital (8-10 mg/Kg), VL spike clusters assumed their known rhythmicity and EEG spindles also became evident in the ipsilateral VL-motor cortex complex, although even in this case the difference remained significant when comparison was made with the normal spindling of the contralateral, intact hemisphere (Fig. 14, C_2). Such an asymmetry was also induced by transections (F 10.0 - 11.5, L 2.0, D 4.0 - 0.5) interrupting a gross part of nonspecific-specific projections, but essentially sparing the medial and lateral nuclei and leaving intact synaptic transmission through the VL relay (73).

The discrepancy between the above asymmetry in the EEG spindling resulted from our experiments and the statement of Andersen et al. (2) according to which the removal of midline and intralaminar nuclei on one side did not interfere with the appearance of the cortical spindles on either side, "all parameters of the spindle activity being the same as before the lesion" (p. 269), has to be explained by two major differences between the experimental conditions. First, the lesions depicted in their Fig. 9 show less complete destruction of the medial thalamus than in our experiments (see again Fig. 14; see also ref. 73), and, more importantly, their lesion also significantly affected the opposite medial thalamus (see especially parts B-C in their Fig. 9), which may be a determinant factor in preventing the appearance of an asymmetry. Secondly, an additional 8 mg/Kg of Surital was enough to change the picture from an almost complete lack of spindling in the ipsilateral motor cortex (Fig. 14, C_1) to the appearance of some spindle waves, despite the fact that even in this case the asymmetry remained obvious (Fig. 14, C_1); the much higher doses of barbiturate used in their experiments might account for an even more developed spindling.

These findings do not imply that spindle activity depends on direct medial ("nonspecific") thalamic projections to cortical areas. Actually, even more drastic changes or complete disappearance of spindle waves in the motor cortex occurred after an elective destruction of the VL nucleus (74), which agree with the lack of spindling in the somatosensory cortical area following removal of the VB complex, as reported by Andersen et al. (2). Thus elective lesions of either medial ("nonspecific") or lateral (specific) thalamic nuclei may prevent normal development of EEG spindling without interfering with 2-5/sec slow waves.

The following steps were an attempt to relate the role of the ascending mesencephalic reticular system and intrathalamic circuitries in the onset and development of synchronized sleep, with special emphasis on spindle activity. The sudden removal of the powerful excitatory impingement realized by the upper brain stem on specific thalamic nuclei induces at the very onset of sleep a disfacilitation, expressed by striking neuronal silence in the VL preceding the EEG signs of synchronization (see again Fig. 8B). Consequently, inhibition of medial thalamic nuclei by specific relays, as indicated by VL-evoked IPSPs in medial thalamic cells (16, 17), will be released and non-

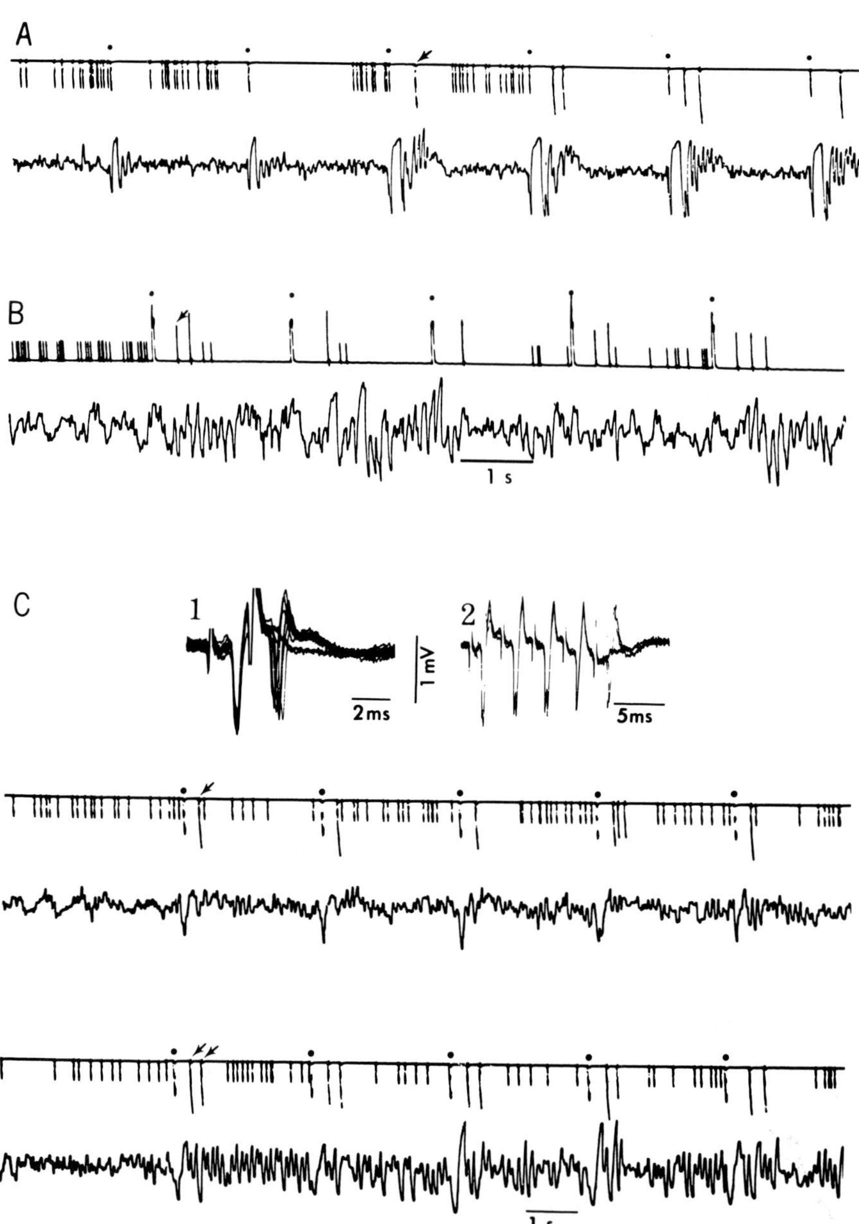

FIG. 16. Relationships between EEG synchronization and inhibition of spontaneous firing with subsequent rebounds in VL cells following motor cortex stimulation. A–C: three different neurons. A: the last four testing shock-trains (dots) were delivered with higher voltages (13 V, 0.1 msec) than the two first ones (8 V, 0.1 msec). Note

specific-specific thalamic projections will in turn set in motion synchronous EPSP-IPSPs sequences in various thalamic nuclear groups (53, 56), partially responsible for EEG spindles and related clustered firing in specific relays. The latter may be regarded as "final common paths" which transfer the spindle activity elaborated in thalamic internuclear loops into appropriate cortical areas, as evidenced by abolition of this activity following an elective specific thalamic destruction. On the other hand, the midline and intralaminar nuclei represent an important prerequisite for the reinforcement of the spindle mechanism, considering the abortive character of spindling in medial thalamic lesioned animals (73).

CORTICALLY ELICITED RHYTHMIC THALAMIC ACTIVITY

Long-lasting suppression of spontaneous discharges, preceded or not by antidromic invasion and/or orthodromic activation of the VL unit under observation, and subsequent rebound activity may be induced by a testing shock-train to the motor cortex. The cortically elicited postinhibitory rebounds,i.e.,one to three bursts of high-frequency discharges, were identical in morphology with the spike clusters developing during spontaneously occurring EEG synchronization (compare Figs. 6, B-D and 15 with Fig. 8C). These unit events elicited in the VL following the long inhibitory period were associated with an 8-12/sec EEG afterdischarge, perfectly mimicking a spontaneous EEG spindle sequence, recorded either in the VL (Fig. 17) or in the immediate vicinity of the cortical stimulating precruciate electrode (Fig. 15). An increase in the cortical stimulation strength usually resulted in a prolongation of the silent period, an increase in the frequency and/or number of spike discharges of the VL postinhibitory rebound, and a greater amplitude (with additional components) of the spindle-like afterdischarge (Fig. 15).

This afterdischarge died out within 700-800 msec following cortical stimulation

---

increased amplitude of the 12-14/sec EEG afterdischarge simultaneous with the appearance of progressive inhibition in VL spontaneous firing and sequences of unit rebounds (arrow). In B, on a background of more "relaxed" EEG, cortical stimulation (dots) resulted in striking silence of the VL neuronal firing, postinhibitory rebounds (arrow) and prolonged periods of spindle waves. In C, a typical VL relay cell. 1: antidromic invasion following precruciate stimulation (first shock) and rubrally evoked monosynaptic activation (second shock). 2: a series of five cortically elicited antidromic spikes (320/sec shocks). Below, the same train of cortical shocks, as depicted in 2, was delivered every 2.75 sec (dots), and spontaneous firing of the cell (top traces, recorded as in the preceding figures) and EEG rhythms of the motor cortex (bottom traces) were simultaneously analyzed. Two different periods of recording, the second one a few minutes later than the first one, when the animal exhibited pupillary and EEG signs of drowsiness. Note the marked and continuous cortically elicited EEG spindling at the bottom of the figure depicting the second period, related to the increase in the number of postinhibitory spike clusters (arrows) following cortical stimulation. C is modified from Steriade, Apostol and Oakson (73).

on the background of an "aroused" EEG activity (Fig. 16A). However, provided that the spontaneous EEG rhythms indicated a tendency to synchronized sleep, with appearance of slow waves, a protracted (Fig. 16B) or continuous (Fig. 16C) spindling could be evoked by 0.3-0.5/sec trains of pulses to the motor cortex, simultaneous with longer inhibition of spontaneous VL firing and more intensive rebound activities (73). The amount of elicited spindles was directly related to duration in cortically induced inhibition and richness of the subsequent spike clusters (Fig. 16C; see also Fig. 15) and both depended upon a reduced reticular drive as seen by a "relaxed" EEG.

Conversely, the desynchronization of EEG rhythms and the related increase in background neuronal firing was accompanied by a decrease in amplitude of the focal slow positive (P) wave following cortical stimulation (11, 74) and a reduction in the frequency and number of spikes in the subsequent rebound (73). Arousal induced by high-frequency pulses to the mesencephalic reticular formation was even more effective, practically erasing the P wave, the cyclic rebound and the associated spindle-like waves elicited by cortical stimulation (Fig. 17C; see also Fig. 19). This reticular inhibition of cortically induced rhythmic inhibitory events in the VL nucleus is in line with the reticular blockade of hyperpolarizing potentials of VL cells triggered by medial thalamic stimulation (55). It might imply that the increased responsiveness, during waking, of the VL principal neurons tested directly (see again Figs. 9-11) is opposite in sign to the behavior of the VL inhibitory interneuronal apparatus inferred from changes in rhythmic sequences following cortical stimulation. Such an assumption is supported by a similar picture found in a sensory (lateral geniculate) thalamic relay where enhancement, during arousal, of synaptic transmission in relay cells (69, 71, 76, 81) was in contrast with inhibition of inhibitory interneurons both during brain stem reticular stimulation (30) and natural waking (62). At the level of the motor cortex, the reduced duration of both recurrent and feed-forward inhibition during reticular arousal in the *encephale isole* cat or behavioral waking in the chronically implanted monkey (77, 79) was shown to be exerted not only simultaneously with an increased spontaneous neuronal firing (suggesting in this case that marked excitation may overwhelm inhibition), but also in those cells where the absence of an increased mean-

---

FIG. 17. Multiunit recordings of four different (A-D) VL neuronal populations. A: more or less regular, continual firing during EEG patterns of waking (W) and clustered firing of all recorded neurons during spontaneously occurring local spindle waves (S). B: similarity between spontaneous spindle sequences with clustered unit firing during sleepiness and cortically (Cx) elicited rhythmic VL activity. Compare also the spontaneous spindle patterns in A and B with the cortically elicited rhythmic activity in C and D. C: erasure of cortically elicited VL spindle-like rhythmic waves and related unit spike clusters by a preceding high-frequency reticular (RF) stimulation (at the arrow). D: contrast between powerful sequences of spindle waves and unit spike clusters triggered by a three shock-train to the precruciate gyrus and lack of such rhythmic VL activity following red nuclear (RN) stimulation with the same parameters; the large spike was identified as a relay cell. See other comments in text.

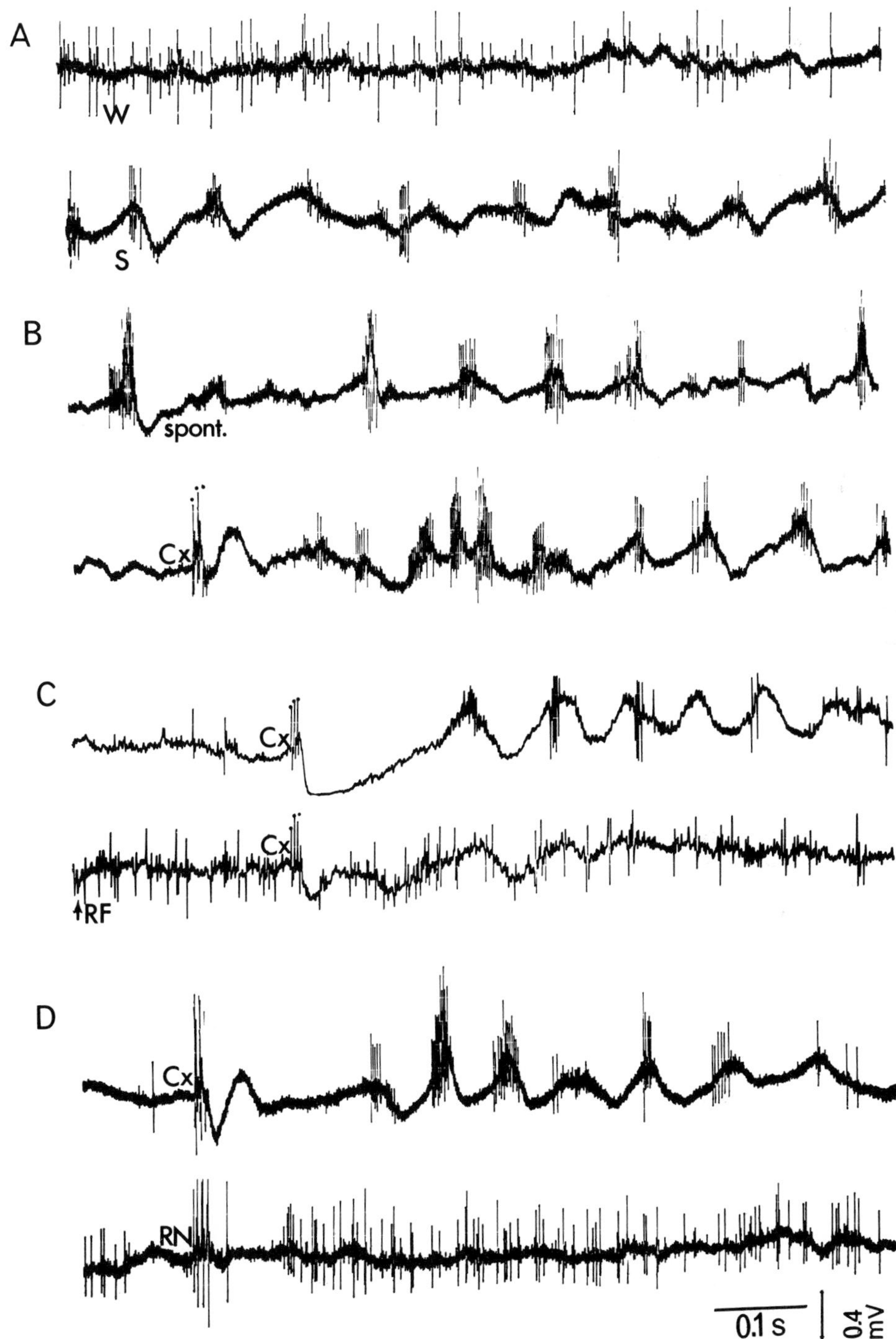

FIG. 17

discharge rate during waking called upon an alternative mechanism involving inhibition of inhibitory interneurons. In the VL, a significant increased frequency of the spontaneous discharges accompanied practically without exception the erasure of inhibition and rhythmic activity during arousal (Fig. 17C) (73), thus showing that, at least at this level, powerful excitatory reticular influences on VL neurons (55, 68, 78) are the essential, if not the unique, mechanism accounting for this phenomenon.

A major question arises concerning the causal relationship between the VL spike clusters and the EEG spindle waves. Some arguments for such a relation appearing within the frame of the spontaneous rhythmic activity during synchronized sleep were exposed in the previous section. Here are further data on cortically elicited spindle-like waves. The objection against such a relation can be raised considering the difference between the number and frequency of EEG waves belonging to the afterdischarge induced by cortical stimulation (7-8 oscillations at 8-10/sec) and those of the spike clusters discharged by individual cells (only 1-3 bursts, usually at 2-5/sec, but sometimes at higher frequencies, as the spontaneously occurring clusters). As already argued, this may be true when single units are studied; in multiple unit recordings, almost all the focal slow negative waves elicited by cortical stimulation (following positive shifts reflecting neuronal inhibition) were superimposed by bursts of high-frequency spikes of one, or another, or all the neurons under observation (Fig. 17, B-D).

The similarity between a focal VL spindle sequence occurring naturally during slow sleep and a cortically elicited sequence in the same neuronal population is depicted in Fig. 17B. Let us also mention that the differences between the oscillation frequencies elicited by cortical stimulation in one or another VL neuronal population (Fig. 17, B-D) are within the range of various frequencies encountered in different cell clusters during naturally occurring spindles, thus again emphasizing that similar basic mechanisms are involved in both these cases. When the cortically induced VL afterdischarge transferred to the appropriate precruciate point was analyzed, a good time-relation could also be found between the negative waves of the spindle-like sequence recorded at the depth in the motor cortex and the spike clusters of several VL neurons. The latter preceded the former, and this time relation was preserved by displacing both (VL and cortical) events with different strengths of testing cortical stimulation (Fig. 15, A1-2). It goes without saying that such a precise topographical relationship is rather

---

FIG. 18. Cortically elicited EEG spindle-like afterdischarge and related spike clusters in two simultaneously recorded VL cells (a and b). Spontaneous firing depicted at the top. The effect of a train of three shocks applied to the precruciate cortical area is seen below; 2, 8 and 10 represent the corresponding sweeps (indicated by arrows), in the wavegram of ten successive sweeps. At the bottom, the activity of cell a was electronically separated from the cell b and it was recorded on the EEG machine (first trace), simultaneous with the EEG rhythms from the motor cortex (second trace); the last four effects of cortical shock-trains (7-10 from the above depicted wavegram; stimuli indicated by dots) are depicted. Full explanation and comments in text. From Steriade, Wyzinski and Oakson (80).

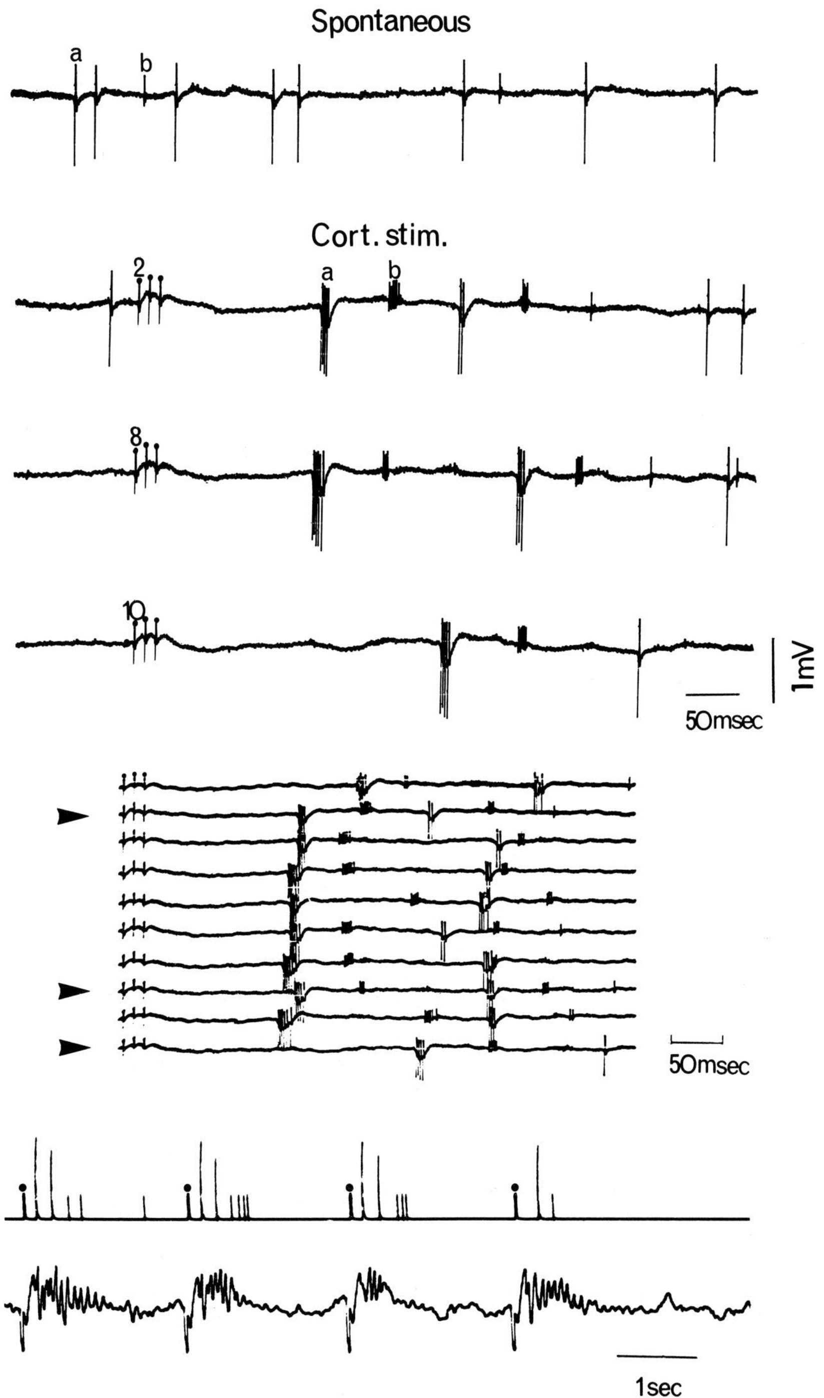

FIG. 18

difficult to find and requires careful positioning of the cortical recording electrode after a thorough mapping of the precruciate area.

Figure 18 shows the spontaneous single spike discharge of two simultaneously recorded VL cells, the temporal course in the sequence of spike clusters discharged by both neurons following the initial inhibitory period elicited by a cortical shock-train, and the related EEG spindle-like afterdischarge recorded from the same cortical area as that used for testing stimulation. The synchronizing neuronal process induced by cortical stimulation is suggested by the fact that different intervals between the clusters of one cell were associated with quite identical differences in the bursts of spikes of the other neuron (compare 2 with 8), and that a contingent, unusually delayed appearance of the first cluster of the cell a, was faithfully associated with the same event in the cell b (see 10). The intercluster intervals were roughly estimated in both neurons at 150-170 msec, indicating a rhythmicity at around 6.5/sec, while the frequency of the associated EEG oscillations reached 12-13/sec. However, in light of the temporal patterns of spike clusters in both cells (and taking into consideration the great number of projection neurons outside the field of the recording microelectrode), their succession (see the wavegram of ten sweeps) fully justifies the assumption that the cortically elicited unit rebounds are behind the appearance of the EEG spindle waves.

Under the experimental condition of barbiturate anesthesia the rhythmic thalamic activity elicited by cortical stimulation was ascribed to a mechanism involving local inhibitory interneurons directly excited by recurrent collaterals of specific thalamocortical axons (1, 3-5). If this were the principal modality of spindle genesis, one would expect that similar patterns of activity could be elicited by afferent (prethalamic) and antidromic (cortical) stimuli in relay neurons. At least for the VL nucleus of the *encéphale isolé*, unanesthetized cat, this was not seen to be the case. The most impressive evidence came from multiunit analysis: powerful cortically elicited spindle sequences related with cyclic period of neuronal silence and subsequent clustered activity in almost all simultaneously recorded neurons contrasted sharply with the scarcity or lack of such phenomena following red nuclear stimulation with identical parameters (Fig. 17D). Rhythmic inhibition in VL cells (and the associated spindle-like afterdischarge) by stimulating the cerebellothalamic pathway at the level of the red nucleus was possible only following barbiturate administration or in a

---

FIG. 19. EEG synchronization and postinhibitory rebounds in VL units following contralateral precruciate cortical stimulation. Two different cells (A and B). In each case, the first trace indicates application of three testing three shocks to the right precruciate gyrus, the second trace is the left VL unit (arrows depict rebounds, as seen at the bottom: 1-3), and the last two traces the EEG rhythms recorded from the right and left motor cortex, respectively; at the bottom, the oscilloscopic records depict three (1-3) typical postinhibitory rebounds in the VL unit (same as in B) elicited by the contralateral cortical shock-train, and reduction of the inhibitory period with erasure of subsequent spike clusters by an arousing train of high frequency pulses to the mesencephalic reticular formation (4-6). From Steriade, Wyzinski and Oakson (80).

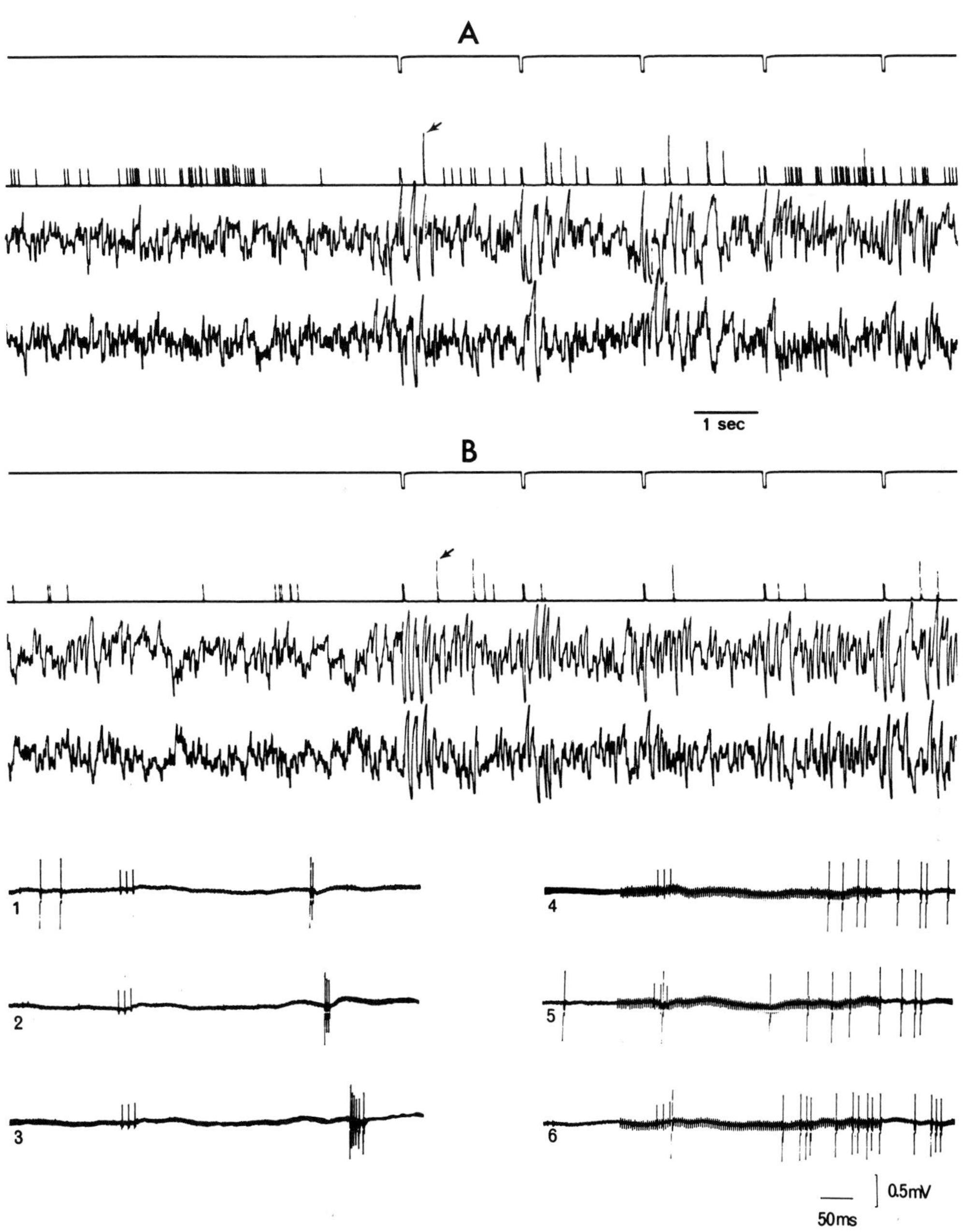

FIG. 19.

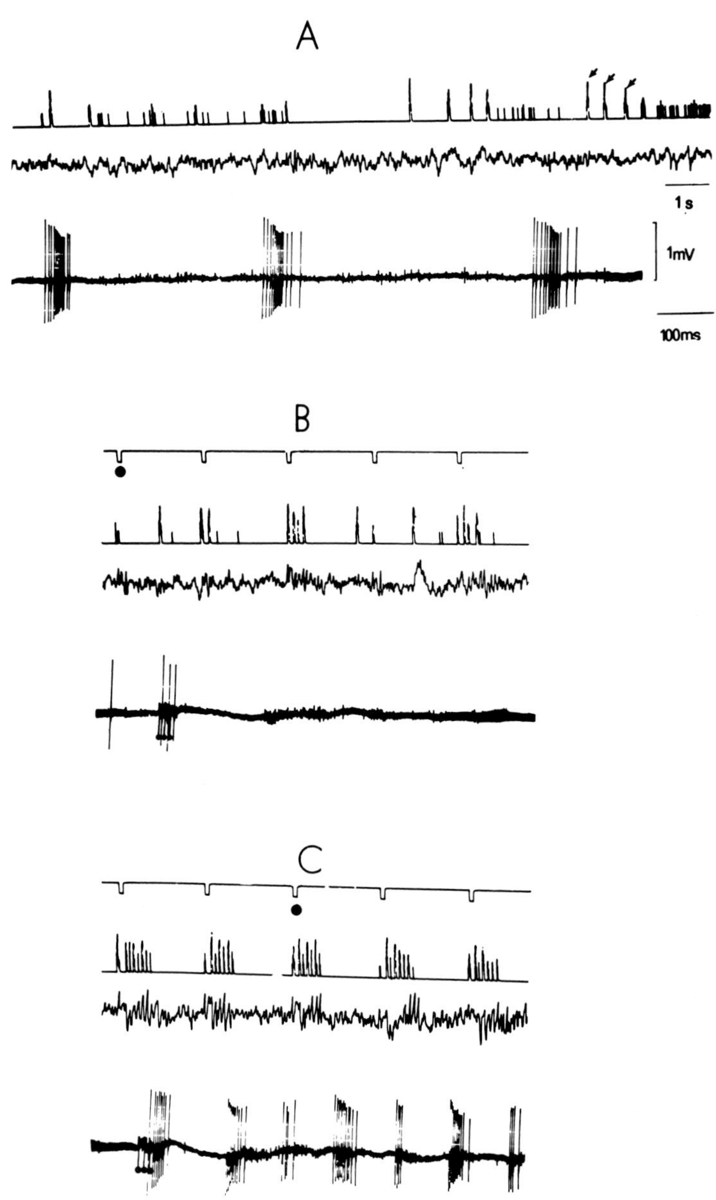

FIG. 20. Spontaneous firing and cortically evoked discharges of a presumed interneuron recorded within the VL anatomical limit (F 11.00, L 3.8, D +1.5). A: ink-written spontaneous unit firing (first trace), EEG rhythms recorded from the ipsilateral

rostropontine preparation exhibiting a marked tendency to spontaneous spindling (80). In all cells found in the VL-VA complex, identified as receiving their input from the cerebellothalamic fibers and projecting their axons to the motor cortical area, this contrast between the effect of cortical and prethalamic stimulation in a vigil preparation was evident. It can not be ascribed to a different degree in setting in motion the presumed inhibitory interneurons by the recurrent collateral pathway, since it did not depend upon the richness of the early excitation in the observed cell, as reflected by the number of spikes evoked by red nuclear synaptic, or cortical antidromic, shock-train stimulation. With regard to the synchronous excitation of the inhibitory interneurons by one or another of the testing volleys, we are inclined to predict that if the recurrent collateral mechanism were essential in the VL, a stimulus applied to a compact bundle of afferent cerebellothalamic fibers which then gives rise to action potentials in a great population of thalamocortical fibers would be more efficient in driving the local VL inhibitory interneurons than a focal cortical stimulus which affects only a small number of axon terminals in the precruciate gyrus; actually, there is no exception in the literature in emphasizing the great number of VL units synaptically driven by cerebellothalamic stimulation and the difficulty in invading antidromically the same neurons from the motor cortex.

The above described contrast between cortically elicited thalamic activity and the absence of such activity in relay neurons following afferent cerebellothalamic stimuli was one of the findings suggesting that the recurrent collateral mechanism may have only a conjoint or even an ancillary role in triggering this activity in specific thalamic nuclei of unanesthetized preparations, and that another system, involving orthodromic corticothalamic projections, may be mainly responsible for eliciting the rhythmic activity by cortical stimulation. As shown in the first section (Fig. 6), the responses due to these projections are highly sensitive to barbiturates in doses as low as 1mg/Kg. It is likely that emphasis on the recurrent collateral mechanism can be ascribable to the use of much larger doses of barbiturate which may have masked the

---

motor cortex (second trace) and original spikes (third trace). Note high-frequency, long-lasting (around 50 msec) spike barrages corresponding to the arrows on the EEG ink-written record; compare these spike clusters with the very dissimilar bursts of discharges occurring during EEG synchronization in the VL principal neuron depicted in Fig. 8C. Below (B-C), the activity evoked in this cell by three shocks to the precruciate gyrus during an "aroused" EEG (B) and a slight EEG synchronization induced by 1 mg/Kg Surital (C) is depicted (the dot indicates the corresponding cortical stimulation on the EEG record). Note the short-latency, single discharges evoked by each of the cortical shocks (B) and augmentation of evoked discharges (but with increased latency) during EEG synchronization (C); compare the very similar responsiveness of this VL interneuron during EEG desynchronizing and synchronizing patterns with that of the reticularis neuron depicted in Fig. 21. Note also the striking rhythmicity at 10/sec of the late spike clusters occurring in close time-relation with spindle waves elicited by the cortical shock train (C). Modified from Steriade, Wyzinski and Oakson (80).

simultaneous cortically evoked synaptic discharges, leaving less affected the antidromic invasion of relay cells. The synaptic activity elicited in thalamic cells by cortical stimulation was also shown in the work of Andersen *et al.* (5), but in their Fig. 4 only short latency discharges (around 1.5-2 msec) were depicted (and again ascribed to collaterals of thalamocortical axons, this time within the frame of a positive feed-back), presumably because responses with longer latencies through plurisynaptic pathways (see again our Figs. 5-6), commonly seen in unanesthetized preparations and representing the bulk of the corticothalamic pathways, are much more affected by barbiturates. This was perhaps the main reason for their dismissing the participation of orthodromic descending pathways in the elicitation of thalamic rhythmic activity. Experiments conducted on unanesthetized (34) or barbiturized (5) preparations led to essentially different conclusions with regard to the role of corticothalamic (34) or antidromic (5) activation in interpreting the results. The fact that the evoked activity in the VB was profoundly influenced (with enhancing and depressing effects on different components of the tested responses) by ablation of the somatosensory cortex in acute experiments seemed to be incompatible with the

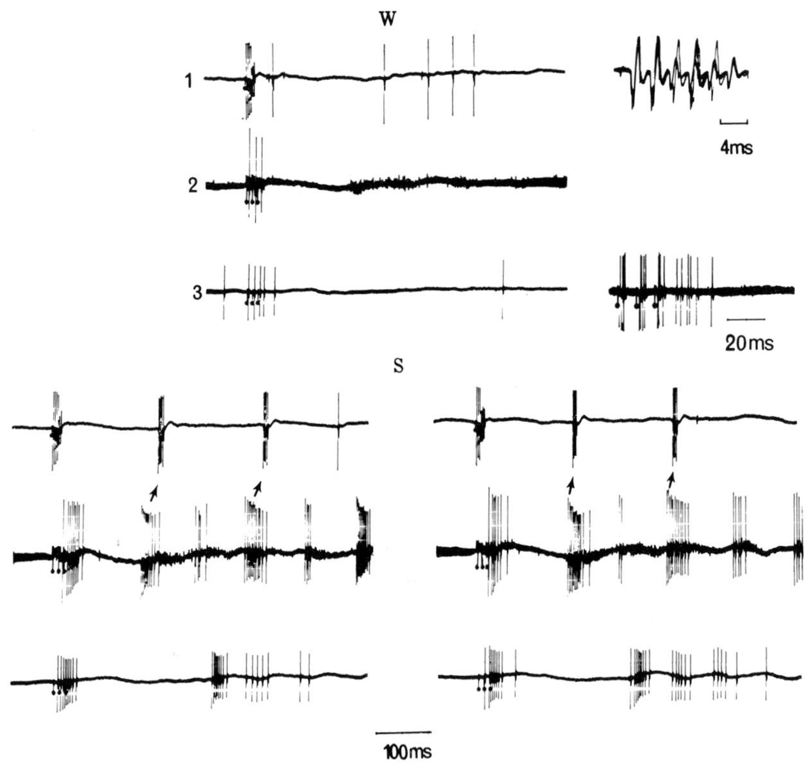

FIG. 21

attempt to explain the effects of cortical stimulation in terms of exclusive antidromic invasion (34). Therefore, in the study which emphasizes the lack of any effects of cortical ablation on rhythmic thalamic activity, thus postulates its independence of corticofugal influences (3), one is puzzled by some data (see their Fig. 3, G-I) which show a clear-cut reduction in amplitude of peripherally elicited rhythmic thalamic waves following an extensive removal of all cortical parts connected with the VB complex.

The role of orthodromic corticothalamic projections in controlling the thalamic rhythmic activity was further shown by EEG spindling (Fig. 19A) and related VL neuronal silence with subsequent spike clusters (Fig. 19, B_{1-3}) following contralateral precruciate stimulation, which avoids the contamination of antidromic invasion of thalamocortical axons. The inhibitory period was shortened and the postinhibitory rebound disappeared with a concomitant arousing high-frequency reticular stimulation (Fig. 19, B_{4-6}). In some experiments, the contralaterally induced synchronizing effects were reproduced following a transection interrupting the cortex from the thalamus in the stimulated hemisphere, to avoid possible interactions between the VL nuclei of both sides, as demonstrated for the VB nuclei (23). Therefore, the rhythmic thalamic waves elicited by contralateral motor cortex stimulation are ascribable to the synaptic drive of VL cells exerted through the callosal and then the cortico-VL pathways, as shown in Fig. 4 and reported in detail elsewhere (80).

Finally, we will attempt to search for the neuronal basis of the postinhibitory spike clusters which, as shown above (see again Figs. 15-18), are behind the spindle

---

FIG. 21. Comparative patterns of cortically evoked discharges in three different neurons, recorded in the VL-VA complex (1 and 2) and in the rostral pole of the thalamic reticularis nucleus (3), during EEG patterns of waking (W) and synchronized sleep (S), to show, tentatively, their possible interactions. Cell 1 was antidromically invaded by a shock train to the lateral part of the precruciate gyrus (see at right the detailed pattern of antidromic invasion, with IS-SD break at successive shocks) and synaptically driven by red nuclear stimulation (not depicted); on the lower speed records, dot indicates the first cortical shock in the train. Cell 2 is a VL interneuron, the same unit as depicted in Fig. 20. Reticularis cell 3 exhibited spontaneous long spike barrages and, during W, was synaptically driven by precruciate stimulation with one impulse discharge to one shock at 0.9 - 1.5 msec latency, as seen in the superimposition depicted at faster speed at the right. Note the very similar behavior of cortically evoked synaptic discharges of cells 2 (VL interneuron) and 3 (reticularis cell) during W and S (two typical records are depicted during S). The two spike clusters following cortical stimulation in the relay cell (compare with identical pattern of activity in other VL relay neurons depicted in Figs. 15 and 16C) are time-related in a ratio of 1:2 to the spike clusters of the VL interneuron, following the rich bursts of discharges in the latter (arrows), but neither the inhibitory pauses nor the subsequent rebounds in the VL relay cell are apparently related to the late events in the reticularis cell. See further comments in text.

waves seen on the EEG. Some experimental data (42) made it difficult to explain the rebound activity based exclusively on postanodal exaltation. One can hypothesize that a delayed, powerful excitatory impingement is exerted on VL projection neurons when they recover from the long-lasting inhibition, thus allowing the initiation of the rebound in the form of a burst of high-frequency discharges. According to this

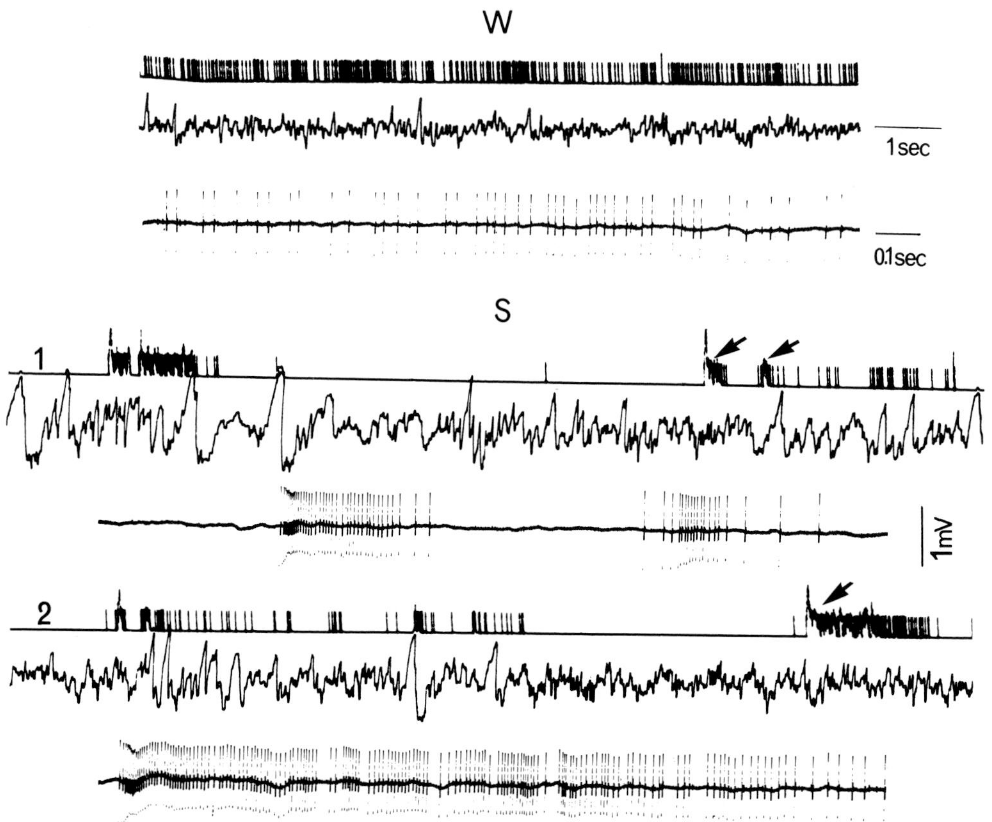

FIG. 22. Spontaneous firing of a neuron recorded from the rostral pole of the thalamic reticularis nucleus during EEG patterns of waking (W) and synchronized sleep (S). In each case, the first trace represents the unit discharges recorded on the ink-writing machine, the second trace the EEG rhythms of the ipsilateral precruciate area, and the third trace the original neuronal spikes (two episodes are depicted during S). Note the continual, more or less regular firing during W; long and irregular bursts of discharges (those marked by arrows on the EEG records are also depicted below with the original spikes) and very long intercluster silent periods during S. The mean-frequency during W was 21.65/sec (a number of 3461 spikes was recorded during 159.8 sec) and it was 11.22/sec during S (1633 spikes during 145.6 sec), the intervals being mainly dispersed between 15 and 45 msec during W, and between 5 and 25 msec during S. See also comments in text.

tentative assumption, the decline of the preceding inhibition creates a favorable condition for the cells which exert the excitatory drive. When both events (the hyperexcitable phase of the membrane following inhibition and the excitation triggered by other elements) are eclectically considered, the completed picture may afford a better understanding of the rebound. The cells exerting a synaptic excitatory drive on VL relay neurons in the declining period of their inhibitory potential were repeatedly envisaged (5, 9, 50), but they were not evidenced. In our experiments, the best candidates for generating the rhythmic sequences of spike clusters in VL principal cells have been proved to be the intrinsic VL interneurons. The cortically evoked short-latency discharges in such neurons, indicating a monosynaptic pathway linking corticofugal fibers with these cells (Fig. 7), was increased during periods of EEG synchronization compared with EEG patterns of waking (Fig. 20, B–C), which stood in contrast to the responsiveness of VL relay neurons (see Figs. 9–11) during the same functional states. On the other hand, the cortically elicited late activity of VL interneurons became far-reaching, exhibiting a striking rhythmicity at around 10/sec, each spike cluster was strictly related to each wave of the spindle sequence; this was observed to this extent only in this class of neurons (Fig. 20C; see also Fig. 7C). When comparing the patterns of rhythmic spike clusters in VL relay cells following cortical stimulation (which implies both activation of corticothalamic fibers and antidromic invasion of the specific thalamocortical axons) with the rhythmic activity elicited in VL presumed interneurons by orthodromic volleys arising in the same cortical focus, and when looking at their time-relation (Fig. 21), we are inclined to regard the much richer interneuronal clusters as a possible source of powerful excitatory impingement on VL relay cells, which is required to allow the initiation of rebound when recovering from the inhibitory period. The one-to-two ratio of grouped discharges in a VL relay cell (1) and a VL interneuron (2) depicted in Fig. 21 may be at least partially due to the alternation in the richness of spikes seen in the 10/sec clusters of the VL interneuron. Thus, the discrepancy between the rhythmicity of spindling at 8–12/sec and the lower frequency of related postinhibitory spike clusters in VL relay cells can be further understood if one considers the possibility that each cortically elicited thalamic spindle wave transferred back to the motor cortex reflects the input from different VL relay neuronal populations (see Fig. 17), triggered by their own equipment of excitatory interneurons.

It is likely that presumed VL interneurons depicted in Figs. 7 and 20–21 do not belong to the category of postulated cells of the pathway from the axon collaterals of thalamocortical axons, since they were synaptically driven only by cortical, and never by cerebellothalamic stimuli. Their "excitatory" or "inhibitory" nature can not be deduced from the pattern of rhythmic bursts of discharges subsequent to the inhibitory period following the early evoked excitation, because such bursts can be considered as representing the effect (and not the cause , as proposed above) of spike clusters in VL relay neurons. Any further inference, concerning a positive feed-back between VL principal cells and interneurons or other possibilities, would be tenuous. Let us say only that we termed some of these interneurons as "excitatory" since the latency of the first burst of high-frequency discharges appearing following the inhibitory period was always shorter in such cells than in VL relay neurons, which suggests that the former precede and may exert a depolarizing pressure on the latter. The inhibition following the early antidromic and/or synaptic excitation elicited by cortical stimulation, and the subsequent sculpturing of the rhythmic spike clusters, may be realized by other types (Renshaw-like) of VL intrinsic interneurons (directly or indirectly engaged by corticofugal fibers, or activated by the recurrent collaterals of thalamo-cortical axons especially under the experimental condition of barbiturate anesthesia) and by cells lying in the thalamic reticularis nucleus which project their axons back to the specific thalamic relays (64) and inferred in some studies (41, 44, 65) to have an inhibitory function on principal cells at these levels. As mentioned in the first section, reticularis neurons could be driven by precruciate shocks at latencies as short as 0.9 msec indicating that they are directly contacted by corticofugal fibers, and the behavior of their cortically elicited discharges was similar to that of cortically evoked discharges in VL interneurons during periods of EEG desynchronization and synchronization (Fig. 21). However, the long spike barrages in reticularis cells during synchronized sleep had no rhythmicity and did not appear as mirror images of rhythmic activity in VL relay cells, which hardly accounts for their inhibitory effect on the latter. Such bursts of discharges in neurons recorded in the reticularis nucleus were interspersed during synchronized sleep with very irregular and long lasting (in some instances more than 3-4 seconds) silent periods, which probably explain the decrease in the mean-rate of discharges during EEG synchronization compared with EEG desynchronization (Fig.22) (80). This was also reported in a comparison of the mean frequency of spontaneous firing in reticularis cells during behavioral slow sleep and waking in freely moving animals (49). We must emphasize that the evolution of reticularis spike clusters and the occurrence of more or less long-lasting intercluster silent periods during EEG synchronization were very variable and, therefore, the increase (41, 65) or decrease (49, 80) in the mean rate of discharge during slow sleep may depend upon the analyzed period, consisting of prevalent spike barrages or long pauses, possibly related with different patterns of EEG rhythms.

The rhythmic activity, appearing as a sign of decreased vigilance, is a basic, intrinsic property of the thalamic neuronal network, since it can be exhibited in the absence of cortical modulating influences. Nevertheless, the cerebral cortex controls this activity in critical thalamic districts through a complex and precise arrangement of corticofugal projections, and it can even reveal the oscillatory mechanism with a pattern perfectly mimicking that of naturally occurring spindle waves. The capacity to trigger this mechanism suggests that the cerebral cortex may actively contribute to the reinforcement of rhythmic inhibitory processes characteristic of the period of falling into sleep.

ACKNOWLEDGMENTS

This work was supported by grants from the Medical Research Council of Canada and the Ministere de l'Education du Gouvernement du Quebec which are gratefully acknowledged. We are greatly indebted to Mr. G. Oakson for his collaboration and continuous assistance in the electronic work.

REFERENCES

1 ANDERSEN, P., and ANDERSSON, S.A. Physiological basis of the alpha rhythm. Appleton, New York, 1968, 235 pp.

2 ANDERSEN, P., ANDERSSON, S.A., and LOMO, T. Some factors involved in the thalamic control of spontaneous barbiturate spindles, J. Physiol. (Lond.), 192 (1967) 257-281.

3 ANDERSEN, O., BROOKS, C. McC., ECCLES, J.C., and SEARS, T.A. The ventrobasal nucleus of the thalamus: potential fields, synaptic transmission and excitability of both presynaptic and postsynaptic components, J. Physiol.(Lond.), 174 (1964) 348-369.

4 ANDERSEN, P., and ECCLES, J.C. Inhibitory phasing of neuronal discharge, Nature (Lond.), 196 (1962) 645-647.

5 ANDERSEN, P., ECCLES, J.C., and SEARS, T.A. The ventro-basal complex of the thalamus: types of cells, their responses and their functional organization, J. Physiol. (Lond.), 174 (1964) 370-399.

6 ANDERSEN, P., JUNGE, K., and SVEEN, O. Cortico-thalamic facilitation of somato-sensory impulses, Nature (Lond.), 214 (1967) 1011-1012.

7 ANDERSEN, P., OLSEN, L., SKREDE, K., and SVEEN, O. Mechanism of the thalamo-cortical rhythmic activity with special reference to the motor system. In F.J. Gillingham and I.M.L. Donaldson (Eds.), Third Symposium on Parkinson's disease, Livingstone, Edinburgh and London, 1969, pp. 112-118.

8 ANDERSON, M.E. Cerebellar and cerebral inputs to physiologically identified efferent cell groups in the red nucleus of the cat, Brain Res., 30 (1971) 49-66.

9 ANDERSSON, S.A., and MANSON, J.R. Rhythmic activity in the thalamus of the unanesthetized decorticate cat, Electroenceph. clin. Neurophysiol., 31 (1971) 21-34.

10 AUER, J. Terminal degeneration in the diencephalon after ablation of the frontal cortex in the cat, J. Anat. (Lond.), 90 (1956) 30-41.

11 BREMER, F. Inhibitions intrathalamiques recurrentielles et physiologie du sommeil, Electroenceph. clin. Neurophysiol., 28 (1970) 1-16.

12 CLARE, M.H., LANDAU, W.M., and BISHOP, G.H. Electrophysiological evidence of a collateral pathway from the pyramidal tract to the thalamus in the cat, Exptl. Neurol., 9 (1964) 262-267.

13 COURVILLE, J., and BRODAL, A. Rubro-cerebellar connections in the cat: an experimental study with silver impregnation methods, J. comp. Neurol., 126 (1966) 471-486.

14 DAGNINO, N. FAVALE, E., MANFREDI, M., SEITUN, A., and TARTAGLIONE, A. Tonic changes in excitability of thalamocortical neurons during the sleep-waking cycle, Brain Res., 29 (1971) 354-357.

15 DEMPSEY, E.W., and MORISON, R.S. The interaction of certain spontaneous and induced cortical potentials, Am. J. Physiol., 135 (1942) 301-308.

16 DESIRAJU, T., BROGGI, G., PRELEVIC, S., SANTINI, M., and PURPURA, D.P. Inhibitory synaptic pathways linking specific and nonspecific thalamic nuclei,

Brain Res., 15 (1969) 542-543.

17 DESIRAJU, T., and PURPURA, D.P. Organization of specific-nonspecific thalamic internuclear synaptic pathways, Brain Res., 21 (1970) 169-181.

18 DORMONT, J.F., and MASSION, J. Duality of cortical control on ventrolateral thalamic activity, Exp. Brain Res., 10 (1970) 205-218.

19 DORMONT, J.F., and OHYE, C. Entopeduncular projection to the thalamic ventrolateral nucleus of the cat, Exp. Brain Res., 12 (1971) 254-264.

20 DUSSER de BARENNE, J.G., and McCULLOCH, W.S. Functional interdependence of sensory cortex and thalamus, J. Neurophysiol., 4 (1941) 304-310.

21 ECCLES, J.C., LLINAS, R., and SASAKI, K. The inhibitory interneurons within the cerebellar cortex, Exp. Brain Res., 1 (1966) 1-16.

22 EVARTS, E.V. Temporal patterns of discharge of pyramidal tract neurons during sleep and waking in the monkey, J. Neurophysiol., 27 (1964) 152-171.

23 FADIGA, E., and MANZONI, T. Relationships between the somatosensory thalamic relay nuclei of the two sides, Arch. ital. Biol., 107 (1969) 604-632.

24 FANARDZHYAN, V.V., and SARKISYAN, D.S. Intracellular investigation of antidromic and synaptic activation of rubral neurons in the cat, Neurosci. Transl., 9 (1969) 66-76.

25 FAVALE, E., SEITUN, A., TARTAGLIONE, A., and TONDI, M. Presynaptic and postsynaptic changes in the ventrolateral thalamic nucleus during natural sleep and wakefulness, Brain Res., 29 (1971) 351-353.

26 FILION, M., LAMARRE, Y., and CORDEAU, J.P. Neuronal discharges of the ventro-lateral nucleus of the thalamus during sleep and wakefulness in the cat. II Evoked activity, Exp. Brain Res., 12 (1971) 499-508.

27 FRIGYESI, T.L., and MACHEK, J. Basal ganglia-diencephalon synaptic relations in the cat. I. An intracellular study of dorsal thalamic neurons during capsular and basal ganglia stimulation, Brain Res., 20 (1970) 201-217.

28 FRIGYESI, T.L., and MACHEK, J. Basal ganglia-diencephalon synaptic relations in the cat. II. Intracellular recordings from dorsal thalamic neurons during low frequency stimulation of the caudato-thalamic projection systems and the nigrothalamic pathway, Brain Res., 27 (1971) 59-78.

29 FRIGYESI, T.L., and PURPURA, D.P. Functional properties of synaptic pathways influencing transmission in the specific cerebello-thalamo-cortical projection system, Exptl. Neurol., 10 (1964) 305-324.

30 FUKUDA, Y., and IWAMA, K. Inhibition des interneurones du corps genouille lateral par activation de la formation reticulee, Brain Res., 18 (1970) 548-551.

31 GJERSTAD, L.I., and SKREDE, K.K. Rhythmic thalamic unit activity in the unanesthetized cat, Acta Physiol. Scand., 79 (1970) 34A-35A.

32 HUMPHREY, D.P. Re-analysis of the antidromic cortical response. I Potentials evoked by stimulation of the isolated pyramidal tract, Electroenceph. clin. Neurophysiol., 24 (1968) 116-129.

33 ITO, M., YOSHIDA, M., and OBATA, K. Monosynaptic inhibition of the intracerebellar nuclei induced from the cerebellar cortex, Experientia, 20 (1964) 575-576.

34 IWAMA, K., and YAMAMOTO, C. Impulse transmission of thalamic somatosen-

sory relay nuclei as modified by electrical stimulation of the cerebral cortex, Jap. J. Physiol., 11 (1961) 169-182.

35 JABBUR, S.J., and TOWE, A.L. Analysis of the antidromic cortical response following stimulation at the medullayr pyramids, J. Physiol. (Lond.), 155 (1961) 148-160.

36 JANSEN, J., and JANSEN, J.K.S. On the efferent fibers of the cerebellar nuclei in the cat, J. comp. Neurol., 102 (1955) 607-623.

37 JASPER, H.H. Diffuse projection systems: the integrative action of the thalamic reticular system, Electroenceph. clin. Neurophysiol., 1 (1949) 405-420.

38 JASPER, H., and STEFANIS, C. Intracellular oscillatory rhythms in pyramidal tract neurones in the cat, Electroenceph. clin. Neurophysiol., 18 (1965) 541-553.

39 JOUVET, M. Recherches sur les structures nerveuses et les mecanismes responsables des differentes phases du sommeil physiologiques, Arch. ital. Biol., 100 (1962) 125-162.

40 KUSAMA, T., OTANI, K., and KAWANA, E. Projections of the motor, somatic sensory, auditory and visual cortices in cat. In T. Tokizane and J.P. Schade (Eds.), Correlative Neurosciences: Fundamental mechanisms, Progress in Brain Research, vol. 21A, Elsevier, Amsterdam, 1966, pp. 292-322.

41 LAMARRE, Y., FILION, M., and CORDEAU, J.P. Neuronal discharges of the ventro-lateral nucleus of the thalamus during sleep and wakefulness in the cat. I Spontaneous activity, Exp. Brain Res., 12 (1971) 480-498.

42 MAEKAWA, K., and PURPURA, D.P. Properties of spontaneous and evoked synaptic activities of thalamic ventrobasal neurons, J. Neurophysiol., 30 (1967) 360-381.

43 MARCO, L.A., BROWN, T.S., and ROUSE, M.E. Unitary responses in ventrolateral thalamus upon intranuclear stimulation, J. Neurophysiol., 30 (1967) 482-493.

44 MASSION, J. Etude d'une structure motrice thalamique, le noyau ventrolateral, et de sa regulation par les afferences sensorielles. These de doctorat d'Etat, Paris, 1968.

45 McLARDY, T. Thalamic microneurons, Nature (Lond.), 199 (1963) 820-821.

46 MINDERHOUD, J.M. An anatomical study of the efferent connections of the thalamic reticular nucleus, Exp. Brain Res., 12 (1971) 435-446.

47 MORISON, R.S., and BASSETT, D.C. The electrical activity of the thalamus and basal ganglia in decorticate cats, J. Neurophysiol., 8 (1945) 309-314.

48 MORISON, R.S., and DEMPSEY, E.W. A study of thalamo-cortical relations, Am. J. Physiol., 135 (1942) 281-292.

49 MUKHAMETOV, L.M., RIZZOLATTI, G. and TRADARDI, V. Spontaneous activity of neurones of nucleus reticularis thalami in freely moving cats, J. Physiol. (Lond.), 210 (1970) 651-667.

50 NAKAMURA, Y., and SCHLAG, J. Cortically induced rhythmic activities in the thalamic ventrolateral nucleus of the cat, Exptl. Neurol., 22 (1968) 209-221.

51 POIRIER, L., and BOUVIER, G. The red nucleus and its efferent nervous pathways in the monkey, J. comp. Neurol., 128 (1966) 223-244.

52 PURPURA, D.P. Operations and processes in thalamic and synaptically related neural subsystems. In F.O. Schmitt (Ed.), The Neurosciences (second study program), The Rockefeller Univ. Press, New York, 1970, pp. 458-470.

53 PURPURA, D.P., and COHEN, B. Intracellular recording from thalamic neurons during recruiting responses, J. Neurophysiol., 25 (1962) 621-635.

54 PURPURA, D.P., FRIGYESI, T.L., McMURTRY, J.G., and SCARFF, T. Synaptic mechanisms in thalamic regulation of cerebello-cortical projection activity. In D.P. Purpura and M.D. Yahr, (Eds.), The Thalamus, Columbia Univ. Press, New York, 1966, pp. 153-172.

55 PURPURA, D.P., McMURTRY, J.G., and MAEKAWA, K. Synaptic events in ventrolateral thalamic neurons during suppression of recruiting responses by brainstem reticular stimulation, Brain Res., 1 (1966) 63-76.

56 PURPURA, D.P., SCARFF, T., and McMURTRY, J.G. Intracellular study of internuclear inhibition in ventrolateral thalamic neurons, J. Neurophysiol., 28 (1965) 487-496.

57 RAMON y CAJAL, S. Histologie du systeme nerveux de l'homme et des vertebres (vol. II). Maloine, Paris, 1911.

58 RENSHAW, B. Central effects of centripetal impulses in axons of spinal ventral roots, J. Neurophysiol., 9 (1946) 191-204.

59 RINVIK, E. A re-evaluation of the cytoarchitecture of the ventral nuclear complex of the cat's thalamus on the basis of corticothalamic connections, Brain Res., 8 (1968) 237-254.

60 RINVIK, E. The corticothalamic projection from the pericruciate and coronal gyri in the cat. An experimental study with silver-impregnation methods, Brain Res., 10 (1968) 79-119.

61 RISPAL-PADEL, L. and MASSION, J. Relations between the ventrolateral nucleus and the motor cortex in the cat, Exp. Brain Res., 10 (1970) 331-339.

62 SAKAKURA, H. Spontaneous and evoked unitary activities of cat lateral geniculate neurons in sleep and wakefulness, Jap. J. Physiol., 18 (1968) 23-42.

63 SAKATA, H., ISHIJIMA, T., and TOYODA, Y. Single unit studies on ventrolateral nucleus of the thalamus in cat: its relation to the cerebellum, motor cortex and basal ganglia, Jap. J. Physiol., 16 (1966) 42-60.

64 SCHEIBEL, M.E., and SCHEIBEL, A.B. The organization of the nucleus reticularis thalami: a Golgi study, Brain Res., 1 (1966) 43-62.

65 SCHLAG, J., and WASZAK, M. Electrophysiological properties of units in the thalamic reticularis complex, Exptl. Neurol., 32 (1971) 79-97.

66 SHIMAZU, H., YANAGISAWA, N., and GAROUTTE, B. Cortico-pyramidal influences on thalamic somatosensory transmission in the cat, Jap. J. Physiol., 15 (1965) 101-124.

67 STEFANIS, C., and JASPER, H. Recurrent collateral inhibition in pyramidal tract neurons, J. Neurophysiol., 27 (1964) 855-877.

68 STERIADE, M. Ascending control of motor cortex responsiveness, Electroenceph. clin. Neurophysiol., 26 (1969) 25-40.

69 STERIADE, M. Physiologie des voies et des centres visuels. Masson, Paris, 1969, 188 pp.

70 STERIADE, M. The cerebello-thalamo-cortical pathway: ascending (specific and unspecific) and corticofugal controls, Int. J. Neurol., 7 (1970) 177-200.

71 STERIADE, M. Ascending control of thalamic and cortical responsiveness. In C.C. Pfeiffer and J.R. Smithies (Eds.), International Review of Neurobiology, Academic Press, New York, 1970 (vol. 12), pp. 87-144.

72 STERIADE, M., APOSTOL, V., and OAKSON, G. Clustered firing in the cerebellothalamic pathway during synchronized sleep, Brain Res., 26 (1971) 425-432.

73 STERIADE, M., APOSTOL, V., and OAKSON, G. Control of unitary activities in cerebellothalamic pathway during wakefulness and synchronized sleep, J. Neurophysiol., 34 (1971) 389-413.

74 STERIADE, M., APOSTOL, V., and OAKSON, G. Systemes de regulation de l'activite spontanee et evoquee des neurones du relais thalamique moteur, Rev. Can. Biol., 1972 (in press).

75 STERIADE, M., and BRIOT, R. Convergences inhibitrices d'influx cerebelleux et corticaux au niveau du noyau rouge et du noyau thalamique ventral lateral, J. Physiol. (Paris), 59 (1967) 298-299.

76 STERIADE, M., and DEMETRESCU, M. Unspecific systems of inhibition and facilitation of potentials evoked by intermittent light, J. Neurophysiol., 23 (1960) 602-617.

77 STERIADE, M., DESCHENES, M., WYZINSKI, P., and HALLE, J.Y. Input-output organization of the motor cortex and its alterations during sleep and waking. In J. Schlag and O. Petre-Quadens (Eds.), The Basic Mechanisms of sleep, Academic Press, New York, 1972 (in press).

78 STERIADE, M., IOSIF, G., and APOSTOL, V. Responsiveness of thalamic and cortical motor relays during arousal and various stages of sleep, J. Neurophysiol., 32 (1969) 251-265.

79 STERIADE, M., WYZINSKI, M., DESCHENES, M., and GUERIN, M. Disinhibition during waking in motor cortex neuronal chains in cat and monkey, Brain Res., 30 (1971) 211-217.

80 STERIADE, M., WYZINSKI, P., and OAKSON, G. Corticofugal impulses eliciting rhythmic activity in the ventrolateral thalamus, (in preparation).

81 SUZUKI, H., and TAIRA, M. Effects of reticular stimulation upon synaptic transmission in cat's lateral geniculate body, Jap. J. Physiol., 11 (1961) 641-655.

82 TOMBOL, T. Short neurons and their synaptic relations in the specific thalamic nuclei, Brain Res., 3 (1966-67) 307-326.

83 TOMBOL, T. Two types of short axon (Golgi 2nd) interneurons in the specific thalamic nuclei, Acta Morphol. Acad. Sci. Hung., 17 (1969) 285-297.

84 TSUKAHARA, N., TOYAMA, K., and KOSAKA, K. Electrical activity of red nucleus neurones investigated with intracellular microelectrodes, Exp. Brain Res., 4 (1967) 18-33.

85 UNO, M., YOSHIDA, M., and HIROTA, I. The mode of cerebello-thalamic relay transmission investigated with intracellular recording from cells of the ventrolateral nucleus of cat's thalamus, Exp. Brain Res., 10 (1970) 121-139.

86 VELASCO, M., and LINDSLEY, D.B. Role of orbital cortex in regulation of thal-

amo-cortical electrical activity, Science, 149 (1965) 1375-1377.
87 VERZEANO, M., LAUFER, M., SPEAR, P., and McDONALD, S. The activity of neuronal networks in the thalamus of the monkey. In K.H. Pribram and D.E. Broadbent (Eds.), Biology of memory, Academic Press, New York, 1970, pp. 239-271.
88 VILLABLANCA, J., and SCHLAG, J. Cortical control of thalamic spindle waves, Exptl. Neurol., 20 (1968) 432-442.
89 WALLER, H.J., and FELDMAN, S.M. Somatosensory thalamic neurons: effects of cortical depression, Science, 157 (1967) 1074-1077.

Corticothalamic Projections and Sensorimotor Activities
T. Frigyesi, E. Rinvik, and M.D. Yahr, editors. © 1972
Raven Press, New York.

Rhythmic Bursting of Unit Potentials in the Ventrolateral Thalamus of the Monkey

Yves Lamarre and A. J. Joffroy

Rhythmic bursting is a dominant feature of neurons in the ventrolateral nucleus (VL) of the thalamus. Spontaneous rhythmic burst discharges have been recorded in cats anesthetized with barbiturate (2) or with chloralose (9, 10) and also in monkeys under light chloralose anesthesia (1). In paralyzed, unanesthetized cats, however, the high frequency bursts occur only during slow wave sleep with EEG synchronization (3, 5, 13). Finally, in chronic monkeys, VL units discharge in bursts at a frequency of about 5 per sec when the animal is immobile and drowsy (6, 7). This rhythmic bursting pattern has been considered a reflection of the action of powerful inhibitory mechanisms which impair transmission of cerebellofugal activities during slow wave sleep (4, 9, 10, 11, 13).

Analysis of Burst Firing

The technique we used for central unit recording in the moving animal has been described elsewhere (8). In normal monkeys, the occurrence of two firing patterns is characteristic of the majority of units recorded in VL. Periods of sustained, irregular firing at 10 to 30 per sec alternate with periods of relative silence, when the activity is always in the form of short duration bursts of high frequency discharges. These bursts occur during relaxation and with the appearance of slow waves on the ECoG. This is illustrated in Fig. 1B where the lower trace is the ECoG from the ipsilateral motor cortex. The cell shows bursting when the animal is relaxed (first half of record B, ECoG slow waves). This pattern of firing changes, together with ECoG desynchronization, while the animal prepares to move (second half of record B). In this instance, the cell fires single spikes at an irregular rate of about 10 per sec.

The short duration bursts (3–20 msec) consist of 2 to 6 discharges at high frequency (200–600 per sec). Figure 2 shows the duration (ordinate) of consecutive intervals within the bursts of a VL cell (90 bursts). The intervals were measured with the help of a PDP-9 computer with a resolution of 0.25 msec. Values for the intervals within each individual burst are joined by a line. The majority of the bursts are composed of 4

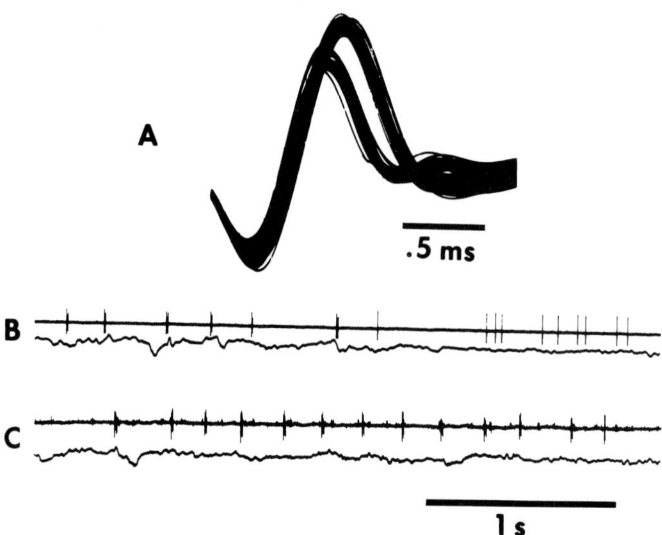

FIG. 1. Spontaneous VL unit activity in the unanesthetized awake monkey. In B and C, the top line is the unit activity and the lower line, the motor cortex ECoG. A: superimposed photographs of the same spike as in B, displayed with a fast time base. The smaller spike is "the first spike" of the bursts which occurs in the left half of record B. The larger spike is from the same cell, which fires single spikes in the right half of record B. The record in C was obtained 8 days after ipsilateral cortical ablation (see Fig. 3). In all records, negativity is upward.

spikes (3 intervals); only two bursts have six spikes. In most instances, the duration of the first interval falls between 2 and 4 msec. The second interval is usually shorter than the first one, particularly when the first interval has a duration of 3 msec or more.

In many instances, we observed that the amplitude of the "first spike" of the burst is smaller than the amplitude of the single spike discharges which occur during arousal. Several superimposed traces from a typical cell which illustrates this phenomenon are shown in Fig. 1A. The larger spike is the one fired during ECoG desynchronization (second half of trace B) while the smaller one is the "first spike" of the bursts occurring during ECoG slow waves (first half of trace B). Thus, the first spikes of the bursts have a negative phase of smaller amplitude and shorter duration. About half of the cells recorded in VL showed this phenomenon and, when recordings were made from such units for several hours, this difference in amplitude was maintained throughout. When we moved the electrode, we always lost the two types of spike at the same time. For these reasons, we think that these two types of discharge are generated by the same neuronal element. With extracellular recordings such as these, it is impossible to dis-

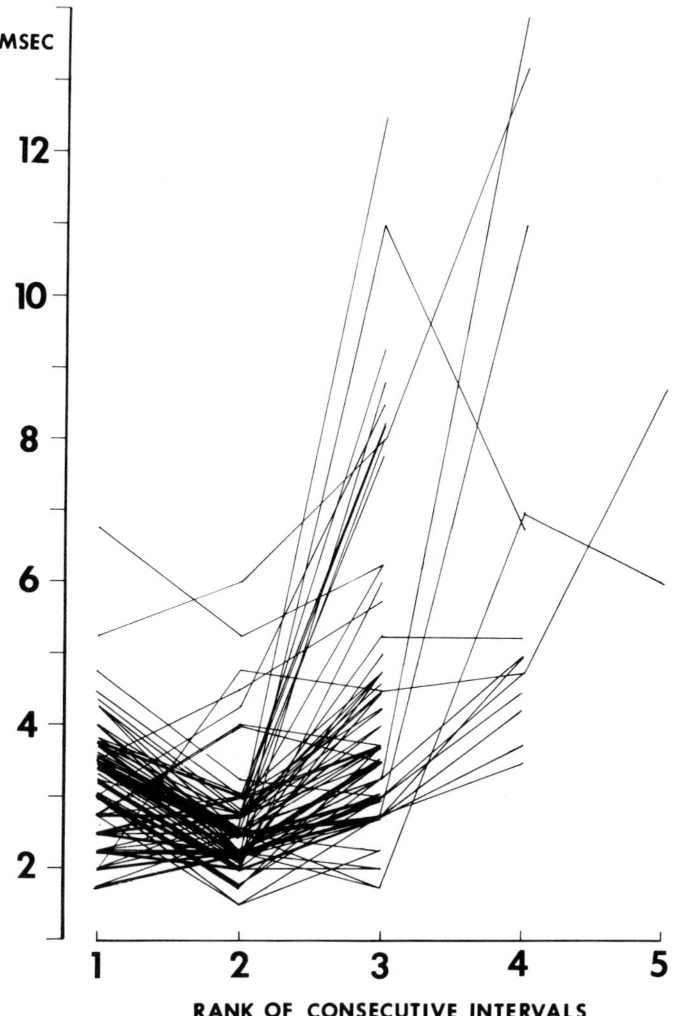

FIG. 2. Duration of consecutive intervals within 90 bursts from a VL unit. The intervals within each burst are joined by a line.

cern the nature of the phenomenon. However, one likely possibility, as stated by Purpura (12), would be that the spike amplitude is smaller because of the shunting action of a persisting increase of membrane conductance during bursting.

The interburst intervals varied from 100 to 400 msec but mostly were of the order of 200 msec. In many instances, there was a progressive shortening of the interburst intervals during a sequence of bursting. When two or more cells were recorded with the same microelectrode, we did not observe synchronization of the bursts of these cells

(Fig. 1C). On many occasions, spontaneous unit bursting and local thalamic slow waves were recorded with the same microelectrode. In these instances, we were unable to establish any clear relationship between these two events. Furthermore, no direct relationship was found between thalamic bursts and cortical spindle waves. Finally, we looked at the possible correlation between some burst parameters (such as duration, number of spikes, intra-burst frequency) and the duration of the intervals preceding or following the burst itself. We did not find any significant correlation.

VL Unit Bursting after Cortical Ablation

Steriade (14) has suggested that corticofugal impulses play a major role in setting up rhythmic activity of VL relay cells, possibly through a direct linkage of corticofugal fibers with interneurons located within the nucleus itself.

However, the fact that electrical stimulation of the motor cortex induces rhythmic excitatory and inhibitory sequences in VL relay elements does not necessarily mean that such a mechanism is responsible for the spontaneous rhythmic bursting of VL cells observed during relaxation and drowsiness in the monkey (6, 7). One way to investigate the function of the corticothalamic fibers to VL is to record the spontaneous behavior of VL neurons after lesion of the sensorimotor cortex. Figure 3 shows the extent of such a lesion centered in the arm area. This lesion resulted in complete paralysis of the contralateral arm. Extracellular recording in the VL nucleus on the side of the cortical lesion was performed 10 days after the cortical ablation.

The findings can be briefly summarized as follows: Most cells encountered in the

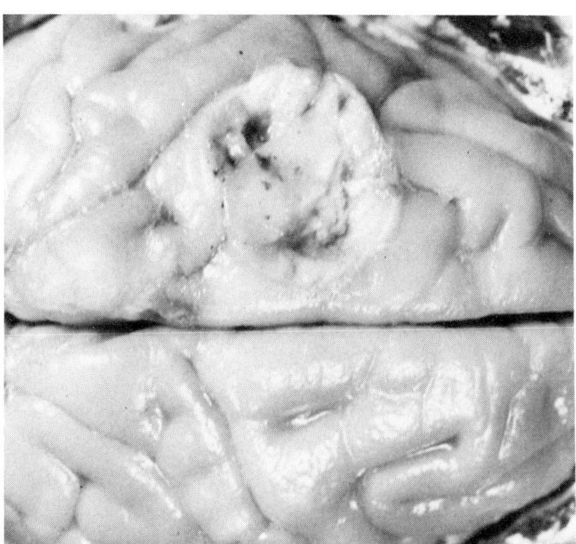

FIG. 3. Photograph showing the extent of a cortical lesion centered in the arm area of the left sensorimotor cortex.

VL region, from which responses could be evoked by stimulation of the paralyzed contralateral arm, showed sustained rhythmic bursting at a frequency of 3 to 5/sec (Fig. 1C). Such rhythmic activity was almost continuous and present even when the animal was strongly aroused. This abnormal pattern of activity contrasts sharply with all our previous recordings obtained in monkeys with intact sensorimotor cortex, where the VL bursting activity is present only when the animal is immobile and drowsy.

These results indicate that corticothalamic impulses are not essential elements for the appearance of the normal spontaneous bursting of VL relay cells. It is more probable that the spontaneous rhythmic bursting of VL elements is mainly, if not exclusively, the result of intra-thalamic mechanisms producing EPSP-IPSP sequences such as have been demonstrated in reciprocal specific - non specific intrathalamic pathways (11). Moreover rhythmic bursting may be enhanced abnormally when VL cells are deprived of the direct corticothalamic input, although this could also be the result of a reduction of proprioceptive input from the paralyzed contralateral limb.

ACKNOWLEDGMENT

Research supported by grant MA-2863, Medical Research Council of Canada.

REFERENCES

1 ALBE-FESSARD, D., GUIOT, G., LAMARRE, Y. and ARFEL, G. Activation of Thalamocortical Projections Related to Tremorogenic Processes. In: The Thalamus, D.P. Purpura and M.D. Yahr, (Eds.), New York, Columbia University Press, 1966, pp. 237-253.

2 ANDERSEN, P. OLSEN, L., SKEDE, K. and SVEEN, O. Mechanisms of Thalamo-Cortical Rhythmic Activity with Special Reference to the Motor System. In: Third Symposium on Parkinson's Disease. F.J. Gillingham and I.M.L. Donaldson, (Eds.), Edinburgh, Livingston, 1969, pp. 112-118.

3 DORMONT, J.F. Activite Unitaire dans le Noyau Ventral Lateral chez le Chat Eveille. J. Physiol. 60, 242, 1968.

4 FILION, M., LAMARRE, Y. and CORDEAU, J.P. Neuronal Discharges of the Ventrolateral Nucleus of the Thalamus during Sleep and Wakefulness in the Cat. II. Evoked Activity. Exp. Brain Res. 12, 499-508, 1971.

5 LAMARRE, Y., FILION, M. and CORDEAU, J.P. Neuronal Discharges of the Ventrolateral Nucleus of the Thalamus during Sleep and Wakefulness in the Cat. I. Spontaneous Activity. Exp. Brain Res. 12, 480-498, 1971.

6 LAMARRE, Y. and JOFFROY, A.J. Thalamic Unit Activity in Monkey with Experimental Tremor. In: D-Dopa and Parkinsonism. A. Barbeau and F.H. McDowell, (Eds.), Philadelphia, Pa., F.A. Davis, 1970, pp. 163-170.

7 LAMARRE, Y. and JOFFROY, A.J. Spontaneous Unit Activity in the Ventrolateral Thalamus of the Chronic Monkey. Int. J. Neurol., (1972) in press.

8 LAMARRE, Y., JOFFROY, A.J., FILION, M. and BOUCHOUX, R. A Stereotaxic Method for Repeated Sessions of Central Unit Recording in the Paralyzed or Moving Animal. Rev. Can. Biol. 29, 371-376, 1970.

9 MASSION, J. Etude d'une Structure Motrice Thalamique, le Noyau Ventrolateral et de sa Regulation par les Afferences Sensorielles. These de doctorat d'Etat es Sciences Naturelles, Faculte des Sciences de Paris, 1968.

10 MASSION, J., ANGAUT, P. et ALBE-FESSARD, D. Activites Evoquees chez le Chat dans la Region du Nucleus Ventralis Lateralis par Diverses Stimulations Sensorielles. II. Etude Microphysiologique. Electroenceph. clin. Neurophysiol. 19. 452-469, 1965.

11 PURPURA, D.P., FRIGYESI, T.L., McMURTRY, J.G. and SCARFF, T. Synaptic Mechanisms in Thalamic Regulation of Cerebello-Cortical Projection Activity. In: The Thalamus, D.P. Purpura and M.D. Yahr, (Eds.). New York, Columbia University Press, 1966, pp. 153-170.

12 PURPURA, D.P. Chapter in this volume.

13 STERIADE, M., APOSTOL, V. and OAKSON, G. Control of Unitary Activities in Cerebellothalamic Pathway during Wakefulness and Synchronized Sleep. J. Neurophysiol. 34, 389-413, 1971.

14 STERIADE, M. Chapter in this volume.

DISCUSSION

PURPURA:

I think Dr. Steriade's extracellular data are critically important in attempts to define the relations of reticularis neuron discharges to inhibitory activities elsewhere. Could you comment on the relationship of the onset of the burst discharges to the stimuli?

STERIADE:

Permit me to present a new slide which will allow me to comment factually on your question. This cell, the same as depicted in Fig. 21 of my presentation, recorded

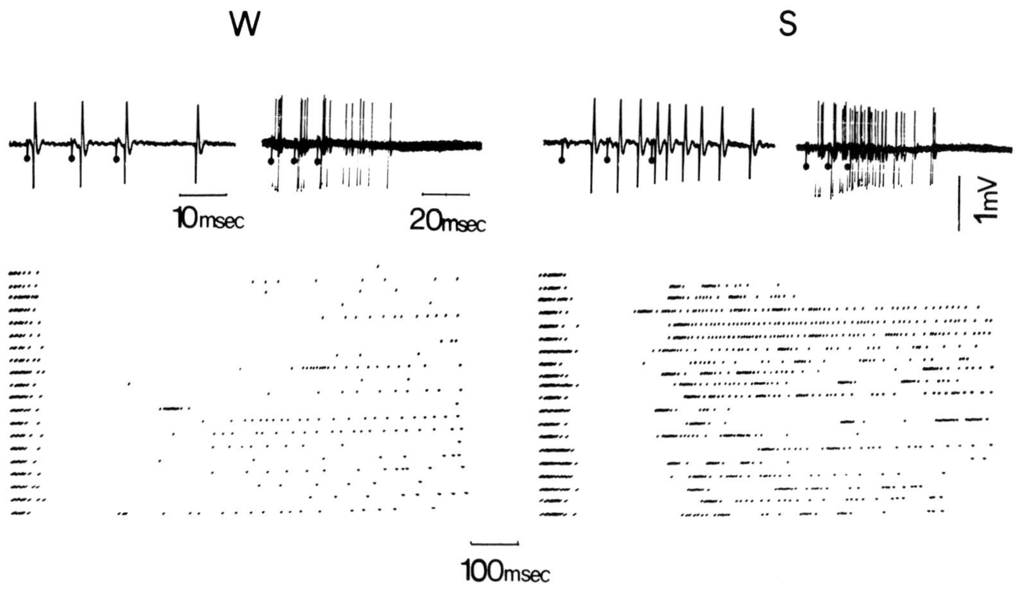

Cortically-evoked activities in a neuron recorded from the rostral pole of the thalamic reticularis nucleus during EEG patterns of waking (W) and synchronized sleep (S). A three-shock train (dots) was applied to the lateral part of the precruciate area. Single sweep at fast speed (at left) and superimposition of several traces (at right). Below, the dotgrams of the same neuronal spikes, at much lower speed, to depict the early cortically evoked excitation, the following period of silence, and the subsequent late events. Full description of latencies of the early responses, burst frequencies and duration in the inhibitory periods during W and S in the text.

in the rostral pole of the thalamic reticularis nucleus, was synaptically driven by precruciate stimuli with the shortest latency at 0.8 msec during waking, and it could follow fast (100/sec) cortical shocks, thus demonstrating a monosynaptic high-security cortico-reticular pathway. During EEG synchronization, the cortically elicited response took the form of a burst with repetitive spikes at 250/sec and the latency of the first discharge reached 5-6 msec. The dotgrams of the same neuronal spikes in the bottom part of the figure depict the inhibition following the early excitation evoked by cortical stimuli and the subsequent late events. The recovery of single spike discharges during EEG patterns of waking (occasionally with a unique barrage) changed during EEG synchronization into multiple, postinhibitory spike barrages at around 300/sec, lasting 30 to 60 msec. Bursting following a period of suppressed firing was also seen in VL neurons after a shock-train to the motor cortex. But such cortically evoked VL spike clusters had a striking rhythmicity which was not seen in reticularis cells, among them the neuron depicted in this slide is a typical example. To infer an inhibitory role of reticularis neurons on VL relay cells within the frame of rhythmic sequences evoked by cortical stimulation, it would be necessary to find a close time-relation between reticularis bursts and periods of firing suppression in VL relay cells, or some relations between bursting in both types of neurons. Such a relation was found between VL relay cells and VL intrinsic interneurons (see again Fig. 21 in my chapter), but the irregularity of spike barrages in reticularis neurons, also evident when considering their spontaneous activity, markedly contrasted with the stereotyped rhythmicity induced by cortical stimuli (and occurring also spontaneously during EEG synchronization) in both VL relay cells and in VL interneurons. Of course, the fact that burst discharges in the reticularis nucleus were not time-locked with the events recorded from the VL has only the value of a negative finding and it has to be restricted to the neurons recorded in the rostral part of the reticularis complex.

PURPURA:

Yes, I thought they weren't time-locked. Now I'd like to comment on the problem of the small spike in Dr. Lamarre's presentation. I wonder if the change in spike height might be due to the increased conductance of the neuronal membrane during the burst because there always seems to be an underlying IPSP in such synchronizing activities upon which the EPSP and burst discharges are superimposed. Hence there might be some shunting of the spike potential. Perhaps Dr. Grundfest can comment on this.

GRUNDFEST:

I would like to ask Dr. Lamarre about that last slide. Do you have direct evidence that the desynchronized spikes that you showed are really the same as the ones in the bursting? They look different to me.

LAMARRE:

Well, they are indeed different and the fast superimposed sweeps were presented to show this. This difference was noticed very often and the superimposed traces always had the same appearance. I could show you many more cells which show exactly the same thing. It would be a very improbable coincidence if whenever a desynchronized cell stops firing we immediately begin to record another cell firing in bursts and vice versa. This hypothesis becomes even more untenable when one finds that both types of spike are lost at the same time. This is our evidence.

STERIADE:

The easiest reply would be to refuse a comparison between cortically elicited rhythmic bursting in cat's VL cells with an intact brain, which represented the bulk of my talk, and spontaneous rhythmic bursting in the monkey's VL with an extensive cortical sensorimotor lesion, as reported by Yves Lamarre. I can't, however, resist from commenting on Yves' discussion and on his own findings. Let's first say that, in spite of my repeated emphasis that VL rhythmic activity at 8-12/sec induced by motor cortex stimulation is certainly not the same as natural spindling but only a mimic, cortically elicited thalamic 8-12/sec waves are very similar, if not identical, in their gross morphology and related unitary events to thalamic spindles spontaneously occurring during EEG synchronization (see again Figs. 16-17 in my chapter). The main methodological reason for using cortical stimulation to induce the rhythmic thalamic bursting was to disclose the synaptic corticothalamic pathways underlying this activity, as hypothesized in our previous papers. Studying natural phenomena and waiting for what the animal is ready to show us are certainly not forbidden, and the results of a simple observation might sometimes be very interesting, but in my feeling using the effects of shocks, which do not occur in the brain during normal life, may have the physiological advantage of modeling a normal function, even if the result is simply a simulation, and to disclose its mechanisms. Why not repeat that delivering low-rate shocks to the medial thalamus and recording mass and especially intracellular activities taught us much more about the intimate basis of EEG synchronization than the profuse clinical observations done in much more natural conditions? Therefore, I believe that rhythmic bursting is an intrinsic property of the thalamic networks, but that in intact brain animals the cerebral cortex controls such activity and, I would say more, the cortex may actualize this pattern of thalamic activity if, under certain circumstances, it remains only virtual.

Now, after these very general things, I would like to comment on two kinds of findings reported by Yves. I already gave in my chapter enough details on the correspondence between unit bursting and slow waves recorded in the VL with the same microelectrode (see my Fig. 17). I also gave my explanation for the lack of correspondence between VL spike clusters and cortical spindle waves: such a lack of time-relation likely depends on the position of cortical recording electrode which has to be checked carefully after a thorough exploration of many cortical foci. When this precaution is taken, one can find such a time-relation between VL rhythmic spike clusters and cortical spontaneous EEG spindles (see Fig. 8A in my chapter), even if the relation becomes even more evident following administration of very small doses of barbiturate (Fig. 8B). In one of the slides presented by Dr. Purpura this afternoon, it was also very obvious that rhythmic EPSP–IPSP sequences in VB neurons (and we know that spike clusters may follow the long-lasting IPSPs) are closely time-related with different components of spontaneously developing spindle waves in the corresponding point of the somatosensory cortex. You will accept that the EEG spindles you are recording in a chronically implanted animal reflect an activity which you are not choosing in function of the position of your VL microelectrode but the activity of a diffuse cortical neuronal population where you implanted for ever your screws, without any subsequent choice of changing according to analytical purposes.

Let's go into your major finding, namely the apparent increase of VL bursting following a cortical sensorimotor lesion. I am unhappy when I have to compare what happens in a VL of a lesioned animal with the events in VL of other animals studied as a control. All of us are aware that different preparations show different susceptibilities to exhibit rhythmic bursting, probably because they are more or less aroused. The crucial proof would be (if "crucial" exists) to compare VL bursting before and after removal of sensorimotor cortex in the same animal. Why not use, Yves, the beautiful technique Professor Jasper is employing studying the effects of reversible cooling of the cerebral cortex, and to observe the VL bursting before, during and after this procedure? The result of such a demonstration would be indeed a pleasure to see.

Corticothalamic Projections and Sensorimotor Activities
T. Frigyesi, E. Rinvik, and M.D. Yahr, editors. © 1972
Raven Press, New York.

Cortical Control of Somatic Inflow to Medial Thalamus

Denise Albe-Fessard, J. M. Besson, G. Guilbaud and A. Levante

Connections through direct pathways between cortical areas and medial-intralaminar thalamic neurons have been shown to exist by the use of anatomical techniques in cats and monkeys (Rinvik; the Scheibels; and Petras, elsewhere in this volume). We ourselves shall examine the possible excitatory or inhibitory roles which these direct connections may play. We shall also discuss other connections, those difficult to study by anatomical techniques because they are comprised of polysynaptic pathways, but which can, however, play an important role in behavior.

The results presented here have been obtained from a large number of experiments on cats and monkeys and with various collaborators, and often from experiments performed for purposes other than searching for cortical projections to thalamic areas. Some of the cats were anesthetized with chloralose or with volatile agents (Ether, Halothane) and maintained thereafter under local analgesia; all these animals were curarized. In another group of cats, bipolar macroelectrodes were implanted in the thalamic regions and stimulating electrodes were placed on the radial nerve. The mean value of the evoked thalamic activities in these animals was evaluated by use of an averager during different phases of sleep. The monkeys were intubated, lightly curarized and maintained under local analgesia; cortical electrodes for stimulation had been implanted in advance. End-tidal CO_2 was monitored in all the curarized animals. Stimulation and recording procedures will be given in the legends of each figure. Special techniques for spinal cord recordings for DRP (1) and for the use of microelectrodes (2).

1. DEMONSTRATION OF DESCENDING CORTICAL INFLOWS TO THE MEDIAL THALAMUS

More than ten years ago, Albe-Fessard and Gillett (3) had searched with macroelectrodes, then microelectrodes, for cortical regions the stimulation of which would demonstrate descending connections with Pf-CM in cats. They found that it is only the motor and inferior SII cortical areas in which stimulation always evoked slow waves or spike activities in these thalamic regions (orbital cortex not then explored). This occurred in cats under chloralose as well as in animals under local analgesia (Fig. 1). The shortest latencies were found after stimulation of the motor cortex and, at unitary level, it was possible to demonstrate that both excitatory and inhibitory phenomena were produced by cortical stimulation (Fig. 2).

However, in this earlier work, it was difficult to determine whether impulses responsible for either excitation or inhibition and coming from cortical areas were

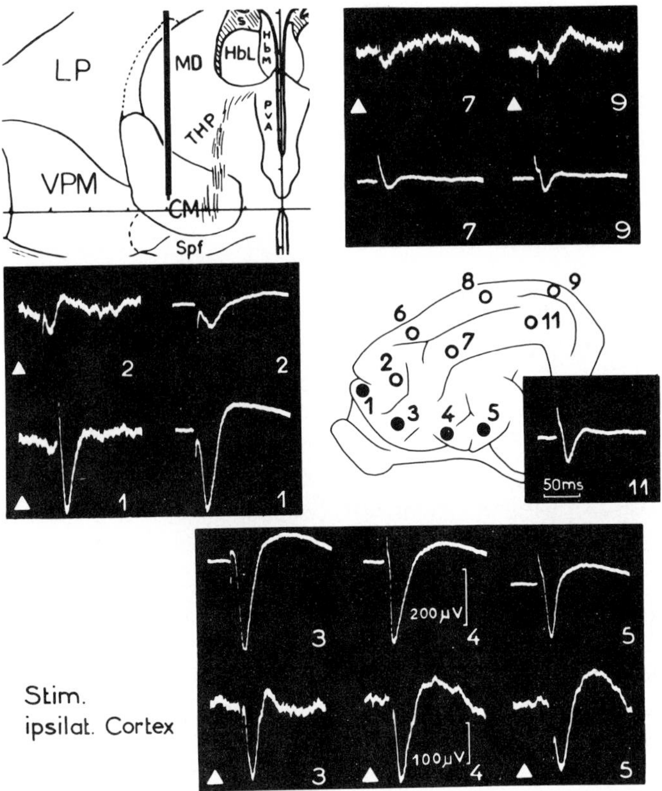

FIG. 1. Responses from cat's CM to stimulation (4 V - 1 ms) of ipsilateral cortical areas, applied to dura mater by two superficial electrodes separated by 4 mm. Recording concentric macroelectrodes stereotaxically implanted (downward deflection= positivity of deeper electrode). Inset, upper left side: schema of stereotaxic anterior plane 7.5. Middle: lateral view of the cat's brain with the 11 selected stimulated places. Responses obtained from two animals under different conditions: one anesthetized with volatile agent and maintained afterwards under local analgesia (triangles); the other anesthetized with chloralose. The numbers refer to the points where stimulations were applied. Responsive stimulated areas (black points) are the same under either condition. (From Albe-Fessard and Gillett, 1961; slightly modified.)

acting directly at the thalamic level or at the level of relays placed on the ascending pathways to this thalamic zone. In particular, an action at reticular level (bulbar or mesencephalic) could not be ignored because some of the impulses are known to relay to the medial thalamus (14) through these structures which are also known to receive cortico-descending pathways from the somato-motor cortex (13, 15, 29, 34-37, 44, 50).

A. DEMONSTRATION OF THE EXISTENCE OF MULTIPLE EXCITATORY CORTICO-THALAMIC CONNECTIONS

In a series of experiments using the technique of antidromic activation and undertaken to search for the cortical sites of projection from cells in the medial thalamus, we were able to find, not only cells of the medial thalamus that were antidromically activated, but also cells orthodromically driven.

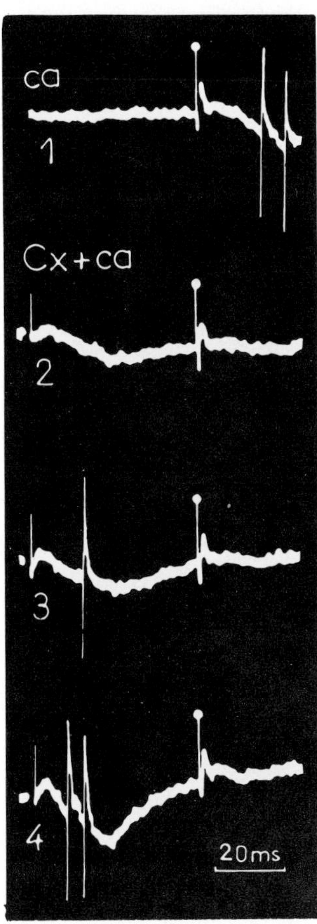

FIG. 2. Microelectrode recordings from a cell in CM (micropipettes filled with KCl; same in Fig. 3, 4, 5). A peripheral stimulation is applied to the contralateral anterior paw (ca), and a cortical one (cx) to the inferior posterior part of the suprasylvian gyrus. 1, Response to the stimulation of the limb alone. 2, 3, 4, The same stimulation of the limb is preceded by a cortical stimulation of increasing intensity. In 2, liminal effect results only in an inhibition, which is preceded in 3 and 4 by an excitatory response when the stimulation is increased. (From Albe-Fessard and Gillett, 1961.)

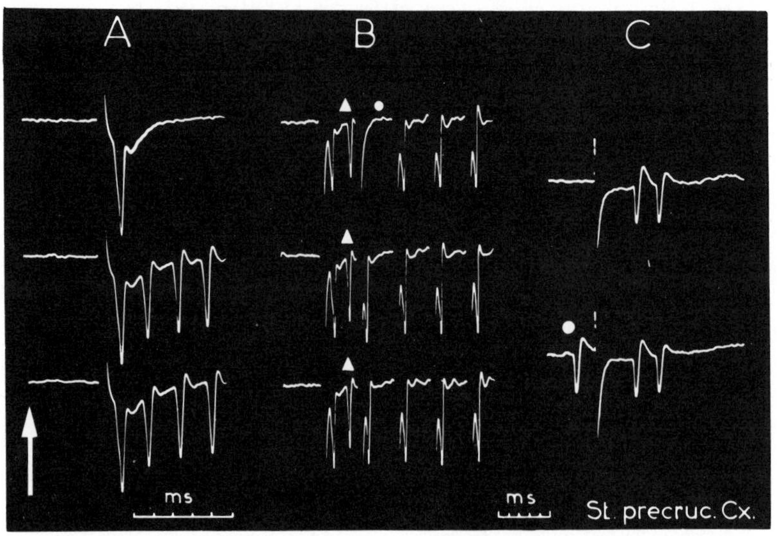

FIG. 3

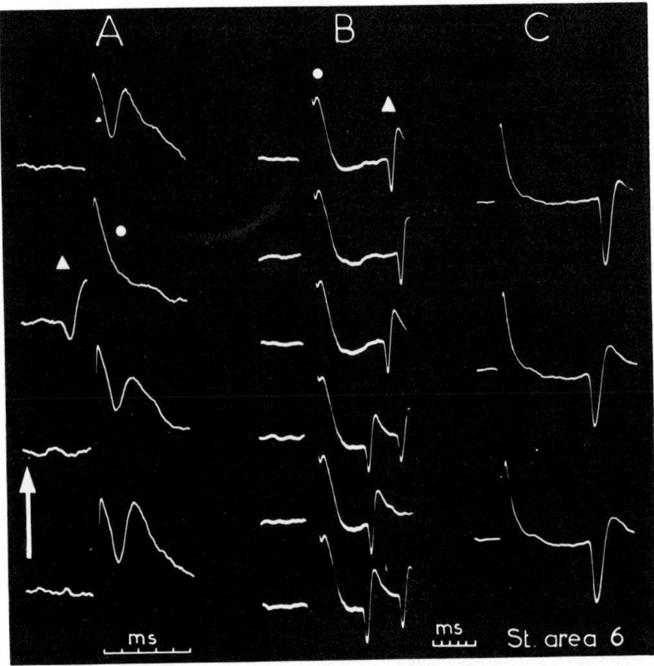

FIG. 4

The stimulations were applied to the precruciate cortex; CM and Pf nuclei as well as the neighboring thalamic structures, n. centralis lateralis (CL) and n. dorsalis medialis (MD) were the thalamic regions explored with glass microelectrodes. These experiments formerly made on the cat (4) were later pursued on the monkey.

Cells of the medial thalamus responding to a cortical stimulation by spikes can be divided into three groups on the basis of the characteristics of their responses.

a- Cells presenting antidromic activation.

The latency of the spikes was short and stable, with a mean value of 1.5 msec. The one-spike responses followed trains of stimulation at high frequency; the collision test was positive. The majority of the cells responding in this way (15 p. 100 among 781 observed in the cat) were located between planes 8 and 9.5, that is, in the anterior part of CM-Pf and CL.

b- Cells presenting antidromic and orthodromic activations.

Frequently, as shown in Fig. 3 and 4, an antidromic response was not the only one presented by cells of the explored region. Spikes were observed, and their fatigability to repetitive stimuli, together with the lack of collision with an orthodromic spike of different origin, demonstrated their orthodromic nature. These orthodromic responses had variable latencies. Some were as short as 2.5 msec, not much

---

FIG. 3. Three examples (A and B, cat under chloralose, C under local analgesia) of units recorded in anterior CM and responding to cortical stimulations (3 V - .2 ms couple of electrodes separated by 4.5 mm, laid on dura mater). Trains of stimulations delivered every second. Tracings in succession from bottom to top. A, Response of one short latency antidromic spike followed by 3 orthodromic ones which disappear with repetition. B, Same response, but rapid repetition of stimulation (270/sec) suppresses the orthodromic responses except the first (Δ). In the upper row (Δ) has a slightly longer latency and by collision suppresses at (o) the following response. C, Orthodromic responses with relatively short latency, the nature of which is demonstrated by the lack of collision with a spontaneous spike (o).

FIG. 4. Tracings from 2 monkeys with chronically implanted cortical stimulating electrodes and maintained under local analgesia during the recording time. Three responsive units are recorded from the superior part of n. centralis lateralis. Tracings in succession from bottom to top. A, Cell antidromically excited only. A spontaneous activity of orthodromic origin (Δ) has a collision effect which suppresses the following antidromic spike (o). B, Two kinds of responses appear, one with very short latency (o) is antidromic, the other spikes (Δ) are of orthodromic origin. C, The responses are orthodromic only. Note, in B and C, the lack of stability of the orthodromic response latencies.

longer than the mean antidromic latency. In these cases, a direct excitatory connection from the cortex was an easy deduction, since anatomists have demonstrated its existence. One cell is generally activated both antidromically and orthodromically from the same cortical zone. Thus a double reciprocal connection between the thalamic and cortical areas can be said to exist.

c- Cells presenting orthodromic activation only.

In these cases, activation most often appears after a latency longer than 5 msec and frequently ranging from 15 to 20 msec. In the cat, 133 cells among the 781 studied responded in this way.

Another group of cells responded after latencies of 100 to 600 msec (34 cells were counted which responded after long latencies only). In general, latencies fluctuated more than the shorter orthodromic ones, and the responses did not follow stimuli given at more than 3/sec. All these facts indicate that these responses are generated by impulses delayed through a polysynaptic pathway. The large margin of the latency values suggests that, in addition to reticular, longer central loops may also be involved.

The antidromic responses could be obtained in cats maintained under local analgesia as well as those anesthetized with chloralose; they were, however, greatly modified by barbiturate anesthesia. The orthodromic responses seem to be more easily obtained under chloralose. As Fig. 4 shows, the same sort of connections can be demonstrated in non-anesthetized monkeys between area 6 and the same medial thalamic zone. These last conclusions are merely preliminary; no statistical analyses were made on the number of cells of each type.

B. EXISTENCE OF A DIRECT INHIBITORY PATHWAY

During the experimental series described above, we had observed a relatively important number of spontaneously firing cells that were merely inhibited by cortical stimulations. Moreover, we had occasion to penetrate into a few cells with the microelectrodes. Among a part of these cells (13 of the total investigated population), hyperpolarizations (of 50 msec duration) were observed exhibiting short latencies (2-5 msec) following cortical stimulation. This sort of intracellular records has been more frequently observed at the limit of inferior dorsalis medialis nucleus and CM or CL nuclei. Two such records are presented in Figure 5. These are similar to the results obtained by Frigyesi (elsewhere in this volume) to capsular stimulations.

In general, the cells presenting this hyperpolarization were not responding antidromically to the same stimulation. Thus, the existence of a descending direct inhibitory pathway originating in the cortex is suggested. However, the duration of the hyperpolarization is shorter than that of inhibitions which could be demonstrated by an extracellular technique (3). Consequently, if a direct inhibitory pathway does exist, we also have to assume the existence of other pathways which inhibit the activating messages in the relays of the afferent pathway. We shall discuss in succession two possible sites of action of these inhibitory effects.

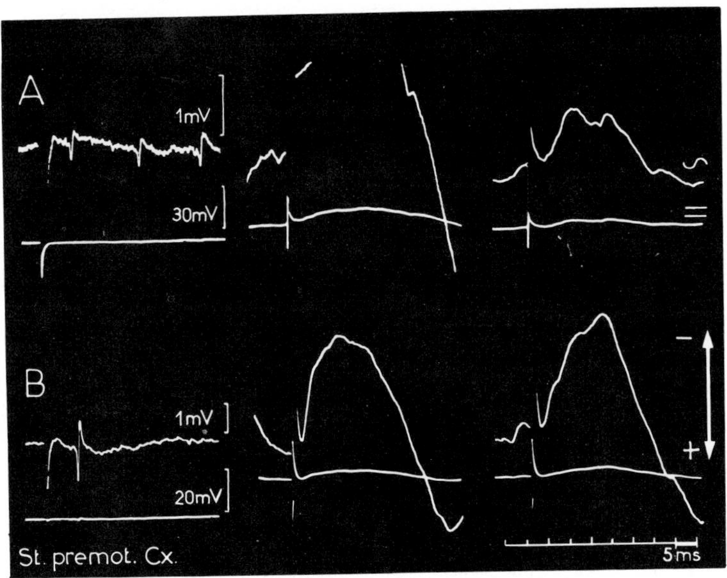

FIG. 5. Tracings from 2 cats (A and B), showing cellular penetrations at the limit of n. dorsalis medialis and CM. Two amplification channels; one, ac, at high gain; the other, dc, at much lower gain. From left to right: just before the penetration, just after it, a moment later. Note the small dc shift and, however, the clear hyperpolarization wave appearing with a relatively short latency after the cortical stimulation.

2. CORTICAL CONTROLS OF AFFERENTS TO MEDIAL THALAMIC NUCLEI IN CHRONICALLY IMPLANTED CATS

The evoked responses observed in the thalamus during one or the other of the two phases of sleep differ considerably. The amplitudes in the primary thalamic relays and in the thalamic nuclei fed through extralemniscal pathways are both affected, but in opposite directions depending on the state of sleep of the animal (5, 6, 21, 24). These modifications can be clearly seen in Fig. 6 where it is shown that, during fast sleep as compared to slow sleep, the amplitudes of responses in the primary thalamic relay are increased, while those in CM nuclei are reduced. This fact and the recognition of the existence of descending inhibitory pathways from the somatomotor cortex which are able to affect different relays along the ascending pathways to medial thalamus induced us to assume that the reduction of the responses in CM, observed during the fast sleep phase, is due to increased activity in the primary cortical areas which was also observed with microelectrodes during fast sleep (6, 20, 31). This hypothesis was confirmed when an ablation of a well delineated precruciate cortical area was shown to suppress the reduction of the CM responses commonly observed in intact animals during the phase of fast sleep (26) (Fig. 7). This was a demonstration that an inhibitory

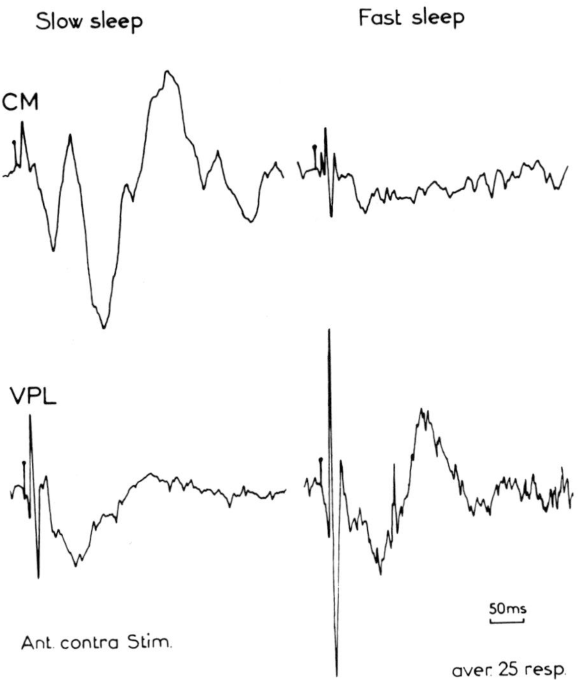
Slow sleep
Fast sleep
CM
VPL
50ms
Ant. contra Stim.
aver. 25 resp.

FIG. 6

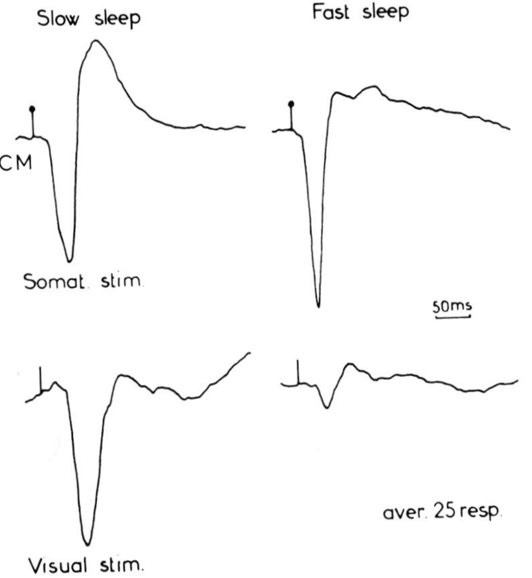
After abl. precruc. Cx.
Slow sleep
Fast sleep
CM
Somat. stim.
50ms
aver. 25 resp.
Visual stim.

FIG. 7

pathway was acting from the precruciate cortex upon the somatic nonspecific afferent pathway. Moreover, these controls are put into action through a specific inflow, since the same workers have found, after chronic sections of the lemniscal pathways, effects similar to those observed after precruciate cortex ablation.

These results are in agreement with the work of several authors (2, 10, 13), mainly obtained in acute experiments, which emphasized the part played by the somatomotor cortex in the control of nonspecific thalamic afferents.

The next step was to specify the site of action of the descending controls during fast sleep. We could show here that this site is certainly not at the CM postsynaptic level. Many cells of these regions in the cat respond to visual and auditory stimulations as well as to somatic ones. If the inhibitory effect exerted by the motor cortex is acting at the CM synaptic level, should it not inhibit the visual and auditory inputs as well as the somatic ones? It must be emphasized that, on the contrary, visual and auditory inputs were shown to be controlled by their respective primary areas of projection, and not by the somatomotor cortex (27). For instance, the removal of precruciate cortex that suppresses the evolution of somatic responses does not suppress the reduction of amplitude observed during fast sleep in response to visual stimulation (Fig. 7). On the contrary, the change of visual responses during fast sleep is suppressed by bilateral removal of the primary visual cortex, while somatic responses are still reduced under these conditions (Fig. 8).

Consequently, it may be said that the cortical descending control acting during fast sleep cannot be exerted at the postsynaptic site in the medial thalamic nuclei; it must be exerted elsewhere, prior to the synapses. The same sort of experiments, made at the level of the bulbar and mesencephalic reticular formation where some of the different sensory afferents are relayed (9, 11, 14, 52) lead to the same conclusion (Fig. 9). Finally, all these experiments indicate that the most important inhibitory controls are not exerted at the heterosensory convergence loci, but prior to it, just presynaptically at reticular relays or at the first synapses of each non-primary inflow pathways, i.e., for the somatic relays, in the spinal cord.

3. CORTICAL CONTROLS OF MEDIAL THALAMUS INFLOW AT SPINAL LEVEL

The synaptic transmission at the level of the first relays of somatic afferent

---

FIG. 6. In a cat implanted with two bipolar electrodes, one in CM, the other in VPL, 25 responses to stimulation of radial nerve were averaged during the two phases of natural sleep. Note the reduction of CM responses during fast sleep and, on the contrary, the increase of VPL ones (namely, the short latency response).

FIG. 7. Same sort of chronic preparation as in Fig. 6, but precruciate cortex was bilaterally removed. Note that the CM responses to somatic stimulation do not undergo a reduction of amplitude during fast sleep, whereas, on the contrary, responses to visual stimulation do.

FIG. 8. Same sort of chronic preparation as in Fig. 6. Responses to somatic and visual stimulations are recorded in CM but this time after bilateral ablation of the primary visual cortex; the precruciate cortex was left intact. Note that, in this case, it is the response to visual stimulation that is the same during either phase of sleep whereas the response to somatic stimulation undergoes a normal reduction of amplitude during fast sleep.

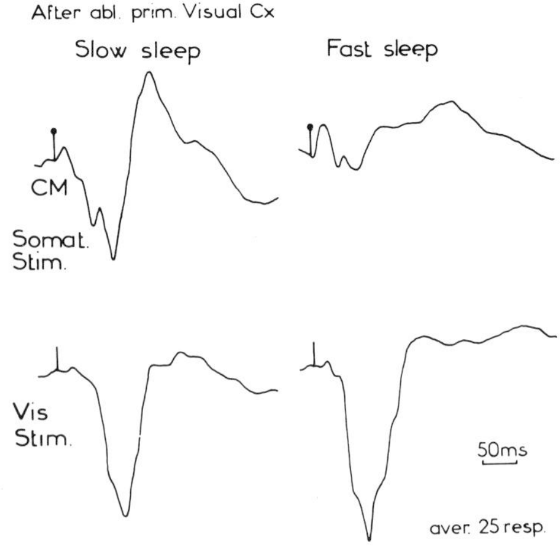

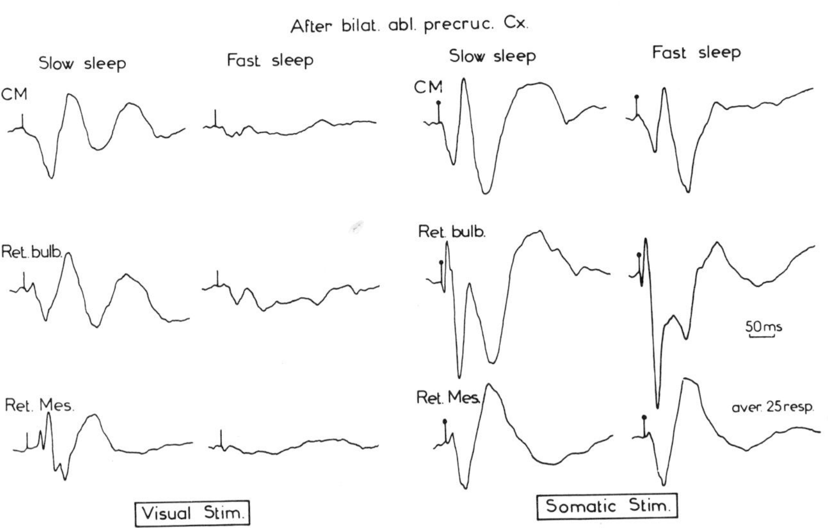

FIG. 9. Same sort of chronic preparation as in Fig. 6. Electrodes have been implanted in CM and in bulbar and mesencephalic reticular formations. Note that at the three levels, after bilateral ablation of both precruciate cortices, the somatic responses (last two columns at right) are barely modified when the state of sleep has changed, while a neat variation is still present for visual stimulation (first two columns at left).

pathways (spinal cord, dorsal column nuclei, trigeminal nuclei) is submitted to controls of various origins and natures. We shall consider primarily the data related to controls exerted by cortical areas at the spinal cord level; for, although the starting point of the anterolateral pathway through which medial thalamus is mainly fed is still unknown, cells of the dorsal horn are likely at the origin of this tract, even if another relay exists in spinal gray before the departure of the fibers of this pathway itself.

In the dorsal horn, the dorsally located cells which correspond mainly to the lamina IV and a part of lamina V (48) are known to be at the origin of the spino-cervical tract (14, 33, 42, 43, 56, 57). This point is confirmed by the fact that about 43 percent of the lamina IV cells and 19 percent of lamina V cells are antidromically activated by the stimulation of dorsolateral columns (23). On the other hand, cells located more ventrally (level of Rexed's laminae VI and V) might be on the trajectory of the anterolateral pathway.

Decisive experiments proving the connection between cells of these two lamiae and reticular or thalamic termination of the anterolateral bundle have not yet been made, and it is the complexity of organization of the spinal cord (47, 51, 55) which is certainly responsible for this failure.

However, that lamina V units play an important part in the nociceptive message transmission is suggested by the fact that they show specific and graduated responses to intense stimulations (30, 53, 54, 58, 59) and may also be driven by afferents from

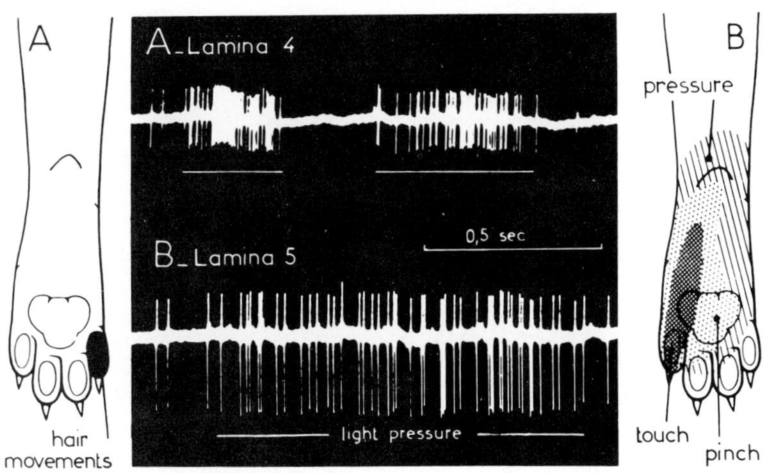

FIG. 10. Records from two cells in the cat's spinal cord (dorsal part of the dorsal horn). A, Small peripheral field, responses to light tactile stimulations; an example typical of lamina IV cells. B, Central zone sensitive to light touch surrounded by a larger zone requesting stronger stimuli; an example typical of lamina V cells.

visceral origin (45, 53, 54). Moreover, when cells of laminae IV and V are recognized by their electrophysiological properties (Fig. 10), our group was able to show (12) that intraarterial injection of Bradykinin at the level of posterior limb (Fig. 11) induced activity in lamina V cells and had practically no effect on lamina IV cells. Bradykinin is a polypeptid which, when intraarterially injected, induces a painful sensation in man and nociceptive reactions in animals (38). Thus, we shall propose here that the interneurons which are the most probable candidates for feeding the anterolateral pathway are located in layers V and VI where they are intermingled with the interneurons which contribute to the flexor reflexes. This hypothesis has been confirmed by the recent investigations of Price and Wagman (46) who showed that the activities of axons from the "controlateral anterolateral quadrant" have characteristics similar to those of cells recorded at the level of Rexed's lamina VI in the cat (59) and in the monkey (58). Consequently it is the controls of laminae V and VI cells by cortical areas which we will consider in this paper. Until now, we have considered only controls on lamina V cells; however, as mentioned by Wall (59), cutaneous impulses activating lamina VI cells are probably relayed from lamina V.

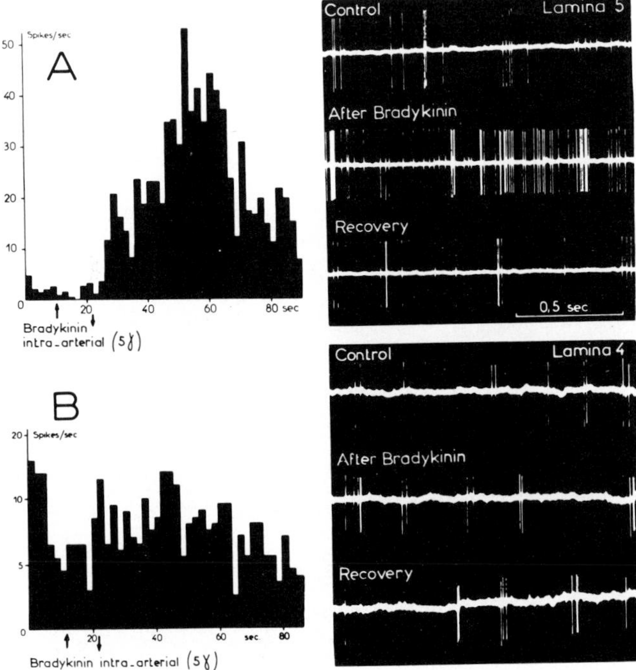

FIG. 11. Comparison between the effects of Bradykinin intra-arterial injection into the popliteal artery: A, on a cell in lamina V; B, on a cell in lamina IV. At left, time-histograms showing the variations of the cell firing frequency before and after an injection. At right, samples of unitary recordings. Modified from Besson et al., 1972.

Controls which act upon the transmission of afferent volleys at spinal level have already been studied by many authors. The first problem concerns the nature of these controls. Without neglecting postsynaptic phenomena (33, 39), we can assert that most of these influences are of presynaptic nature. These influences are subdivided into segmental and supraspinal controls; we shall consider here only the supraspinal one. We shall examine the results obtained by two techniques: first, the existence of dorsal root potentials considered as the sign of presynaptic inhibition and provoked by cortical stimulation; second, the modification of activities of cells in the dorsal horn provoked by cortical stimulation.

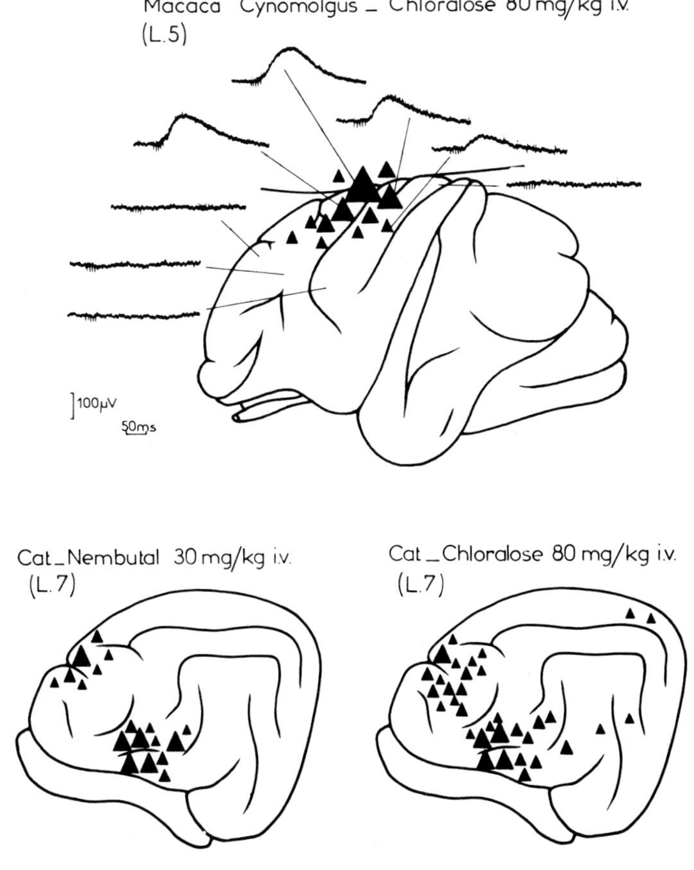

FIG. 12. Schematic representation in monkey and cat of cortical areas the stimulation of which induces dorsal root potentials at lumbar spinal level (L5 in the monkey, L7 in the cat). Monkey dorsal root recordings at L5 are presented with the sites of stimulation.

A. DORSAL ROOT POTENTIALS

The first observations of inhibitory descending influences were made by Hagbarth and Kerr (28) and Magni and Oscarrson (40) who showed that stimulation of the sensorimotor cortex induced a depression in transmission of the activity conveyed by the ascending spinal tracts. The presynaptic nature of these controls was demonstrated by Andersen et al. (7, 8) and Carpenter et al. (18, 19) who obtained dorsal root potentials (DRPs) by cortical stimulation. The effective areas include the pre- and postcruciate gyri and area SII, to which, in the cat, the orbital cortex must be added (1) (Fig. 12). The regions studied induce bilateral DRPs and the ipsilateral effect is not suppressed by section of the corpus callosum. The organization was shown to be somatotopic for area SI (7, 8), but not for SII or the orbital cortex. However, by comparing the cortical areas inducing DRPs in cats and monkeys, Abdelmoumene et al. (1) have encountered a preferential organization in the former species, while in the latter, they have found a strict somatotopic organization (Fig. 12).

These cortical effects do not affect the afferent terminals of fibers Ia, but are exerted on fibers Ib and on the flexor reflexes afferents (8, 19). The latency of the cortical effects varies from 20 to 30 msec; the maximal effect is at about 40-50 msec and its total duration around 150-200 msec. Carpenter et al. (19) had shown that DRPs induced by sensorimotor cortex stimulation were provoked primarily through the medium of the pyramidal tract. However when the animals are under chloralose anesthesia, these phenomena remain after bilateral pyramidectomy, a fact which indicates that other pathways, especially the rubrospinal and probably the reticulospinal tracts are also involved (32). These latter results must be compared to those of Carpenter et al. (18, 19), who showed that DRPs could be obtained at lumbar level by stimulation of wide regions in the brain stem.

From a functional point of view, as many authors have suggested, the presynaptic inhibition of cortical origin would act in the primary system as a negative feedback loop which increases localization of the active stimulation. In the present study, its function is different since this control is exerted by the centers of specific projection upon extralemniscal afferents. The interesting fact is that a part of the cortical areas that produces DRPs were shown (see preceding paragraph) to inhibit CM cellular activities.

B. UNITARY RECORDINGS AT DORSAL HORN LEVEL

These data are in consonance with those just quoted. In 1964, Andersen et al. (8) reported that cortical stimulation provokes an inhibition of the dorsal horn interneurons, and that the time course of inhibition corresponds to that of the DRP. In the decerebrate animal, cells within laminae IV, V, VI (59) and cells which are at the origin of the spinocervical tract (17) were shown to be dependent on descending controls which are suppressed by section or cooling of the spinal cord.

Units belonging to laminae IV, V and VI and recognized by their electrophysiological characteristics (Fig. 10) as described by Wall (59) were studied in animals

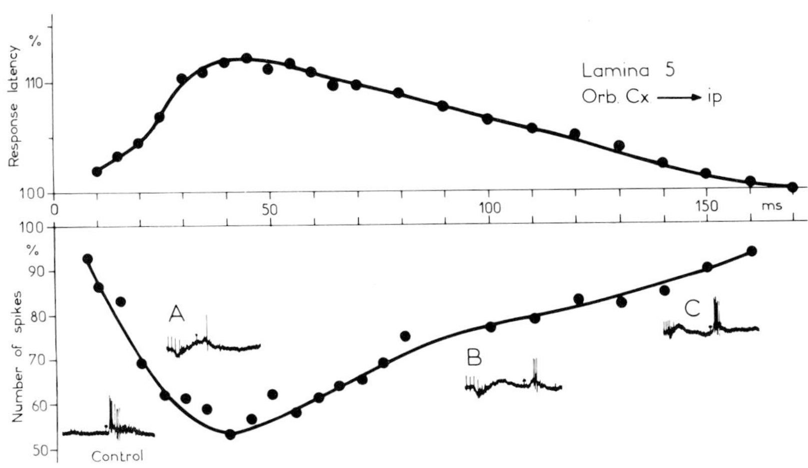

FIG. 13. Cat under light chloralose anesthesia. Average effects on lamina V cells (28 cells) of a stimulation applied to orbital cortex (short trains of shocks, 300/sec, 2 msec, bipolar electrodes separated by 2 mm) and intervening at different intervals prior to stimulation of the ipsilateral posterior limb. This results in an increase of the response latency (upper curve) and in a reduction of the number of spikes (lower curve). A, B, C, samples of response at different moments. Control: response to posterior limb stimulation alone.

with spinal sections. Cells from lamina IV are affected by the most powerful inhibitory controls since two thirds of its units are inhibited by stimulation of the pyramidal tract (23) while in lamina V, 40 percent of the cells are inhibited (23).

In the intact animal, we found an important effect of cortical area stimulation, of orbital gyrus in particular, on the cells of both layers of IV and V: 80 p. 100 are inhibited in laminae IV, 60 p. 100 in layer V (Fig. 13).

These results, compared to the ones of Fetz (23), show again that the pyramidal tract is not the only one which conveys descending inhibitory messages and that indirect pathways through reticular formation, nucleus ruber and possibly caudate nucleus (22) also have to be considered.

Due to the lack of intracellular recordings, it has not been possible to eliminate completely the eventuality of postsynaptic mechanisms. However, by comparing the time courses of inhibition and DRP obtained by pyramidal stimulation (23) and by stimulation of the orbital cortex (41), the hypothesis that these phenomena are largely dependent on a mechanism of presynaptic inhibition can be put forward.

Such inhibitory controls of cortical origin most probably act by means of interneurons located in Rexed laminae VI and VII (49). These interneurons themselves are activated by stimulations of the sensorimotor cortex (Fig. 14) and also by heterotopic and heteromodal stimulations; moreover there is a close parallelism between acceleration of unitary discharges in these interneurons and the appearance of corresponding DRPs (Fig. 14).

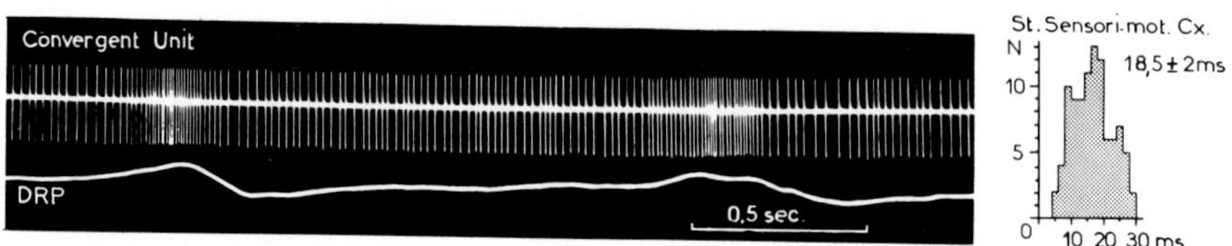

FIG. 14. Cat under chloralose anesthesia. Simultaneous records of the spontaneous activity of cell in lamina VII and of spontaneous DRPs derived from a rootlet at the same level. Such interneuron cells in laminae VI and VII are excited when the sensorimotor cortex is stimulated. Latencies vary from 4 to 30 msec (see histogram at right).

In conclusion, we want to emphasize that the different actions on the sensory afferents to medial thalamus as presented here are certainly only a part of the complex story of the controls exerted by primary cortical areas on these inflows to thalamic regions which receive convergent heterotopic and heterosensorial messages.

SUMMARY

Stimulation of the precruciate cortex has shown that fibers arising in this region can evoke orthodromic responses at the level of medial thalamus. The orthodromic pathways involved may be either excitatory or inhibitory in nature. For either of them, direct as well as indirect connections do exist.

1) The multiplicity of excitatory pathways was deduced from the wide range of latency measurements on spikes recorded with microelectrodes.

2) A multiplicity of inhibitory pathways was demonstrated by using three sorts of data:

a) Hyperpolarizations, recorded intracellularly at the thalamic level, which had short latencies, suggest direct inhibitory synapses.

b) In chronic cats with implanted electrodes, during the phase of fast sleep, an inhibition was shown to act on the sensory afferents converging onto the cells of the CM-Pf nuclei. This inhibition appeared to be differentially produced by the specific primary cortical area to which the corresponding afferent messages are projected. From this, it follows that the inhibitory action takes place prior to the level of convergence, i.e., before the thalamic or reticular regions of neuronal convergence.

c) Since it is known that the main afferent pathways to the medial thalamus are in the anterolateral region of the cord, it is at this level, on the cells which feed the anterolateral bundle, that the first inhibitory effects must be sought. It is possible that the cells of laminae V and VI are at the origin of the anterolateral fibers, even if their impulses are once more relayed by interneurons in deeper laminae. Former experiments which demonstrate that the somato-motor cortex has a powerful inhibitory control on cells of lamina V have been reviewed. Supplementary evidence is based on dorsal root potentials as well as unitary spinal recordings.

REFERENCES

1 ABDELMOUMENE, M., BESSON, J.M. et ALEONARD, P. Cortical areas exerting presynaptic inhibitory action on the spinal cord in cat and monkey. Brain Res., 20 (1970) 327-329.

2 ADEY, W.R., SEGUNDO, J.P. and LIVINGSTON, R.B. Influence des stimulations corticales sur la "conduction" dans le tronc cérébral. J. Neurophysiol., 20 (1957) 1-16.

3 ALBE-FESSARD, D. and GILLETT, E. Convergences vers le Centre Median. Electroenceph. clin. Neurophysiol., 13 (1961) 257-269.

4 ALBE-FESSARD, D., LEVANTE, A. et ROKYTA, R. Cortical projections of cat medial thalamic cells. Intern. J. Neuroscience, 1 (1971) 327-338.

5 ALBE-FESSARD, D., MASSION, J., HALL, R. and ROSENBLITH, W. Modifications au cours de la veille et du sommeil des valeurs moyennes des reponses nerveuses corticales induites par des stimulations somatiques, chez le chat libre. C.R. Acad. Sci. Paris, 258 (1964) 353-356.

6 ALLISON, T. Cortical and subcortical evoked responses to central stimuli during wakefulness and sleep. Electroenceph. clin. Neurophysiol., 18 (1965) 131-139.

7 ANDERSEN, P., ECCLES, J.C. and SEARS, T.A. Presynaptic inhibitory action of cerebral cortex on spinal cord. Nature (Lond.), 194 (1962) 740-743.

8 ANDERSEN, P., ECCLES, J.C. and SEARS, T.A. Cortically evoked depolarization of primary afferent fibres in the spinal cord. J. Neurophysiol., 27 (1964) 63-77.

9 BACH Y RITA, P. Convergent and long latency unit responses in the reticular formation of the cat. Exp. Neurol., 9 (1964) 327-344.

10 BAUMGARTEN, R.V., MOLLICA, A. and MORUZZI, G. Influence of the

motor cortex on the spike discharges of bulbo-reticular neurons. Electroenceph. clin. Neurophysiol., Sup. 3 (1953) pp. 68.

11 BELL, C., SIERRA, G., BUENDIA, N. and SEGUNDO, J.P. Sensory properties of neurons in the mesencephalic reticular formation. J. Neurophysiol., 27 (1964) 961-987.

12 BESSON, J.M., CONSEILLER, C., HAMANN, K.-F. and MAILLARD, M.C. Modifications of dorsal horn cell activities in the spinal cord, after intra-arterial injection of Bradykinin. J. Physiol. (London), 221(1972) 189-205.

13 BORENSTEIN, P. et BUSER, P. Observations sur les projections du cortex dans la formation réticulée mésencéphalique chez le chat. C.R. Soc. Biol. (Paris), 154 (1960) 38-42.

14 BOWSHER, D., MALLART, A., PETIT, D. and ALBE-FESSARD, D. A bulbar relay to the Centre Median. J. Neurophysiol., 31 (1968) 288-300.

15 BREMER, F. et TERZUOLO, C. Contribution à l' étude des mécanismes physiologiques du maintien de l'activité vigile du cerveau. Interaction de la formation reticulée et de l' écorce cérébrale dans le processus du réveil. Arch. int. Physiol., 42 (1954) 157-178.

16 BRODAL, P. and REXED, B. Spinal afferents to the lateral cervical nucleus in the cat. An experimental study. J. comp. Neurol., 98 (1953) 179-212.

17 BROWN, P.B. Descending control of the spinocervical tract in decerebrate cats. Brain Res., 17 (1970) 152-155.

18 CARPENTER, D., LUNDBERG, A. and NORRSELL, U. Effects from the pyramidal tract on primary afferents and on spinal reflex actions to primary afferents. Experientia (Basel), 18 (1962) 337-338.

19 CARPENTER, D., LUNDBERG, A. and NORRSELL, U. Primary afferent depolarization evoked from the sensorimotor cortex. Acta physiol. scand., 59 (1963) 126-152.

20 EVARTS, E. Temporal patterns of discharge of pyramidal tract neurons during sleep and waking in the monkey. J. Neurophysiol., 27 (1964) 151-171.

21 FAVALE, E., LOEB, C. and MANFREDI, M. Somatic responses evoked by central stimulation during natural sleep and during arousal. Arch. int. Physiol. Biochem., 71 (1963) 229-235.

22 FELTZ, P., KRAUTHAMER, G. and ALBE-FESSARD, D. Neurons of the medial diencephalon. I. Somatosensory responses and caudate inhibition. J. Neurophysiol., 30 (1967) 55-80.

23 FETZ, E.E. Pyramidal tracts effects in the cat lumbar dorsal horn. J. Neurophysiol., 31 (1968) 69-80.

24 GUILBAUD, G. Evolution au cours du sommeil des réponses somatiques evoquées aux differents niveaux corticaux et sous-corticaux chez le chat. Thesis (Paris) (1968) pp. 93.

25 GUILBAUD, G. Essai de classification des structures centrales au moyen des variations d'amplitude évoqués somatiques au cours des cycle veille-sommeil. Electroenceph. clin. Neurophysiol., 28 (1970) 340-350.

26 GUILBAUD, G. et MENETREY, D. Rôle joué par les voies et aires de projection lemniscales dans le contrôle des afferences extralemniscales au cours du sommeil

naturel chez le chat. Electroenceph. clin. Neurophysiol., 29 (1970) 295-302.

27 GUILBAUD, G., MENETREY, D., KREUTZER, M. and OLIVERAS, J.L. Control exerted during sleep by primary sensory cortical areas upon the different sensory afferents. Proc. of the Int. Union Physiol. Sci., Vol. IX (XXV Int. Congress of Physiol. Sci., Munich), (1971).

28 HAGBARTH, K.E. and KERR, D.I.B. Central influences on spinal afferent conduction. J. Neurophysiol., 17 (1954) 295-307.

29 HERNANDEZ-PEON, R. and HAGBARTH, K. Interaction between afferent and cortically induced reticular responses. J. Neurophysiol., 18 (1955) 44-45.

30 HILLMAN, P. and WALL, P.D. Inhibitory and excitatory factors influencing the receptive field of lamina 5 spinal cord cells. Exp. Brain Res., 9 (1969) 284-304.

31 HODES, R. Lower cortical threshold in rapid eye movement periods than during sleep. Fed. Proc., 23 (1964) 208.

32 HONGO, T. and JANKOWSKA, E. Effects from the sensorimotor cortex on the spinal cord in cats with transected pyramids. Exp. Brain Res., 3 (1967) 117-134.

33 HONGO, T., JANKOWSKA, E. and LUNDBERG, A. Post-synaptic excitation and inhibition from primary afferents in neurones of the spinocervical tract. J. Physiol. (London) 199 (1968) 569-592.

34 HUGELIN, A., BONVALLET, M. et DELL, P. Topographie des projections cortico-motrices au niveau du telencephale, du tronc cerebral et du cervelet chez le Chat. Revue Neurol., 89 (1953) 419-425.

35 KUYPERS, H.G.J.M. An anatomical analysis of cortico-bulbar connexions to the pons and lower brain stem in the cat. J. Anat. (Lond.) 92 (1958a) 198-218.

36 KUYPERS, H.G.J.M. Some projections from the peri-central cortex to the pons and lower brain system in monkey and chimpanzee. J. comp. Neurol., 110 (1958b) 221-255.

37 KUYPERS, H.G.J.M. Central cortical projections to motor and somato-sensory cell groups. Brain, 83 (1960) 161-184.

38 LIM, R.K.S. Neuropharmacology of pain and analgesia. In: Pharmacology of Pain, R.K.S. Lim, D. Armstrong & E.G. Pardo (Eds.) Pergamon Press, London, (1968), pp. 169-217.

39 LUNDBERG, A. Supraspinal control of transmission in reflex path to motor-neurones and primary afferents. Prog. Brain Res., 12 (1964) 197-221.

40 MAGNI, F. and OSCARSSON, O. Cerebral control of transmission to the ventral spinocerebellar tract. Arch. ital. Biol., 99 (1961) 369-396.

41 MAILLARD, M.C., BESSON, J.M., CONSEILLER, C. et ALEONARD, P. Effets provoqués par la stimulation du cortex orbitaire sur les cellules des couches IV et V de la corne dorsale de la moelle chez le Chat. C.R. Acad. Sci. Paris, 272 (1971) 729-732.

42 MORIN, F. and CATALANO, J.V. Central connections of a cervical nucleus (nucleus cervicalis lateralis of the cat). J. comp. Neurol., 103 (1955) 17-32.

43 OSWALDO-CRUZ, E. and KIDD, C. Functional properties of neurons in the lateral cervical nucleus of the cat. J. Neurophysiol., 27 (1964) 1-14.

44 PETERSON, E.W. and BICKERS, D. Projection of cortical area 6 to brain stem in monkey. J. Neurophysiol., 15 (1952) 87.
45 POMERANZ, B., WALL, P.D. and WEBER, W.V. Cord cells responding to fine myelinated afferents from viscera, muscle and skin. J. Physiol. (London) 199 (1968) 511-532.
46 PRICE, D.D. and WAGMAN, I.H. Characteristics of two ascending pathways which originate in spinal horn of M. mulatta. Brain Res., 26 (1971) 406-410.
47 RETHELYI, M. and SZENTAGOTHAI, J. The large synaptic complexes of the substantia gelatinose. Exp. Brain Res., 7 (1969) 258-274.
48 REXED, B. The cytoarchitectonic organization of the spinal cord in the cat. J. comp. Neurol., 96 (1952) 415-495.
49 RIVOT, J.P., BESSON, J.M., ABDELMOUMENE, M. et ALEONARD, P. Relations entre les decharges de certains interneurones spinaux et les potentiels radiculaires dorsaux. J. Physiol. (Paris), 62 (1970) 440.
50 ROSSI, G. et BRODAL, A. Corticofugal fibres to the brain stem reticular formation. An experimental study in the cat. J. Anat. (Lond) 90 (1956) 42-52.
51 SCHEIBEL, M.E. and SCHEIBEL, A.B. Terminal axonal patterns in cat spinal cord. II. The dorsal horn. Brain Res., 9 (1968) 32-58.
52 SCHEIBEL, M.E., SCHEIBEL, A.B., MOLLICA, A. and MORUZZI, G. Convergence and interaction of afferent impulses on single units of reticular formation. J. Neurophysiol., 18 (1955) 309-331.
53 SELZER, M. and SPENCER, W.A. Convergence of visceral and cutaneous afferent pathways in the lumbar spinal cord. Brain Res., 14 (1969a) 331-348.
54 SELZER, M. and SPENCER, W.A. Interactions between visceral and cutaneous afferents in the spinal cord: reciprocal primary afferent fibre depolarization. Brain Res., 14 (1969b) 349-366.
55 SZENTAGOTHAI, J. Neuronal and synaptic arrangement in the substantia gelatinose Rolandi. J. comp. Neurol., 122 (1964) 219-230.
56 TAUB, A. Local, segmental and supraspinal interaction with a dorsolateral spinal cutaneous afferent system. Exp. Neurol., 10 (1964) 357-374.
57 TAUB, A. and BISHOP, P.O. The spinocervical tract, dorsal column linkage, conduction velocity, primary afferent spectrum. Exp. Neurol., 13 (1965) 1-21.
58 WAGMAN, I.H. and PRICE, D.D. Responses of dorsal horn cells of Macaca mulatta to cutaneous and sural nerve A and C fibre stimuli. J. Neurophysiol., 32 (1969) 803-817.
59 WALL, P.D. The laminar organization of dorsal horn and effects of descending impulses. J. Physiol. (London) 188 (1967) 403-423.

DISCUSSION

PURPURA:

I want to congratulate you on your fine presentation and at the same time ask you to clarify a point of some importance. You have interpreted your findings as demonstrating a direct inhibition of a CM cell by cortical stimulation. This would be of historical significance since as you know there is no evidence at this time that pyramidal neurons of neocortex emit corticofugal axons that are directly inhibiting to postsynaptic elements. I am also somewhat puzzled by the multiphasic nature of the hyperpolarization you found in CM cells following cortical stimulation. Do you have satisfactory latency measurements?

ALBE-FESSARD:

When the electrode has just impaled the cell, the hyperpolarization is not multiphasic. The multiphasicity seems to be due to a progressive destruction of the membrane. These cells seem to be relatively small because they are rapidly destroyed. For the latency, it is difficult to be more precise. The smallest latency are difficult to measure because of the short stimulation artifact; the smallest are of 1.5-2 msec. I looked to this latency because I was not convinced also of the existence of a direct inhibition.

PURPURA:

Well, you know they are fine fibers.

ALBE-FESSARD:

I begin to think of an orthodromic inhibition because the antidromic activation is of the order of 1.5 to 2.5 msec in the surrounding cells so latencies of orthodromic and antidromic activation are of the same order of magnitude. The majority of the inhibited cells were not in CM itself, but in the part of the dorso-medial nucleus just adjacent to CM.

KUYPERS:

In respect to what you just said, the direct projections from the area which you are talking about to the motor cortex, let's define that sort of loosely: Do they come from the CM itself or from the adjacent part of the dorso-medial nucleus?

ALBE-FESSARD:

The direct projection going from thalamus to cortex comes from the anterior part of CM and in majority from the n. centralis lateralis. If, for example, as in the cat, the largest part of the CM nucleus is comprised between anterior planes 7-8.5, it is from planes 8.5 to 9 that you can find cells being at the origin of this pathway.

Corticothalamic Projections and Sensorimotor Activities
T. Frigyesi, E. Rinvik, and M.D. Yahr, editors. © 1972
Raven Press, New York.

Chairman's Summary

Herbert H. Jasper

I would like to begin this summary by making some general comments which may apply to other parts of this symposium as well as to this particular session, though well illustrated in this session, particularly in the papers by Purpura and Steriade.

With the refinements in both anatomical and electrophysiological techniques, many of which are apparent in this symposium, it becomes necessary to refine also the precision of our terminology and the conceptual framework used in the interpretation of our results. I would like first to question continued use of the term "non-specific" to describe relatively "unspecified" parts of the "mesial thalamus". Are these terms correct or sufficiently precise today, even though they may have served a useful purpose a generation ago?

The designation "non-specific" has been used in both a topographic and functional sense. A neuronal system with a convergent multisensory input, or/and with a diffusely ramifying axonal projection not exclusively related to local areas of cortex, specific thalamic nuclei, or to topographically organized motor pathways is called "non-specific". Presumably also it should have a generalized function such as "arousal", regulation of states of sleep and wakefulness or degree of generalized motor activity (hypokinesis, hyperkinesis, akinetic mutism). Generalized emotional states such as level of anxiety, mood, or emotional drive when not related to a "specific" behavioural pattern such as fear, rage, sex, or hunger may be also included under the functional designation "non-specific". A wide variety of neuronal systems can, therefore, be classified as "non-specific". In some respects one might even include the association areas of the cerebral cortex and their respective thalamic nuclei, since they too may have a multisensory convergent input and no clear topographically organized efferent connections. The limbic system has often been included with the non-specific reticular activating system, because of its multisensory afferent supply and its projections to the brain stem reticular system. Corticofugal projections to thalamic or brain stem reticular systems have also been considered "non-specific".

There can be no doubt, it seems to me, that the broad conceptual framework of the non-specific reticular system, including the so-called intralaminar system of the thalamus, has directed our attention toward important new principles in the search for anatomical and neurophysiological substrata for the central integrative action of the brain as a whole. However, with more refined histochemical, anatomical, and microphysiological studies it should be possible now, and in the near future, to describe the various parts of this heterogeneous interneuronal network in more precise terms and to attribute to them more "specific" integrative or regulatory functions.

To return to the subject of this symposium, and in particular the communications presented in this session, they have served to give us some more precise information with regard to thalamo-cortical, corticothalamic, and intrathalamic relationships. Dr. Petras has shown important projections of frontal cortex to mesial portions of the intralaminar thalamus, but no apparent projections from parietal cortex to the intralaminar thalamus. Parietal cortex appears to project only to dorsal thalamus, in the Lateralis Posterior Pulvinar complex. Motor cortex appears to send some fine fibers to Centre Medianum and intralaminar thalamus, but mostly it seems to project to substantia nigra, subthalamus and red nucleus. Ventralis Anterior appears to receive no corticofugal projections, and likewise for the medial portion of Ventralis Lateralis (VLM). Ventralis Lateralis Oralis appears to receive converging afferents from many sources, including the motor cortex. A similarly large degree of convergence is apparent in the lateral wings of the intralaminar system, Centralis Lateralis, including projections from motor and frontal cortex, but not parietal.

I was particularly impressed by the large areas of thalamus which apparently do not receive corticothalamic projections from Dr. Petras' studies. It is obvious that thalamocortical projections are highly organized with respect to their selective cortical origin and to specific parts of the thalamus, including areas of convergence. These areas of convergence may also subserve relatively specific integrative functions, as for example in VLO for the integration of coordinated motor activities.

Dr. Purpura has presented a most interesting summary of his extensive studies of intrathalamic and thalamo-cortico-thalamic interrelationships at the unitary level. Particularly valuable are his intracellular microelectrode studies showing a strong reciprocal synaptic interaction between cells of n. Ventralis Lateralis and cells of the mesial thalamus belonging to the recruiting system. However, the nature of synaptic organization is not the same in both directions, since the latency, duration, and pattern of synaptic potentials in mesial thalamic cells in response to VL stimulation is different (and stronger) than the E—I sequences of VL cells in response to mesial thalamic stimulation.

Corticofugal fibers converge with direct VL fibers in the control of excitatory and inhibitory synaptic potentials in mesial thalamic cells. The mesial thalamic system then provides widely distributed modulating, gaiting, or timing (synchronizing) effects upon many forebrain structures, including cerebral cortex as well as intrathalamic and extrathalamic structures. In this process, long lasting inhibitory post-synaptic potentials play a leading role but Purpura believes that they are not due to axon collateral inhibition, in most instances, but rather to a more direct "feed forward" inhibition in which convergence in common interneuronal pools may be important. The relative lack of axo-somatic synapses from anatomical studies would suggest that these synaptic events occur largely on dendrites, and that dendro-dendritic synaptic contacts may be important at the thalamic level.

Purpura was unable to find similar relationships to exist between "mesial thalamus" and cells of the ventrobasal nuclear complex, and for those of the Lateral Geniculate projecting to visual cortex. This may be due to failure to appreciate the fine structure and topographic organization of the thalamic recruiting system itself. It has long been known from physiological studies, and more recently from anatomical evidence as well, that different parts of the intralaminar recruiting system project primarily to different areas of cortex, and that the mesial portions project forward to frontal and motor areas, the lateral portions (such as the lateral wings of CL) project to more posterior cortical areas, including parietal and visual cortex.

It may be that sensory relay nuclei, such as VB and LG do have different relationships with the recruiting system than does VL, but this will have to be studied with more attention to the topographical organization of the thalamic recruiting system itself. Corticothalamic projections to sensory relay nuclei may be also of a different character, as judged by other studies presented at this symposium, especially with regard to corticofugal projections to the Lateral Geniculate Body.

Dr. Steriade has presented rather convincing evidence for the importance of corticofugal projections from the motor area in the cat to the n. Ventralis Lateralis and also to n. Reticularis of the thalamus with particular reference to mechanisms underlying rhythmic repetitive discharge, spindle waves and after-discharge, and as affected by states of slow wave synchronized sleep or "desynchronized" arousal. He has shown that in animals without barbiturate general anaesthesia indirectly activated orthodromic projections from the cruciate sulcus to VL induce long lasting periods of inhibition with repetitive "spindle" like bursts in VL relay cells which differed in important respects from the apparently collateral inhibition which followed excitation of the same cells by stimulation of the red nucleus. Other cells were encountered, presumable interneurones, which were activated to short latency rapid repetitive discharge by a corticothalamic volley, firing during the period of silence or inhibition of the relay cells. Excitatory corticothalamic projections on VL cells were also found to converge, in some instances, with excitatory effects arriving over the cerebellothalamic pathway. It would appear that corticofugal impulses play an important role in the control of the pattern of repetitive discharge, "spindle waves", and synaptic transmission through the VL nucleus, inhibitory effects via interneurones being the most prominent effect. However, one cannot conclude that corticofugal projections are necessary for rhythmic unit bursts and spindle like waves in VL since they may be even more prominent after decortication, as was pointed out by Lamarre in the discussion. It should also be pointed out that there are several forms and mechanisms underlying "spindle like waves" in cortex or thalamus with rhythmically repeated burst discharge in cortical or thalamic cells. Different degrees of control may arise from different potential pacemaker systems (mesial thalamus, striatal, reticular, or cortical) depending upon the physiological state of the animal (sleep or waking and arousal) and upon the intensity of activity in a given system.

Dr. Fessard has described evidence for a well organized modality specific corticofugal projection system to sensory relay nuclei of the thalamus as well as to portions of the intralaminar system (CM and CL). Slow wave sleep as compared to fast wave or paradoxical sleep serve to differentiate synaptic mechanisms of cortical projections to VPL as compared to CM; having opposite effects. This differential reciprocal relationship to states of sleep is abolished with cortical sensory ablation which causes a marked increase in evoked responses in CM to sensory stimulation. She concludes that these effects are most probably of a presynaptic character. Stimulation of orbital frontal cortex produced inhibitory effects in units at the mesencephalic and spinal levels which were also considered to be presynaptic in nature. It would appear, therefore, that both pre- and postsynaptic inhibitory mechanisms may be involved in the important and well organized control exerted by corticofugal projection systems to sensory relay nuclei, as well as to intralaminar regions of the thalamus.

Corticothalamic Projections and Sensorimotor Activities
T. Frigyesi, E. Rinvik, and M.D. Yahr, editors. © 1972
Raven Press, New York.

Neurophysiological Evidence of Vestibular Projections to Thalamus, Basal Ganglia, and Cerebral Cortex

Paula Copack, Nachum Dafny and Sid Gilman

A series of behavioral, anatomical and physiological investigations initiated in the early parts of this century has suggested that activity generated in vestibular receptors ascends to the thalamus, basal ganglia, and cerebral cortex, and there exerts an important influence on postural and equilibratory functions. However, there is little known about the precise conduction pathways, the extent to which vestibular activity engages these structures, and the degree to which activity initiated in other neural structures interacts with and thereby modifies ascending vestibular responses.

Muskens (40) was among the first to point out the importance of vestibular activity ascending to the basal ganglia. He proposed the important concept that the globus pallidus is a vestibular "end-station" from the finding that circling behavior resulted from lesions along the neuraxis extending from the vestibular nucleus to the globus pallidus (41). Several years later, Bergouignan and Verger (3) reported that natural vestibular stimulation could alter the motor responses induced by basal ganglia lesions. Circling movements to the side of unilateral caudate nucleus lesions in dogs were accentuated by rotation to the side of the lesion and stopped by rotation to the opposite side. Subsequently, Mettler and Mettler (36) found that removal of the heads of the caudate nuclei bilaterally in cats reduced the duration of the behavioral effects of labyrinthine stimulation by rotation. In addition, abnormalities of posture and gait produced by labyrinthectomy were abolished by ablation of the heads of the caudate nuclei bilaterally.

Recent behavioral studies have reopened the problem of vestibular effects on postural and movement disorders in animals and humans with lesions in the basal ganglia. Studies on the effects of lesions in the globus pallidus of monkeys led Denny-Brown (13) to the conclusion that the thalamo-striate and thalamo-pallidal fibers are essential for the integrity of the vestibular righting reflexes. Although, as pointed out by Magnus (32), some tonic vestibular effects appear after high midbrain section, Denny-Brown (13) concluded that vestibular responses interact with cutaneous reflexes at the level of the basal ganglia and that interference with these interactions by basal ganglia lesions lead to characteristic postural abnormalities. Richter (46) had previously reported similar postural abnormalities in monkeys with symmetrical necrosis of the globus pallidus resulting from exposure to carbon disulfide gas. Martin (33, 34) carried the analysis of vestibular effects on basal ganglia to the level of the human by devising methods of testing a series of tilting reactions which depend chiefly upon vestibular function. The reactions were lost in patients with diseases of basal ganglia in association with the loss of other postural reflexes leading to the conclusion that the tilting reactions depend physiologically on these nuclei.

Anatomical studies of the projection of vestibular fibers to the upper brainstem have shown consistent findings, but there have been conflicting reports concerning the extension of vestibular fibers to thalamus and basal ganglia (5, 6, 7). Ascending fibers originating in the vestibular nuclei traverse the medial longitudinal fasciculus, terminating in or providing collaterals to the abducens, trochlear, and oculomotor nuclei (8, 17, 21, 29, 40, 45). In addition some fibers continue rostrally beyond the oculomotor nuclei, ending in the interstitial nuclei of Cajal, the nuclei of Darkschewitsch, and the nuclei of the posterior commissure (6, 10, 15, 45, 54).

However, it has not been established that ascending vestibular fibers project to regions rostral to the posterior commissure. Carpenter and Strominger (12) reported finding vestibulothalamic fibers ascending in the medial longitudinal fasciculus which terminate in the ventral posterior inferior (VPI), ventral posterior medial (VPM), parafascicular (PF), centromedian (CM), and reticular nuclei of the thalamus. In addition, Hassler (22, 23) states that a vestibulothalamic lemniscus passes through the dorsolateral tegmentum and projects to the thalamic nucleus ventralis intermedius externa. Additional older studies, such as that of Whitaker and Alexander (58), have also provided evidence that secondary vestibular fibers reach the thalamus. In contrast to these positive studies, Brodal and Pompeiano (6) could not find evidence of projections from the vestibular nuclei to the thalamus, in agreement with several previous studies (8, 15, 21, 45, 53). These findings led Brodal, Pompeiano, and Walberg (7) to conclude that the existence of a vestibulothalamic pathway must be considered unproved. In support of this conclusion, Tarlov (54) found no evidence of vestibulothalamic fibers in material studied with silver stains after extensive lesions of the vestibular nuclei. In addition, Tarlov (54) personally examined the material upon which Carpenter and Strominger (12) based their conclusions and stated that the material does not provide evidence sufficient to prove that vestibulothalamic projections exist.

There is no conclusive anatomical evidence that fibers originating in the vestibular nuclei ascend to the level of the basal ganglia, but Locke (30, 31) reported an anatomical study suggesting that the magnocellular portion of the medial geniculate body (MGB) may serve as a relay in an ascending vestibular pathway to the globus pallidus (31) and to the cortex (30). However, Tarlov (54) has criticized strongly the evidence upon which Locke (30, 31) based his conclusions.

Despite these conflicting anatomical studies, there is good evidence from neurophysiological experiments that ascending vestibular activity engages nuclei of the thalamus, basal ganglia, and cerebral cortex. Evoked potentials following stimulation of the vestibular nerve or nuclei have been recorded in the MGB (52), CM (52), ventral lateral (VL) (48), and ventral posterior lateral (VPL) (48) nuclei.

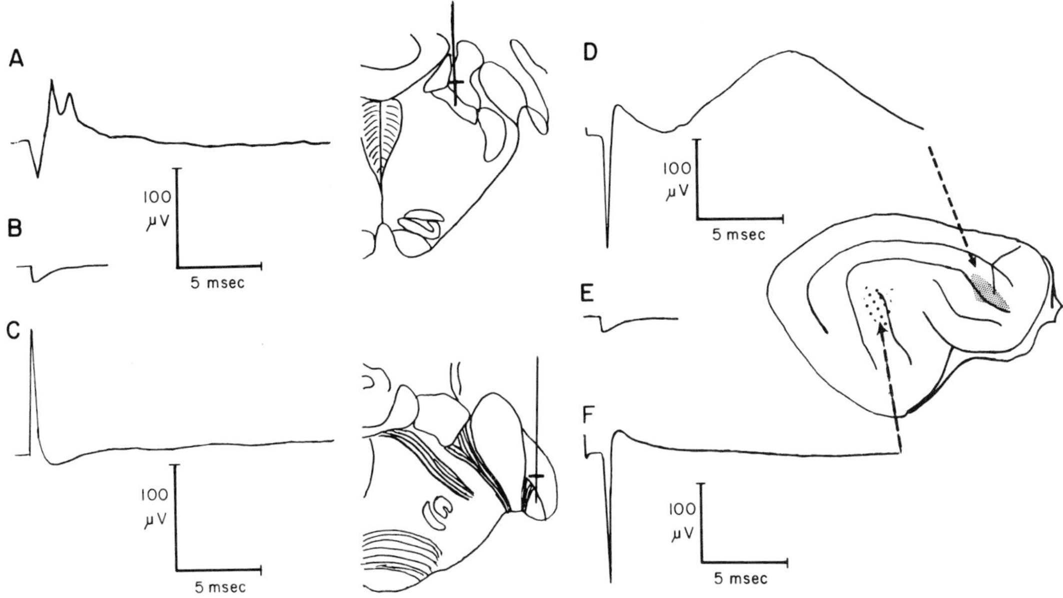

FIG. 1. Averages of 32 bipolar recordings to vestibular nerve stimulation from ipsilateral (A) lateral vestibular and (C) dorsal cochlear nuclei and monopolar recordings from the contralateral (D) cortex of the suprasylvian fold and (F) posterior ectosylvian gyrus. Stimulus artifacts in (B) and (E). In this and subsequent illustrations, upward deflection indicates positivity unless otherwise indicated.

Responses to stimulation of the vestibular nerve or nuclei have been recorded in the caudate nucleus (42, 52), putamen (52), and globus pallidus (52). Evoked responses have been recorded in cerebral cortex following stimulation of the vestibular nerve (1, 4, 16, 27, 28, 37–39, 42, 48, 55) and vestibular nuclei (35, 52).

Although these studies give ample evidence of ascending vestibular projections to higher centers, there are many contradictory findings in the reports. Thus, Gernandt (18) and later Spiegel, Szekely and Gildenberg (52) recorded vestibular responses in the MGB, but Mickle and Ades (38) localized the responses to a point somewhere between MGB and VPL, though not within either nucleus. Spiegel et al. (52) concluded that the magnocellular MGB is an important relay station for vestibular activity ascending to cortex. Recently, Sans, Raymond, and Marty (48) found vestibular responses in the VL and VPL nuclei and suggested that the VPL is an important relay station in conducting vestibular activity to cortex.

Many investigators have recorded vestibular responses from an area limited to the cortex of the anterior suprasylvian and anterior ectosylvian gyri (1, 27, 28, 37, 55). Thus, the existence of this vestibular projection area of cortex is well substantiated. Two new vestibular projection areas in cortex have been described recently but there is debate concerning their existence. Milojevic and St. Laurent (39) found projections from vestibular nerve to the posterior portion of the middle ectosylvian and

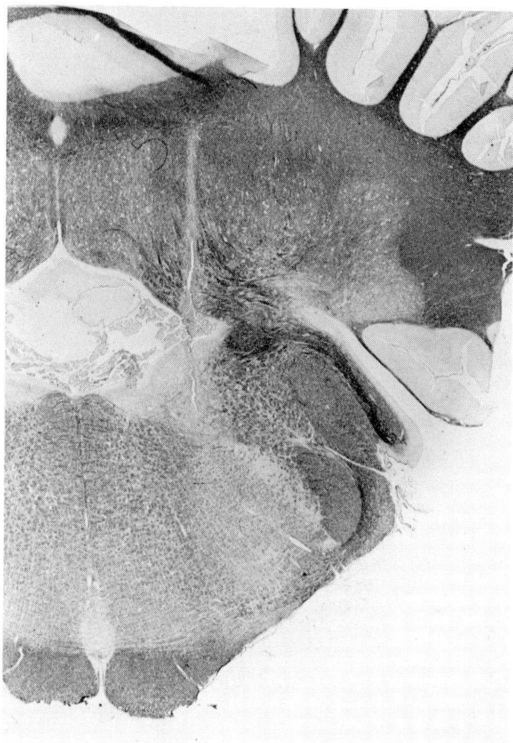

FIG. 2. Histological section showing electrode tract in the lateral vestibular nucleus. Luxol fast blue stain.

anterior portion of the posterior ectosylvian gyri. However, this region of cortex receives a strong input from the auditory system and Landgren et al. (28) suspect that the above findings may have resulted from current spread to cochlear nerve branches. Sans, Raymond, and Marty (48) described a vestibular projection to the posterior sigmoid gyrus, at the level of the postcruciate dimple. In contrast, Landgren et al. (28) specifically stated that they found no projection to this area.

Some of the discrepancies in the above studies may be attributed to the spread of current to the nearby cochlear and facial nerve branches during vestibular nerve stimulation in the bulla (28) or to nearby brainstem structures during stimulation of the vestibular nuclei. Accordingly, the present study was initiated to establish whether responses to stimulation of the vestibular nerve can be recorded in the thalamus and basal ganglia when careful measures are taken to prevent current spread to cochlear and facial fibers. In addition, the experiments were designed to 1. determine the ascending vestibular pathway in the brainstem which relays activity to the thalamus, basal ganglia and cortex,and 2. determine whether the magnocellular portion of the MGB is an essential relay for vestibular activity ascending to basal ganglia and cerebral cortex, as suggested by the anatomical studies of Locke (30, 31).

METHODS

Surgical Preparation.

The present material was obtained from experiments on 22 cats anesthetized with Surital (sodium thiamylal) 15-20 mg intravenously. Doses of 2.5-5.0 mg were administered periodically when dilatation of the pupils indicated that additional anesthesia was required. A tracheal canula was inserted, the preparations were paralyzed with gallamine triethiodide (Flaxedil), and respirations were maintained with a pump. The body temperature, measured rectally, was maintained at 37-38°C. Blood pressure, monitored through a catheter in the femoral artery, was held above 100 mm Hg by an intravenous drip of Dextran (dextran 75) when needed.

Vestibular and cochlear nerve exposure and stimulation.

The vestibular branches of the eighth nerve were exposed in the left bulla according to the technique of Andersson and Gernandt (1). The ipsilateral cochlear branch was exposed near the apex of the cochlea, as described by Landgren, Silfvenius, and Wolsk (28). The stimulating electrode consisted of a semi-micro (100μ) stainless steel bipolar electrode (David Kopf) or twisted strands of enameled silver wire (50μ) chlorided at the tips, both with a tip separation of 0.25-0.5 mm. The electrode was lowered with a micromanipulator until it touched the vestibular nerve near the junction of the branches from the superior and lateral canals and the utricle. An identical electrode was placed on the cochlear branch and both electrodes were fixed to the cut edge of the bulla with dental cement, then the bulla was filled with petroleum jelly to form an insulated chamber. The nerves were stimulated with single rectangular pulses of 0.1 msec duration through a photon-coupled stimulus isolation unit at a frequency of 0.33 Hz. A bipolar concentric insulated steel recording electrode of 0.5 mm diameter was positioned stereotaxically, then lowered in steps of 0.5 mm, beginning 2 mm dorsal to the calculated center of the lateral vestibular nucleus, using the atlas of Snider and Niemer (50). When an optimum response to vestibular nerve stimulation was recorded from the vestibular nucleus, the electrode was fixed in position. A similar procedure was followed in positioning another recording electrode in the dorsal or ventral cochlear nucleus while stimulating the cochlear nerve.

Prevention of current spread.

To prevent current spread from vestibular to cochlear nerves in the bulla, the voltage and polarity of the vestibular stimulus were adjusted to give a response in the vestibular nucleus without evoking a response in the cochlear nucleus. In some experiments, after it had been ascertained that current spread in the bulla could be monitored satisfactorily by cortical recordings, the optimal stimulation parameters were determined by recording with cotton wick electrodes from the contralateral (right) vestibular (the cortex of the anterior suprasylvian fold) and auditory (the cortex of the posterior and middle ectosylvian gyri) projection areas. In these experiments the parameters of the vestibular nerve stimulus were adjusted to evoke a maximal response in the vestibular projection area with no response in the auditory area. In addition, the animals were permitted to emerge periodically from the gallamine induced paralysis, the face was examined for twitching in response to vestibular nerve stimulation, and none was found, indicating that current spread to facial nerve had not occurred. At the termination of 2 experiments, the responses to vestibular nerve stimulation recorded from the contralateral MGB and the cortex of the suprasylvian fold were abolished by intracranial section of the eighth nerve, thus excluding the possibility that the responses resulted from current spread from the bulla diffusely into the brainstem. Thus, in the conditions of the present experiments spread of stimulating current to nerve fibers other than the vestibular or into the brainstem did not occur.

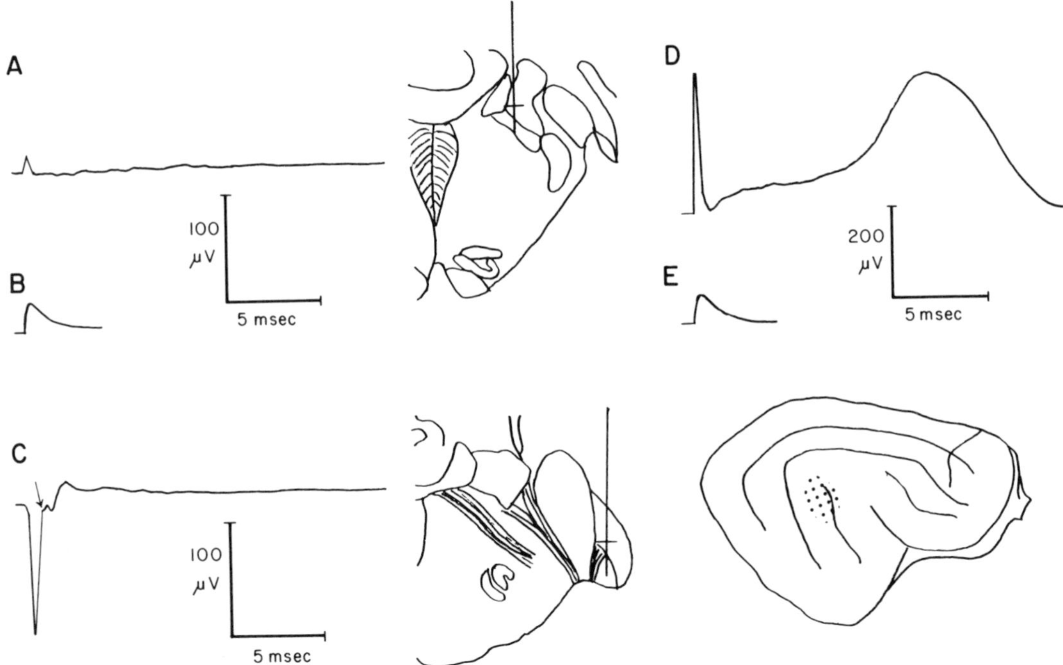

FIG. 3. Averages of bipolar recordings to cochlear nerve stimulation from ipsilateral (A) lateral vestibular and (C) dorsal cochlear nuclei and monopolar recordings from (D) contralateral posterior ectosylvian gyrus. Stimulus artifacts in (B) and (E).

Subcortical recordings.

Either a single concentric bipolar insulated steel electrode of 0.5 mm diameter or an array of 2-4 of these electrodes was lowered stereotaxically into various parts of the thalamus and basal ganglia. Stereotaxic coordinates were obtained from the atlas of Jasper and Ajmone-Marsan (26). Recordings were begun 2 mm dorsal to the calculated center point and continued at 0.5 or 1.0 mm intervals through the depth of the structure under investigation. Monopolar recordings were made using both inner and outer poles as the active electrode, with a steel needle in the temporalis muscle serving as the indifferent electrode. Bipolar recordings were made between the inner and outer poles.

In experiments designed to study interactions between responses to vestibular and cortical stimulation in medial geniculate body, the vestibular projection area of cortex was mapped initially using the vestibular nerve stimulation parameters described above. Then a bipolar concentric insulated stainless steel electrode of 0.5 mm diameter was inserted into the cortex at the site of the maximal vestibular response. Rectangular pulses of 0.1 msec duration were applied between the two poles of this electrode and the stimulating voltage was increased until a response was recorded with an electrode positioned in the MGB. Then interactions between the responses evoked by vestibular nerve stimulation and cortical stimulation in MGB were studied.

Responses were amplified, monitored on an oscilloscope, and stored on tape. A Fabritek Model 1072 Multichannel Signal Averaging Computer was used to average the responses which were plotted by an x-y recorder. 256 addresses were used with bin widths of 40, 80, 160, 800 or 1600 μsec, depending upon the recording situation, and 32, 50 or 64 responses were summated algebraically ("averaged"). At the termination of most experiments, electrocoagulation was used to mark the sites in which maximum amplitude responses were recorded. The preparation was sacrificed with intravenous Surital and then perfused intracardially with normal saline followed by 10% formalin. The brain was removed, stored in 10% formalin for several days, and cut at 40μ for frozen sections or at 10μ for paraffin sections. Alternate sections were stained with cresyl violet and luxol fast blue.

RESULTS

Responses to Vestibular and Cochlear Nerve Stimulation in Vestibular and Cochlear Nuclei.

Figure 1 (A) illustrates responses to vestibular nerve stimulation recorded bipolarly from the ipsilateral lateral vestibular nucleus. The stimulus artifact appears in (B) and recordings taken simultaneously from the ipsilateral dorsal cochlear nucleus are shown in (C). The traces in (A–C) represent the average of 32 successive recordings. The positions of the recording electrodes in the vestibular and cochlear nuclei, established from reconstructions of the histological specimens, are shown diagrammatically next to the respective recorded potentials. In the diagrams the vertical line indicates the electrode tract, the short intersecting horizontal line the site of recording. The strength of stimulation to the vestibular nerve was sufficient to evoke a response in the vestibular nucleus (A) without eliciting a response in the cochlear nucleus (C). The vestibular response in this bipolar recording consists of two positive waves with a latency to onset of 0.7 msec. Monopolar recordings taken from the lateral vestibular nucleus in several animals have shown consistently an initial positive wave with a latency to onset of 0.6–1.1 msec, followed by a negative component with a latency to onset of 1.0–1.4 msec and a second negative wave with a latency of

1.7-1.9 msec. The average of 32 responses to vestibular nerve stimulation recorded from the cortex of the suprasylvian fold is shown in (D). The area in the anterior suprasylvian and anterior ectosylvian gyri from which responses could be recorded in other experiments is shown with stippling in the diagram of cortex. As shown in (F) a response could not be recorded from the middle or posterior ectosylvian gyri when the stimulus strength to the vestibular nerve was adjusted to give a maximum response in the vestibular nucleus and no response in the cochlear nucleus. Figure 2 illustrates a histological specimen documenting the position of the recording electrode in the lateral vestibular nucleus.

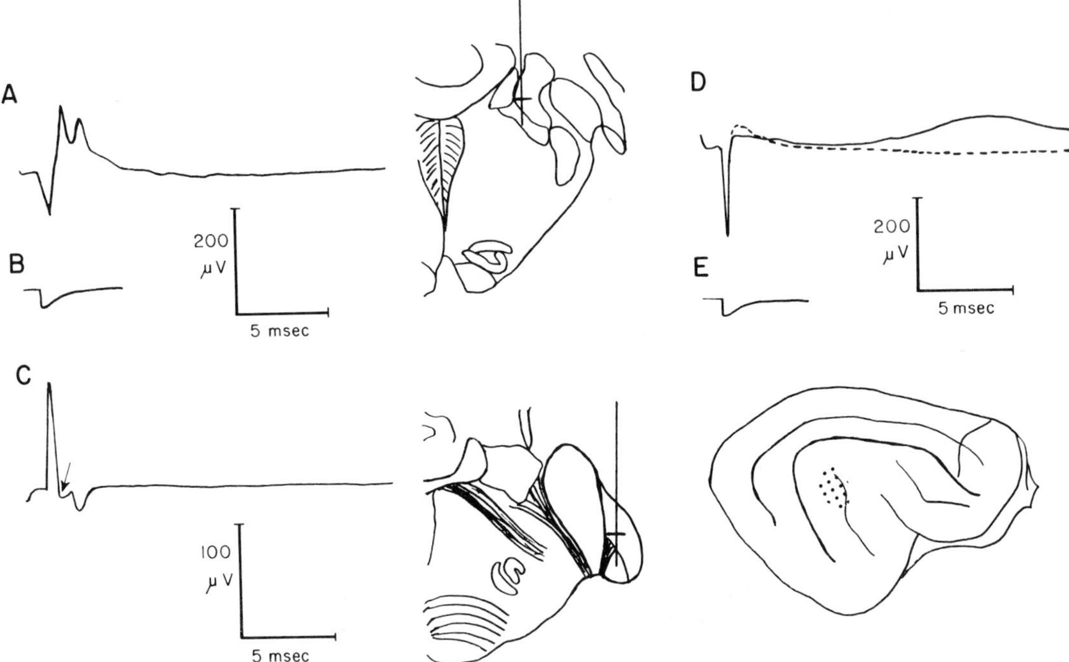

FIG. 4. Averages of bipolar recordings to vestibular nerve stimulation from ipsilateral (A) lateral vestibular and (C) dorsal cochlear nuclei and monopolar recordings from (D) contralateral posterior ectosylvian gyrus. Vestibular stimulus increased so that spread of current to cochlear branches occurs, as shown by the response in cochlear nucleus, indicated by arrow (C) and posterior ectosylvian gyrus, indicated by solid line (D). Dotted line in (D) indicates the recording from cortex when stimulus is reduced so that no response occurs in the cochlear nucleus. Stimulus artifacts in (B) and (E).

Figure 3 shows the averages of 32 responses to stimulation of the left cochlear nerve recorded bipolarly from the ipsilateral vestibular (A) and dorsal cochlear (C) nuclei. The positions of the recording electrodes are shown diagrammatically next to the respective responses. The stimulus evokes in the cochlear nucleus a response, marked by an arrow in (C), with an onset latency of 0.8 msec. Monopolar recordings of the cochlear nucleus response in several other experiments have shown the same latency to the onset of an initial positive wave. As shown in (A) of Figure 3, the intensity of the stimulus applied to the cochlear nerve is insufficient to evoke a response in the vestibular nucleus, but sufficient to evoke a response in the posterior ectosylvian gyrus (D). Thus, the appearance of a short latency response in the recording from the cochlear nucleus during stimulation of nerves in the bulla indicates that the stimulus activates cochlear nerve fibers. Consequently, during vestibular nerve stimulation in each experiment of the present series, it was necessary to reduce the stimulus voltage if a short latency response could be detected in recordings from the cochlear nucleus, since this response would indicate current spread to cochlear fibers. The data from a representative experiment in which a spread of current from vestibular to cochlear fibers was detected is shown in Figure 4. At this strength of stimulation applied to the vestibular nerve, a response could be recorded in the cochlear nucleus as shown in (C) and also in the posterior ectosylvian gyrus as shown in (D). Averaging the responses on-line has permitted the detection and prevention of even the slightest spread of current shown by the responses in (C) and (D) of Figure 4. The above techniques have provided a systematic method of controlling current spread between nerves in the bulla.

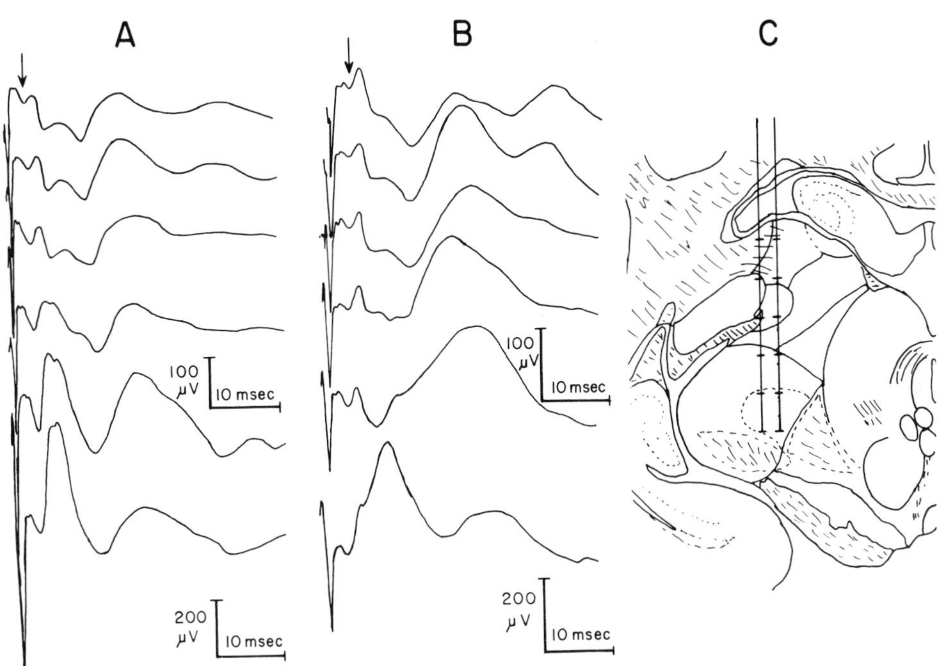

FIG. 5. Averaged responses to vestibular stimulation recorded monopolarly from six sites in contralateral thalamus with a pair of electrodes. Responses shown in (A) and (B) correspond, respectively, to the left and right electrode tracts in (C). Arrows indicate onset of responses.

Responses to vestibular nerve stimulation in cerebral cortex.

In experiments in which spread of the vestibular stimulus to cochlear nerve branches could be ruled out, an evoked response was found in a small region of cortex within 1-2 mm on either side of the vertical portion of the suprasylvian fold contralateral to the side of stimulation, as described by several previous investigators (28, 37, 42, 48, 55). The response usually consisted of a positive wave with a latency to onset ranging from 3.4 to 6.4 msec and an amplitude of 30 to 600μV (see D of Figure 1). In previous studies from this laboratory using encèphale isolé preparations, without use of averaging techniques, the latency to onset was 3-7 msec (42). The cortex of the middle and posterior ectosylvian gyri was explored carefully during vestibular stimulation and responses were found only when current had spread to cochlear fibers, as indicated by a response in the cochlear nucleus. In four animals, as the stimulus voltage applied to the vestibular nerve was gradually increased, a response appeared initially in the ipsilateral vestibular nucleus, and then, with a further increase of voltage, in the dorsal or ventral cochlear nucleus, but a response was not detected in the cortex of the suprasylvian fold. Only a further increase in stimulus strength could evoke a cortical response. It was assumed that the vestibular stimulus was spreading to the cochlear branches because of fluid accumulation in the bulla and the experiments were terminated.

Responses to vestibular nerve stimulation in thalamus.

Responses to stimulation of the left vestibular nerve were recorded from the right MGB monopolarly or bipolarly in 10 cats. In monopolar recordings, when the electrode was placed in the magnocellular portion of the nucleus, the shortest latency and largest amplitude responses were recorded. In the representative experiment shown in Figure 5, a pair of electrodes was lowered successively through the posterior thalamic nuclei and responses in both electrodes were recorded monopolarly from each of six sites as shown in (A) and (B), which correspond, respectively, to the left and right electrode tracts in (C). The electrodes were lowered successively through the pulvinar (top two traces in A and B), the lateral posterior and posterior nuclei (third traces), the parvocellular portion of the MGB (fourth traces), and the magnocellular portion of the MGB (bottom two traces). The responses recorded during the descent through the posterior nuclei consisted of an initial positive wave with a latency to onset of 3.0 msec (marked by the arrows) followed by two negative components and a later slow positive wave. Little change in configuration developed until the electrodes entered the magnocellular portion of MGB, when a large amplitude (about 500μV) initial positive wave appeared, with a latency to onset of 3.0 msec, followed by a negative component with a latency of 10 msec and then a slow positive wave with a latency of 14 msec. The bottom two traces in (B) show a reversal in polarity of the initial negative component, indicating that the electrode had passed through a current source. In other animals, monopolar recordings from the magnocellular portion of MGB revealed similar response configurations with latencies to onset as short as 2.0 msec. As shown in Table 1, the minimum latency to onset in parvocellular MGB

TABLE I

RECORDING SITE	LATENCY (msec) MONOPOLAR	BIPOLAR
Vestibular nucleus	0.6-1.1	0.7*
MGB (magnocellular)	2.0-3.0	2.0-5.0
MGB (parvocellular)	2.9-3.7	3.0-5.3
VL	---	2.3-2.5
VPL	3.4**	3.9*
Globus pallidus	3.0-3.4	5.5*
Caudate	3.2-4.0	---
Cortex (Suprasylvian fold)	3.4-6.4	---

Range of latencies to onset of averaged responses to vestibular nerve stimulation. * Data from single experiments in different animals. ** Data from two animals.

was greater than in magnocellular MGB. In addition, in most experiments in which monopolar recordings were taken from both portions of MGB, the response in the magnocellular portion had the shorter latency. When recordings were taken simultaneously from magnocellular MGB and the cortex of the suprasylvian fold, the MGB response showed a latency to onset 1.5 to 2.1 msec shorter than the cortical response.

In order to ensure that the responses recorded monopolarly in MGB were localized to this structure, bipolar recordings were also made in several animals. These recordings were taken first from the parvocellular portion and, with descent of the electrode into the magnocellular portion, the responses increased in amplitude and shortened in latency. Reversal of polarity of the response occurred during further descent through magnocellular MGB in one experiment. An example of a response recorded bipolarly from magnocellular MGB is shown in Figure 11(B). In three experiments the latencies in magnocellular MGB were 2.0, 2.3, and 5.0 msec whereas the corresponding latencies in parvocellular MGB were 3.7, 3.0, and 5.3 msec. Thus, in bipolar as well as in monopolar recordings, shorter latency responses were recorded in magnocellular MGB.

Responses to vestibular stimulation were also recorded from the ventral lateral (VL) nucleus. During descent of the electrode through the ventral anterior (VA) nucleus, a response could not be detected. Upon entry into the VL, a response of 2.3 msec latency appeared and showed a reversal of polarity with further electrode descent. Responses to vestibular stimulation were also recorded from ventral posterior lateral (VPL) nucleus, both monopolarly and bipolarly. The responses recorded monopolarly consisted of an initial positive wave with a latency to onset of 3.4 msec followed by two negative components and a positive wave. Potentials recorded bipolarly from VPL are shown in Figure 6. No response is evident in (A). In (B) a response with a latency to onset of 3.9 msec occurs. The response reverses in polarity in (C)

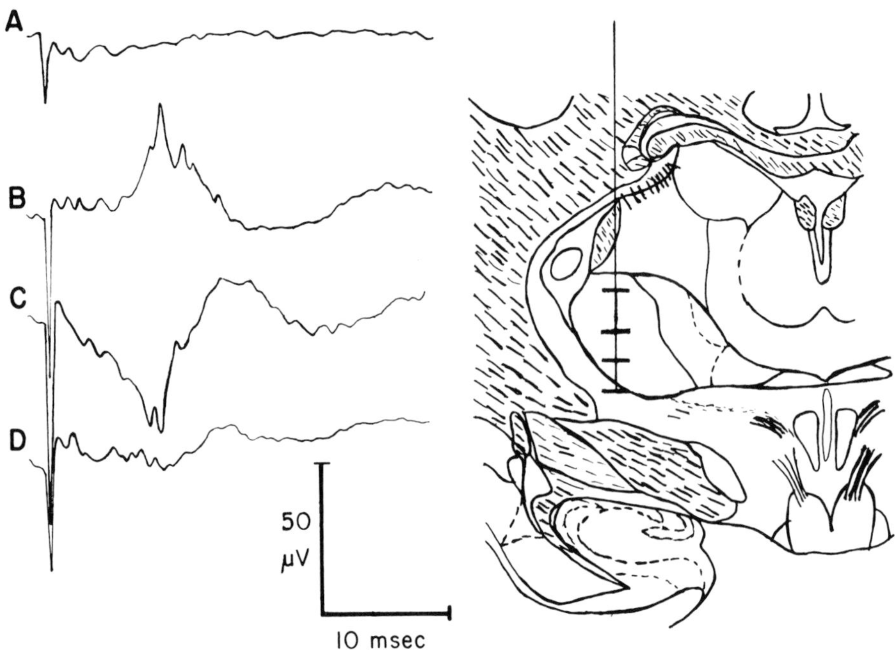

FIG. 6. Averaged responses to vestibular stimulation recorded bipolarly from contralateral VPL nucleus.

and no response can be detected with certainty in (D).

Responses to vestibular nerve stimulation in basal ganglia.

1. Caudate nucleus. In previous experiments (42), responses to vestibular nerve stimulation were recorded bipolarly with macroelectrodes in locally anesthetized encèphale isolé preparations. Response characteristics were evaluated from recordings of single oscilloscope traces. Responses to unilateral vestibular or cochlear nerve stimulation were recorded in the heads of the caudate nuclei bilaterally. The responses showed a minimum latency of 4 msec, and in individual experiments no latency difference was found between responses recorded from comparable regions of contralateral and ipsilateral caudate. In order to determine the locus of generation of these potentials, reversals in polarity of the evoked potentials were noted as the recording electrode was lowered through the caudate (Figure 7). Most of the reversal points on the contralateral side were confined to the lateral one-third of the caudate; the ipsilateral points were all found on the dorsal border of the caudate. Over all experiments, responses to vestibular stimulation were concentrated in the dorsolateral portion of the contralateral caudate and the dorsomedial portion of the ipsilateral caudate (Figure 8). These responses were usually found in areas also responding to stimulation of the ipsilateral cochlear nerve or to click stimuli applied to the intact

(right) ear. At some sites in the caudate, vestibular responses were opposite in polarity to cochlear responses. Furthermore, in several cats sites were found in the caudate from which responses could be evoked to vestibular but not to auditory (cochlear or click) stimulation. One of these areas and the responses recorded from it are shown in Figure 7. Thus, vestibular and cochlear responses show specific topographic localizations in caudate nucleus.

In the present experiments, using Surital anesthesia and response averaging techniques, responses to vestibular stimulation were recorded from caudate nucleus with a minimum latency of 3.2 msec, though in most recordings the latencies have been 3.4-4.0 msec. The responses recorded monopolarly consisted of an initial positive wave followed by a negative component and then a late positive wave.

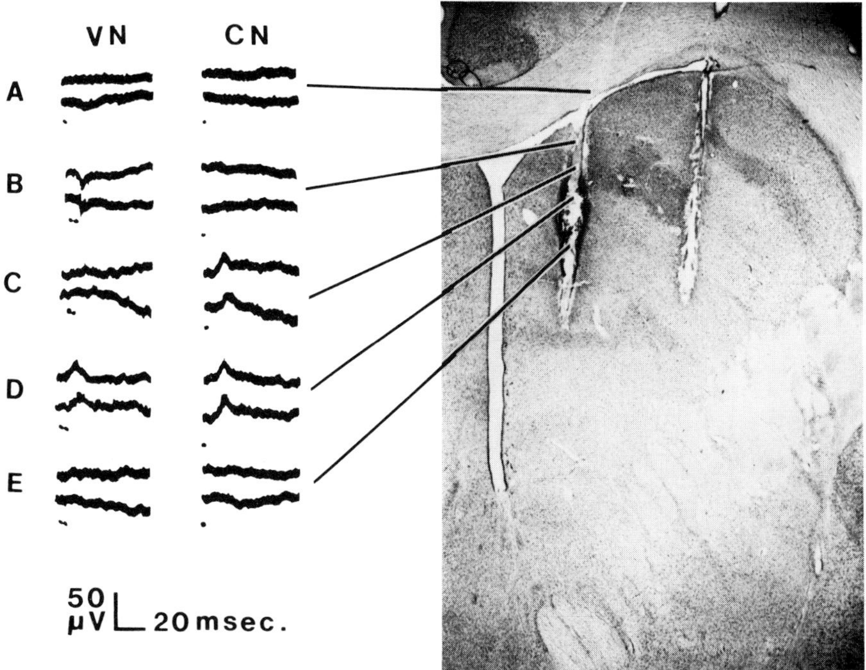

FIG. 7. Single bipolar recordings from caudate nucleus showing responses to vestibular nerve (VN) and cochlear nerve (CN) stimulation. The histological section shows the region of the medial portion of the ipsilateral caudate nucleus from which recordings (A-E) were taken. Downward deflection indicates positivity. Reproduced by courtesy of the Editor of Experimental Neurology. Copyright held by Academic Press.

2. Globus pallidus. Responses to vestibular nerve stimulation were recorded from the globus pallidus both monopolarly and bipolarly. The responses recorded monopolarly showed a latency to onset of 3.0-3.4 msec. Figure 9 shows monopolarly recorded potentials in the globus pallidus of one of these animals and Figure 10 veri-

fies histologically the recording site. The bipolar recordings showed a latency to onset of 5.5 msec and confirmed that the response was localized to the globus pallidus.

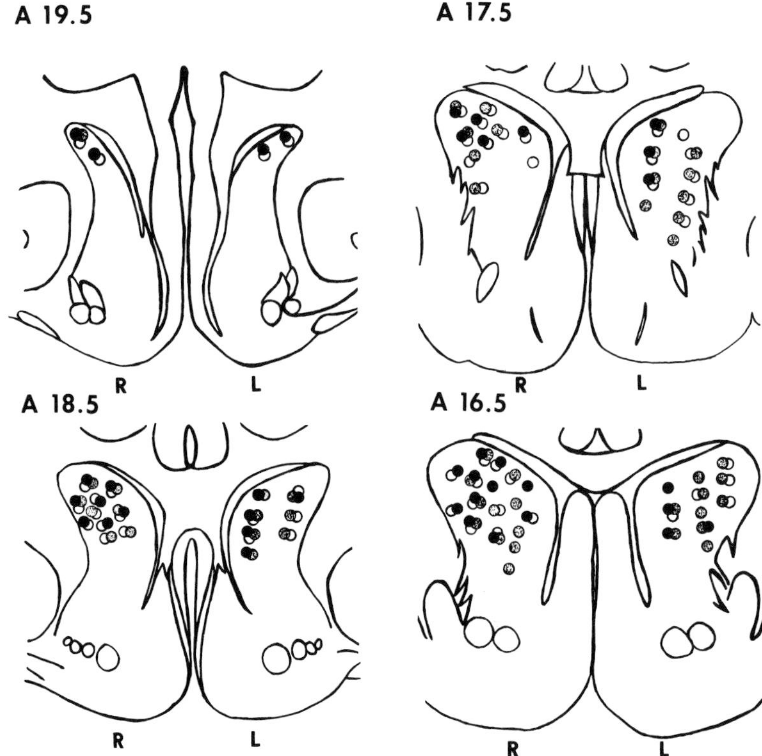

FIG. 8. Distribution of responses in ipsilateral and contralateral caudate nuclei to stimulation of left vestibular nerve (filled circles), left cochlear nerve (dotted circles) and clicks to the right ear (open circles). Data compiled from nine experiments. Numbers correspond to stereotaxic planes in the Snider and Niemer Atlas (50). R signifies the right hemisphere, L the left. Reproduced by courtesy of the Editor of Experimental Neurology. Copyright held by Academic Press.

Vestibular ascending pathways to thalamus and basal ganglia.

Three sets of experiments were carried out to study the effects of lesions in cerebellum and brainstem on the responses to vestibular nerve stimulation recorded contralaterally in the magnocellular portion of MGB and the cortex of the suprasylvian fold. In the first of these experiments, complete removal of the cerebellum by subpial aspiration had no effect on the responses. As a next step in the same experiment, the medial longitudinal fasciculus (MLF) was completely transected rostral to the superior vestibular nuclei at approximately the level of the mid-portion of the inferior colliculus. This procedure also did not alter the response. The lesion, subsequently verified histologically, extended 2 mm laterally and ventrally into the dorsal tegmentum on each side of the midline. As a final procedure in the same experiment, the eighth nerve on the side of vestibular nerve stimulation was transected intracranially, and both the thalamic and the cortical responses were abolished. In a second set of experiments, after removal of the cerebellum and transection of the MLF, the MLF lesion was extended 1 mm laterally on both sides of the brainstem. This procedure did not alter the responses although the section extended sufficiently far laterally to transect the vestibulothalamic tract described by Hassler in the dorsolateral tegmentum. As a final procedure the eighth nerve was sectioned, which again completely abolished the responses. Results from the third set of experiments are shown in Figure 11. In (A) and (B) are depicted the control responses recorded from cortex and magnocellular MGB, respectively. The responses persisted following complete cerebellectomy (C, D) and transection of the MLF (E, F). The MLF lesion extended 2 mm lateral to the midline bilaterally. Further extension of the lesion an additional 2 mm laterally on each side resulted in a severe decrease in amplitude of both the cortical (G) and magnocellular MGB (H) responses. This lesion included the dorsolateral tegmentum and the most medial portion of the lateral lemniscus. Extension of the lesion completely through the lateral lemniscus bilaterally resulted in complete loss of both responses (I, J). These findings suggest that either the medial portion of the lateral lemniscus or some other pathway just medial to the lemniscus in the dorsolateral tegmentum conveys vestibular activity to MGB and cortex.

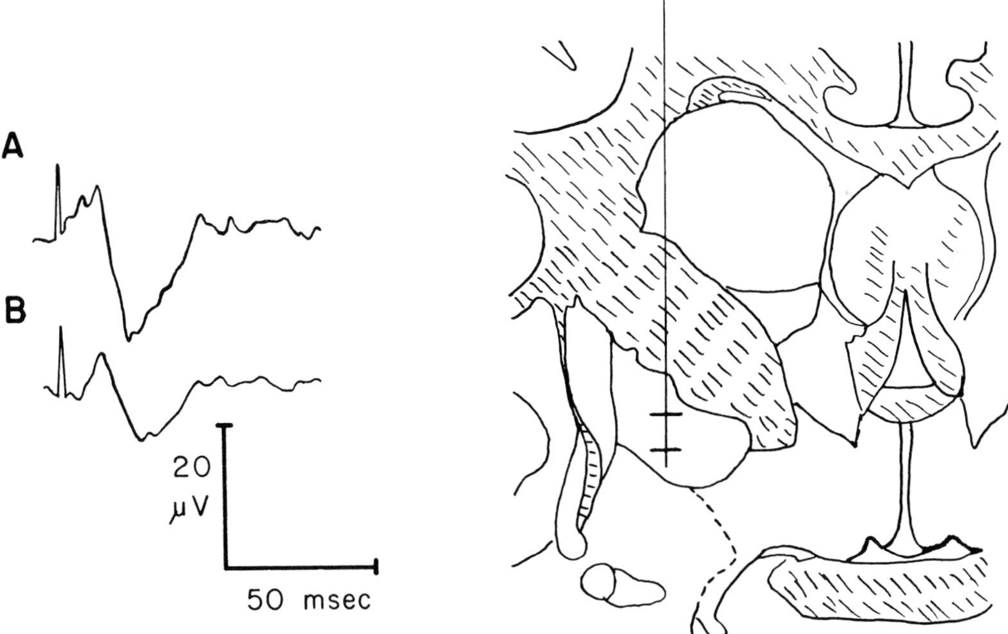

FIG. 9. Averaged responses to vestibular stimulation recorded monopolarly from contralateral globus pallidus.

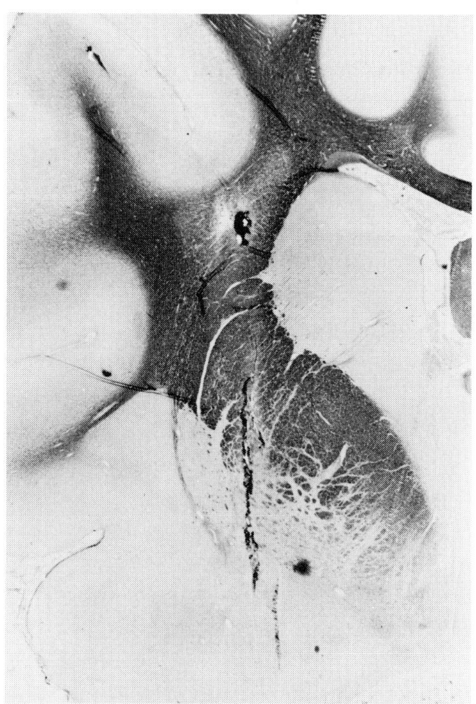

FIG. 10. Histological section showing electrode trajectory in the globus pallidus. Luxol fast blue stain.

In a study reported previously (42), it was found that large but incomplete bilateral lesions of the magnocellular portion of the MGB depressed the amplitude of cortical and caudate responses to vestibular and cochlear nerve stimulation by an average of 80%. Examples of the effects on the evoked responses in an encèphale isolé

FIG. 11. Averaged responses to vestibular stimulation recorded monopolarly from cortex of suprasylvian fold (left row) and bipolarly from magnocellular MGB (right row). (A,B) control; (C,D) after cerebellectomy; (E,F) after section of MLF; (G,H) after extension of MLF lesion in dorsolateral tegmentum including medial portion of lateral lemniscus (LL); (I,J) after complete section of LL.

FIG. 12. (A-C) single responses to stimulation of left vestibular nerve; (D-F) single responses to stimulation of left cochlear nerve. Recordings from cortex of suprasylvian fold (each upper trace) and right caudate (each lower trace). (A,D) control; (B,E) after lesion of magnocellular portion of MGB ipsilateral to side of recording; (C,F) after subsequent lesion of contralateral magnocellular MGB. Downward deflection indicates positivity. Reproduced by courtesy of the Editor of Experimental Neurology. Copyright held by Academic Press.

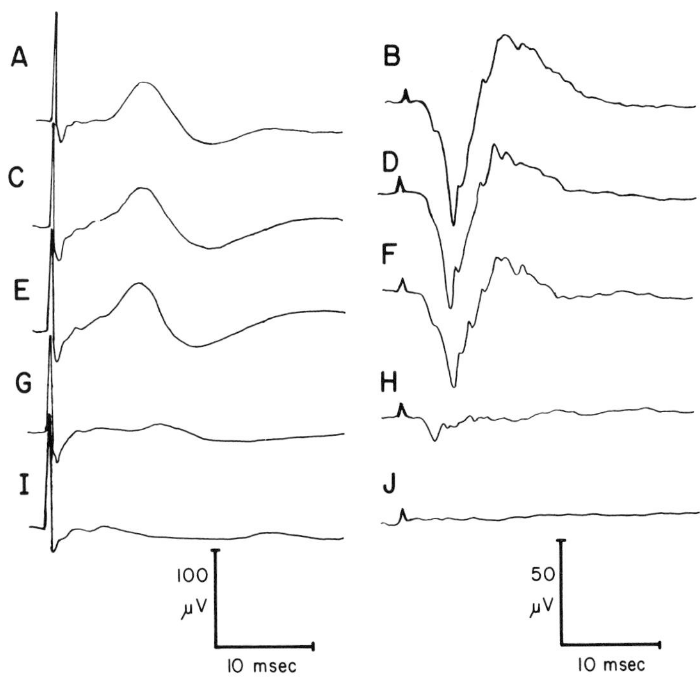

FIG. 11

EFFECT OF GENICULATE LESIONS

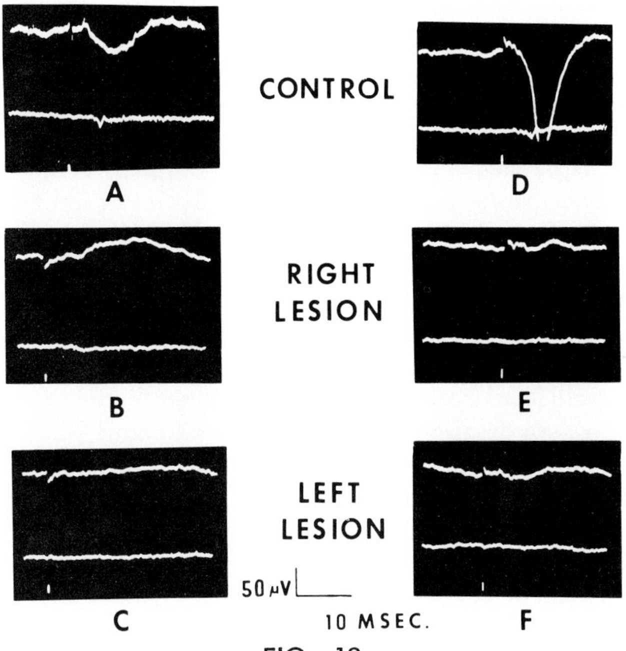

FIG. 12

preparation are shown in Figure 12, with the vestibular responses recorded from cortex (upper trace) and caudate (lower) shown in A–C, the cochlear responses in D–F. The lesions of the MGB that resulted in the abolition of these responses are shown in Figure 13. Lesions of the parvocellular portion of the MGB which included the dorsolateral one-fourth of the magnocellular MGB reduced the caudate and cortical responses by an average of 50%. Lesions of the magnocellular portion of the MGB on the side of cortical or caudate recording produced a more substantial decrease in response amplitude (about 50%) than lesions on the opposite side (about 30%).

Corticovestibular interactions in thalamus and basal ganglia.

Responses to stimulation of the vestibular projection area in the cortex of the anterior suprasylvian fold were recorded from the magnocellular and parvocellular portions of the MGB. At each site the response consisted of a positive wave with a latency to onset of about 4 msec. Interactions between the responses to cortical and vestibular stimuli were studied in recordings from the magnocellular portion of MGB. The cortical stimulus was adjusted to a just—threshold intensity for a response in the MGB, then applied preceding the vestibular stimulus at varying intervals. The amplitude variations of the second positive to second negative component of the vestibular evoked response were measured peak-to-peak. These components were selected for measurement because they were the most stable elements of the response. In Figure 14, which illustrates data from a representative experiment, each point represents the average of 32 conditioned responses expressed as a percentage of the unconditioned responses which were recorded alternately. The result was a marked depression of the vestibular evoked response at close intervals, with a delayed recovery toward control amplitude at wide intervals.

DISCUSSION

The present experiments provide electrophysiological evidence that vestibular activity generated peripherally ascends to several nuclei of the thalamus and basal ganglia as well as to a restricted region of the cerebral cortex. The evidence is based upon monopolar and bipolar recordings using strict control of current spread from vestibular to cochlear nerves by monitoring from the vestibular and cochlear nuclei. By adjusting vestibular nerve stimulus strength to a level sufficient to provide a response in the vestibular but not in the cochlear nucleus, it has been possible to confirm the existence of the small focal cortical projection around the suprasylvian fold in the contralateral hemisphere described by previous investigators (28, 37, 48, 55). However, we did not find responses in the region of the middle ectosylvian gyrus as described by Milojevic and St. Laurent (39), leading to the conclusion that their findings are attributable to current spread from vestibular to cochlear fibers in the bulla. Indeed, it was possible in the present experiments to record a response in the region they described only when responses appeared in the cochlear nucleus during increasing strength of vestibular stimulation. In the present studies, the cortex of the pericruciate sulcus was not explored for vestibular responses. However, Sans,Raymond and Marty

(48) found vestibular responses in cortex of the postcruciate depression observing precautions to prevent current spread similar to those used in the present experiments. In addition, Boisacq-Schepens and Hanus (4) have reported evidence from microelectrode recordings of vestibular responses from single cells in the postcruciate dimple, some of which have been identified as pyramidal tract neurons.

The recordings from the vestibular and cochlear nuclei in the present experiments were taken for the purpose of detecting and preventing current spread; consequently the components of the responses were not analyzed with high-frequency stimulation or pharmacological agents. The bipolar recordings exhibited a sharp localization. The responses recorded monopolarly showed latencies and configurations similar to those described by Precht and Shimazu (43) who recorded focal potentials with microelectrodes in vestibular nuclei to ipsilateral vestibular nerve stimulation. In their studies the responses also consisted of an early positive wave (P), with a latency to onset of 0.6-0.14 msec, a large sharp negative wave (N_1) and a delayed negative component (N_2).

As pointed out above, there is conflicting anatomical evidence concerning the existence of secondary vestibular fibers projecting directly to the thalamus. In addition, the extensive projections to cerebellum of both primary and secondary vestibular fibers (7, 11) raise the possibility that vestibular activity may reach the MGB (11) of the thalamus by means of a circuit through the cerebellum. Price and Spiegel (44) have previously reported that changes in the electrocorticogram (increase of the amplitude of the fast oscillations and abolition of the slow waves) induced by rotational vestibular stimuli persisted after cerebellar ablation combined with section of the MLF in the pons. Several other investigators, using similar techniques, have also concluded that vestibular responses in cortex persist after section of the MLF (2, 19, 20, 51). Price and Spiegel suggested that ascending vestibular activity may be mediated by vestibulo-reticulo-thalamic fibers, such as the bundle of Held (25) or by the ascending cochlear system. Evidence in favor of the latter possibility was provided by Gerebtzoff (19, 20), who found that section of the lateral lemnisci or the brachia of the inferior colliculi abolished the electrical activity of the cerebral cortex responsive to labyrinthine stimulation. However, the regions of cortex responsive to vestibular stimuli reported by these investigators do not correspond to the areas currently considered to represent the cortical vestibular projection areas. In addition, the previous investigators did not explore the effects of the lesions on vestibular responses in subcortical nuclei. Consequently, it was of interest in the present experiments to find no alteration of vestibular evoked responses in MGB, or cerebral cortex following complete ablation of the cerebellum and subsequent section of the MLF in the mesencephalon, confirming the prior investigations cited above. In addition, the present investigation supports Gerebtzoff's (19, 20) conclusion, since lesions in the medial portion of the lateral lemniscus or just medial to this tract severely decreased the vestibular responses in MGB and cortex following cerebellar ablation and section of the MLF. A complete loss of the responses in cortex and MGB when the cut is extended out laterally to completely sever the lateral lemniscus further supports this conclusion. These findings are in accord with the general conclusion of Mickel and Ades (38) that the pathway utilized by vestibular impulses to cortex follows closely the central auditory pathway. In the present experiments no evidence was provided implicating in the transmission of ascending vestibular activity the pathway described by Hassler (22, 23) in the dorsolateral tegmentum, since lesions at the presumed site of this tract bilaterally did not alter the responses in MGB or cortex. More rostrally, this tract is found in the region of Forel's Haubenfaszikel (22, 23). In the experiments of Spiegel, Szekely, and Gildenberg (52) lesions of MLF and of Forel's tract also failed to abolish the responses in cortex and caudate nucleus to stimulation of the vestibular nuclei. It should be emphasized that the present experiments do not rule out the possibility that ascending vestibular activity may also be transmitted by reticulo-thalamic connections.

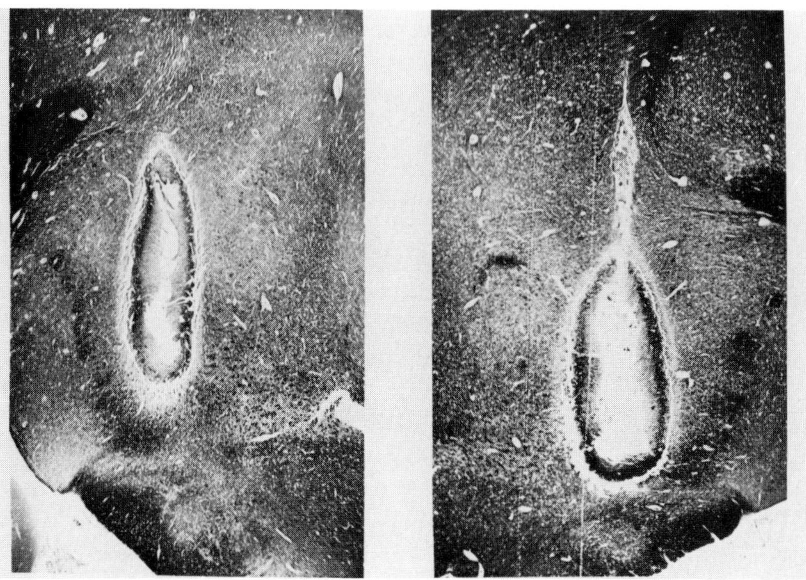

FIG. 13. Coronal sections through centers of lesions in MGB from experiment in Figure 12, ipsilateral (left photograph) and contralateral (right) to the side of the recording. Lesions include a large part of the magnocellular and encroach slightly on the parvocellular portion of MGB. Luxol fast blue stain. Reproduced by courtesy of the Editor of Experimental Neurology. Copyright held by Academic Press.

Evidence was provided in the present study that vestibular activity projects to several thalamic nuclei, including MGB, VL, and VPL, since responses were recorded in these nuclei using both monopolar and bipolar techniques. During descent of the recording electrodes through these nuclei, alteration of wave form in monopolar recordings and reversal of potentials in bipolar recordings provided evidence that the responses were picked up from these nuclei. In addition, Sans, Raymond and Marty (48) recorded vestibular responses in VL and VPL using microelectrode recordings and precautions to prevent current spread from vestibular to cochlear fibers. The present experiments supply evidence suggesting that vestibular activity projects to some of the posterior thalamic nuclei, such as pulvinar and lateral posterior nucleus, but systematic study of the responses in these regions was not attempted.

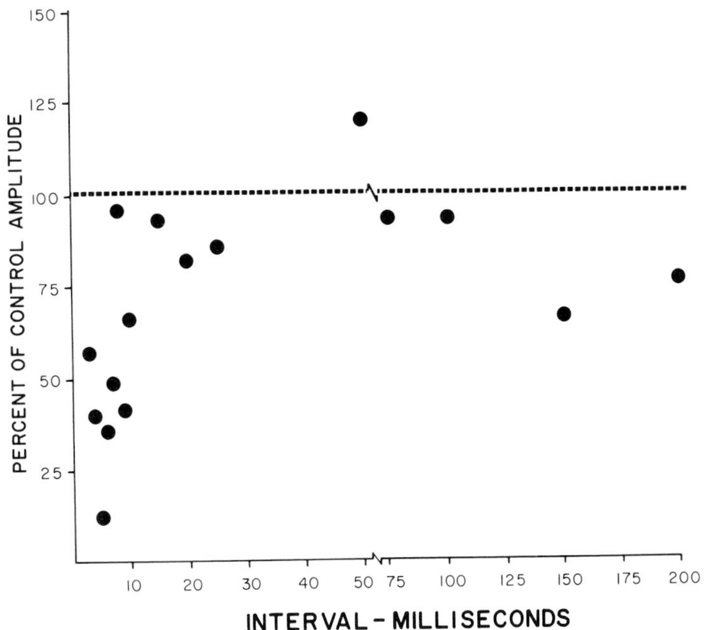

FIG. 14. Interactions between responses to stimulation of vestibular projection area of cortex and vestibular nerve recorded from magnocellular MGB. Each point represents the amplitude of the averaged vestibular test response, expressed as a percentage of the amplitude of the unconditioned response when preceded by a conditioning cortical stimulus.

There are several strong indications that the magnocellular MGB alone or in combination with the suprageniculate nucleus constitutes an important relay station for vestibular activity ascending to the cortex of the anterior suprasylvian fold. Butler, Diamond and Neff (9) and Locke (30) found partial degeneration in the magnocellular MGB when lesions of the auditory cortex extended forward across the anterior ectosylvian gyrus into the anterior suprasylvian gyrus. Heath and Jones (24) found that lesions restricted to the magnocellular MGB produced, in Nauta stains, heavy degeneration of the part of the suprasylvian fringe occupying the upper part of the anterior suprasylvian sulcus. Woolsey (59) found that electrical stimulation of the magnocellular MGB evokes responses in the suprasylvian fringe. Spiegel, Szekely and Gildenberg (52) recorded responses to stimulation of the vestibular nuclei in magnocellular MGB and the cortex of the anterior suprasylvian fold and found that lesions of MGB, which included the suprageniculate nucleus, abolished the cortical responses. However, Mickle and Ades (38), on the basis of depth macroelectrode recordings of responses to vestibular nerve stimulation, localized the thalamic relay site for ascending cortical activity to a histologically indistinct location between the MGB and the VPL.

In the present experiments, responses to vestibular nerve stimulation were recorded from the magnocellular MGB with a latency to onset shorter than for any of the other thalamic nuclei, the basal ganglia, or the cerebral cortex. In two experiments simultaneous recordings revealed a latency-to-onset of about 1.5-2.1 msec shorter for the vestibular responses in MGB than in the cortex of the anterior suprasylvian fold. In addition, previous experiments (42), reviewed briefly, demonstrated loss of the cortical response to vestibular nerve stimulation following bilateral lesions of the magnocellular MGB. Consequently, we are led to the conclusion that the magnocellular MGB constitutes an essential relay for mediating ascending vestibular activity to the cortex of the suprasylvian fold.

It has been appreciated for some time (18) that the MGB serves not only as a relay station for polysensory activity (56) but also as a site for mechanisms of integration and coordination. In addition, it has been established that the magnocellular MGB receives corticofugal fibers from cortex bordering upon the vestibular projection area (14, 47). Accordingly, it was of interest in the present study to find that activation of corticofugal fibers by stimulation of the vestibular projection area of cortex could influence strongly the responses to vestibular stimulation recorded in the magnocellular MGB. The type of influence disclosed in the present study was of the nature of occlusive or inhibitory interaction, suggesting that corticothalamic projections to MGB may serve to control the information to be relayed upward. Since the influence is derived from the cortical receptive area for vestibular responses, it is conceivable that the corticofugal connections serve as a feed-back loop for modulating upcoming vestibular activity.

The present findings of responses to vestibular nerve stimulation in caudate nucleus and globus pallidus complement the earlier similar findings of Spiegel, Szekely and Gildenberg (52), who found responses in these nuclei from stimulation of the vestibular nuclei. Segundo and Machne (49) had earlier demonstrated alteration of unitary activity in globus pallidus and putamen from stimulation through an electrode inserted into the ear, presumably providing vestibular stimulation. The pathway for mediation of vestibular activity to the basal ganglia is only partly established with certainty. Spiegel, Szekely and Gildenberg (52) found that lesions of the magnocellular MGB, also including the suprageniculate body, abolished the responses to stimulation of the vestibular nuclei recorded in the caudate nucleus. The responses in the pallidum were diminished but not abolished. In the studies of Potegal et al. (42), the responses in caudate were severely decreased by ablation of the magnocellular portion of the MGB. Consequently, it may be assumed that the MGB is an essential relay in conduction of vestibular responses to caudate. The experiments of Potegal et al. (42) ruled out the possibility that vestibular responses may reach the caudate by means of a circuit through the cortex, since complete ablation of the vestibular projection area of cortex as well as a considerable extent of surrounding cortex failed to alter the caudate responses to vestibular nerve stimulation. Connections between the MGB and the caudate nucleus have not been described, but there is both anatomical (31) and physiological (57) evidence of connections between magnocellular MGB and the pallidum. Spiegel, Szekely and Gildenberg (52) presented suggestive evidence that the centrum medianum may transmit vestibular activity to the caudate nucleus. They recorded responses to vestibular nerve stimulation consistently from the centrum medianum, and found that lesions in this nucleus at least transitorily, in most experiments, depressed the responses to vestibular nuclear stimulation in caudate nucleus without altering the responses in cortex. Accordingly, it is possible that CM constitutes a second relay nucleus for vestibular conduction to caudate, the first being the magnocellular MGB. Despite the evidence for connections between MGB and pallidum (31, 57), in the studies of Spiegel et al. (52), lesions of MGB did not consistently or completely abolish vestibular nucleus evoked responses in pallidum. Further studies are needed to establish the precise conduction pathway from thalamus to the basal ganglia.

SUMMARY

In Surital-anesthetized cats, areas of cerebral cortex and nuclei of the thalamus and basal ganglia were explored with macroelectrodes for responses to stimulation of the vestibular nerve in the bulla. Spread of stimulating current to cochlear nerve branches was prevented by monitoring from the ipsilateral vestibular and cochlear nuclei in brainstem and adjusting stimulus strength to provide responses in the former but not in the latter nuclei. Responses were recorded contralaterally in the cortex bordering the suprasylvian fold but not in the middle or posterior ectosylvian gyri. Responses were recorded contralaterally in the magnocellular medial geniculate body (MGB), ventral lateral (VL) and ventral posterior lateral (VPL) nuclei of the thalamus. Responses were recorded in the caudate nucleus and globus pallidus. The responses in the caudate nucleus showed a specific topographic distribution.

Responses in magnocellular MGB and in cortex persisted following cerebellectomy, transection of the medial longitudinal fasciculus and the tract described by Hassler in the dorsolateral tegmentum, but were abolished by lesions of the lateral lemniscus. The responses recorded in magnocellular MGB showed a shorter latency to onset than responses recorded in the other thalamic or basal ganglia nuclei, and were decreased by preceding stimulation of the vestibular projection area of cortex. Lesions of magnocellular MGB abolished responses in caudate nucleus and cortex.

It is concluded that vestibular activity ascends to the thalamus by way of the classical auditory pathway and makes synaptic connection in the magnocellular MGB where occlusive or inhibitory interaction with corticofugal activity may take place. The magnocellular MGB is an essential relay in the conduction of vestibular activity to caudate nucleus, cortex and possibly to other thalamic and basal ganglia structures.

ACKNOWLEDGMENTS.

This work has been supported by the Clinical Research Center for Parkinson's and Allied Diseases NS 05184, and by US Public Health Service Grants NS 52431, NS 2552, and MH 10315.

REFERENCES

1 ANDERSSON, S., and GERNANDT, B.E. Cortical projection of vestibular nerve in cat, Acta. Otolar., Stockh., Supp. 116 (1954) 10-18.

2 ARONSON, L. Conduction of labyrinthine impulses to the cortex, J. Nerv. Ment. Dis., 78 (1933) 250-259.

3 BERGOUIGNAN, M., and VERGER, P. Les réactions labyrinthiques chez le chien après lésion d'un noyau caude, C.R. Soc. Biol.(Paris), 118 (1935) 1539-1541.

4 BOISACQ-SCHEPENS, N., and HANUS, M. Macro- and microelectrode studies of motor cortex vestibular responses, Proc. Intern. Union of Physiol. Sciences, XXV Intern. Congr., Vol. IX (1971) 72.

5 BRODAL, A. Fiber connections of the vestibular nuclei. In G.L. Rasmussen and W.F. Windle (Eds.) Neural Mechanisms of the Auditory and Vestibular Systems, Charles C Thomas, Springfield, 1960, pp. 224-246.

6 BRODAL, A., and POMPEIANO, O. The origin of ascending fibers of the medial longitudinal fasciculus from the vestibular nuclei. An experimental study in the cat, Acta Morph. Neerl-Scand., 1 (1957) 306-328.

7 BRODAL, A., POMPEIANO, O., and WALBERG, F. The Vestibular Nuclei and Their Connections, Anatomy and Functional Correlations, Oliver and Boyd, London, 1962, pp. 42-51 and 129-134.

8 BUCHANAN, A.R. The course of the secondary vestibular fibers in the cat, J. Comp. Neurol., 67 (1937) 183-204.

9 BUTLER, R.A., DIAMOND, I.T., and NEFF, W.D. Role of auditory cortex in discrimination of changes of frequency, J. Neurophysiol., 20 (1957) 108-120.

10 CAJAL, S.R. Histologie du Système Nerveux de L'Homme et des Vertébrés. Tome I et II, Maloine, Paris, 1909-1911.

11 CARPENTER, M.B. Experimental anatomical-physiological studies of the vestibular nerve and cerebellar connections. In G.L. Rasmussen and W.F. Windle (Eds.), Neural Mechanisms of the Auditory and Vestibular Systems, Charles C Thomas, Springfield, 1960, pp. 297-323.

12 CARPENTER, M.B., and STROMINGER, N.L. The medial longitudinal fasciculus and disturbances of conjugate horizontal eye movements in the monkey, J. Comp. Neurol., 125 (1965) 41-66.

13 DENNY-BROWN, D. The Basal Ganglia and Their Relation to Disorders of Movement, Oxford Univ. Press, London, 1962, pp. 108-121.

14 DIAMOND, I.T., JONES, E.G., and POWELL, T.P.S. The projection of the auditory cortex upon the brain stem and diencephalon in the cat, Brain Res., 15 (1969) 305-340.

15 FERRARO, A., PACELLA, B.L., and BARRERA, S.E. Effects of lesions of the medial vestibular nucleus. An anatomical and physiological study in Macacus Rhesus monkeys, J. Comp. Neurol., 73 (1940) 7-36.

16 FREDRICKSON, J.M., FIGGE, U., SCHEID, P., and KORNHUBER, H.H. Vestibular nerve projection to the cerebral cortex of the Rhesus monkey, Exp. Brain Res., 2 (1966) 318-327.

17 GEHUCHTEN, P. VAN, Les voies nerveuses du nystagmus, Rev. Neurol., 2 (1928) 849-869.

18 GERNANDT, B. Midbrain activity in response to vestibular stimulation, Acta Physiol. Scand., 21 (1950) 73-81.

19 GEREBTZOFF, M.A. Des effets de la stimulation labyrinthique sur l'activité électrique de l'écorce cérébrale, C.R. Soc. Biol., Paris, 131 (1939) 807-813.

20 GEREBTZOFF, M.A. Récherches sur la projection corticale du labyrinthe. 1. Des effects de la stimulation labyrinthique sur l'activite electrique de l'écorce cérébrale, Arch. Int. Physiol., 50 (1940) 59-99.

21 GRAY, L.P. Some experimental evidence on the connections of the vestibular mechanism in the cat, J. Comp. Neurol., 41 (1926) 319-364.

22 HASSLER, R. Forels Haubenfaszikel als vestibuläre Empfindungsbahn mit Bemerkungen über einige andere sekundäre Bahen des Vestibularis und Trigeminus, Arch. Psychiat. Z. ges. Neurol., 180 (1948) 23-53.

23 HASSLER, R. Die zentralen Apparate der Wendebewegungen. II. Die neuronalen Apparate der vestibulären Korrekturwendungen und der Adversivbewegungen, Arch. Psychiat. Z. ges. Neurol., 194 (1956) 481-516.

24 HEATH, C.J., and JONES, E.G., An experimental study of ascending connections from the posterior group of thalamic nuclei in the cat, J. Comp. Neurol., 141, (1971) 397-426.

25 HELD, H. Die anatomische Grundlage der Vestibularisfunktionen, Beitr. Anat. Physiol. Path. Ther. d. Ohres, d. Nase u.d. Halses, 19 (1923) 305-312.

26 JASPER, H.H., and AJMONE-MARSAN, C. A Stereotaxic Atlas of the Diencephalon of the Cat, Nat. Res. Council of Canada, Ottawa, 1954.

27 KEMPINSKY, W.H. Cortical projection of vestibular and facial nerves in cat, J. Neurophysiol., 14 (1951) 203-209.

28 LANDGREN, S., SILFVENIUS, H., and WOLSK, D. Vestibular, cochlear, and trigeminal projections to the cortex in the anterior suprasylvian sulcus of the cat, J. Physiol. (Lond.), 191 (1967) 561-573.

29 LEIDLER, R. Experimentelle Untersuchungen über das Endigungsgebeit des Nervus vestibularis, Arb. Neurol. Inst. Univ. Wien, 21 (1914) 151-212.

30 LOCKE, S. The projection of the magnocellular medial geniculate body, J. Comp. Neur., 116 (1961) 179-193.

31 LOCKE, S. Subcortical projection of the magnocellular medial geniculate body of monkey, J. Comp. Neur., 138 (1970) 321-328.

32 MAGNUS, R. Körperstellung, Springer, Berlin, 1924.

33 MARTIN, J.P. Tilting reactions and disorders of the basal ganglia, Brain, 88 (1965) 855-874.

34 MARTIN, J.P. The Basal Ganglia and Posture, Lippincott, Philadelphia, 1967.

35 MASSOPUST, L.C., Jr., and DAIGLE, H.J. Cortical projection of the medial and spinal vestibular nuclei in the cat, Exp. Neurol., 2 (1960) 179-185.

36 METTLER, F.A., and METTLER, C.C. Labyrinthine disregard after removal of the caudate, Proc. Soc. Exp. Biol. Med., 45 (1940) 473-475.

37 MICKLE, W.A., and ADES, H.W. A composite sensory projection area in the cerebral cortex of the cat, Amer. J. Physiol., 170 (1952) 682-689.

38 MICKLE, W.A., and ADES, H.W. Rostral projection pathway of the vestibular system, Amer. J. Physiol., 176 (1954) 243-252.

39 MILOJEVIC, B., and ST. LAURENT, J. Cortical vestibular projection in the cat, Aerospace Med., 37 (1966) 709-712.

40 MUSKENS, L.J.J. An anatomico-physiological study of the posterior longitudinal bundle in its relation to forced movements, Brain 36 (1913-14) 352-426.

41 MUSKENS, L.J.J. The central connections of the vestibular nuclei with the corpus striatum and their significance for ocular movements and for locomotion, Brain, 45 (1922) 454-478.

42 POTEGAL, M., COPACK, P., DEJONG, J.M.B.V., KRAUTHAMER, G., and GILMAN, S. Vestibular input to the caudate nucleus, Exp. Neurol., 32 (1971) 448-465.

43 PRECHT, W., and SHIMAZU, H. Functional connections of tonic and kinetic vestibular neurons with primary vestibular afferents, J. Neurophysiol., 28 (1965) 1014-1028.

44 PRICE, J.B., and SPIEGEL, E.A. Vestibulo-cerebral pathways. A contribution to the central mechanism of vertigo. Arch. Otolaryng., Chic., 26 (1937) 658-667.

45 RASMUSSEN, A.T. Secondary vestibular tracts in the cat, J. Comp. Neurol., 54 (1932) 143-171.

46 RICHTER, R. Degeneration of the basal ganglia in monkeys from chronic carbon disulfide poisoning, J. Neuropath. Exp. Neurol., 4 (1945) 324-353.

47 RINVIK, E. The corticothalamic projection from the second somatosensory cortical area in the cat. An experimental study with silver impregnation methods, Exptl. Brain Res., 5 (1968) 153-172.

48 SANS, A., RAYMOND, J., and MARTY, R. Réponses thalamiques et corticales à la stimulation électrique du nerf vestibulaire chez le Chat, Exp. Brain Res., 10 (1970) 265-275

49 SEGUNDO, J.P., and MACHNE, X. Unitary responses to afferent volleys in lenticular nucleus and claustrum, J. Neurophysiol., 19 (1956) 325-339.

50 SNIDER, R.S., and NIEMER, W.T. A Stereotaxic Atlas of the Cat Brain, Univ. of Chicago Press, Chicago, 1961.

51 SPIEGEL, E.A. Rindenerregung (Auslösung epileptiformer Anfälle) durch Labyrinthreizung. Versuch einer Lokalization der corticalen Labyrinthzentren, Z. ges. Neurol. Psychiat., 138 (1932) 178-196.

52 SPIEGEL, E.A., SZEKELY, E.G., and GILDENBERG, P.L. Vestibular responses in midbrain, thalamus and basal ganglia, Arch. Neurol. (Chic.), 12 (1965) 258-269.

53 SZENTÁGOTHAI, J. Die zentrale Innervation der Augenbewegungen, Arch. Psychiat. Nervenkr., 116 (1943) 721-760.

54 TARLOV, E. The rostral projections of the primate vestibular nuclei: An experimental study in macaque, baboon and chimpanzee, J. Comp. Neurol., 135 (1969) 27-56.

55 WALZL, E.M., and MOUNTCASTLE, V.B. Projection of vestibular nerve to cerebral cortex of the cat, Amer. J. Physiol., 159 (1949) 595.

56 WEPSIC, J.G. Multimodal sensory activation of cells in the magnocellular medial geniculate nucleus, Exp. Neurol., 15 (1966) 299-318.
57 WEPSIC, J.G., and SUTIN, J. Posterior thalamic and septal influence upon pallidal and amygdaloid slow wave and unitary activity, Exp. Neurol., 10 (1964) 67-80.
58 WHITAKER, J.G., and ALEXANDER, L. Die Verbindungen der Vestibulariskerne mit dem Mittel- und Zwischenhirn, J. Psychol. Neurol., 44 (1932) 253-376.
59 WOOLSEY, C.N. Electrophysiological studies on thalamocortical relations in the auditory system. In: A. Abrams, H.H. Garner, and J.E. Toman (Eds.), Unfinished Tasks in the Behavioral Sciences, Williams and Wilkins, Baltimore, 1964, pp. 45-57.

DISCUSSION

COHEN:

Drs. Gilman, Copack and Dafny's work confirms other studies which show that gross potential changes and unit activity are induced in the anterior suprasylvian gyrus by vestibular nerve stimulation. Evoked potentials have also been recorded in the anterior ectosylvian gyrus, and cells which respond to vestibular stimulation in a direction-specific manner are present in the motor cortex (3). The primary vestibular projection area of the monkey is in the parietal lobe (2). Differences in distribution of cortical evoked responses reported in various studies are probably dependent on a number of factors including the method of stimulation, the state of alertness, and some individual variation among animals. There is still some question as to whether or not there is a specific receiving area for each of the semicircular canals and for utricle and saccule over the cortex as originally suggested by Andersson and Gernandt (1).

Projection nuclei in the thalamus for ascending vestibulocortical activity have been reported in various studies to include MGB, VPL, and VL. MGB appears to be the major projection nucleus for activity ascending in the brainstem, and gross potential changes over the cortex are markedly attenuated after MGB lesions (7). MGB is a multimodal sensory receiving area, and has been shown to respond to somatosensory, auditory, and vestibular stimuli (4, 8). The pathways which carry vestibular information to the thalamus are not entirely clear. Cortical responses to vestibular nerve stimulation are not affected by MLF and para-MLF lesions (7), nor do the pathways utilize the trapezoid body. Presumably the fibers ascend in the reticular formation. Activity in VL probably reaches the thalamus by way of the cerebellum (6).

When vestibular areas of the cerebellum (flocculus, nodulus, and uvula) are electrically stimulated, gross potential changes are induced over regions of the cerebral cortex which were activated by vestibular nerve stimulation (5). This suggests that there is a common projection area for vestibular information over the cerebral cortex, regardless of whether vestibular information ascends through the brainstem or cerebellum.

One caveat is that it may be difficult to restrict effects of axonal reflexes in stimulation studies. Some primary afferent fibers in the vestibular nerve send one axon to the vestibular nuclei and a branch to the cerebellum. Thus both vestibular nuclei and cerebellum would be activated by stimulation anywhere along this axon.

Findings by Gilman and co-workers that vestibular projections reach the caudate nucleus also agree with work of Spiegel *et al.* (7). They induced gross potential changes in the caudate, putamen, pallidum and centromedian nucleus of the thalamus by vestibular nucleus stimulation. In both studies the potential changes were small and were recorded with monopolar electrodes using averaging techniques. Therefore, some caution must be exercised in making statements about the precise distribution of these responses. It would be of interest to know whether these projections are specific or non-specific. This information can best be obtained by unit studies with adequate vestibular stimulation.

An unanswered question is the functional use of the ascending vestibular information. It seems reasonable to suppose that the cortex, thalamus and basal ganglia receive information about head position and movement of the head in space from the vestibular system and cerebellum. Nevertheless, there are few vestibular defects in humans with cortical lesions. This suggests that the vestibulocortical information is not vital for maintenance of balance or posture. Presumably its function is to bias the activities of the motor cortex in non-stereotyped motor behavior.

REFERENCES

1 ANDERSSON, S., and GERNANDT, B.E. Cortical projection of vestibular nerve in cat, Acta oto-laryng. Suppl. (Stockh.) 116 (1954) 10-18.

2 FREDRICKSON, J.M., FIGGE, U., SCHEID, P., and KORNHUBER, H.H. Vestibular nerve projection to the cerebral cortex of the rhesus monkey, Exp. Brain Res., 2 (1966) 318-327.

3 KORNHUBER, H.H., and DA FONSECA, J.S. Optovestibular integration in the cat's cortex. In M.B. Bender (Ed.), The Oculomotor System, Harper & Row (Hoeber Medical Division), New York, 1964, pp. 239-277.

4 MEULDERS, M., COLLE, J., and GODFRAIND, J.M. Evoked sensory responses of somatic origin in the lateral geniculate body, Arch. int. Physiol., 72 (1964) 346-348.

5 RUWALDT, M.M., and SNIDER, R.S. Projection of vestibular areas of cerebellum to the cerebrum, J. comp. Neurol., 104 (1956) 387-401.

6 SANS, A., RAYMOND, J. and MARTY, R. Reponses thalamiques et corticales a la stimulation electrique du nerf vestibulaire chez le chat, Exp. Brain Res., 10 (1970) 265-275.

7 SPIEGEL, E.A., SZEKELY, E.G., and GILDENBERG, P.L. Vestibular responses in midbrain, thalamus and basal ganglia, Arch. Neurol. (Chic.), 12 (1965) 258-269.

8 WEPSIC, J.G. Multimodal sensory activation of cells in the magnocellular medial geniculate nucleus, Exp. Neurol., 15 (1966) 299-318.

SCHWARTZ:

We possess some data on the primate (rhesus monkey) which is of considerable importance with Dr. Gilman's findings. We did some isolated stimulation of the vestibular nerve and recorded from the thalamus and cortex. The projection field in the parietal lobe, which was presumed to lie within area 2, is now known not to lie within area 2. Considering the projections via or to the magnocellular portion of the medial geniculate body, we have some data of considerable interest. We recorded field potentials in this area. As a matter of fact, we mapped out with microelectrodes the whole thalamus of the primate after vestibular stimulation and found, as Dr. Gilman, short latency activation in the medial geniculate body. But a few millimeters rostral, that is in the Vpi nucleus, we found clear evidence of cell activation with short latency after vestibular nucleus stimulation. Whereas for the short latency activation within MGB we could not find evidence for cell activation, so we concluded that the activation there was fiber activation transversing rostrally. The latency of these responses were 3-4 msec, which is a little bit longer than in the cat; but the brain of the monkey is a little bit larger too. Cells within this nucleus could be antidromically invaded by stimulation of the cortex. The lowest threshold of this area was again the vestibular projection field. Other areas of the thalamus yielded a little longer latency responses. Among those were CM, MGB and the whole extent of VP and an area caudal to VL, which Hassler described yesterday as the intermediate nucleus in that area. This area particularly seems to yield some focal activation but the latency again is somewhat longer than within Vpi. It is some 6-8 msec in the primate. There is another point which is of considerable interest, that is single cells with the shortest latency activation by vestibular nerve stimulation in the thalamus as well in the cortex respond not only to vestibular stimulation but also to kinesthetic stimulation. The activation pattern is always direction specific; sometimes the cells mimic complex positions of the whole body so there is a convergent activation of many joints. So it appears that the shortest latency ascending vestibular projection ends in the parietal cortex of the primate. We think that this corresponds to the ascending pathway Dr. Gilman just now reported.

HASSLER:

I want to speak first about this magnocellular part of the medial geniculate body. This magnocellular part is the subcortical projection nucleus of the composite area in the anterior ectosylvian gyrus; I think it was first described by Miglan in 1951. One should not say that this is a real vestibular nucleus but it is a multisensory nucleus because fiber afferents from the visual system (I can say this based on my own studies), the acoustic system, the vestibular system, and the somatosensory system are convergent to this nucleus. The other very important point is that Dr. Gilman found, and Dr. Schwartz mentioned also, the region of VPL but Dr. Cohen quoted Sans et al. who related this vestibular reaction to the VL nucleus. We have new studies with Nauta-Gygax method after vestibular nuclei lesions in the cat. It is quite clear that only the medial part of the intermediate ventral nucleus, at the border between the VL and the

VPL, a very small restricted region, has direct vestibular afferents. Dr. Gilman is completely right if one looks at the anatomical literature that this anatomical pathway is controversial. But I think from these new studies, and it is quite clear from the physiological studies, that there is a real anatomical, a real primary, place in the thalamus which receives direct vestibular fibers. They are not going through the posterior longitudinal bundle but they are projecting through the dorsal lateral tract of the tegmentum. Another projection from the vestibular nuclei is going to the centre médian nucleus. It is quite clear that these findings of Dr. Gilman in the caudate and putamen are indirect projections from this place going through the centre médian nucleus. Perhaps I may mention that Guttenberg is publishing now in Experimental Brain Research another study about the cortical influences on the vestibular nucleus activity. He did extracellular recordings in the vestibular nucleus and stimulated all the cortex of the cat; there were only two places from which he could have direct influences on vestibular cell activity: the anterior ectosylvian gyrus and a very small place in the cruciate sulcus belonging to area 6. This is the same place from which one can have by the Hess method of direct stimulation ipsiversive turning in the unanesthetized animal. I think this pathway goes through the ViM to the area 6, and is the real vestibular pathway and is not mixed up with other sensory modalities.

SCHWARTZ:

There are some data corresponding to what Dr. Hassler just now said and some of the details corresponding to what Dr. Albe-Fessard told us yesterday; namely about dorsal root potentials after motor cortex stimulation. After stimulation of the somewhat more caudal part of area 6, we could record slow potentials from the vestibular nerve which looked very similar to the dorsal root potentials.

PURPURA:

Several problems of interpretation arise in consideration of the data presented by Dr. Gilman. Many of the responses look rather homogeneous and of short latency. It is difficult to understand how the latency of evoked activities in CM and caudate can be the same since studies have shown that stimulation in CM generally elicits a relatively long-latency response in the caudate. The same may apply to the question of the relationship of cortical evoked responses to activities in the basal ganglia. If the cortex is the source of entry fibers into the basal ganglia in these studies then it can be expected that there will be even greater discrepancies in latencies from available data on the subject.

GILMAN:

I wish to thank the discussants for their interesting and provocative thoughts. As Dr. Cohen pointed out, at least four thalamic nuclei have been implicated in the conduction of vestibular activity to cortex, but considerable controversy exists about the importance of each nucleus. For example, Gernandt (1950) found vestibular responses in MGB and Spiegel, Szekely, and Gildenberg (1965) provided evidence indicating that the magnocellular portion of the MGB is the essential relay nucleus for conduction to the vestibular projection area in the anterior suprasylvian fold of cortex. The present studies support this view. However, Mickle and Ades (1954) suggested that the important thalamic relay station in the conduction pathway to cortex was somewhere between MGB and VPL, though not within either nucleus. Recently, Sans, Raymond, and Marty (1970) have stated that vestibular impulses are mediated by way of the VPL nucleus to the vestibular projection area in the anterior suprasylvian fold and also to the cortex of the postcruciate dimple. In addition, they found vestibular activity in the VL nucleus and suggested that the responses may be mediated there by way of the cerebellum. They did not have evidence indicating that the VL transmits vestibular activity to the cortex, and had no direct evidence of a route through cerebellum. Finally, Dr. Schwartz's interesting comments about his experiments in monkey raise the possibility that the VPI nucleus is an important thalamic relay station for ascending vestibular activity in primates. Accordingly, there are many important problems to explore with respect to the vestibular projections through thalamus to cortex.

In response to Dr. Hassler's interesting comments, our evidence indicates that the responses to vestibular nerve stimulation persist in the magnocellular MGB and suprasylvian fold after cerebellectomy and lesions in the dorsolateral tegmentum. We believe that the lesions interrupt the vestibulothalamic pathway he described in his publications in 1948 and 1956 and conclude that the vestibular projections ascend to the thalamus through some other route, possibly in association with the classical auditory projection or possibly through reticulothalamic fibers. Dr. Purpura raised several pertinent issues. His first question related to the latencies of our responses. The short latency from vestibular nerve to cortex is surprising, but similar latencies have been reported by other investigators, including Landgren, Silfvenius, and Wolsk (1967), who suggested that there may be only two synapses between the vestibular nerve and the cortical projection area. We were also interested to determine whether there may be a vestibular projection from cortex to the caudate nucleus, but have ruled out that possibility. The experiments are described in detail in the publication of Potegal, Copack, DeJong, Krauthamer, and Gilman (1971). In that study it was found that caudate responses to vestibular stimulation persisted despite extensive ablations of the vestibular projection area of cortex and surrounding regions. Although we do not know with certainty the route from vestibular nerve to caudate, we are inclined to believe the explanation provided by Spiegel, Szekely, and Gildenberg (1965), also mentioned by Dr. Hassler, that vestibular responses are relayed from magnocellular medial geniculate to centrum medianum and then to the caudate nucleus. However, we did not record from CM and have no definitive experiments to settle this issue.

Corticothalamic Projections and Sensorimotor Activities
T. Frigyesi, E. Rinvik, and M.D. Yahr, editors. © 1972
Raven Press, New York.

Activity in the Thalamus, Calcarine Cortex and Pontine Reticular Formation Associated with Rapid Eye Movement

Bernard Cohen

It was shown in the previous chapter that vestibular stimulation induces potential changes in thalamus, basal ganglia, and cortex at short latencies. These are the direct vestibular projections. However, the vestibular system also activates other ascending pathways from the reticular formation to the thalamus and cortex. For example, vestibular nucleus stimulation causes enhancement of optic tract responses induced by lateral geniculate body (LGB) stimulation (27). Similar enhancement is produced by changes in alertness (9). In the absence of direct vestibulo-geniculate pathways, these effects are probably mediated over reticulo-thalamic pathways which are known to powerfully affect transmission in visual pathways (1, 3, 9, 14, 26, 30, 37).

In addition, if nystagmus or other rapid eye movements are evoked by vestibular stimulation in the alert monkey two other types of potential changes are found in thalamus and cortex. The first of these potential changes reflects efferent activity of the oculomotor system (2, 4, 5, 7, 9, 16, 24, 25). The second is a light-evoked response generated in the retina by the movement of the eyes (4, 8, 15, 18, 20, 21, 23, 32, 34, 35, 40). A third type of potential change is induced in the cerebellum by eye muscle proprioceptors (17), but will not be considered further here.

Figure 1A shows an example of the first type of potential change. It was induced in LGB by stimulation of the left lateral semicircular canal nerve (16). It was associated with a biphasic eye movement which consisted of an initial deviation and a second "return" eye movement. The latter is a rapid eye movement similar to saccades or quick phases of nystagmus (10, 19). At the end of the trace in Fig. 1A a spontaneous saccade occurred which was also associated with a similar potential change in LGB.

The animal was in darkness during these eye movements so that the LGB responses were not light-evoked responses due to movement of the eyes. When the animal was drowsy, only the initial deviation was induced (Fig. 1B). There was no rapid return eye movement, and no potential change in LGB was associated with the vestibular stimulus. An LGB potential change associated with a quick phase of caloric nystagmus is shown in the top trace of Fig. 1C. These potential changes were recorded from the dorsal (small cell) layers of the lateral geniculate body (Fig. 2, black dots).

Light-evoked responses to eye movement are also widely distributed in LGB. In dorsal regions they are manifested as small positive deflections (Fig. 1D, upward arrow) which precede the previously described negative LGB potential changes (16). Regions where the only response to rapid eye movement was a light-evoked potential change were limited to ventral (large cell) areas of LGB. Several of these recording sites are indicated by the open circles in Fig. 2, A5.

Both types of potential changes associated with eye movement are found in other regions of the thalamus which are related to the visual system. In posterior portions

---

FIG. 1. A, Potential change in LGB induced by stimulation of left lateral semicircular canal nerve. The stimulus was a 50 msec train of 0.5 msec square waves at an in tratrain frequency of 500 Hz. The period of stimulation is shown by the artifact parallel to the EOG. The upper trace is a bipolar recording from LGB, the middle trace is the bitemporal EOG, and the bottom trace the differentiated EOG showing eye velocity. A spontaneous saccade occurred at the end of the trace in A and was also associated with an LGB potential change. B is the same as A except that the time base is slower and the animal was drowsy. Although an initial deviation of the eyes to the right was induced by the left lateral canal stimulus, no return eye movement was induced nor was there an associated LGB potential change. A small saccade at the end of the movement was again associated with an LGB potential change. C, Recordings from LGB, top trace; PPRF, middle trace; EOG, bottom trace during quick phase of caloric nystagmus to left. The potential change in PPRF preceded the quick phase of nystagmus and the LGB potential change. D, Saccadic eye movement in light. Note initial positive deflection (upward arrow) which disappeared during a saccade in darkness, E. Toward the end of trace in E the PPRF was electrically stimulated with a short train of pulses and an LGB potential change was induced without an eye movement. The vertical bars show 200 μV for LGB recordings, 100 μV for PPRF recording; 45° of horizontal deviation for A, B, 15° for C, and 30° for D, E. The horizontal bars show the time base which is 100 msec for A, 200 msec for B, D and E, and 40 msec for C. (From Feldman & Cohen, J. Neurophysiol., 31 (1968) 455-466 and, Cohen & Feldman, J. Neurophysiol., 31 (1968) 806-817.)

FIG. 2. Black dots show recording sites in LGB from which potential changes associated with rapid eye movements in dark were recorded. Responses were plotted on sections of left LGB in vertical stereotaxic planes from A8 to A3. Pgn and pulv are pregeniculate nucleus and pulvinar, respectively. 21 monopolar and 80 bipolar recording points are shown. Open circles show recording sites where there was no response to eye movement in darkness, but at which potentials were recorded during rapid eye movements in light. (From Feldman & Cohen, J. Neurophysiol., 31 (1968) 455-466.

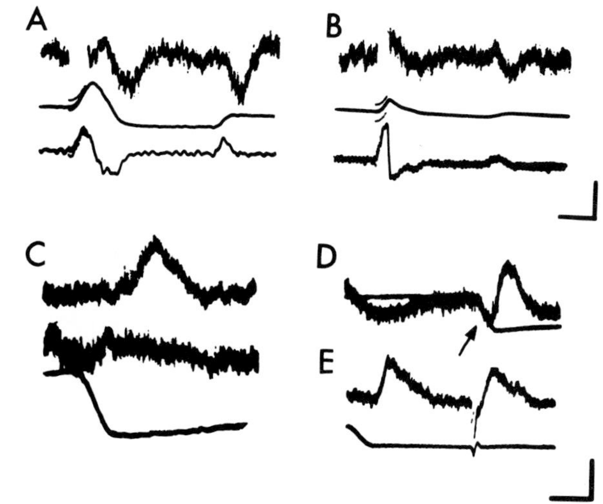

FIG. 1

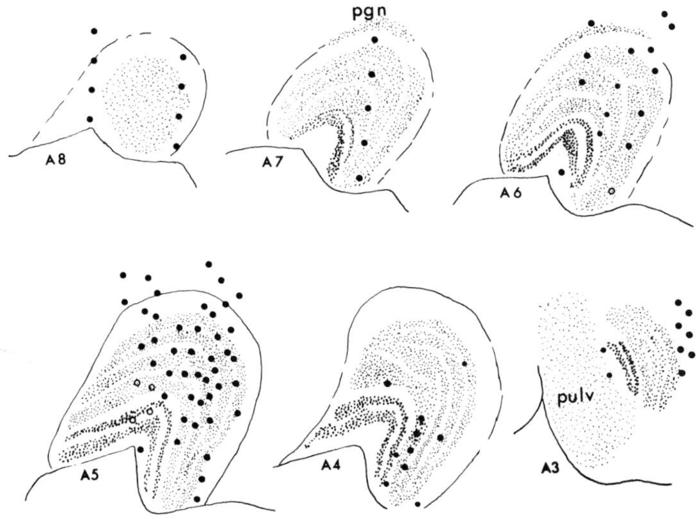

FIG. 2

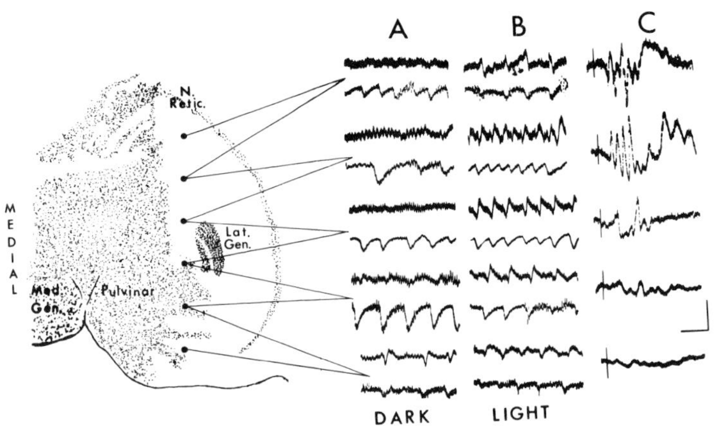
A
B
C
N.
Retic.
Lat.
Gen.
MEDIAL
Med.
Gen.
Pulvinar
DARK
LIGHT

FIG. 3

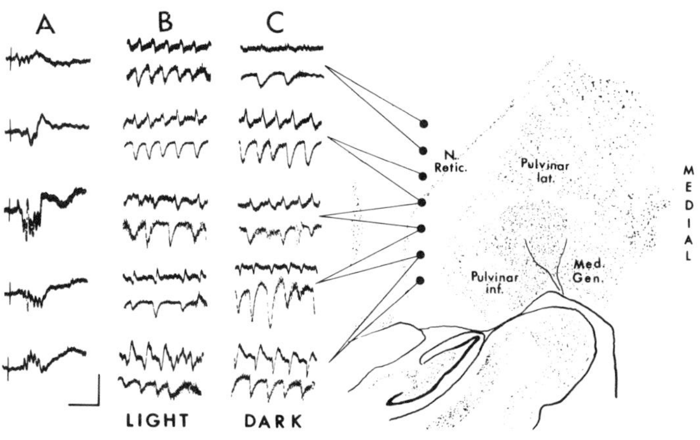
A
B
C
N.
Retic.
Pulvinar
lat.
MEDIAL
Pulvinar
inf.
Med.
Gen.
LIGHT
DARK

FIG. 4

of the thalamus between LGB and the pulvinar, there was a prominent potential change associated with each rapid eye movement in light (Fig. 3B). This was predominantly a light-evoked response since it disappeared when the animal was in darkness (Fig. 3A). In lateral parts of the posterior thalamus, on the other hand, in the region of nucleus reticularis (Fig. 4), there was no difference in the potential changes whether the animal was in light (Fig. 4B) or in darkness (Fig. 4C). These potential changes more closely reflected efferent activity of the oculomotor system. In both thalamic regions the potential changes were independent of the direction of eye movement, and were similar regardless of whether the eyes had moved spontaneously during saccades or during induced nystagmus.

In the calcarine cortex of the monkey the major events associated with eye movement are light-evoked responses similar to those induced by light flash (8, 23). An example of a potential change in the calcarine cortex induced by a quick phase of nystagmus in light is shown in the middle trace of Fig. 5A. It disappeared when the animal was in darkness (Fig. 5B). Similar potential changes are induced by saccades or quick phases of OKN (Fig. 5C), but not by pursuit movements (Fig. 5D). These light-evoked potential changes can be the most prominent activity in the calcarine cortex during induced nystagmus (Fig. 6 B,C), and have very little dependence on contrast in the external visual fields (8).

The electrode locations from which these responses were recorded are shown in Fig. 6A. These portions of the calcarine cortex receive afferent information from the periphery of the retina (11). Coded into the latency of these potential changes is the absolute level of illumination, while the amplitude reflects the amount of light which reaches the retina and the size and velocity of the rapid eye movement which induced these potential changes (8). Potential changes called lambda waves (15, 18, 20, 23, 32, 34, 35) and unit activity (40) associated with eye movement are

---

FIG. 3. Eye movement-associated potential changes in posterior thalamus, just medial to posterior portions of LGB. The top trace of each pair records the potential changes between points indicated on diagram and the bottom trace shows the horizontal EOG. The response to light flash is also shown. The time base is the horizontal bar which is 200 msec for recordings during caloric nystagmus and 40 msec for recordings during light flash. The vertical bar is 100 μV for the top trace and about 30° of horizontal deviation for the EOG. Note the absence of response in darkness at all recording locations except the bottom pair. Responses in light were prominent at each recording site in this electrode track. (From Feldman & Cohen, J. Neurophysiol., 31 (1968) 455-466.)

FIG. 4. Scheme similar to that of Fig. 3. Note the prominent potential changes in darkness at points in and close to nucleus reticularis. The potential changes in darkness reversed polarity between the 3rd and 4th set of recordings, suggesting that the source was located in this region.

present over lateral portions of the occipital lobes which receive projections from the fovea (11). Contrary to calcarine potential changes, this activity is dependent on strong contrast in the external visual fields. It disappears if the external contrast is reduced, even though the eyes move in light (20, 34, 40).

Potential changes which reflect efferent activity of the oculomotor system in the visual cortex are much more prominent in the cat (4, 5, 24, 25, 29), but also occur in the monkey. An example is shown in Fig. 7. The top trace is a recording from an electrode located in the cross-hatched area of Fig. 6A. The second trace is from LGB and the third trace is the horizontal EOG. Similar potential changes were induced in LGB and calcarine cortex by saccades whether animals were in light (Fig. 7A) or darkness (Fig. 7B). Potential changes associated with caloric stimulation were similar before (Fig. 7C) and after (Fig. 7D) the animal was paralyzed. This shows that the potential changes were not dependent on afferent activity arising in eye muscle proprioceptors.

Potential changes shown in Fig. 1 A-D, Fig. 4 and Fig. 7 are believed to have been generated by activity which originated in medial portions of nucleus reticularis magnocellularis in the paramedian zone of the pontine reticular formation (PPRF)(7). This region is shown by the cross-hatched area in Fig. 8A. Oculomotor function is strongly represented in the PPRF and horizontal eye movements appear to be generated in this region (6). Potential changes and unit activity in the PPRF lead every rapid eye movement (7). Fig. 8B shows the sequence of activity during a saccade to the left. First there was activity in the PPRF (top trace), then the left lateral rectus muscle was activated (bottom trace), then the eye moved to the left (middle trace).

FIG. 5. A, Calcarine potential changes associated with eye movement in light. Upper trace is EOG, middle trace is bipolar recording from calcarine cortex, and lower trace from optic tract. B, Schema as in A except that animal was in darkness. Note absence of activity in optic tract and calcarine cortex. C, Calcarine potential change associated with quick phase of OKN. D, Pursuit eye movement of similar amplitude did not induce a calcarine potential change. (From Cohen & Feldman, Exp. Neurol., 31 (1971) 100-113.)

FIG. 6. A, Dots show location of electrode sites in calcarine cortex from which potential changes were recorded which were associated with eye movement in light. Potential changes associated with eye movement in darkness were infrequently encountered. Electrodes which recorded the potential changes in Fig. 7 were lateral to the calcarine cortex in the cross-hatched area. B, Light-dependent calcarine potential changes during OKN to right, and C, during OKN to left. (From Cohen & Feldman, Exp. Neurol., 31 (1971) 100-113.)

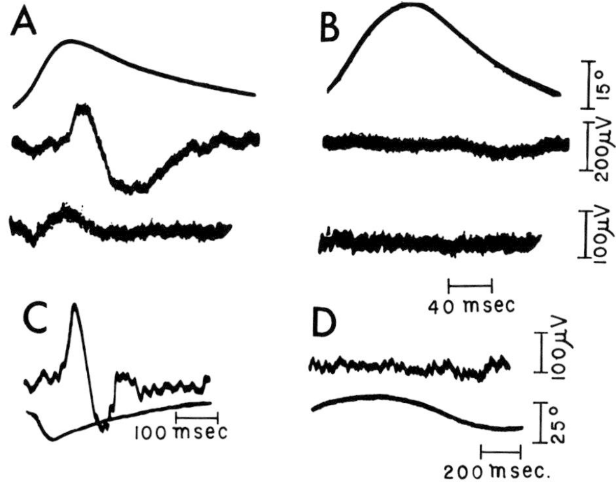
A
B
C
D
15°
200μV
100μV
40 msec
100 msec
100μV
25°
200 msec.

FIG. 5

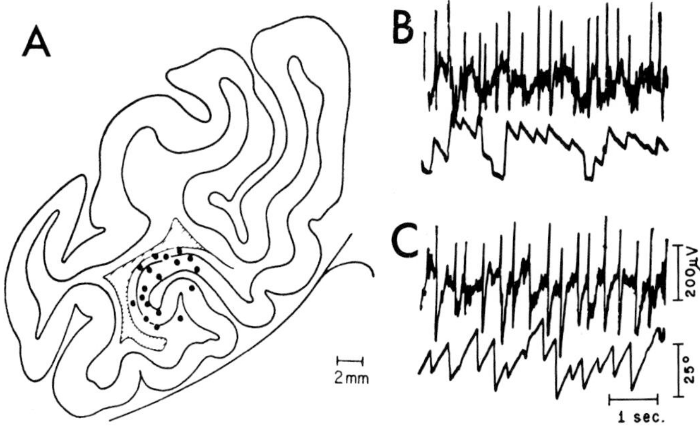
A
B
C
2mm
200μV
25°
1 sec.

FIG. 6

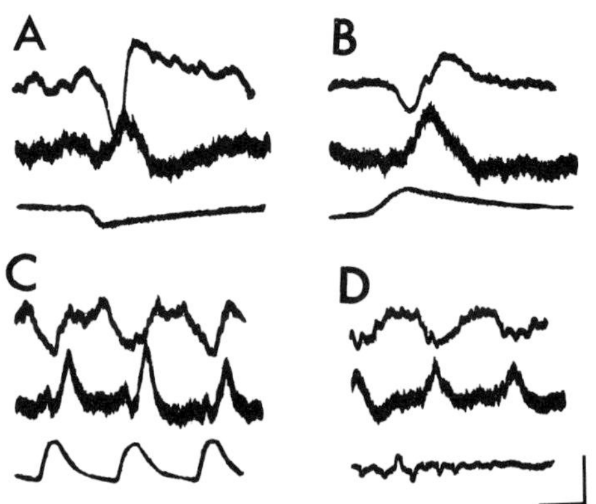

FIG. 7

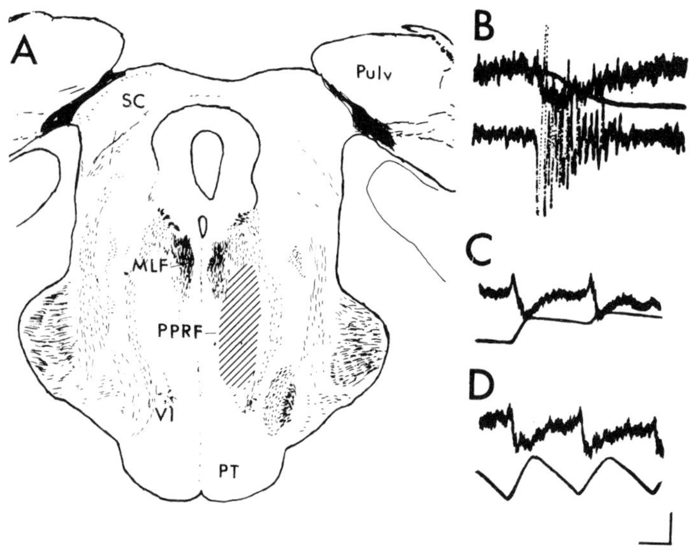

FIG. 8

The comparative latencies of PPRF and LGB potential changes are shown in Fig. 1C. If the PPRF is electrically stimulated, potential changes are induced in LGB and surrounding regions which are similar to those which occur naturally (Fig. 1E) (2, 7, 9). The ascending pathway for this activity is probably through the MRF since similar LGB potentials can be induced by MRF stimulation (7, 9).

Thus vestibular stimuli cause complex changes in the thalamus and cortex as a result of activity which arises in such disparate places as the retina and the pontine reticular formation. As demonstrated, the potential changes are primarily associated with rapid eye movement and were only secondarily evoked by vestibular stimuli. Similar potential changes can be induced by other sensory stimuli, even when there is no eye movement (16, 28), or during sleep (2, 5, 25, 29). In alert animals, however, the correspondence between potential changes and rapid eye movements in portions of the reticular formation, thalamus and cortex is high. Consequently, they or waveforms associated with body movement (12) could contribute importantly to potential changes found in these regions during complex problem solving which might involve vision and eye movement (22, 31, 33).

The functional significance of eye movement-associated responses is not entirely clear. In the pons, at least part of the potential change probably reflects activity which generated the eye movements and the light-independent potentials in other parts of the nervous system. It is possible that the thalamic and cortical potentials may be responsible for saccadic suppression (21, 38, 41). In one study there was no change in transmission through LGB during rapid eye movement (9), but changes in evoked potentials over the visual cortex have been reported in other studies (21, 41). How-

---

FIG. 7. A, B, Calcarine (upper traces) and LGB potential changes (middle traces) associated with rapid eye movements in light (A) and in darkness (B). C, Repetitive calcarine and LGB potential changes associated with quick phases of caloric nystagmus in darkness. D, Caloric stimulation after animal was paralyzed induced similar LGB and calcarine potential changes. The EOG gain was increased 10x in D to demonstrate the absence of eye movement. Vertical bar is 30° for the EOG, and 200 μV for LGB and calcarine recording. Horizontal bar is 40 msec for A, B and 200 msec for C, D.

FIG. 8. A, Diagram of brainstem showing location of PPRF on one side (cross-hatched area). This section is through the mid-pons in the P 0.5 vertical stereotaxic plane. SC, superior colliculus; MLF, median longitudinal fasciculus; pulv, pulvinar; PPRF, paramedian zone of the pontine reticular formation; VI, sixth nerve rootlets; PT, pyramidal tract. B, Potential change in left PPRF (top trace) during saccadic eye movement to left (middle trace). EMG of left lateral rectus muscle is shown in bottom trace. C, D, Potential changes in right PPRF during saccades (C) and during quick phases of caloric nystagmus (D). The time base is 20 msec for B and 100 msec for C, D. The vertical bar is 100 μV for PPRF recordings and 30° of deviation for the EOG. (From Cohen & Feldman, J. Neurophysiol., 31 (1968) 806-817.)

ever, the temporal sequence seems wrong since saccadic suppression begins before the onset of eye movement (36, 39) and the LGB and calcarine potential changes occur only after a rapid eye movement has begun.

Another possibility is that these responses are part of a mechanism by which the reticular formation signals to the thalamus and visual cortex that a rapid eye movement has occurred (36, 39). It is of interest that slow eye movements, i.e., pursuit movements or slow phases of nystagmus, do not induce these potential changes. Presumably the visual system has adequate incoming information during slow eye movements which precludes the necessity for this type of response.

ACKNOWLEDGMENTS

Supported by NINDS Research Grants NS-00294 and 1K3-34,987. These experiments were done in conjunction with Martin D. Feldman, M.D.

REFERENCES

1 ARDEN, G.B., and SODERBERG, U. The transfer of optic information through the lateral geniculate body of the rabbit. In: Principles of Sensory Communication, W. Rosenblith (Ed.), Cambridge Technology Press, Cambridge, Massachusetts, 1961, pp. 521-544.

2 BIZZI, E., and BROOKS, D.C. Functional connections between pontine reticular formation and lateral geniculate nucleus during deep sleep, Arch. ital. Biol., 101 (1963) 666-680.

3 BREMER, F., and STOUPEL, N. Facilitation et inhibition des potentiels évoques corticaux dans l'eveil cerebral, Arch. int. Physiol. Biochem., 67 (1959) 240-275.

4 BROOKS, D.C. Localization and characteristics of the cortical waves associated with eye movement in the cat, Exp. Neurol., 22 (1968) 603-613.

5 BROOKS, D.C. Waves associated with eye movement in the awake and sleeping cat, Electroenceph. clin. Neurophysiol., 24 (1968) 532-541.

6 COHEN, B. Vestibulo-ocular relations. In: The Control of Eye Movements, P. Bach-y-Rita and C.C. Collins (Eds.), Academic Press, New York, 1971, pp. 105-148.

7 COHEN, B., and FELDMAN, M. Relationship of electrical activity in pontine reticular formation and lateral geniculate body to rapid eye movements, J. Neurophysiol., 31 (1968) 806-817.

8 COHEN, B., and FELDMAN, M. Potential changes associated with rapid eye movement in the calcarine cortex, Exp. Neurol., 31 (1971) 100-113.

9 COHEN, B., FELDMAN, M., and DIAMOND, S.P. Effects of eye movement, brainstem stimulation, and alertness on transmission through lateral geniculate body of monkey, J. Neurophysiol., 32 (1969) 583-594.

10 COHEN, B., GOTO, K., and TOKUMASU, K. Return eye movements, an ocular compensatory reflex in the alert cat and monkey, Exp. Neurol., 17 (1967) 172-185.

11 COWEY, A. Projection of the retina on to striate and prestriate cortex in the squirrel monkey, Saimiri Sciureus, J. Neurophysiol., 27 (1964) 366-392.

12 DEECKE, L., SCHEID, P., and KORNHUBER, H.H. Distribution of readiness potential, pre-motion positivity, and motor potential of the human cerebral cortex preceding voluntary finger movements, Exp. Brain Res., 7 (1969) 158-168.

13 DODGE, R. The illusion of clear vision during eye movement, Psychol. Bull., 2 (1905) 193-199.

14 DOTY, R.W., KIMURA, D.S., and MOGENSON, G.J. Photically and electrically elicited responses in the central visual system of the squirrel monkey, Exp. Neurol., 10 (1964) 19-51.

15 EVANS, C.C. Spontaneous excitation of the visual cortex and association areas. Lambda waves. Electroenceph. clin. Neurophysiol., 5 (1953) 69-74.

16 FELDMAN, M., and COHEN, B. Electrical activity in the lateral geniculate body of the alert monkey associated with eye movements, J. Neurophysiol., 31 (1968) 455-466.

17 FUCHS, A.F., and KORNHUBER, H.H. Extraocular muscle afferents to the cerebellum of the cat, J. Physiol. (Lond.), 200 (1969) 713-722.

18 GASTAUT, H., ALVIN-COSTA, C., GASTAUT, Y., and ALVIN-COSTA, M.R. Méchanisme des potentiels occipitaux évoques par les mouvements saccadés des yeux, Acta physiol. pharmacol. neerl. 6 (1957) 515-525.

19 GOTO, K., TOKUMASU, K., and COHEN, B. Return eye movements, saccadic movements, and the quick phase of nystagmus, Acta oto-laryng. (Stockh.), 65 (1968) 426-440.

20 GROETHUYSEN, U.C., and BICKFORD, R.G. Study of the lambda-wave response of human beings, Electroenceph. clin. Neurophysiol., 8 (1956) 344.

21 GROSS, E.G., VAUGHAN, H.G., and VALENSTEIN, E. Inhibition of visual evoked responses to patterned stimuli during voluntary eye movements, Electroenceph. clin. Neurophysiol., 22 (1967) 204-209.

22 HOREL, J.A., and VIERCK, C.J. Jr. Average evoked responses and learning, Science 158 (1967) 394.

23 HUGHES, J.R. Responses from the visual cortex of unanesthetized monkeys, Int. Rev. Neurobiol., 7 (1964) 99-152.

24 JEANNEROD, M., and SAKAI, K. Occipital and geniculate potentials related to eye movements in the unanesthetized cat, Brain Research, 19 (1970) 361-377.

25 JOUVET, M. Recherches sur les structures nerveuses et les méchanismes responsables des differéntes phases du sommeil physiologique, Arch. ital. Biol., 100 (1962) 125-206.

26 MAFFEI, L., MORUZZI, G., and RIZZOLATTI, G. Influence of sleep and wakefulness on the response of lateral geniculate units to sinewave photic stimulation, Arch. ital. Biol., 103 (1965) 596-608.

27 MARCHIAFAVA, P.L., and POMPEIANO, O. Enhanced excitability of intrageniculate optic tract endings produced by vestibular volleys, Arch. ital. Biol., 104 (1966) 459-479.

28 MEULDERS, M., COLLE, J., and GODFRAIND, J.M. Evoked sensory responses of somatic origin in the lateral geniculate body, Arch. int. Physiol., 72 (1964)

346-348.
29 MOURET, J., JEANNEROD, M., and JOUVET, M. L'activité électrique du système visuel au cours de la phase paradoxale du sommeil chez le chat, J. Physiol. (Paris), 55 (1963) 305-306.
30 OGAWA, T. Midbrain reticular influences upon single neurons in lateral geniculate nucleus, Science, 139 (1963) 343-344.
31 PRIBRAM, K.H., SPINELLI, D.N., and KAMBACK, M.C. Electrocortical correlates of stimulus response and reinforcement, Science, 157 (1967) 94-96.
32 ROTH, M., and GREEN, J. The lambda wave as a normal physiological phenomenon in the human electroencephalogram, Nature (Lond.), 172 (1953) 864-866.
33 RUCHKIN, D.S., and JOHN, E.R. Evoked potential correlates of generalization, Science, 153 (1966) 209-211.
34 SCOTT, D.F., GROETHUYSEN, V.C., and BICKFORD, R.G. Lambda responses in the human electroencephalogram, Neurology (Minneap.), 17 (1967) 770-778.
35 SCOTT, D.F., LICHTENHELD, F.R., and BICKFORD, R.G. Lambda-wave studies on the EEG of animals, Arch. Neurol. (Chic.), 18 (1968) 574-582.
36 SPERRY, R.W. Neural basis of the spontaneous optokinetic response produced by visual inversion, J. Comp. physiol. Psychol., 43 (1950) 482-489.
37 SUZUKI, H., and TAIRA, M. Effect of reticular stimulation upon synaptic transmission in cat's lateral geniculate body, Jap. J. Physiol., 11 (1961) 641-655.
38 VOLKMANN, F.C. Vision during voluntary saccadic eye movements, J. opt. Soc. Am., 52 (1962) 571-578.
39 VON HOLST, E., and MITTELSTEDT, H. Das Reafferenzprincip., Naturwissenschaften, 37 (1950) 464-476.
40 WURTZ, R.H. Response of striate cortex neurons to stimuli during rapid eye movements in the monkey, J. Neurophysiol., 32 (1969) 975-986.
41 ZUBER, B.L., and STARK, L. Saccadic suppression: elevation of visual threshold associated with saccadic eye movements, Exp. Neurol., 16 (1966) 65-79.

DISCUSSION

PURPURA:

I would like to ask Dr. Cohen a question concerning the PGO waves, a component of which is recordable from the geniculate. What cellular elements are involved in their production? It would seem that the principal cells of the lateral geniculate are not the source of these waves in view of negative findings following stimulation of lower brain stem reticular regions and recording intracellularly from LGB neurons. Bowsher has described a pathway to the LGB from more rostral brain stem regions and perhaps this is where such a direct pathway to LGB arises. Of course there could be multisynaptic pathways ascending in the brain stem to this site. The question remains, however, what does the PGO wave mean in relation to transmissional characteristics in the relay projection system at the LGB level?

COHEN:

This is an important question because LGB is the most obvious place where extra-visual structures might influence transmission of visual information before it reaches the visual cortex. If the LGB responses associated with eye movement have functional importance, then they should be associated with changes in neural activity. There are at least two distinct influences which ascend to LGB from the brain stem reticular formation (1). One is associated with alerting, the other with rapid eye movement. A wealth of evidence shows that processes associated with alerting modify transmission through LGB. Recently Fukuda and Iwama (2) have demonstrated that facilitation caused by arousal is probably due to inhibition of inhibitory interneurons in LGB which in turn causes dysinhibition of geniculo-calcarine relay cells.

There have been conflicting reports on the effects of eye movements on activity of LGB neurons or on transmission of visual information through LGB. Michael and Ichinose (5) found no effect of eye movement on LGB units. However, other authors disagree (4, 6, 9), and I will mention two of these studies in greater detail.

Jeannerod and Putkonen (4) have recently demonstrated that 42 of 81 LGB neurons which were studied in the cat changed firing rates 40-200 msec after the onset of eye movements in darkness. Fig. 1A, from their paper, shows a phasic increase in activity in an LGB neuron. The top trace is the EOG and the second trace is the integrated neuronal discharge. Other LGB neurons were inhibited at the same time (Fig. 1B). Montero and Robles (9) found similar effects of eye movement on LGB neuronal activity in the rat. There was a partial decrease in activity of concentric cells to stationary or moving light stimuli from 30-40 msec to 120-200 msec after the onset of eye movement. Such a change in cellular response is shown by the bar histo grams in Fig. 1C. 0 denotes the onset of the saccades. Shortly thereafter there was a decrease in the amount of activity (downward arrow). Two on-off units which were studied showed an increase in discharge frequency at that time. The histogram of one of these units is shown by the solid black portion of Fig. 1C, and the increase in discharge frequency by the white upward arrow. Two cells which gave high frequency on-responses throughout the receptive fields and were dependent on light intensity were unaffected by saccades.

These results indicate that activity associated with rapid eye movements does modify the behavior of various types of LGB cells. Moreover, it apparently does so in different ways. Those cells which are directly involved in the transmission pathway from retina to visual cortex appear to have a reduction in activity during eye movements, whereas cells which are most likely inhibitory interneurons in LGB are activated.

Thus, there are probably two separate mechanisms by which changes in visual threshold are effected during saccades. Movements of images at certain velocities on the retina causes inhibition of cells in the visual pathway (3), and an increase in threshold of light perception (7, 8). Secondly, it would appear that there is also activation of inhibitory interneurons in LGB, probably under control of the brain stem,

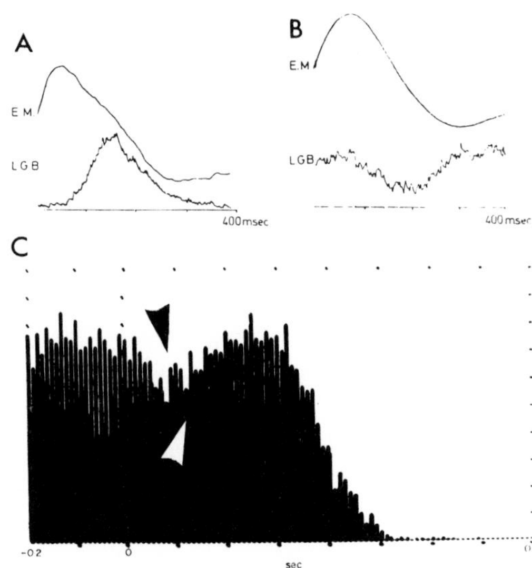

FIG. 1. A, Phasic increase in discharge rate of a lateral geniculate neuron associated with saccades in the dark. The upper trace shows the averaged EOG's of 30 saccades and the lower trace the lower trace the integrated spike discharges. B, Phasic decreases in another LGB neuron during 30 saccades in darkness. (Adapted from M. Jeannerod and P.T.S. Putkonen, Exp. Brain Res., 13 (1971) 533-546. Courtesy Springer-Verlag.)

C, Superimposed post fast-phase histograms obtained from responses of an on-center LGB unit (lighter region) and an on-off LGB unit (darker region). These graphs show the reciprocal relationship between the firing patterns of both responses. The black downward arrow points to the decrease in response of the concentric cell and the white upward arrow to the concurrent increase in activity of the on-off cell. (Adapted from V.M. Montero and L. Robles, Vision Res., Suppl., 3 (1971) 253-268. Courtesy Pergammon Press.)

which may cause post-synaptic inhibition of geniculo-calcarine relay cells (9). More work is necessary, however, before we understand how important these mechanisms are in reducing perception of rapid eye movements or in producing saccadic suppression. It is clear that activity associated with eye movements also reaches the visual cortex and affects neuronal activity there as well (10).

REFERENCES

1 COHEN, B., FELDMAN, M., and DIAMOND, S.P. Effects of eye movement, brain stem stimulation, and alertness on transmission through lateral geniculate body of monkey, J. Neurophysiol., 32 (1969) 583-594.

2 FUKUDA, Y., and IWAMA, K. Reticular inhibition of internuncial cells in the rat lateral geniculate body, Brain Research, 35 (1971) 107-118.

3 HAYASHI, Y. Terminal depolarization of intrageniculate optic tract fibers produced by moving visual stimulus, Brain Research, (1972, in press).

4 JEANNEROD, M., and PUTKONEN, P.T.S. Lateral geniculate unit activity and eye movements: Saccade-locked changes in dark and in light, Exp. Brain Res., 13 (1971) 533-546.

5 MICHAEL, J.S., and ICHINOSE, L.Y. Influence of oculomotor activity on visual processing, Brain Research, 22 (1970) 249-253.

6 LOMBROSO, C.T., and CORAZZA, R. Central visual discharge time-locked with spontaneous eye movements in the cat, Nature (Lond.), 230 (1971) 464-467.

7 MACKAY, D.M. Elevation of visual threshold by displacement of retinal image, Nature (Lond.), 225 (1970) 90-92.

8 MACKAY, D.M. Interocular transfer of suppressive effects of retinal image displacement, Nature (Lond.), 225 (1970) 872-873.

9 MONTERO, V.M. and ROBLES, L. Saccadic modulation of cell discharges in the lateral geniculate nucleus, Vision Res., Suppl., 3 (1971) 253-263.

10 NODA, H., FREEMAN, R.B. Jr., and CREUTZFELDT, O.D. Neuronal correlates of eye movements in the visual cortex of the cat, Science, 175 (1972) 661-663.

Corticothalamic Projections and Sensorimotor Activities
T. Frigyesi, E. Rinvik, and M.D. Yahr, editors. © 1972
Raven Press, New York.

Differential Control of Motor Cortex and Sensory Areas on Ventrolateral Nucleus of the Thalamus

J. Massion and L. Rispal-Padel

The ventrolateral nucleus of the thalamus (VL) is known to be the main relay for the pallidal and cerebellar efferents to the motor cortex. It has been shown in the cat that this nucleus is controlled by two types of cortical areas. Some cortical areas affect the VL only ipsilaterally, whereas others have bilateral effects (6).

The cortical area which exerts an ipsilateral effect on the VL nucleus, i.e., the pericruciate motor cortex, is also the receiving area for projections from the VL (16, 35). Fibers originating in the same area end in VL (2, 12, 13, 23-25). Excitatory as well as inhibitory effects are induced by stimulation of this area, as has been shown by many physiological studies (3, 6, 8, 11, 21, 22, 26, 27, 34, 37).

The areas with bilateral effects on VL correspond roughly to the cortical sensory areas. These areas exert an excitatory as well as inhibitory control, with some degree of topographic organization. The pathway for these effects is indirect and includes at least one intermediary relay. The connections which are shown to exist between the sensory areas and VL represent one of the possible pathways by which sensory messages could act on the motor cortex and from there influence the musculature.

The present topic will be restricted primarily to the study of the relations between the motor area and VL. Despite the fact that many studies have been devoted to this problem, it seemed to be of some interest to investigate one relatively neglected aspect, namely, the organization of corticothalamic relations with respect to different parts of the motor area controlling axial, proximal and distal muscles. This study was based on a theoretical approach similar to that of Kuypers (14), who examined the control exerted by cortical and subcortical structures on axial, proximal and distal muscles.

METHODS

The experiments were performed on over 80 adult cats anesthetized with chloralose (80 mg/Kg) and paralyzed with Flaxedil. In most of the experiments, extracellu-

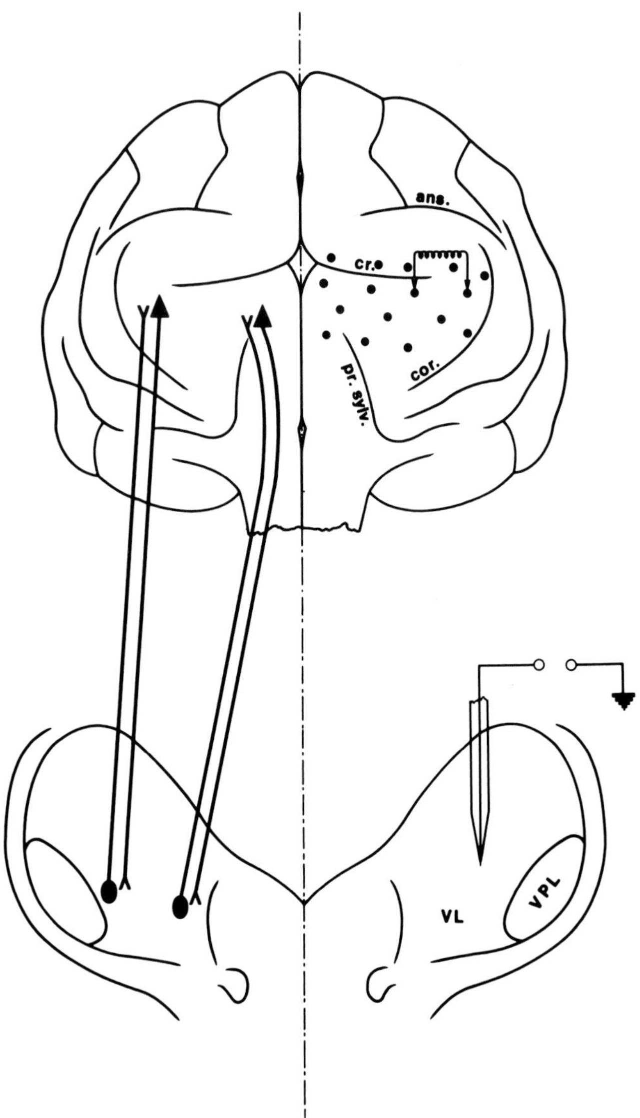

FIG. 1. Schematic representation of the experimental procedure. cr.: cruciate sulcus; cor.: sulcus coronalis; ans.: ansate sulcus; pr. sylv.: presylvian sulcus; VL: ventrolateral nucleus; VPL: ventroposterolateral nucleus.

lar recording of unitary activity of VL was obtained by means of tungsten microelectrodes with an impedance of 15-20 MΩ.

In order to stimulate the different parts of the motor cortex, nickel-chrome electrodes, varnished except at their tips, were placed intracortically at a depth of 1.5 mm, through tiny trephine holes separated from each other by 2 mm. Ten such electrodes were implanted in a first series (26), and 16 in a second series of experiments. In the second series, of the 16 electrodes used, twelve were placed in the precruciate and four in the postcruciate area (Fig. 1). Each electrode was cemented to the bone. The stimulation (3 shocks of 0.5 msec., 300 /sec., 150 μA) was applied by means of a constant current stimulator to the electrodes, connected in pairs; an electrode was successively cathode and anode. When a thalamic response was evoked by stimulation through a pair of electrodes, the stimulating current was progressively reduced until the response disappeared to determine the weakest current which could elicit the response (i.e., the threshold). Only responses with a threshold lower than 120 μA were retained for these experiments.

To test the inhibitory effect induced by cortical stimulation, a test shock was applied to the brachium conjunctivum, the nucleus interpositus posterior or to the dentate nucleus. The threshold as well as the latency of the inhibitory effect were systematically measured. Responses with a threshold lower than 120 μA and a latency shorter than 10 ms were used for this mapping study. Recordings were made in the first series of experiments (20 cats) with fine concentric bipolar electrodes to obtain a rough idea of the distribution of the inhibitory effects within the nucleus. In the second series of experiments (15 cats), the inhibitory effects were tested at the unitary level.

After each experiment, the brain was perfused with formalin and photographed to localize with precision the sites of the cortical stimulating electrodes. Electrolytic lesions were made at the points of the deepest penetration of the microelectrodes and at the tips of the cerebellar stimulating electrodes, and histological sections stained with Nissl method were prepared.

RESULTS

Three aspects of the relations between motor cortex and VL nucleus were considered: 1. the organization of the projections from VL to motor cortex; 2. the organization of the excitatory projections from motor cortex to VL; and 3. the organization and the mechanisms of the inhibitory corticothalamic effects.

1. Organization of the Thalamocortical Projections.

The organization of the thalamocortical projections was determined by recording in VL antidromic spikes induced by stimulation of the axon terminals at the cortical level. Three tests were used to differentiate antidromic invasion from orthodromic effects (Fig. 2). First, a fixed latency of the spike, even after three shocks at 300/sec; second, the presence of partial spikes; third, a collision between orthodromic and antidromic spikes (5).

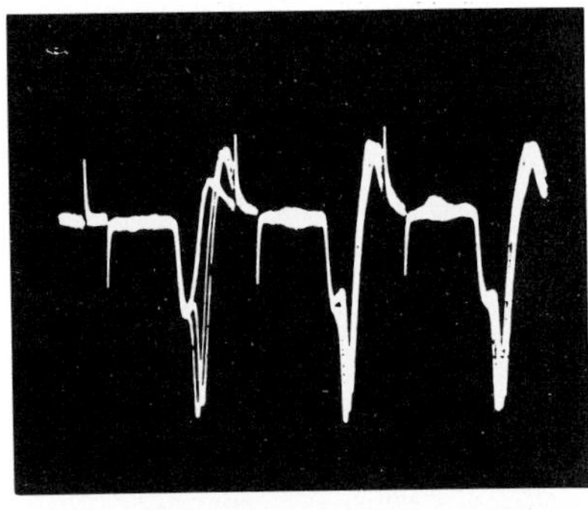

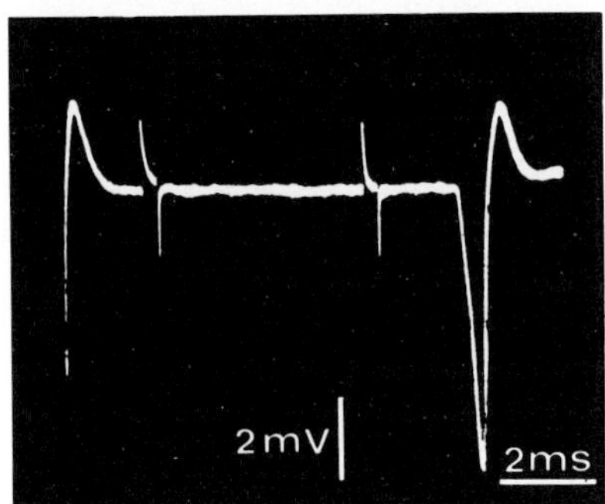

FIG. 2. Antidromic spike criteria. Extracellular unitary response of a VL neuron to stimulation of a cortical area. Five sweeps have been superimposed. Upper sweeps: cortical stimulation at 300/sec. The response after each shock is followed by a spike with a constant latency. Notice the presence of partial spikes. Lower sweep: a "spontaneous" spike triggers both the sweep and the stimulator. The stimulator delivers, with some delay, two cortical shocks. The response to the first is occluded by collision, whereas the antidromic spike follows the second shock with a constant latency. These recordings and those in the following figures were obtained from cats anesthetized with chloralose.

Positive results on the first and at least on one of the two other tests were considered a sufficient criterion for identification of antidromic spikes.

The proportion of identified thalamocortical neurons was found to be very small (1/40), even taking into account the second series of experiments when 16 instead of 10 cortical electrodes were used.

These experiments were designed to answer two questions. First, are the neurons projecting from the VL nucleus to the motor cortex arranged in a topographically distinct way for the control of axial, proximal and distal muscles? Second, is the projecting area of an individual VL neuron very restricted or somewhat diffuse?

With regard to the first question, a rough mediolateral topography of the projecting neurons has been demonstrated. The medial neurons project mainly to area 6 (axial, neck and face motor areas) and the adjacent part of area 4; the most lateral ones project to the part of area 4 which controls the distal muscles. But there is an important overlapping (Fig. 3 and 4). Our results are in consonance with the anatomical findings of Strick (35).

Although most of the VL neurons were found to project to one point in the motor area, 8 of the 29 neurons were shown to project to two, three or even four cortical sites. In our opinion, these neurons with bifurcating axons could be much more numerous than indicated by our results, because they were much more easily found in experiments where 16 cortical stimulating electrodes were used than in experiments in which

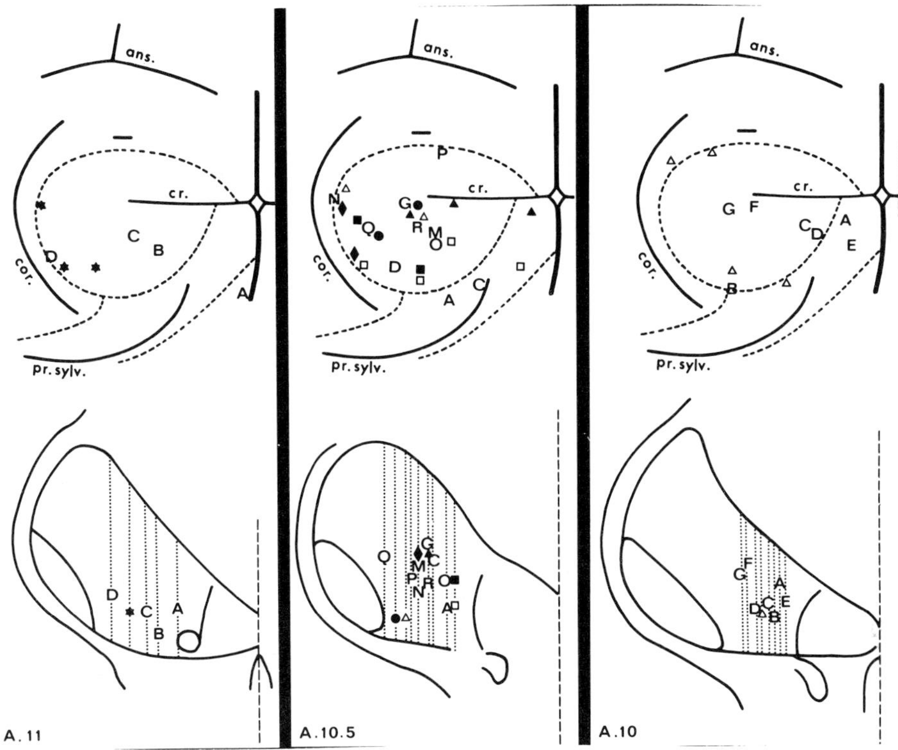

FIG. 3. Topography of the thalamocortical projections. The localization of each thalamic unit from which an antidromic response was recorded is represented by a letter when only one cortical projecting site was identified, and with a symbol for the cells with branching axons. Corresponding letters or symbols on the diagram of the cortex indicate the location of the stimulating electrodes responsible for the antidromic spike. The dotted lines on the thalamic diagram indicate the electrode tracts for each exploration when an antidromic spike was recorded.

only 10 electrodes were used. Moreover, an important part of area 4 and 6, in the depth of the cruciate sulcus (10), has not been explored. In a comparison of the distribution of axonal branching to the organization of cortical motor control according to Woolsey (38), VL units were found to project simultaneously to motor areas for axial and proximal muscles, proximal and distal muscles, neck (or face) and proximal, and neck (or face) and distal muscles (Fig. 5).

These cells with branching axons are not an unexpected finding. As shown by Strick (35), the projecting area from one restricted part of the VL is relatively large. From a functional point of view, these cells should play an important role in motor

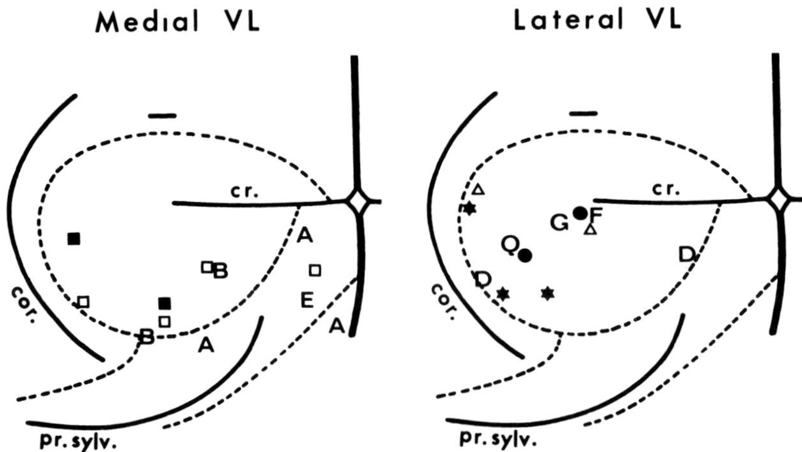

FIG.4. Mediolateral topography of the thalamocortical projections. Two diagrams of the motor area are presented, in which area 6 (anteromedial) and area 4 (around the cruciate sulcus) are delimited by stripped lines according to Hassler and Muhs-Clement (10). On the left the cortical projections for the most medial neurons of each thalamic stereotaxic plane, (2 for A 11, 3 for A 10.5 and 3 for A 10) have been represented with the same letters or symbols as in figure 3. On the right, the projections are for the most lateral thalamic neurons (2 for A 11, 3 for A 10.5 and 3 for A 10). Notice that the projection areas for the lateral and medial neurons are different but show some overlap. The cortical area covered by the lateral neurons corresponds mainly to the forelimb area (to be compared with the cortical motor representation of figure 5), whereas the area covered by the medial neurons covers area 6 and the adjacent part of area 4 (axial, neck, face, and proximal limb)motor areas.

function. Since connections between VL and motor cortex are obviously involved in the central organization of movement, these branching axons represent an anatomical substrate for the organization of complex movements involving the participation of muscles of different segments of the same limb or even of different parts of the body.

2. Corticothalamic Excitatory Effects.

Various authors have shown that stimulation of motor cortex evokes short-latency excitatory responses at the level of VL (vide supra). In our study, the corticothalamic excitatory effects were reexamined in the population of cells identified as projecting to the cortex to determine whether the corticothalamic responses parallel the thalamo-

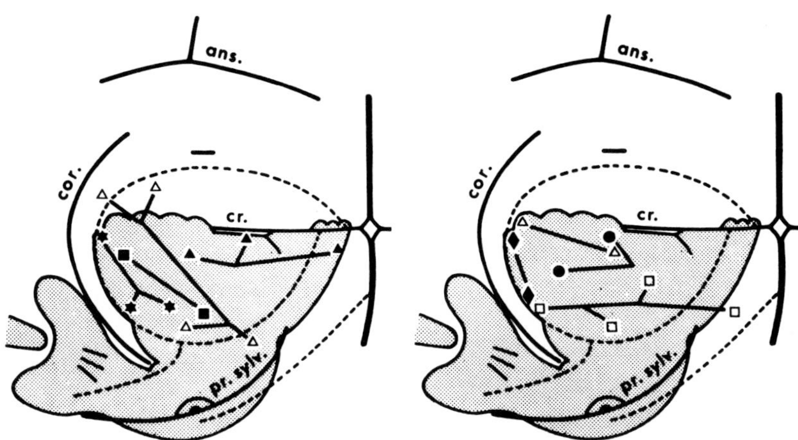

FIG.5. Extension of axonal branching. Eight identified neurons with branching axons are shown. The cortical sites from which antidromic spikes could be evoked for the same cell are indicated by the same symbols and linked by a line. The limits of areas 6 and 4 are indicated by interrupted lines as in Fig.4. Ans.:ansate sulcus; cor.:coronal sulcus;cr.:cruciate sulcus; pr.sylv.:presylvian sulcus. The shadowed area indicates a map of cortical motor representation following Woolsey(38): the neck and face areas are located in front of the cruciate sulcus in the vicinity of the presylvian sulcus, the forelimb motor area can be seen between the lateral end of the cruciate sulcus and the coronal sulcus, a restricted part of the hindlimb area is located behind the cruciate sulcus, near the midline, and the axial motor area can be seen in the median precruciate area(an important part of the motor area lies in the depth of the cruciate sulcus).

cortical projections.

The distribution of the corticothalamic responses (frequently a short burst of spikes) was shown to parallel exactly the distribution of the thalamocortical projections and the orthodromic responses of the cells were always (except in two cases) preceded by an antidromic spike (Fig. 6). These observations suggest that the orthodromic responses are produced by way of axonal recurrent collaterals inside VL (Fig. 7 A).

Our results differ slightly from those of Sakata et al. (27) and Uno et al. (37), on the VL and of Shimazu et al. (32), on the ventroposterolateral nucleus. These authors obtained post-synaptic spikes by stimulation of cortical points which induced antidromic spikes as well as by stimulation of the surrounding cortical areas. The discrepancies might be due to the fact that these authors used subcortical instead of intracortical stimulating electrodes, exciting a relatively greater number of corticothalamic fibers from adjacent or distant cortical areas. This suggests that some degree of spatial summation is needed to provoke an efferent spike discharge of VL cells by way of the corticothalamic fiber system. Thus it is highly probable that two excitatory systems coexist; one, the recurrent collateral excitatory system, the other, the corticothalamic excitatory fiber system (Figs. 7 A and B).

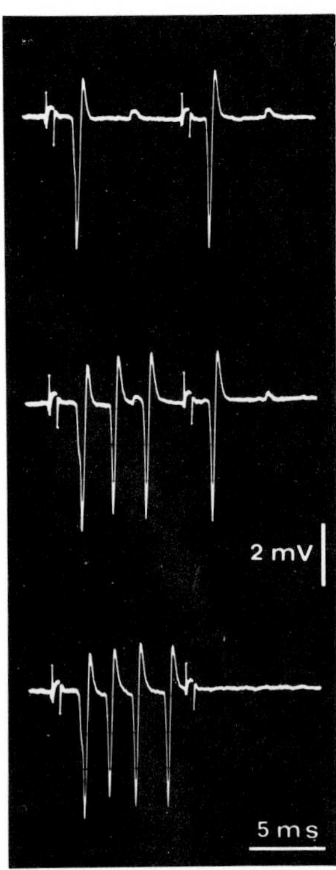

FIG. 6. Orthodromic response. Two stimulations of one point in the motor area; each evokes an antidromic spike in a VL unit (upper sweep). The first antidromic spike is followed by an orthodromic response (middle sweep). The last orthodromic spike prevents (by collision) the appearance of the second antidromic spike (lower sweep).

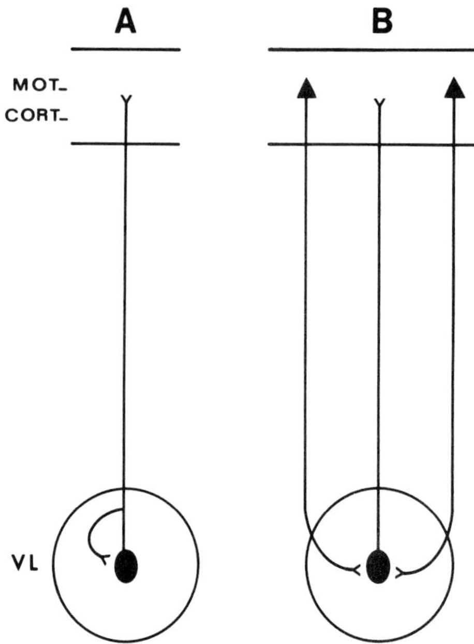

FIG. 7. Possible mechanisms for orthodromic activation of VL neurons.

The functional significance of the excitatory corticothalamic effects is still a matter of speculation. As far as the recurrent collateral excitatory system is concerned, it is suggested that it could play a role in producing the short burst of spikes which, in alternation with long lasting hyperpolarization, characterizes the rhythmic activities of thalamic cells. On the other hand, the corticothalamic excitatory fiber system represents a positive feedback mechanism, similar to that observed in other structures, such as in the cerebellar nuclei (36). This kind of circuit may favor some tonic activity at the VL level and also at the level of the pyramidal cells. Such a circuit may also play a role in phasic activity by prolonging the duration of the activation induced by a brief triggering afferent message. Since spatial summation seems to be required to excite the VL neurons by way of the corticothalamic fiber system, it is suggested that two distinct regions in the motor area must be activated at the same time to initiate the activity of a given VL unit through this fiber system. The activity of the unit would then be associated with a given pattern of motor cortical activation and, thus, with a given pattern of movement.

Figure 8 explains the theoretical basis of the mechanism proposed (which also applies to the corticothalamic inhibitory effects). Let us consider, for instance, a cell

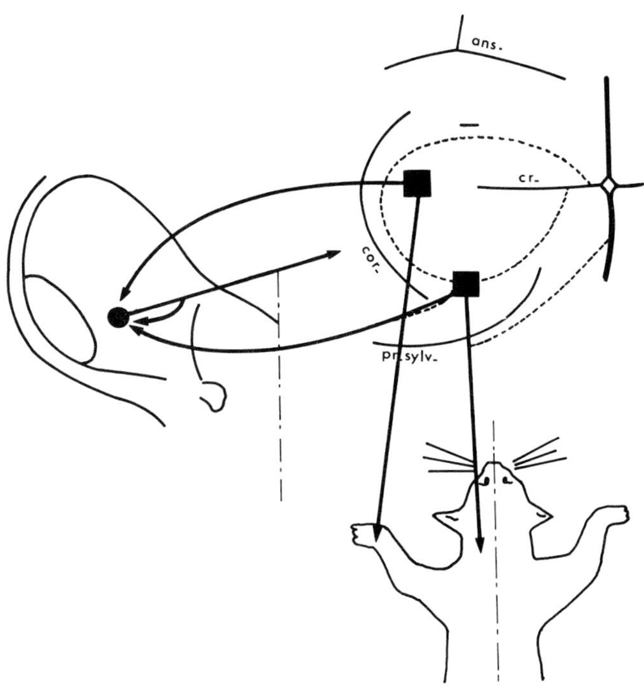

FIG. 8. Spatial convergence of corticothalamic influences. Its possible action on VL unit activity (see text).

in VL projecting to some part of the motor cortex, and receiving corticothalamic fibers from distal limb and neck motor area. If an isolated distal movement occurs, the corticothalamic effects from the corresponding part of the motor area would be insufficient to excite the VL cell. This would be obtained if only a neck movement is produced. But during simultaneous movements of the distal limb and the neck, spatial summation of the corticothalamic effects from both parts of the motor area would be effective in activating the VL neurons. In this way, the activity of a given VL neuron would depend on a given pattern of cortical activation and thus a given pattern of movement.

3. Corticothalamic Inhibitory Effects.

Stimulation of the motor cortex induces in VL inhibitory as well as excitatory effects as we have seen (see Introduction). When intracellular recordings are made, the response consists of long lasting hyperpolarizations rhythmically recurring in alternation with brief bursts of spikes. This kind of effect has been described for cats anesthetized with chloralose or with nembutal and for unanesthetized preparations.

Our present study of corticothalamic inhibitory effects was centered on two problems. First, are the corticothalamic inhibitory effects topographically organized? Second, what could be the anatomical substrate for the inhibitory effect?

In answer to the first question, it was shown that the corticothalamic inhibitory effects are not diffusely distributed throughout the VL. However, there is significant spatial convergence. An example of spatial convergence of the inhibitory effects was shown in a previous work (6, Fig. 3), where an intracellular, long lasting hyperpolarization was induced by stimulation of two distinct areas of the precruciate cortex. In the present experiments, the inhibitory effects induced by cortical stimulation were tested through the responses of VL units to cerebellar stimulation (see Methods). Figure 9 shows an example of the cortical distribution of the inhibitory point for various VL units recorded during the same penetration. Despite the fact that the inhibitory points occupied a wide area of the motor cortex, none of them was found in the medial part of the precruciate cortex.

The inhibitory effects on VL cells can be graded by two factors, i.e., the intensity of cortical stimulation and the spatial convergence from different points in the motor area. It seems, therefore, highly probable that the inhibition of a given VL neuron will depend on the pattern of activation of the motor area and thus on the pattern of movement.

The second problem was the anatomical substrate of the inhibitory effects on VL neurons. Different mechanisms have been proposed: local inhibitory interneurons (1), neurons from the intralaminar nuclei sending collaterals to VL and neurons of the nucleus reticularis thalami. With regard to the last, Scheibel and Scheibel (28, 29) have shown with Golgi material that the axons of this nucleus do not project to the cortex, but branch inside the thalamus. Using a retrograde degeneration technique, Minderhoud (19) recently confirmed the Scheibels' evidence concerning the course and topographical arrangement of the projections from the n. reticularis to the dorsal thalamus.

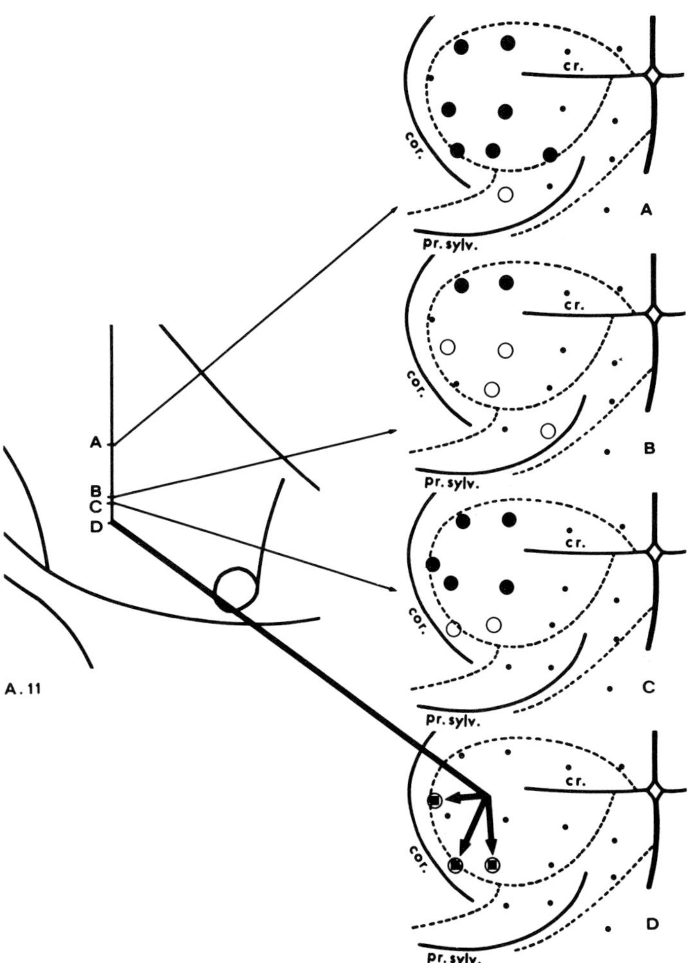

FIG. 9. Cortical distribution of sites eliciting inhibitory effects in various VL neurons.
During an exploration of VL, 4 units responding to cerebellar stimulation were recorded. Their locations within the nucleus are shown on the left part of the figure. On the right, four diagrams of the cat's motor area indicate the locations of the stimulating electrodes (dots) for each of the 4 cells shown on the left. The location of the inhibitory effects occurring with a latency shorter than 10 msec (black circles) and the location of the inhibitory effects with a latency of 10–15 msec (white circles) are also indicated. Neuron D was identified as projecting to 3 cortical points (black squares). The large distribution of the inhibitory effects can be compared to the location of the axon terminals of neuron D, and the lack of effect from the medial part of the precruciate cortex noted.

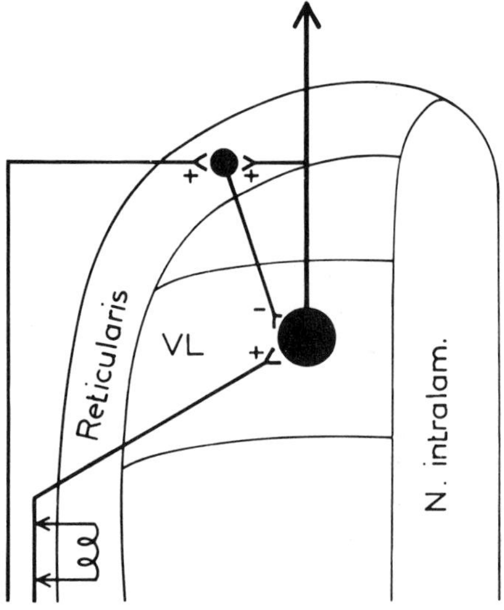

FIG. 10

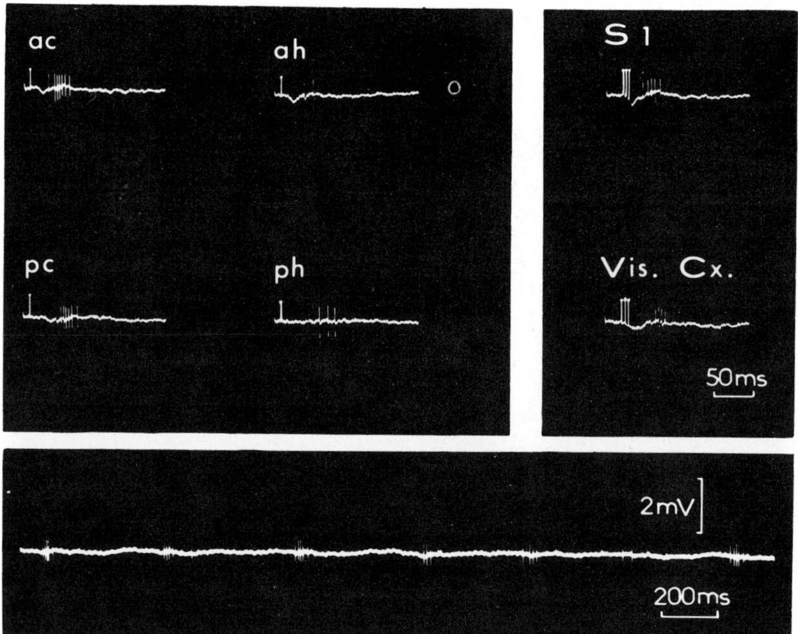

FIG. 11

The concept that the n. reticularis could serve as an inhibitory relay for the thalamic cells was proposed by Scheibel and Scheibel (28) and by one of us (17, 18). The physiological evidence was indirect and based on the fact that cells in n. reticularis are active at the time when VL cells should be inhibited (Fig. 10). The first suggestive evidence comes from observations of the spontaneous activity of VL and n. reticularis cells under chloralose anesthesia. The VL cells show a low frequency (2-5/sec) rhythmic activity (alternation of long lasting hyperpolarizations and short bursts of spikes) (18). The cells in nucleus reticularis also show a rhythmic activity of a similar frequency (2-5/sec) (Fig. 11). Moreover the pattern of discharge resembles the activity expected from inhibitory neurons, and could be responsible for the long lasting rhythmic hyperpolarization of VL neurons. The second argument is derived from the effect of sensory or cortical stimulation on the neurons of both nuclei. Hyperpolarization of VL cells, rhythmically recurring in alternation with short bursts of spikes can be elicited by sensory stimulation or by stimulation of cortical sensory areas (6, 18). The activity of the inhibitory neurons responsible for these rhythmic hyperpolarizations should be a short latency train of spikes, rhythmically recurring, in response to sensory or cortical stimulation. This is in fact the case (Fig. 11). Figure 12 suggests a close relation between a cell in n. reticularis and an adjacent cell in ventroposterolateral nucleus. Both responded selectively to stimulation of the same limb. The cell in n. reticularis showed a train of spikes with short latency. The cell in VPL responded with a long-latency burst of spikes which is known to be preceded by short-latency long lasting hyperpolarization, only seen in intracellular records.

With regard to the inhibitory effects induced by stimulation of the motor area on VL cells, some arguments can be presented which also favor the notion that cells in n. reticularis inhibit VL cells. Notably, one of the cells recorded in the anteroventral part of the reticularis responded with a short-latency train of spikes to stimulation of three of the 16 cortical points, one located in the medial part of area 4, and two in the adjacent part of area 6 (Fig. 13). These topically arranged cortical effects are consonant with the topical arrangement of the inhibitory effects evoked by

---

FIG. 10. N. reticularis as an inhibitory relay for VL neurons. Diagram shows the possible actions of an afferent input to VL neurons, directly or indirectly, by way of n. reticularis.

FIG. 11. Spontaneous and evoked activity of a unit in n. reticularis. This unit (recorded in n. reticularis) presents a spontaneous rhythmic activity (lower trace) of the same order as the rhythmicity of VL cells. Nevertheless, the bursts of spikes are of much longer duration than those of VL units. The unit shows a short-latency response to electrical stimulation of the anterior and posterior contralateral limbs (ac, pc) and a similar but weaker response to stimulation of the homolateral limbs (ah, ph) indicating some preferential somatotopy (17, 18). The same type of short-latency response occurs to stimulation of SI and the visual cortex (Vis. Cx).

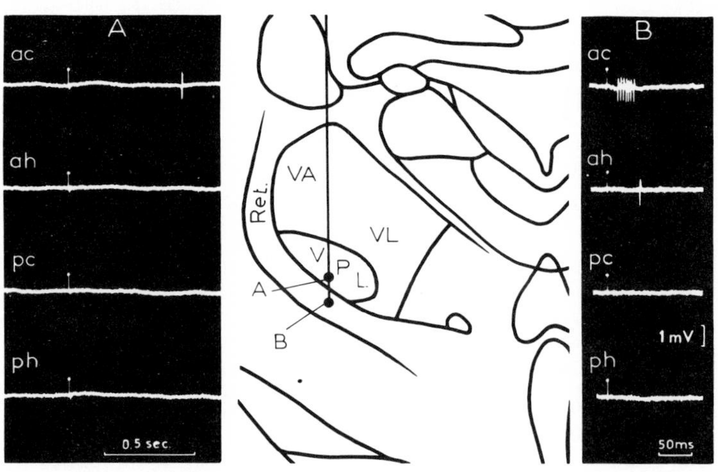
A
ac
ah
pc
ph
0.5 sec.
Ret.
VA
VL
V
P
L.
A
B
B
ac
ah
pc
1 mV
ph
50ms

FIG. 12

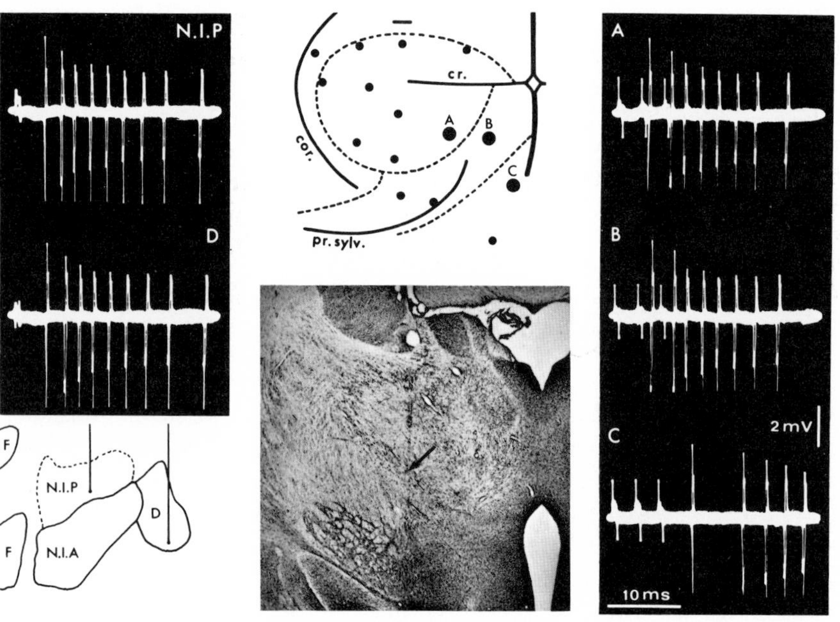
N.I.P
D
F
N.I.P
D
F
N.I.A
cr.
cor.
A
B
C
pr. sylv.
A
B
2 mV
C
10 ms

FIG. 13

cortical stimulation of VL cells and with the anatomical data on the corticoreticular connections (4).

The hypothesis concerning the inhibitory action of cells in reticularis on VL cells has now received further experimental support from various authors (7, 9, 15, 20, 30, 31, 33).

SUMMARY

Three aspects of the corticothalamic relations between the motor cortex and VL were observed in cats anesthetized with chloralose.

1. A mediolateral topography of the thalamocortical projections was observed, in which the medial VL neurons project preferentially to motor areas for axial, neck and facial musculature and the most lateral neurons project to the distal limb motor area.

2. Whereas most of the neurons project to one site within the motor cortex, some show bifurcating axons reaching two, three or even four cortical sites in distinct parts of motor areas which control different segments of one limb or even different parts of the body.

3. The orthodromic responses of VL neurons evoked by cortical stimulation were generally associated with and preceded by the antidromic invasion of the neuron. It is thought that they depend on recurrent excitatory collaterals within VL. It is our hypothesis that the corticothalamic excitatory fiber system demonstrated by other authors needs some spatial summation to be effective.

4. The inhibitory effects induced by cortical stimulation are topographically organized. Spatial summation of the inhibitory effect is thought to be an important factor in determining the degree of inhibition of a given VL neuron. This summation should occur during given patterns of movement. Various arguments have been pre-

---

FIG. 12. Evoked activity of a unit in n.reticularis in the vicinity of VPL.
The same micropipette recorded a unit in the ventroposterolateral nucleus in A, and a unit in n. reticularis in B. The unit in A (VPL) responded selectively to stimulation of the anterior contralateral leg (ac) with a long-latency burst. The unit in B which was found in n. reticularis showed a short-latency burst of spikes to stimulation of the same contralateral leg.

FIG. 13. Unit in n.reticularis responding to cortical and cerebellar stimulation.
The location of the unit recorded in n. reticularis, indicated by arrow, was determined from histological sections. Two discrete coagulations were made, one at the end of the electrode tract, the other 4 mm above. No appreciable shrinkage of the brain was found. This unit responded selectively to stimulation three of the 16 stimulating electrodes (points A, B, C). The unit responded also to a single shock applied to either n. interpositus posterior (N.I.P.) or dentate nucleus (D).

sented which suggest that n. reticularis is the locus of inhibitory neurons for VL cells.

It is obvious from these results that the VL nucleus cannot be considered as a simple relay for cerebellar and pallidal impulses to motor cortex. The elaborate patterns of relations between the motor cortex and the VL nucleus seem to be organized much less for the control of single muscles than for the control of integrated movements. However, the functioning of this complex network during movement remains to be analyzed.

ACKNOWLEDGMENT

The authors are grateful to A.M. Smith for his advice and criticism during the preparation of the manuscript. They acknowledge the technical assistance of Mrs. Devigne, Mrs. Zakarian, Mr. Haour, Mr. Massarino, and Mr. Quilici.

REFERENCES

1 ANDERSEN, P., ECCLES, J.C., and SEARS, T.A., The ventrobasal complex of the thalamus: types of cells, their responses and their functional organization, J. Physiol. (Lond.), 174 (1964) 370-399.

2 AUER, J., Terminal degeneration in the diencephalon after ablation of frontal cortex in the cat, J. Anat. (Lond.), 90 (1956) 30-41.

3 BREMER, F., Inhibitions intrathalamiques récurrentielles et physiologie du sommeil, Electroenceph. clin. Neurophysiol., 28 (1970) 1-16.

4 CARMAN, J.B., COWAN, W.M., and POWELL, T.P.S., Cortical connections of the thalamic reticular nucleus, J.Anat. (Lond.), 98 (1964) 587-598.

5 DARIAN-SMITH, I., PHILLIPS, G., RYAN, R.D., Functional organization in the trigeminal main sensory and rostral spinal nuclei of the cat, J. Physiol. (Lond.), 168 (1963) 129-146.

6 DORMONT, J.F., and MASSION, J., Duality of cortical control on ventrolateral thalamic activity, Exp. Brain Res., 10 (1970) 205-218.

7 FILION, M., LAMARRE, Y., and CORDEAU, J.P., Neuronal discharges of the ventrolateral nucleus of the thalamus during sleep and wakefulness in the cat. II. Evoked activity, Exp. Brain Res., 12 (1971) 499-508.

8 FRIGYESI, T.L., and MACHEK, J., Basal ganglia-diencephalon synaptic relations in the cat. I. An intracellular study of dorsal thalamic neurons during capsular and basal ganglia stimulation, Brain Res., 20 (1970) 201-217.

9 FRIGYESI, T.L., and SCHWARTZ, R., Cortical control of thalamic sensorimotor relay activities in the cat and squirrel monkey. In: Corticothalamic projections and sensorimotor activities, T.L. Frigyesi, E. Rinvik, and M.D. Yahr (Eds.) Raven Press, New York, 1972.

10 HASSLER, R., and MUHS-CLEMENT, K., Architektonischer Aufbau des sensomotorischen und parietalen Cortex der Katze, J. Hirnforsch., 6 (1964) 377-420.

11 HIROTA, I., YOSHIDA, M., and UNO, M., Antidromic and orthodromic responses of the thalamic ventrolateral nucleus by cortical stimulation. Cited by Eccles, J.C., Ito, M., and Szentagothai, J. The cerebellum as a neuronal

machine, p. 291. Berlin-Heidelberg-New York; Springer, 1967.
12 KAWANA, E., and KUSAMA, T., Projections from the anterior part of the coronal gyrus to the thalamus, the spinal trigeminal complex and the nucleus of the solitary tract in cats, Proc. Jap. Acad., 44 (1968) 176-181.
13 KUSAMA, T., OTANI, K., and KAWANA, E., Projections of the motor, somatic sensory, auditory and visual cortices in cats. In: Progress in Brain Research, Vol. 21, Correlative neurosciences. Part A: Fundamental mechanisms, pp. 292-322. T. Tokizane and J.P. Schadé, Eds. Amsterdam: Elsevier 1966.
14 KUYPERS, H.G.J.M., The descending pathways to the spinal cord, their anatomy and function. In: Progress in Brain Research, Vol. 11, Organization of the spinal cord, pp. 178-202. J.C. Eccles and J.P. Schadé, Eds. Amsterdam: Elsevier 1964.
15 LAMARRE, Y., FILION, M., and CORDEAU, J.P., Neuronal discharges of the ventrolateral nucleus of the thalamus during sleep and wakefulness in the cat. I. Spontaneous activity, Exp. Brain Res. 12 (1971) 480-498.
16 MACCHI, G., Organizzazione morfologica delle connessioni thalamocorticali. Atti Soc.ital.Anat. 18e Convegno sociale. Arch. ital. Biol.,Suppl. 66 (1958) 25-124.
17 MASSION, J., Le noyau ventrolatéral, structure motrice thalamique, Laval medical, 40 (1969) 411-421.
18 MASSION, J., ANGAUT, P., and ALBE-FESSARD, D., Activités évoquées chez le chat dans la région du nucleus ventralis lateralis par diverses stimulations sensorielles; II. Étude microphysiologique, Electroenceph. clin. Neurophysiol., 19 (1965) 452-469.
19 MINDERHOUD, J.M., An anatomical study of the efferent connections of the thalamic reticular nucleus, Exp. Brain Res., 12 (1971) 435-446.
20 MUKHAMETOV, L.M., RIZZOLATTI, G., and TRADARDI, V., Spontaneous activity of neurons of nucleus reticularis thalami in freely moving cats, J. Physiol. (Lond.), 210 (1970) 651-667.
21 NAKAMURA, Y., and SCHLAG, J., Cortically induced rhythmic activities in the thalamic ventrolateral nucleus of the cat, Exp. Neurol., 22 (1968) 209-221.
22 PURPURA, D.P., FRIGYESI, T.L., McMURTRY, J.G., and SCARFF, T., Synaptic mechanisms in thalamic regulation of cerebello-cortical projection activity. In: The Thalamus, Ed. by D.P. Purpura and M.D. Yahr. Columbia University, New York. 1966. pp. 153-172.
23 RINVIK, E., A re-evaluation of the cytoarchitecture of the ventral nuclear complex of the cat's thalamus on the basis of cortico-thalamic connections, Brain Research., 8 (1968) 237-254.
24 RINVIK, E., The corticothalamic projection from the pericruciate and coronal gyri in the cat. An experimental study with silver-impregnation methods, Brain Res., 10 (1968) 79-119.
25 RINVIK, E., The corticothalamic projection from the gyrus proreus and the medial wall of the rostral hemisphere in the cat. An experimental study with silver impregnation methods, Exp. Brain Res., 5 (1968) 129-152.
26 RISPAL-PADEL, L., and MASSION, J., Relations between the ventrolateral nu-

cleus and the motor cortex in the cat, Exp. Brain Res., 10 (1970) 331-339.

27 SAKATA, H., ISHIJIMA, T., and TOYADA, Y., Single unit studies on ventrolateral nucleus of the thalamus in cat: its relation to the cerebellum, motor cortex and basal ganglia, Jap. J. Physiol., 16 (1966) 42-60.

28 SCHEIBEL, M.E., and SCHEIBEL, A.B., The organization of the nucleus reticularis thalami: a Golgi study, Brain Res., 1 (1966) 43-62.

29 SCHEIBEL, M.E., and SCHEIBEL, A.B., Structural organization of nonspecific thalamic nuclei and their projection toward cortex, Brain Res., 6 (1967) 60-94.

30 SCHLAG, J., and WASZAK, M., Characteristics of unit responses in nucleus reticularis thalami, Brain Res., 21 (1970) 286-288.

31 SCHLAG, J., and WASZAK, M., Electrophysiological properties of units of the thalamic reticular complex, Exp. Neurol., 32 (1971) 79-97.

32 SHIMAZU, H., YANAGISAWA, N., and GAROUTTE, B., Cortico-pyramidal influence on thalamic somatosensory transmission in the cat. Jap. J. Physiol., 15 (1965) 101-124.

33 STERIADE, M., Alterations in activities of reciprocal synaptic pathways between the thalamic ventrolateral nucleus and the motor cortex during sleep and waking, In: Corticothalamic projections and sensorimotor activities. Eds. T.L Frigyesi, E. Rinvik, and M.D. Yahr. Raven Press, New York, 1972.

34 STERIADE, M., APOSTOL, V., and OAKSON, G., Control of unitary activities in cerebellothalamic pathway during wakefulness and synchronized sleep, J. Neurophysiol., 34 (1971) 389-413.

35 STRICK, P.L., Cortical projections of the feline thalamic nucleus ventralis lateralis, Brain Res., 20 (1970) 130-134.

36 TSUKAHARA, N., A reverberating circuit between cerebellar nucleus and pontine nucleus, Proc. XXV Internat. Congress of Physiol. Sc. Munich 1971.

37 UNO, M., YOSHIDA, M., and HIROTA, I., The mode of cerebello-thalamic relay transmission investigated with intracellular recording from cells of the ventrolateral nucleus of cat's thalamus, Exp. Brain Res., 10 (1970) 121-139.

38 WOOLSEY, C.N., Organization of somatic sensory and motor areas of the cerebral cortex. In: Biological and biochemical basis of behaviour, Ed. by H.F. Harlow and C.N. Woolsey. Madison. The University of Wisconsin Press 1958, pp. 63-81.

Corticothalamic Projections and Sensorimotor Activities
T. Frigyesi, E. Rinvik, and M.D. Yahr, editors. © 1972
Raven Press, New York.

Electrical Cytoarchitectural Study of the Cat's Motor Cortex

Hiroshi Asanuma and Ingmar Rosén

Following the presentation of Dr. Massion's beautiful results on the projection of VL to the cortex, we discuss how these impulses are processed within the cerebral cortex.

We have already reported that there are discrete neuron colonies within the depth of the motor cortex which when stimulated produce contraction of a particular muscle or muscles (1). Each colony extends along the direction of radial fibers within the gray matter and constitutes a columnar structure. It is well known that the motor cortex receives powerful inputs from VL in addition to the inputs from VP and other cortical areas. It is highly likely that these inputs from various parts of the brain are processed in a specific way within each columnar organization and subsequently send corticofugal impulses to a specific motoneuron pool to contract a particular muscle.

To examine how information is processed within the gray matter, the following experiments were performed on cats lightly anesthetized with Nembutal and immobilized with Flaxedil. A closed chamber which permits installation of two manipulators and independent manipulation of each was attached on the skull surrounding the exposed motor cortex. One of the manipulators was used for insertion of tungsten electrodes to stimulate the depth of the cortex and the other was used for glass pipette microelectrodes filled with 2 Mol. K-Cit. or 3 Mol. K-Cl to record from inside of cortical neurons. The tungsten electrode could also be used for recording extracellular unit spikes as described elsewhere (2). Intracortical microstimulation (ICMS) of 0.2 msec duration and up to 4 μa was delivered through the tungsten electrode and postsynaptic potentials (PSP's) in response to the ICMS were recorded through the other electrode. At each spot where PSP's were recorded, a current of 10 μa was passed for 10 sec through the tungsten electrode to make a lesion, and this lesion was used to determine the location of the electrode tip in the later histological examination. The location of the pipette electrode tip in relation to the lesion was calculated by using the depth readings of the manipulators as well as the distance between two electrodes.

Intracellular recordings were successfully obtained from more than 100 cortical neurons. Minimum latency of PSP's produced by ICMS was 0.8 msec at a distance of 0.2 mm between the electrodes. When the electrodes were closer, ICMS frequently produced direct excitation of the cell without synaptic delays. Latency distribution of PSPs showed two distinct peaks at around 1.0 msec and 1.5 msec. From these results, the group of cells which produced PSPs at around 1.0 msec are classified as activated by monosynaptic connections. When intracellular recordings were stable, thresholds for producing PSPs were examined. The minimum value obtained was 0.5 μa and at threshold stimulation, the PSPs produced were unitary in character. They appeared in all or nothing fashion and the size was the same as the size of spontaneous miniature synaptic potentials which appeared constantly in the resting neurons.

A total of 24 cells responded monosynaptically to ICMS's and distribution of them is shown in Fig. 1. The depth of the cortex was arbitrarily divided into superficial, middle and deep layers. Stimulation within superficial and middle layers produced monosynaptic PSPs in the cells located within restricted areas. The horizontal spread of monosynaptic connections throughout the cortex were always less than 1.0 mm, as shown in Fig. 1. A surprising observation was that a considerable

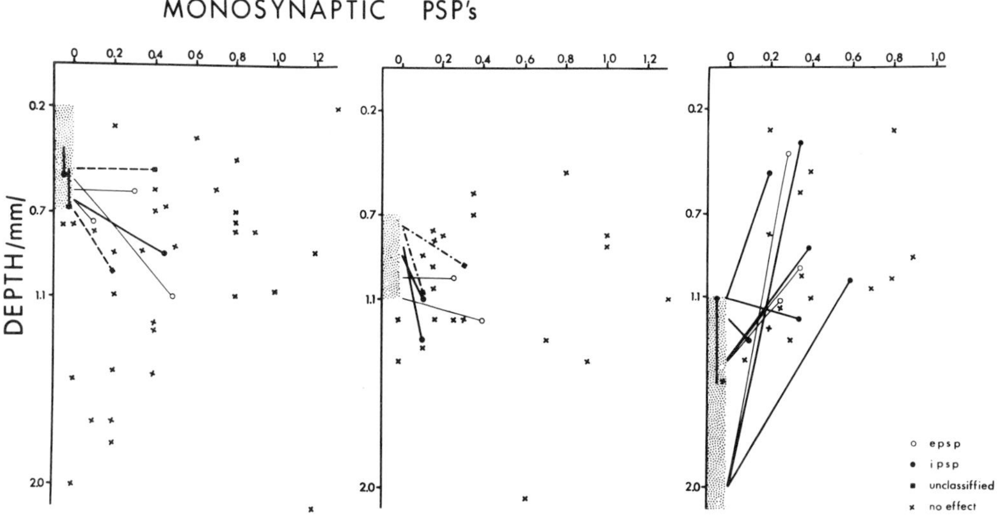

FIG. 1. Neuronal network within the motor cortex. Gray matter is arbitrarily divided into superficial, middle and deep layers. Intracortical microstimulation of 3-4 μa was delivered through a tungsten electrode and postsynaptic potentials were recorded through a pipette electrode filled with K-Cit. or K-Cl. PSPs recorded through K-Cl electrodes were grouped as unclassified. ICMS's within superficial and middle layers produced monosynaptic PSPs in a small number of neurons located within a short distance from the stimulating site whereas the effect of ICMS's in the deep layer travelled back to the superficial layers. Further details are in the text.

number of neurons located within short distances from the stimulating site did not receive monosynaptic inputs. The strength of ICMS used throughout the experiments was 3-4 μa which was likely to have excited more than 10 neurons around the electrode. The results indicate that these groups of cells around the electrode did not send axons diffusely to the neighboring cells. The likely interpretation is that each cortical neuron sends axons to a specific cell or cell group and the secondary cell or cell group then send impulses to the third group and the impulses gradually descend to deep layer cells. In view of the short horizontal spread of the connections, it is likely that these groups of cells constitute a columnar organization along the direction of radial fibers. Once the impulses reach the deep layers, corticofugal impulses are initiated to activate motorneurons and, at the same time, send impulses back to the superficial layers. Clarification of functional significance of this elaborate network waits for further elucidation.

REFERENCES

1 ASANUMA, H. and SAKATA, H. Functional organization of a cortical efferent system examined with focal depth stimulation in cats. J. Neurophysiol., 30 (1967) 35-54.

2 STONEY, S.D. Jr., THOMPSON, W.D. and ASANUMA, H. Excitation of pyramidal tract cells by intracortical microstimulation: Effective extent of stimulating current. J. Neurophysiol., 31 (1968) 659-669.

Corticothalamic Projections and Sensorimotor Activities
T. Frigyesi, E. Rinvik, and M.D. Yahr, editors. © 1972
Raven Press, New York.

Some Subcortical Projections of the Association Cortex in the Cat

Janos Szabo and Peter Cobus

The nucleus ventralis lateralis of the thalamus (VL) occupies a key position in the delicate control of motor mechanisms, owing to its direct projections to the motor cortex. It is in turn under the influence of substantial inputs from some extrathalamic, thalamic and cortical sites.

One of the most powerful afferent systems to the VL is originating in the deep cerebellar nuclei. When unimpeded, the impulses are readily transmitted by the relay cells of the VL to the motor cortex and the corticospinal neurons. The VL neuron discharges, however, are followed by a relatively long period of depression of spontaneous activity, resulting in a cyclic variation of firing. In order to explain the periodic changes of excitability, different mechanisms have been postulated. It appears, that the inhibition might be related to the activation of the interneurons (12, 24) brought into play either directly by afferent collaterals or indirectly by the axon collaterals of the VL relay cells (17). The powerful modulating influence of the nonspecific thalamic system on the transmission of the cerebello-thalamo-cortical projection may be equally important in this respect (6, 16, 17).

The medial segment of the globus pallidus and its feline equivalent, the entopeduncular nucleus, has also been shown to send a substantial projection to the VL (15, 22, 23). The apparent overlap of the projection fields of the cerebellar and pallidal afferents strongly indicate a possible interaction between these inputs either presynaptically or more probably postsynaptically, affecting the activity of local neurons.

It is now well documented that the cerebral cortex is not only a recipient of thalamic afferents but sends a significant projection back to the relay and some other thalamic nuclei. There is general agreement that the motor cortex projects heavily upon the VL neurons and exerts a strong influence on the firing pattern of the VL elements through a combination of facilitatory and inhibitory effects (3, 5, 7, 9, 14, 18, 19). The end result is that the cortex can regulate its own input (11). The mechanisms underlying these effects are not yet fully understood. For the inhibitory effect, however, the participation of three thalamic elements have been implicated: local interneurons, cells of the nonspecific system and the reticular nucleus.

The pericruciate cortex and the surrounding areas also send projections to the intralaminar nuclei (18) and some extrathalamic structures such as the zona incerta (ZI) red nucleus (NR), reticular formation (RF) pontine nuclei (Pons) (4, 10, 18). Since all these structures are directly or indirectly related to the cerebello-thalamo-cortical and the corticospinal systems, the question arises whether the cortex is utilizing these pathways and connections to influence impulse transmission directed rostrally at these sites. It would also be of interest to know, if the effect would be transmitted and expressed at the thalamic level via such alternate routes in the VL nucleus.

The association cortex, occupying in the cat the greater part of the suprasylvian gyrus and the anterior portion of the lateral gyrus (21), is known to have a multisensory input and that parallel processing of different sensory modalities takes place in these cortical areas (2, 25, 26). Physiological studies have also revealed an intimate relationship between the association cortex and the intralaminar thalamic nuclei (1, 8).

While the efferent connections of the sensorimotor cortex have been worked out in some detail, little attention has been paid so far to the subcortical projections of the association cortex.

The aim of the present study was to investigate the possible structural links between these cortical areas and different thalamic nuclei on one hand and extrathalamic structures on the other.

In a series of experiments, lesions of various sizes were placed either on the anterior lateral gyrus (Fig. 1A, A) or on the crown of the middle suprasylvian gyrus of cats (Fig. 1A, B), areas that have unique cyto- and myeloarchitectural characteristics. The animals were allowed to survive 3 to 6 days. The resulting fiber degeneration was studied on sections impregnated with the Nauta technique or its modification by Fink and Heimer. A further modification of the latter method by Wiitanen was also extensively used.

Thalamic Projections

The quantitatively most significant fiber degeneration was observed in the n. lateralis posterior (LP) and to a lesser degree in the pulvinar (Pul). In most instances, a dense network of degenerating fibers could be seen laterally in the LP, along the border of the pulvinar (Fig. 1D). This was particularly evident in animals with suprasylvian gyrus lesions. In other parts of LP and in the pulvinar the fibers were distributed in a more scattered manner (Fig. 1E).

Degeneration in the intralaminar nuclei, excluding the centrum medianum, was most frequently found in the n. centralis lateralis (CL) (Fig. 1B). The n. paracen-

---

FIG. 1. A, two areas of the association cortex are indicated. B-E, degeneration in the n. centralis lateralis; n. ventralis lateralis; n. lateralis posterior and the pulvinar, respectively. Wiitanen method, counterstained with cresyl-violet. Mag., B,D,E, 250X; C, 160X.

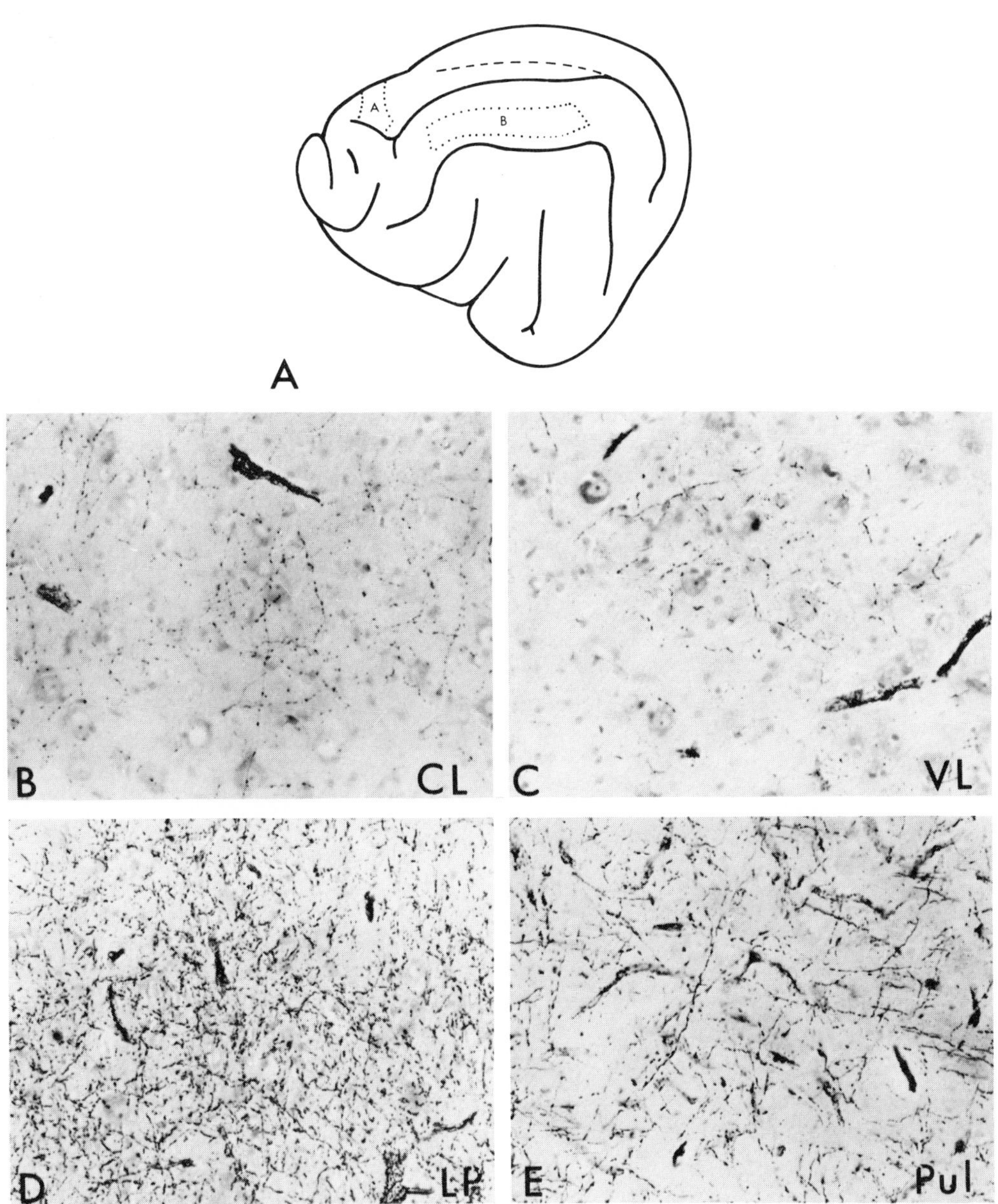

FIG. 1

tralis and the n. centralis medialis showed only a small amount of degenerating elements.

The preterminal arborizations of degenerating fibers in the n. ventralis lateralis were mainly found in paralaminar locations (Fig. 1C). In both nuclei (CL and VL), the amount and distribution of fibers depended on the size and site of the cortical lesion, indicating some degree of topographical relationship.

Extrathalamic Projections

Following lesions of the association cortex, a large amount of degenerating fibers could be traced to the zona incerta (ZI), prerubral field (FF) and the rostral parvocellular part of the red nucleus, in a continuum. In their course, the fibers arborized profusely, indicating terminations in all three structures (Fig. 2A-C).

At the meso-diencephalic junction, the heaviest terminal degeneration was found in the pretectal region, especially in the anterior pretectal nucleus (Fig. 2, D). The mesencephalic reticular formation received a modest amount of degeneration. The degenerating elements were most readily detectable in the dorsolateral vicinity of the red nucleus (Fig. 2E) and in the central tegmental field, ventromedial to the anterior pretectal nucleus.

Summary and Conclusions

The present observations indicate that architectonically and functionally different cortical areas project to common targets in the thalamus and some extrathalamic structures.

Thus the sensorimotor cortex and the association areas are both capable of influencing the transmission in the n. ventralis lateralis directly and also indirectly through intralaminar neurons.

A similar parallelism seems to exist regarding the subthalamic, rubral, reticular and pontine connections in the cat (Fig. 2F). It is interesting to note that comparable findings have been recently reported in the monkey, including modest projections from the parietal lobules to the mesencephalic reticular formation and the parvocellular part of the red nucleus (10).

From a quantitative point of view, it should be mentioned that the projections from the sensorimotor cortex to the VL and CL thalamic nuclei, as well as to the RF and NR, are more numerous than those from the association cortex. This is evident from the relevant literature (10, 20) and is supported by our observations in control animals with pericruciate lesions. In contrast, the association cortex sends additional and heavy projections to the nucleus lateralis posterior and the pulvinar. The func-

FIG. 2. A-F, degeneration in the zona incerta, prerubral field, parvocellular nucleus ruber, anterior pretectal nucleus, mesencephalic reticular formation and pons, respectively. Wiitanen method, counterstained with cresyl-violet. Mag., A,B, 160X; C, D, E, 250X; F, 40X.

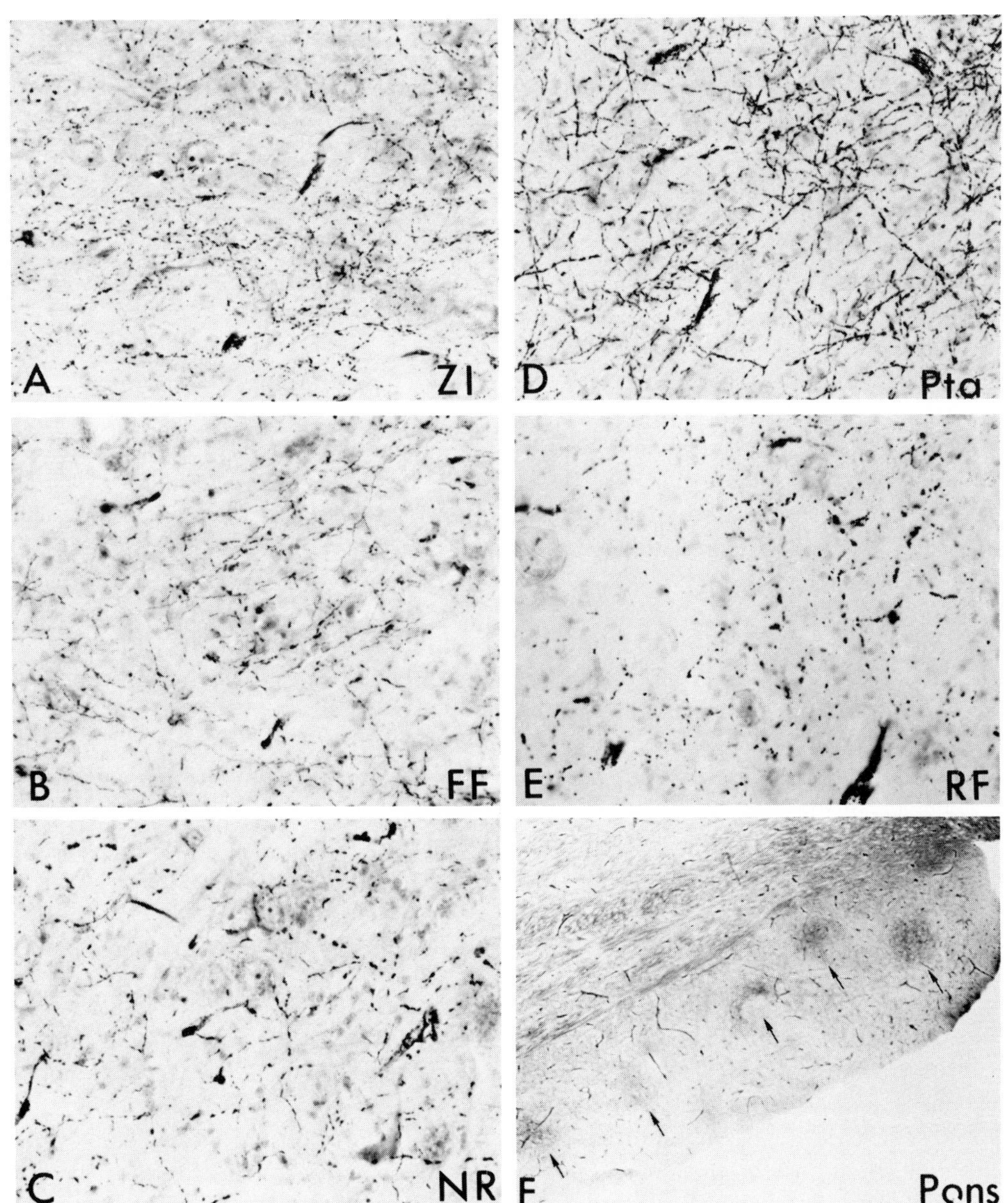

FIG. 2

tional significance of these differences in anatomical organization cannot at present be evaluated. The convergence of projections from different cortical areas in the thalamus and other sites, on the other hand, must have a profound effect on the neuronal activity of the various nuclei in particular and on the sensorimotor mechanisms in general. Further physiological studies are necessary to elucidate the role of the association cortex in this regard.

REFERENCES

1 ALBE-FESSARD, D., and ROUGEUL, A. Activités d'origine somesthésique évoquées sur le cortex nonspecifique du chat anesthesié au chloralose: rôle du centre median du thalamus, Electroencephalog. Clin. Neurophysiol., 10 (1958) 131-151.

2 AMASSIAN, V. Studies on organization of a somesthetic association area, including a single unit analysis, J. Neurophysiol., 17 (1954) 39-58.

3 AUER, J. Terminal degeneration in the diencephalon after ablation of the frontal cortex in the cat, J. Anat. (Lond.), 90 (1956) 30-41.

4 BRODAL, P. The corticopontine projection in the cat. I. Demonstration of a somatotopically organized projection from the primary sensorimotor cortex, Exp. Brain Res., 5 (1968) 210-234.

5 DORMONT, J.F., and MASSION, J. Duality of cortical control on ventrolateral thalamic activity, Exp. Brain Res., 10 (1970) 205-218.

6 FRIGYESI, T.L., and PURPURA, D.P. Functional properties of synaptic pathways influencing transmission in the specific cerebello-thalamocortical projection system, Exp. Neurol., 10 (1964) 305-324.

7 HIROTA, I., YOSHIDA, M., and UNO, M. Antidromic and orthodromic responses in the relay neurons of the thalamic ventrolateral nucleus by cortical stimulation, Cited in: The Cerebellum as a Neuronal Machine, J.C. Eccles, M. Ito, and J. Szentagothai (Eds.) Springer, New York, 1967, p. 291.

8 JASPER, H., NAQUET, R., and KING, E.E. Thalamocortical recruiting responses in sensory receiving areas in the cat, Electroencephalog. Clin. Neurophysiol., 7 (1955) 99-114.

9 KUSAMA, T., OTANI, K., and KAWANA, E. Projections of the motor, somatic sensory, auditory and visual cortices in cats, In: Correlative Neurosciences: Fundamental Mechanisms, Progress in Brain Research, vol. 21A, T. Tokizane and J.P. Schade (Eds.), Elsevier, Amsterdam, 1966, pp. 292-322.

10 KUYPERS, H.G.J.M. and LAWRENCE, D.G. Cortical projections to the red nucleus and the brain stem in the rhesus monkey, Brain Res., 4 (1967) 151-188.

11 LEBLANC, F.E., and CORDEAU, J.P. Modulation of pyramidal tract cell activity by ventrolateral thalamic regions. Its possible role in tremorogenic mechanisms, Brain Res., 14 (1969) 255-270.

12 MARCO, L.A., BROWN, T.S., and ROUSE, M.E. Unitary responses in ventrolateral thalamus upon intranuclear stimulation, J. Neurophysiol., 30 (1967) 482-493.

13 MARCO, L.A., and BROWN, T.S. Rubrally evoked unitary potentials in ventro-

lateral thalamus of cat, Electroencephalog. Clin. Neurophysiol., 21 (1966) 239-248.

14 NAKAMURA, Y., and SCHLAG, J. Cortically induced rhythmic activities in the thalamic ventrolateral nucleus of the cat, Exp. Neurol., 22 (1968) 209-221.

15 NAUTA, W.J.H., and MEHLER, W.R. Some efferent connections of the lentiform nucleus in monkey and cat, Anat. Record, 139 (1961) 260.

16 PURPURA, D.P., McMURTRY, J.G., and MAEKAWA, K. Synaptic events in ventrolateral thalamic neurons during suppression of recruiting responses by brain stem reticular stimulation, Brain Res., 1 (1966) 63-76.

17 PURPURA, D.P., SCARFF, T., and McMURTRY, J.G. Intracellular study of internuclear inhibition in ventrolateral thalamic neurons, J. Neurophysiol., 28 (1965) 487-496.

18 RINVIK, E. The corticothalamic projection from the precruciate and coronal gyri in the cat. An experimental study with silver-impregnation methods, Brain Res., 10 (1968) 79-119.

19 RINVIK, E. The cortico thalamic projection from the gyrus proreus and the medial wall of the rostral hemisphere in the cat. An experimental study with silver impregnation methods, Exp. Brain Res., 5 (1968) 129-152.

20 RINVIK, E., and WALBERG, F. Demonstration of a somatotopically arranged cortico-rubral projection in the cat. An experimental study with silver methods, J. Comp. Neurol., 120 (1963) 393-407.

21 SANIDES, F., and HOFFMANN, J. Cyto- and myeloarchitecture of the visual cortex of the cat and of surrounding integration cortices, J. Hirnforsch., 11 (1969) 79-104.

22 SZABO, J. Synaptic arrangements in the VA-VL thalamic nuclei, Proc. Intern. Congr. Anat. Wiesbaden, (1965) 117.

23 SZABO, J., and RENAUD, L. Cerebello- and pallidothalamic projections in cat, Proc. Can. Fed. Biol. Soc., 7 (1964) 50-51.

24 SZENTÁGOTHAI, J. The nuclear efferents of the cerebellum, In: The Cerebellum as a Neuronal Machine, J.C. Eccles, M. Ito and J. Szentágothai (Eds.), Springer, New York, 1967, pp. 262-267.

25 THOMPSON, R.F., JOHNSON, R.H., and HOOPES, J.J. Organization of auditory, somatic sensory and visual projection to association fields of cerebral cortex in the cat, J. Neurophysiol., 26 (1963) 343-364.

26 WOOLSEY, C.N. Organization of cortical auditory system: a review and a synthesis. In: Neural mechanisms of the auditory and vestibular systems. G.L. Rasmussen and W. Windle (Eds.), Thomas, Springfield, Ill. 1961, pp. 165-180.

Corticothalamic Projections and Sensorimotor Activities
T. Frigyesi, E. Rinvik, and M.D. Yahr, editors. © 1972
Raven Press, New York.

The Pulvinar and Ventrolateral Nucleus of the Human Thalamus

Irving S. Cooper

I am grateful for the opportunity of discussing Dr. Massion's interesting and thought provoking paper.

There is a crucial difference between the experimentalist and the surgical clinical investigator in that the former seeks information concerning mechanisms neutrally at work in the ideal brain, whereas the latter works with the human brain, which in each individual is immeasurably different from another by virtue of aging, experience, and disease. However, these are in fact two approaches to the same problem, and far from being mutually exclusive, each converges on the same questions. It seems logical therefore that the experimentalist and clinician join forces in the solution of a common problem.

To this end I shall mention a few observations in humans following thalamic surgery which appear germane to Dr. Massion's experimental findings and conclusions.

First, surgical experience confirms that there is a mediolateral topography of the thalamocortical projections from VL to cortex. To lessen hypertonus in the lower extremity of man, a lateral posterior lesion in VL is necessary, while a more medial lesion affects the arm, and a still more medial lesion overlapping into DM or centrum medianum is necessary for a lasting effect on nuchal musculature (1). Stimulation in the conscious patient confirms the mediolateral topography described by Dr. Massion.

I was particularly interested in Dr. Massion's observation concerning indirect bilateral pathways from VL to the cortical sensory areas, and his suggestion that VL influences muscle tone, in part by this sensory connection as well as by its direct effect on motor cortex. It is our experience in humans that cooling and freezing within the classical VL nucleus does not effect an evoked potential in sensory cortex. However, extension of cooling into VPL can reversibly diminish a sensory evoked response and, in many instances, extension of the therapeutic lesion posteriorly from VL into VPL will augment the effect on muscle tone produced by the VL lesion alone (Fig. 1). This may support the suggestion of Dr. Massion that there is an indirect contribution of VL to muscular control via a relay through the somesthetic sensory

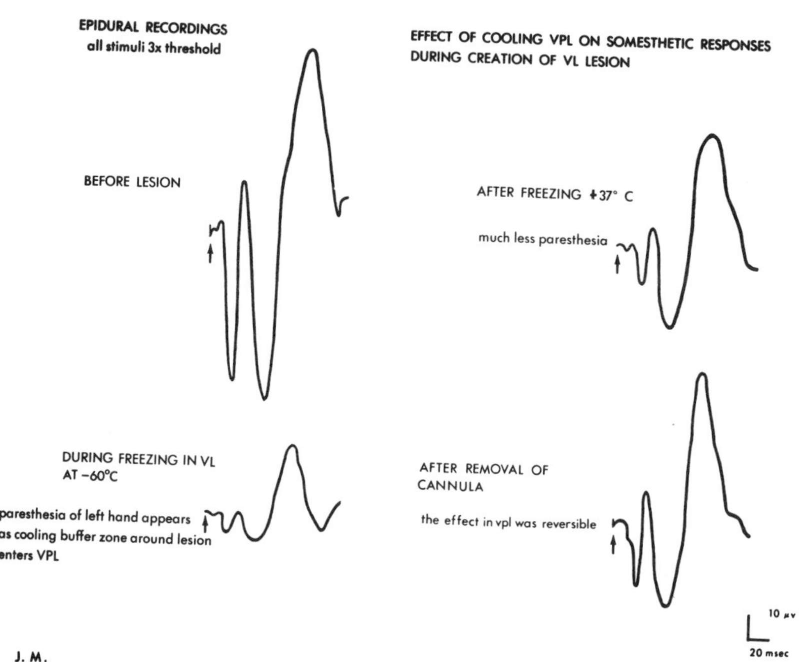

FIG. 1. Demonstration of the effect of cooling in the anterior portion of VPL of the human thalamus upon an evoked potential in ipsilateral sensory cortex. As cooling inhibited function in this portion of VPL, not only was the sensory evoked potential diminished, but the decrease of contralateral motor tone, produced by the VL lesion, was augmented.

nucleus to sensory cortex.

In this regard we have recently learned that another thalamic region, namely the pulvinar, may influence muscle tone, and probably does so indirectly by its connec-

---

FIG. 2A. Cryopulvinectomy at the present time is carried out stereotactically by producing two overlapping lesions, each approximately 11 mms. in diameter, in the pulvinar. The black circles diagrammatically illustrate the stereotactically placed cryosurgical lesions.

FIG. 2B. Anatomic confirmation of lesion placement in the pulvinar in an operation carried out on human cadaver. In this case the site of the lesion has been stained by India ink.

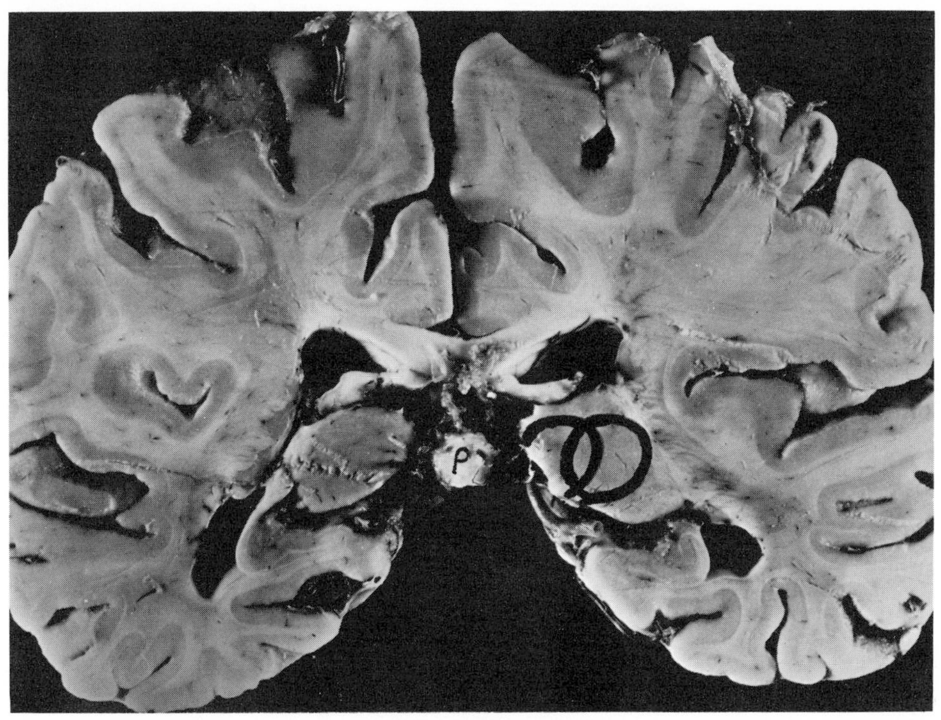

FIG. 2 A

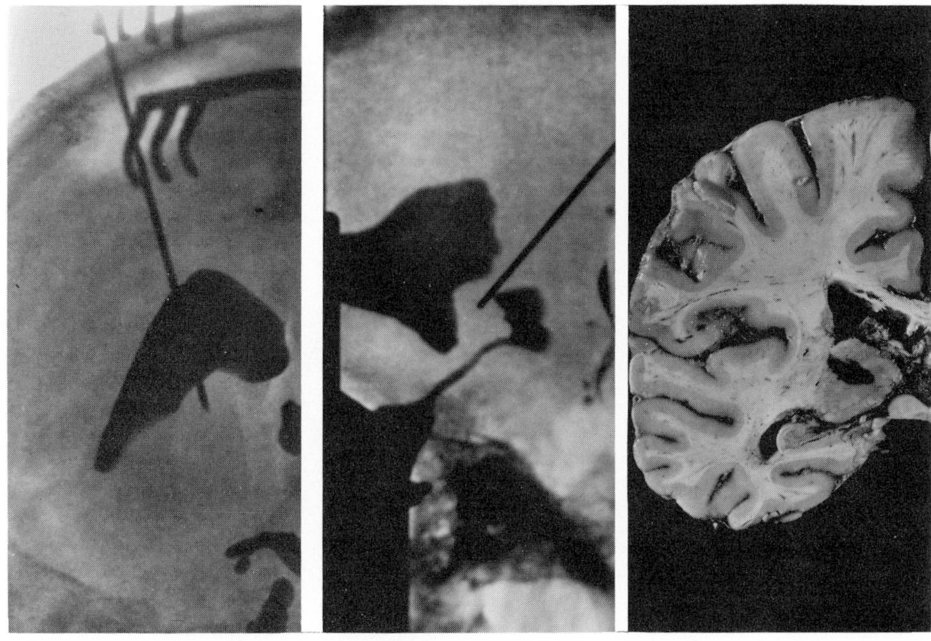

FIG. 2 B

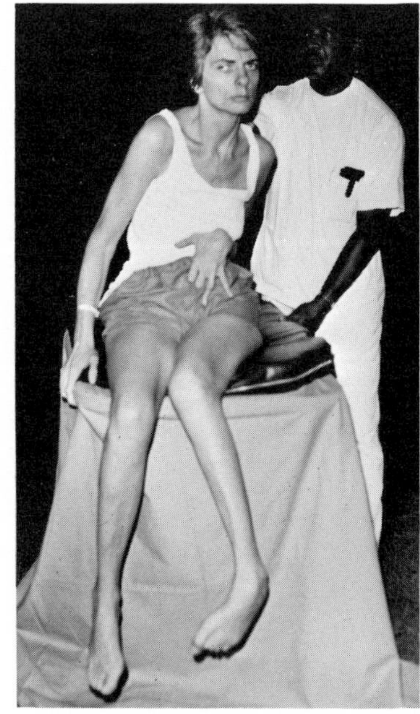

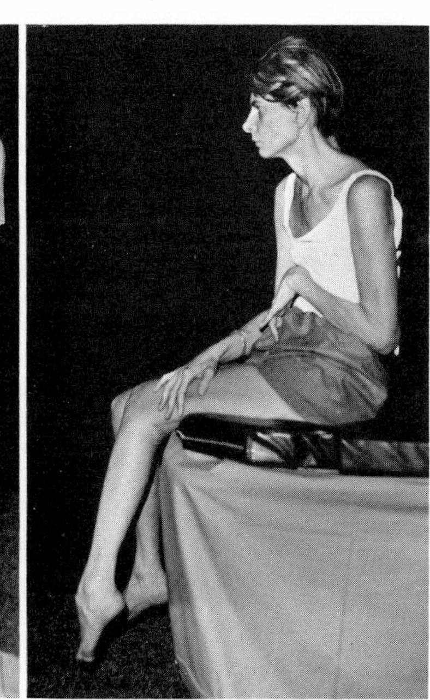

FIG. 3 A

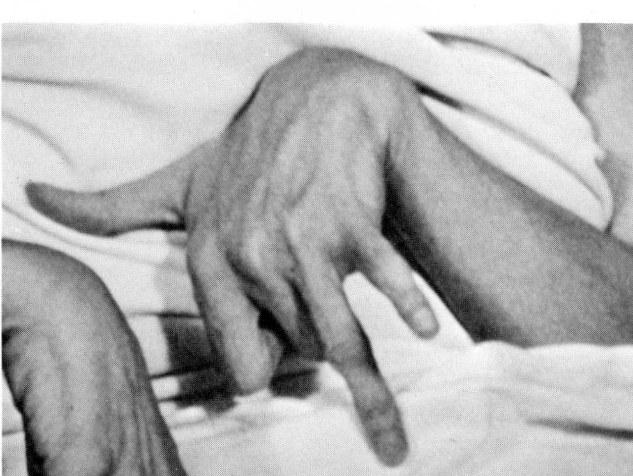

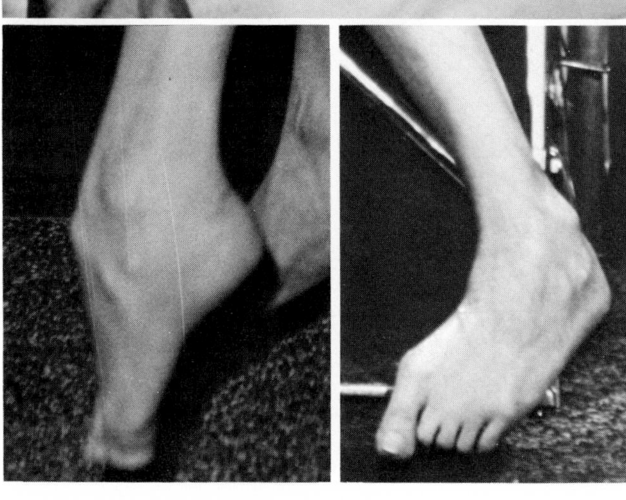

FIG. 3 B

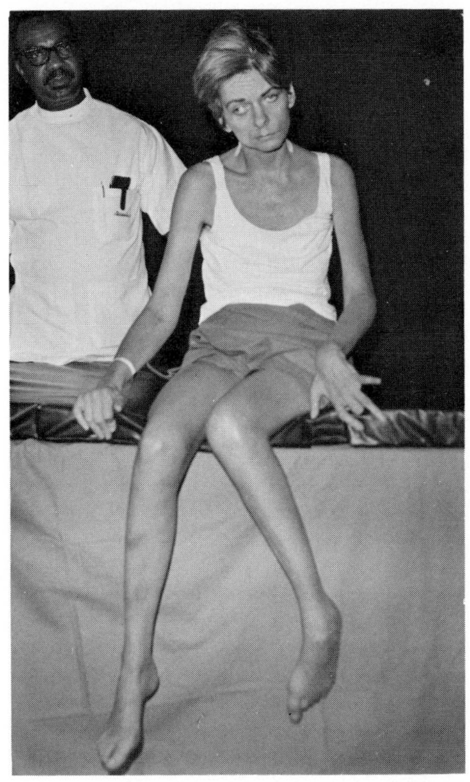

FIG. 3 C. The same patient 24 hours following left cryogenic dentate nucleus ablation. There has been obvious lessening of spasticity of the left upper extremity.

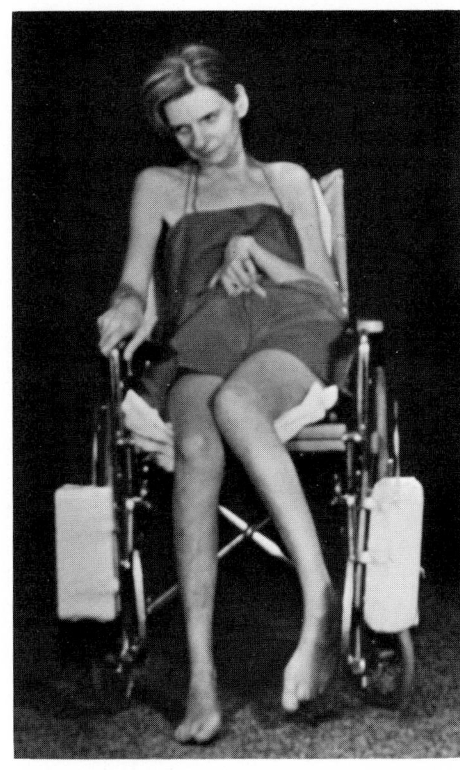

FIG. 3 D. Two weeks following left dentate nucleus surgery, the spasticity had returned to its preoperative state.

tions with sensory cortex (Fig. 2). A large lesion within pulvinar had markedly diminished spasticity, (that is, hypertonus accompanied by increased deep tendon reflexes, clonus and a positive Babinski sign) in 50% of 14 patients totally incapacitated by this symptom (2). An example is illustrated in Figure 3. I should like to ask Dr.

FIG. 3 A. A 47 year old woman demonstrating complete spastic left hemiplegia 2 years following a cerebral vascular accident involving the right side of the midbrain. FIG. 3 B. A close up demonstrating the fixed spastic deformities at the left wrist and left ankle of this patient.

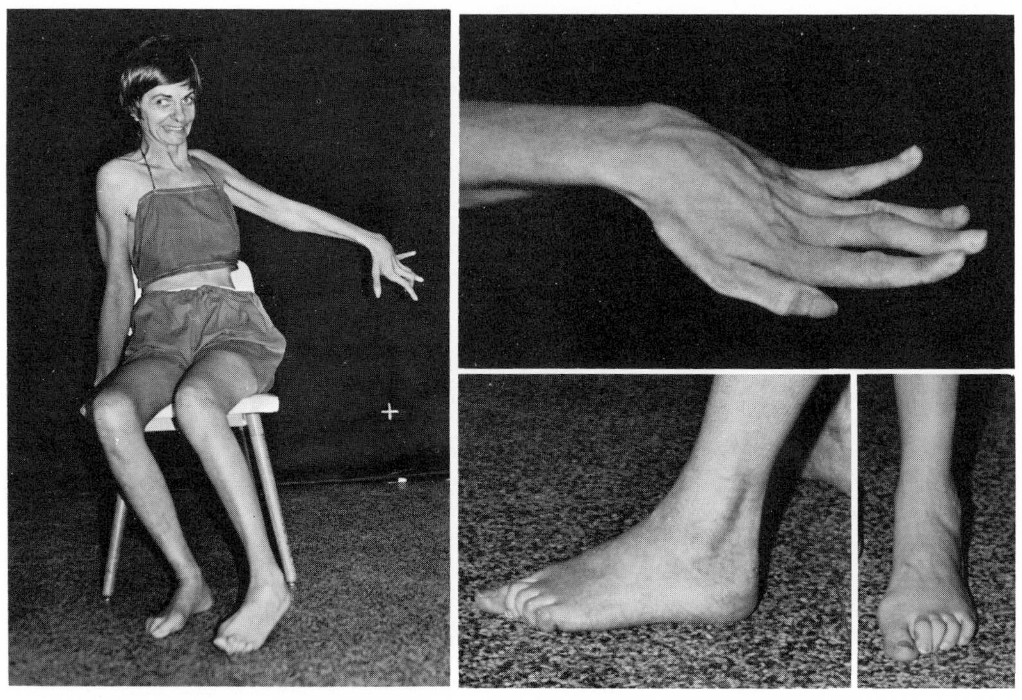

FIG. 3 E

FIG. 3 G

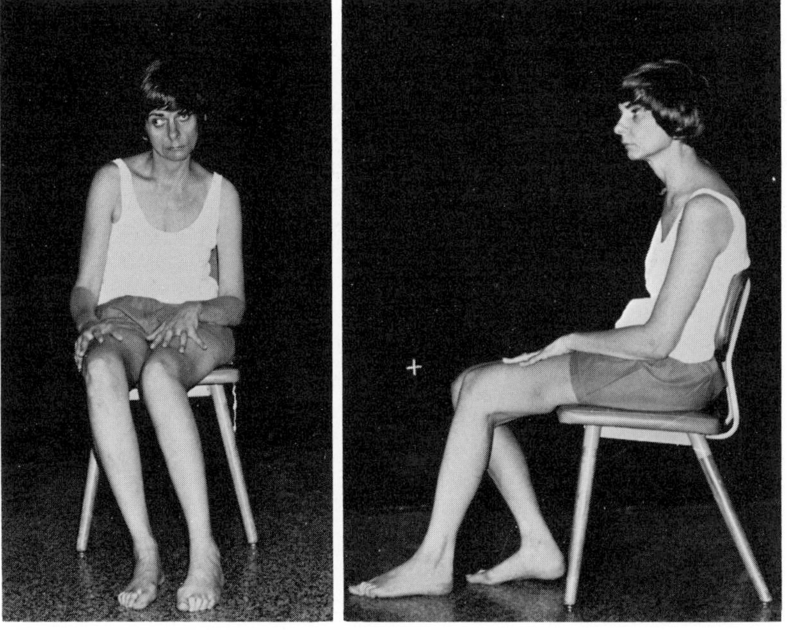

FIG. 3 F

Massion whether he has any data relating to differential control of cortex upon pulvinar, similar to that which he has presented for VL.

In relation to Dr. Purpura's discussion of specific and nonspecific thalamic nuclei, there is evidence that the pulvinar is a polysensory nucleus in which visual auditory and somatic afferents converge to the same neuronal pools (3). The pulvinar, in turn, projects to both association and primary neocortical areas. Our data from surgical studies in humans, as well as the material presented by Dr. Massion and Dr. Purpura during this conference, suggest that VL contributes to so-called nonspecific thalamocortical relations, although it is primarily a specific relay nucleus. On the other hand, although the pulvinar complex is a complex integrator of polysensory stimuli, it acts synergistically with VL in the control of muscle tone and movement.

There is some suggestion in the results of our investigation that VL sensorimotor integration may predominantly affect the muscle tone of more proximal musculature of the extremities and the pulvinar, the more distal, as exemplified by the reversal of the spastic wrist and ankle deformities following the pulvinar lesion in Figure 3.

Finally, I should like to add one observation that is the crux of the clinical problem of thalamic surgery in humans, and which relates directly to the complex question of corticothalamic relationships and sensorimotor activities. In a human with evidence of a relatively intact cortex, either VL or pulvinar or both can be sacrificed, producing a profound effect on muscle hypertonus without incurring a sensorimotor or behavioral abnormality.

Can Dr. Massion suggest how the cortex compensates for these intricate corticothalamic mechanisms when ventrolateral thalamus is ablated therapeutically, since VL and sensorimotor cortex appear to function normally as a unit?

REFERENCES

1 COOPER, I.S. Involuntary Movement Disorders, Harper and Row, N.Y. 1969 pp. 402.

2 COOPER, I.S., WALTZ, J.M., and AMIN, I. Pulvinectomy—A preliminary report, Journal of American Geriatrics Society, 19 (1971a) 553-555.

3 KREINDLER, A., CRIGHEL, E., and MARINESCHESCU: Integrative Activity of the Thalamic Pulvinar Lateralis Posterior Complex and Interrelations with the Neocortex, Experimental Neurology, 22 (1968) 423-435.

FIG.3 E. A right cryothalamectomy, with destruction of a portion of the ventrolateral nucleus was performed. This resulted in moderate lessening of rigidity of the left arm and leg, abolition of intention tremor, and some return of motor power. Spasticity and the deformities at the wrist and ankle, however, persisted.

FIG.3 F. Right cryopulvinectomy, ablation of the pulvinar, was performed which resulted in alleviation of spasticity of the left extremities, marked improvement in voluntary motor power, and reversal of the spastic deformities at the foot and ankle.

FIG.3 G. Close up of the foot and ankle illustrating reversal of the spastic deformities.

Corticothalamic Projections and Sensorimotor Activities
T. Frigyesi, E. Rinvik, and M.D. Yahr, editors. © 1972
Raven Press, New York.

Cerebellothalamocortical Interrelations in Contact Placing and Other Movements in Cats

Vahé E. Amassian, Richard Ross,

Christian Wertenbaker and Herbert Weiner

INTRODUCTION

The tactile placing reaction (contact placing) was initially described by Rademaker (39). In a dog with a hood over its eyes, contact of the dorsum of the unsupported paw with the edge of a table was followed by placing the paw on top of the table. Because it could not be elicited in decorticate dogs, contact placing (CP) was considered to be a postural reaction dependent on cerebral cortex. CP was only transiently lost following cerebellectomy. Subsequently, Bard (11) observed that removal of the sensorimotor cortex in cats led to permanent loss of CP of the contralateral limbs. Removal of all neocortex except the sigmoid gyrus spared CP. In monkeys (12), removal of area 4 or area 3-1-2 led to loss of CP of the stimulated contralateral limb, but removal of area 4 alone spared placing of the corresponding limb on the unstimulated side (cross-placing). Bard supposed that the postcentral gyrus, "on receiving afferent impulses originating at the surface of the contralateral half of the body, somehow brings into action the motor cortex of the opposite hemisphere," thus leading to cross-placing. However, section of the corpus callosum did not abolish cross-placing, which was (and still is) unexplained. Following Bard's important analysis, CP has generally been held to depend on the sensorimotor cortex and has frequently been used in testing the functions of such cortex and related input and output systems, e.g., dorsal columns (23, 29), pyramidal tract (27, 45), cerebral peduncle (13) and cerebellar nuclei (14, 15). However, little attempt was made to measure the parameters, describe the sequence of muscle activities, or to account for the overall neural circuitry subserving CP.

Our interest in CP arose incidentally following a study of monosynaptic and polysynaptic activation of large PT neurons by thalamic N. ventralis lateralis and anterior (VL-VA), and polysynaptic activation by ventralis posterior (VP) (7). In later experiments, the function of these synaptic arrangements in the awake cat was studied by destroying either of the above thalamic nuclei and observing the effects on both the behavior of the cat and the activity of individual PT neurons. Consistent with the important role attributed to the postcentral gyrus (and its homologue in the cat), destruction of VP led to loss of CP. However, destruction of VL-VA also affected CP, abolishing it temporarily; this seemed inconsistent with the notion that a circuit from postcentral gyrus→ precentral gyrus→ corticofugal pathways→ lower motor centers was adequate for CP, as might have been inferred from the work of Bard (12) and from the finding (36) that a stimulus to the postcentral gyrus led to powerful transsynaptic discharge of large PT neurons originating in the precentral gyrus. Furthermore, the involvement in CP of the VL-VA projection system suggested a relationship to the temporary or permanent loss of CP following lesions of cerebellar nuclei dentatus and interpositus, respectively (14, 15). It seemed to us that CP could serve as a model response for analyzing the neural components of higher motor control, leading eventually to an overall synthesis.

Our approach includes: 1) Describing the pattern of muscular activity in CP, 2) observing the effect on CP of permanent lesions or reversible block (e.g., by cooling) of neural structures to define those required for CP and 3) recording, during CP, the activity of individual neurons in neural structures defined by 2), initially to distinguish a dynamic from a steady state role of such structures. Preliminary reports of these findings (4, 5, 6) and an initial synthesis (9) are presented elsewhere.

Methods

The series includes 70 cats, most of them female, with body weights of 2.5-3.5 kg. (Larger or male cats presented greater difficulties if struggling occurred during CP testing.) Under pentobarbital anesthesia, bipolar, polyethylene insulated nichrome wires (interpolar distance 10-15 mm) were implanted within the appropriate forelimb muscles or onto shoulder girdle muscles; the EMG leads emerged through a midline incision between the scapulae and were connected to a multiple socket plug which was attached to a shoulder harness. In preparation for recording from individual neurons in awake cats, a guide consisting of a Delrin cup narrowing to a cylinder with a 19 gauge central bore was placed on the upper part of a snuggly fitting glass-insulated electrode (Fig. 1-left). The electrode was stereotaxically inserted into the dorsal part of the tract or nucleus to be recorded from, accuracy of placement being confirmed by appropriate physiological criteria, e.g., for bulbar PT recording, demonstrating a D response to a motor cortical stimulus (36) or, for N. interpositus recording, demonstrating antidromic invasion of an interpositus neuron following a stimulus at the level of caudal VL (43). (To record from N. interpositus, the electrode was inserted at an angle of 35° to the horizontal.) The lower end of the guide was then allowed to slide down the electrode into the craniotomy and was cemented to the skull. The electrode was withdrawn and the height of the top of the guide was noted for use as a depth reference. The guide was then capped. Subsequently, to record in the awake cat, a microdrive that extruded, without rotating, an eccentric glass-insulated, tungsten microelectrode from a protective 19 gauge hypodermic tube, was screwed into and appropriately oriented by the guide (Fig. 1-right). Prior to extrusion of the microelectrode, the microdrive could be rotated and fixed in any desired position, which permitted a number of

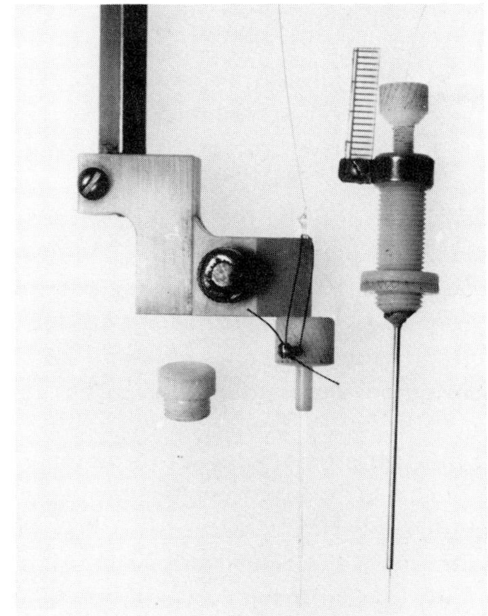

FIG. 1. Apparatus for subcortical unit recording in awake cat. The assembly for stereotaxic implantation of the microdrive guide is shown loaded on a glass-insulated, tungsten electrode at left. Microdrive containing an eccentric glass-insulated tungsten microelectrode shown at right. Dual ring locks microdrive at the desired point of rotation. Cap for guide shown to left of guide.

penetrations to be made in a cylinder of brain tissue. Construction of the microelectrodes is described elsewhere (3). However, in this study, the final stage of electropolishing with cathodal current was omitted. We have found such microelectrodes excellent for chronic unit recording because their properties can be predicted prior to insertion into the brain. Electrode protrusions of 25-65μ beyond the glass are desirable when recording from individual PT axons; recording from nuclear regions requires less protrusion (e.g., 15-30μ) to resolve adequately spikes from closely packed somata. In selected penetrations, cathodal current (20 μamps for one minute) was passed through the microelectrode tip to mark its position.

Insulated bipolar or tripolar nichrome wires, fixed together and cut on a slant, were stereotaxically implanted for stimulating deep structures, e.g., red N., internal capsule and cerebellothalamic pathways. The pulse durations were usually 50 or 100 μ sec; stimulating current was measured with a Tektronix input probe (Type P 6016). Troublesome shock artefacts, such as those observed during antidromic invasion at latencies of 0.5-1.0 msec, were reduced by a bridge. Bipolar nichrome wires on a small Delrin ring were implanted epidurally over motor cortex to elicit D or I discharges (36) in bulbar PT units or antidromic invasion of VL projection neurons (41, 43). When the behavioral state was to be studied, a third electrode on the ring was used for recording the ECoG and other electrodes were implanted for recording the electro-orbitogram and nuchal electromyogram (47). Stimulating and population recording leads were usually connected to separate plugs attached to the shoulder harness.

Lesions were made in thalamic or cerebellar roof nuclei by passing RF current through a stereotaxically placed glass-insulated silver electrode with 1-2 mm of metal protruding. A reversible block of deep nuclei by cooling was done through a stereotaxically implanted probe within the exposed tip of which Freon or ethyl chloride was evaporated. The evaporant entered a fine hypodermic tube extending down the lumen of the probe to its tip and was removed at the top by a tube connected to room air or to a vacuum source. Alternatively, to cool a subcortical nucleus from which a previous recording had been made, a small cooling probe could be inserted through the 19-gauge bore of the microelectrode guide. However, the damage created by the probe prevented further unit recording.

Terminally, the cat was anesthetised with pentobarbital and the functional effects of lesions were usually assayed by appropriate physiological tests; e.g., the extent of "deafferentation" of VL by a lesion made caudal to VL was assessed by comparing the amplitudes of the summed pericruciate responses (usually 20 or 50) on each side to stimulation of contralateral N. interpositus and brachium conjunctivum (24, 41) at current intensities of 4-8 mA. Other physiological observations served as controls for lack of involvement of neural structures near those deliberately destroyed; e.g., demonstrating unimpaired primary responses in somatosensory cortex to peripheral stimuli after VL or red N. lesions implied that the specific somatosensory projections had been spared. The placement of the EMG recording electrodes was confirmed by injecting brief trains of stimuli through them and observing the movements of the limb. Cats were perfused with buffered 10% formalin. Brains were frozen sectioned at 40μ and stained with cresyl violet for anatomical localization of lesions and electrode tracks.

Testing and Measuring CP

The testing procedure is an important parameter in measuring CP. Early in the series, 4 cats were restrained by a harness attached to a frame, and a platform mounted on a swivel was swung in a wide arc, until it contacted the unsupported paw (Fig. 2). This procedure had the advantage of eliminating premonitory cues associated with movement of the cat. However, restraint by a harness was abandoned because it often led to struggling which, although temporary, was sometimes followed by a reduced probability of CP. In the rest of the series, the cat was moved to a stationary platform; such movement often results in an increase in activity of the long extensors of the digits with dorsiflexion of the digits and wrist prior to contact. This increased extensor activity provides a useful background against which to observe an inhibition occurring during the initial withdrawal phase of CP. However, premature activation of biceps may also occur, which is troublesome because biceps is one of the earliest muscles activated in CP. Although with practice premature movements can usually be detected visually, they are much more reliably identified in EMG recordings.

Our standard method of holding the cat for testing CP in one forelimb is to insert the right hand between the right fore- and hindlimbs and then grasp firmly and retract posteriorly the other forelimb; simultaneously, the head is firmly held with the fingers of the left hand below the jaw and the thumb behind the junction of the head and neck, and tilted upwards so that the platform cannot be seen by the cat. In testing for cross-placing, the unstimulated forepaw is not held. Intact cats do not usually place both unsupported forepaws when only one is contacted, i.e., they do not usually exhibit cross-placing. However, if the stimulated forepaw is firmly held to prevent CP, the unstimulated forepaw may then cross-place. Holding the cat

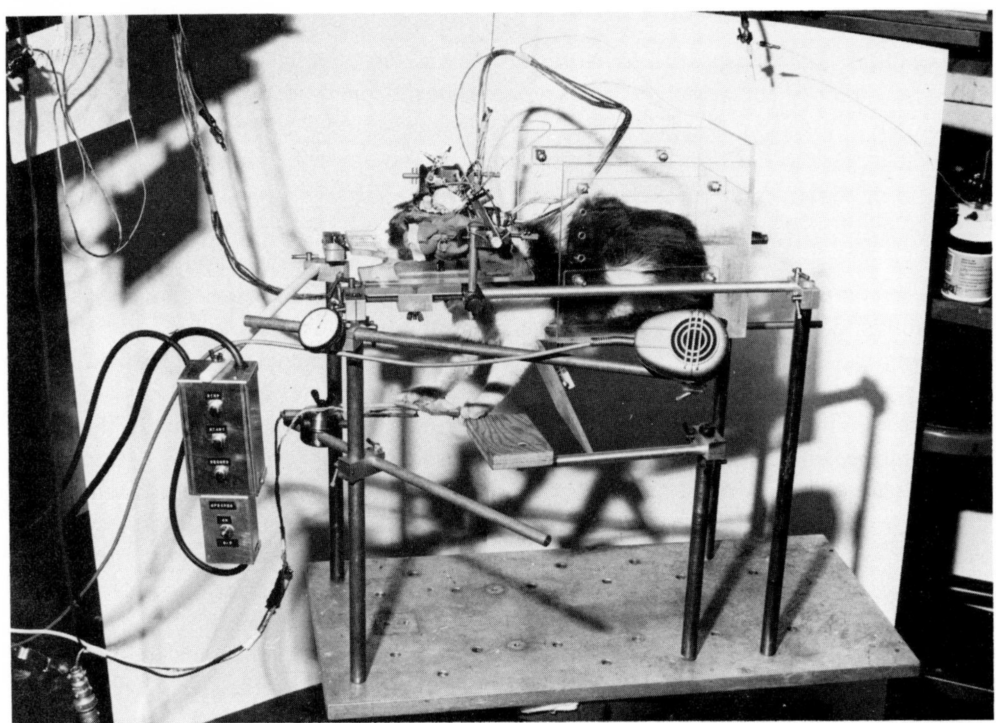

FIG. 2. Restraining apparatus used in testing for CP. Thorax supported by a plastic harness attached at back of neck to a horizontal rod clamped to the frame. Head is unable to look down because of an adjustable plastic halter around the neck. Initially, all four limbs rest on the floor of the plastic box (at right) which is subsequently raised to the level shown. Opening the trap door under front of cat permits forepaw to hang down for CP testing. Left forepaw rests on the edge of an adjustable wooden support; right forepaw rests on platform which is swung into contact with the unsupported forepaw during CP testing. The cat has a solid state input clamped to a head screw and a probe oriented to cool the dentate nucleus.

for testing for CP of the hindpaw tends to be clumsy. A useful procedure is to pass the right hand between the hindlimbs, grasping both forelimbs, while the left hand holds the head as described above.

The importance of testing several cutaneous fields became apparent early in the series. It cannot be overemphasized that merely testing the effect of contact with the dorsum of the paw is inadequate; e.g., following lesions of VL-VA, the deficit in CP to stimulation of the ulnar aspect of the forepaw is far more prolonged than that to stimulation of the dorsal aspect.

Following a lesion, the absence of CP with conventional testing raises the possibility, among others, than an essential component in a 'reflex' circuit has been removed; therefore it is important to determine if CP can be restored by increasing the area of contact, by rubbing the hairs against the placer, or by performing extraordinary maneuvers. Rapidly lowering the cat several times prior to testing is often a useful device. Slowly permitting the left hand to slip forwards under the chin, with retroflexion of the head, prior to contact of the forepaw also promotes CP. In general, procedures that arouse or that appear to anger the cat may make CP more likely. More drastic measures include the administration of d-amphetamine (1-2 mgm/kg, i.m.), or 100/sec tonic stimulation of the red N. (see Results). Both measures may result in a remarkable temporary return of CP, even following removal of the sensorimotor cortex.

Measuring the placing reaction requires that transducers signal at least the following events: 1) The contact of the hairs of the limb with the side of a solid, 2) the clearing of the top edge of the contacted surface during the lifting-withdrawal phase and 3) the landing on top of the solid. In addition, 4) measuring the extent of horizontal displacement of the paw is desirable after cerebellar roof nuclear lesions, which are followed by hypermetria. Signalling the incidence of contact of the hairs ideally requires a transducer sensitive to very small forces. Initially, a piezoelectric crystal and a strain gauge operated at high sensitivity were each tested, but were abandoned because of difficulty in differentiating between the signals generated by the movement of the transducer towards the cat, and those resulting from the contact. Furthermore, a transducer sensitive to direct contact is apt to be damaged if the cat makes sudden violent or clawing movements. Interruption of a light beam incident on a photocell by the hairs of the paw avoids all of the above disadvantages, but introduces an uncertainty as to the exact time of contact because outlying hairs start to occlude the light beam before contacting the solid. Another error is introduced by the delay between the interruption of the light beam and the attainment of the final output level of the overall system. This delay is conveniently measured by interrupting the light beam with a microphone; contact with the solid is signalled by the output of the microphone. The magnitude of the delay depends on the characteristics of the photocell used, but even with the 'fastest' (FPT-100), contact of the microphone occurred *prior* to attainment of the final output level. Therefore, contact occurs at some point during the rising phase of the system output. The duration of the rising phase and hence the magnitude of the uncertainty are inversely related to the velocity of the paw or microphone relative to the solid. With practice, swift stimulation of the paw can be secured without significant bending of the limb. Thus, most of the rising phase of the photocell output in 27 summed CP trials in Fig. 26-right is contained in one 10 msec bin. By contrast, a "slow" photocell system was used in the earlier experiments, e.g., Fig. 21, where most of the rising phase is contained within three 10 msec bins. Calibration of this system, using a microphone to interrupt the light beam, yielded with swift stimulation an interval of 8-12 msec between initial changes in photocell and microphone outputs, the latter corresponding to the attainment of 20-40% of the maximum change in the photocell output. (With slow interruption of the light beam, the values for the interval and percentage both increased.) By this criterion, contact in Fig. 21 would have occurred not at the start of the bin indicated but either late in this bin or early in the following bin, leading to an overestimate of the latency of neuronal discharge. However, because a microphone is manifestly more effective in occluding the outer edge of the light beam than an uneven thicket of hairs, contact probably occurred early in the bin indicated.

A more useful analysis of contact uncertainty is provided by electrical recording at intermediate positions in the somatosensory inflow where the latency of response is unambiguous. Recordings from the superficial radial nerve above the elbow in an anesthetized cat, or population recording, during CP, from the tactile portions of thalamic VP nucleus permitted a "biological" calibration of the transducers used (see Results). It should be noted that the above discussion relates only to the errors in estimates of absolute latency and does not affect intervals between responses, e.g., neuronal and EMG activities.

The clearing of the top edge of the contacted surface during withdrawal is conveniently signalled by return of the output of a photocell placed near the edge to its initial state. Subsequent landing of the paw was signalled in the earlier experiments by a strain gauge attached to a horizontal platform, but this did not permit measuring the extent of horizontal displacement of the paw. The strain gauge assembly was replaced by an assembly of 8 strips ("placer keys"), each 1.5 cm wide with long axis perpendicular to the horizontal component of movement (Fig. 3). Each key signalled through a switch a level of displacement. If two keys were depressed by the paw, the level signalled corresponded to the key furthest from the contacted edge.

To study plasticity of CP, a dual chambered device for testing placing either into water (usually at 19—26° C) or onto a moist metal surface was used. Landing at either site was signalled by current flow generated by dissimilar electrode potentials.

Data Recording, Processing and Analysis

All population electrical recordings were fed through cathode follower inputs and conventionally amplified. Recordings from individual neurons were fed through a solid state input attached to the head and amplified with very short coupling time constant (0.2-0.7 msec). The amplified signals, the outputs of the CP transducers and a

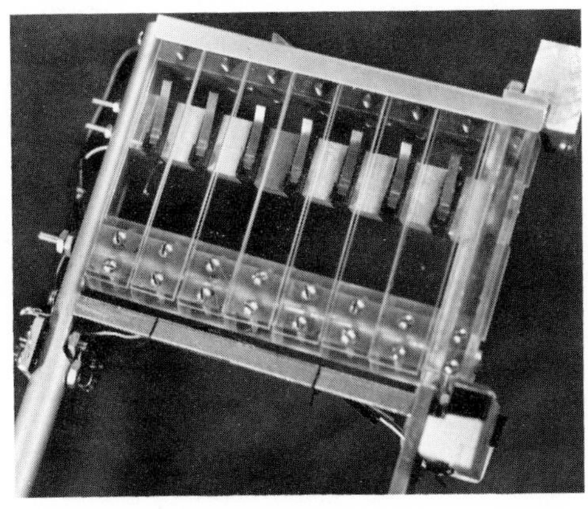

FIG. 3. Apparatus for transducing CP, viewed from above. Emerging light beam at upper right falls on slit before four photocells in housing at lower right. (In this photograph, light source and photocell to signal lower contacts are not attached to apparatus). First placer key at right is more opaque than seven at left and is attached to a vertically oriented contact plate. Other details in text.

voice monitor were recorded on 7 channel analog tape at 15 inches/sec. Subsequently, discharges by individual neurons were converted into standard rectangular pulses and re-recorded (with the original continuous voltage data) on analog tape. When discharges by two or, exceptionally, three distinguishable neurons were recorded, these were separated by standard logical procedures and re-recorded onto separate channels of the analog tape. The data were then recorded on digital tape. The incidences of neuronal discharges on up to 3 channels were each sampled at 2 Kc/sec and the six-bit A/D conversions of, e.g., 2 CP transducer and 2 EMG channels were sampled through a multiplexer at one-fourth the rate used for the spike channels. Although the sampling rate was adequate for handling neuronal discharges, multiplexing reduced the sampling rate and could have resulted in a loss of individual muscle action potentials. Therefore, prior to A/D conversion, EMG activity was led through a 'leaky' integrator with a time constant of decay of 10 msec. An "event" detection computer program permitted combing long runs of digital tape for samples of CP transducer output or EMG that met a preset criterion of change in amplitude. Such samples were "tagged" and individual samples on each of the 7 channels prior to or after this event, or the cumulative distributions of many CPs were available (see Fig . 13). Regardless of the bin width displayed, the event ordinate ('0' time) is placed at the start of the sample at 2 Kc which meets the criterion. Corresponding to each event, spike incidences and transducer or EMG samples were each separately summed between bin limits defined after visual inspection of the cumulative distributions. A rank order correlation test was performed on these sums to determine the relationship between, e.g., spikes and EMG during CP.

RESULTS

Movements and EMG Patterns of Normal CP of the Forepaw

When the support is removed from under one or both forepaws of an awake cat that is prevented from seeing both its limbs and the support, the following patterns of motor behavior may be observed: Initially, after a variable latency, 'searching' movements of the unsupported forepaw may occur which, after repeated CP testing, tend to be in the direction of the previous position of the support. The occurrence of such searching movements is related to the degree of alertness of the cat; they may be absent in a purring cat with relaxed muscles, but are so frequent in cats with tensed muscles as to interfere seriously with CP testing. Either between such searching movements or in their absence, gentle contact of hairs of the radial, dorsal or ulnar aspects of the forelimb with a vertically oriented surface results initially in a *lifting — withdrawal* movement until the top edge of the surface has just been cleared, followed by a *landing* movement directed to bring the plantar surface of the paw onto the horizontal support. CP can be elicited regardless of whether the limb is initially flexed or extended. The lifting-withdrawal phase results from flexion at the elbow and shoulder joints and ventroflexion at the wrist with flexion of the digits. (Contact with the ventral aspect of the digits results in flexion at the elbow, but dorsiflexion at the wrist). The relative contributions of flexion at each joint to the overall movement

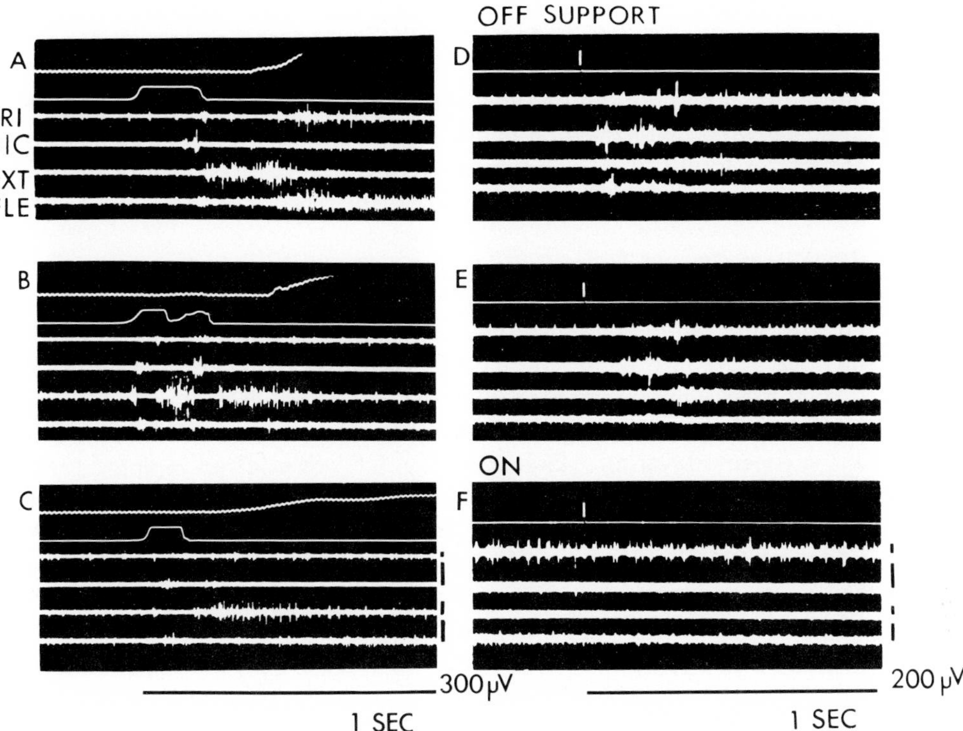

FIG. 4. EMG responses to stimulation only of forepaw hairs. (A–C) show three positive CPs; in each, from above downward, are shown strain gauge output (deflection up indicates downthrust onto platform), photocell output (deflection up indicates interruption of light beam by hairs), EMGs from triceps, biceps, long extensors of digits and flexor mass of forearm. In (D–F), hairs tapped by a probe activated by a 5 msec pulse (indicated on top trace by white line). Position of EMGs unchanged. Forelimb unsupported in (D and E), but supported in (F) where triceps tone increased. EMG amplification at left and right differ; calibrations at right of (C) and (F), respectively.

have not been quantitatively assayed, but, in addition to the usual pattern described above, two extremes may be noted: in some cats, for a few days after EMG recording electrodes have been implanted in forelimb muscles, the limb shows reduced flexion at the elbow and wrist and appears to be lifted mainly by shoulder girdle muscles. By contrast, during the initial phase of CP, occasional cats show marked ventroflexion at the wrist with reduced flexion at the elbow. Another rare pattern, seen especially following a gentle contact, consists of repetitive withdrawals (Fig. 4, B) prior to the final landing phase.

In the above descriptions, contact of the forepaw occurs close to the top edge of a vertically oriented plate. If, however, contact occurs far below the top of a tall structure such as a door, the forepaw may be lifted rapidly for several centimeters, pause in contact with the surface, then be lifted again, and this sequence is repeated up the door. Such vertical "skipping" suggests that the withdrawal phase is not continuously under sensory feedback but has both ballistic and sensory control components (see below).

During the landing phase, extension occurs at the elbow and shoulder joints with dorsiflexion at the wrist and extension of the digits. In addition, the paw is carried medially, forward or laterally following contact with its radial, dorsal or ulnar aspect respectively. Normally, the horizontal displacement rarely exceeds 3 cm (2 placer keys).

The latency of CP is the sum of the latency of withdrawal plus the interval between clearing the top edge and landing; it varies greatly between cats and even in the same cat with successive contacts. Factors contributing to this variability include: 1) The behavioral state of the cat, the shortest latencies being observed in alert cats with tensed body musculature and erect vibrissae and which are attending to the environment. With reduced alertness, the latency of CP increases and CP may become negative during repeated testing. Exceptionally, CP was elicited in one cat that was behaviorally asleep, but it was noted that the spindling ECoG became desynchronized when the forepaw was lifted off the support prior to testing. It should be noted that a few cats fail to exhibit CP when initially tested in a novel environment, but may do so on subsequent days. Such negative tests are often associated with a crouched posture and may reflect "fear." 2) The velocity-intensity relations of the contact stimulus. In general, swift stimulation over a wide area of skin results in the fastest CPs. Displacement of hairs is an adequate stimulus for CP (Fig. 4, A–C), but under the conditions usually used in collecting data it is likely that touch receptors are also stimulated and perhaps contribute to the effective afferent input. However, a smart blow to the forelimb, although resulting in tendon jerk reflexes in biceps and the long extensors of the digits, may inhibit or delay CP. No essential contribution to CP by deep receptors, e.g., those located in muscle, joint or interosseous membrane could be identified. Thus, section under light ether anesthesia of the superficial radial nerve above the elbow resulted subsequently in the loss of CP to stimulation of a small area at the base of digit I, but CP was retained to stimulation elsewhere on the forepaw. Similarly, CP was temporarily lost to stimulation of the dorsum of the forepaw following local subcutaneous injection of 1% procaine. 3) The site of stimulation on the forelimb. The shortest latencies for CP followed contact close to the tips of the digits: swift stimulation at this site in an aroused cat resulted in latencies of withdrawal typically in the range of 80–200 msec. Under similar conditions, the interval for landing was 100–350 msec. When the point of contact was moved half way up the forelimb, the latency of withdrawal increased fivefold but the interval for landing fell slightly.

Biceps and the flexor digitorum mass are both activated early in CP, contributing to the lifting-withdrawal phase. Anterior shoulder girdle muscles also contribute to this phase (see Fig. 32), but do so no earlier than biceps. The contributions made by the individual members of the set of muscles causing lifting-withdrawal may differ in CPs elicited even a few seconds apart, as manifested by the variability in latency and amount of activation of each muscle. Responses may show complex relationships; e.g., withdrawal occurs faster in Fig. 4, C than A, presumably because biceps activation, although smaller, occurs sooner. Nevertheless, the rank order correlation between the amount of integrated biceps activity and the latency of withdrawal may be both high (-.73) and significant ($p < .02$).

Normal patterns of biceps activation include: 1) An early onset (latency 20-40 msec) with maintained discharge leading to fast withdrawal as in Figs. 7-right and 23-8. 2) An early onset with one or more distinguishable later phases of discharge as in Figs. 17-B, 23-2, and 24-1 first CP. 3) A late onset of discharge as in Figs. 4-A and 17-C. The relationship of patterns (2) and (3) to latency of withdrawal is shown in Fig. 5. First episodes of biceps activity with latencies of less than 50 msec in duration are essentially unrelated, while first episodes occurring later than 50 msec and second episodes tend to increase in latency with increasing latency of withdrawal. Such findings imply dual processes of biceps activation, the transition occurring at approximately 50 msec latency. It must be emphasized that both early and later phases of biceps activation can be evoked by stimulation of hairs alone. Interrupting the cutaneous input either by local anesthesia or by nerve section not only abolishes CP from the appropriate skin areas (see above), but also all phases of biceps activation. Even transient stimulation of forepaw hairs by an electromagnetically actuated probe activates biceps (and other muscles), provided that the forepaw is unsupported (cf. Fig. 4, D-E and F).

Any activity present in the long extensors of the digits or in triceps prior to contact often abruptly diminishes at some stage during withdrawal (Figs. 7, 23-2 and -8). A precontact increase in extensor digitorum tone is a convenient byproduct of moving the cat towards a stationary placer; such an increase presumably reflects the vestibular

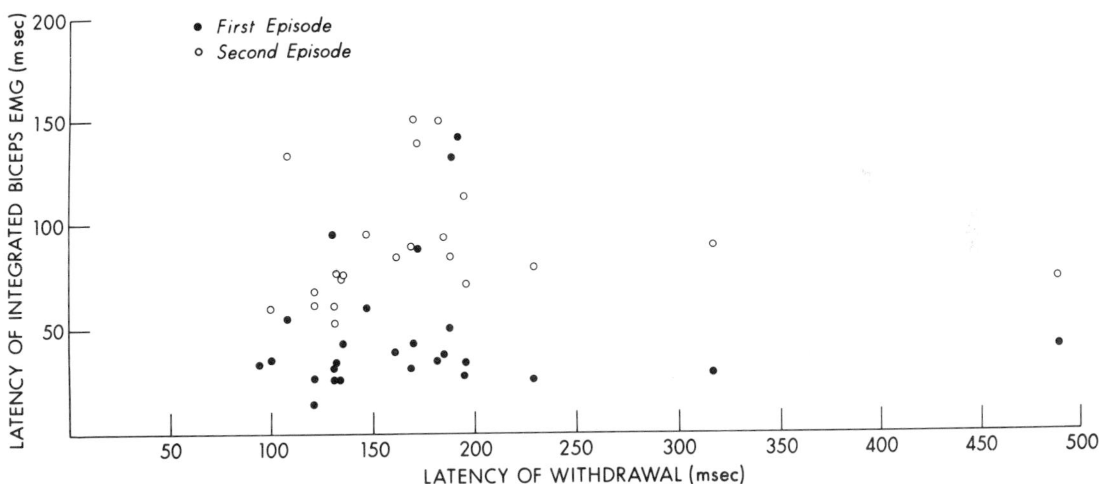

FIG. 5. Relationship of integrated biceps EMG activity to latency of withdrawal during CP. Latency of withdrawal measured from mid-point between start and finish of fast rising phase of photocell output to start of fast return to precontact state. Middorsum and radial-dorsal aspects of forepaw contacted. Not all first episodes of BIC activity followed by distinguishable later episodes of activity.

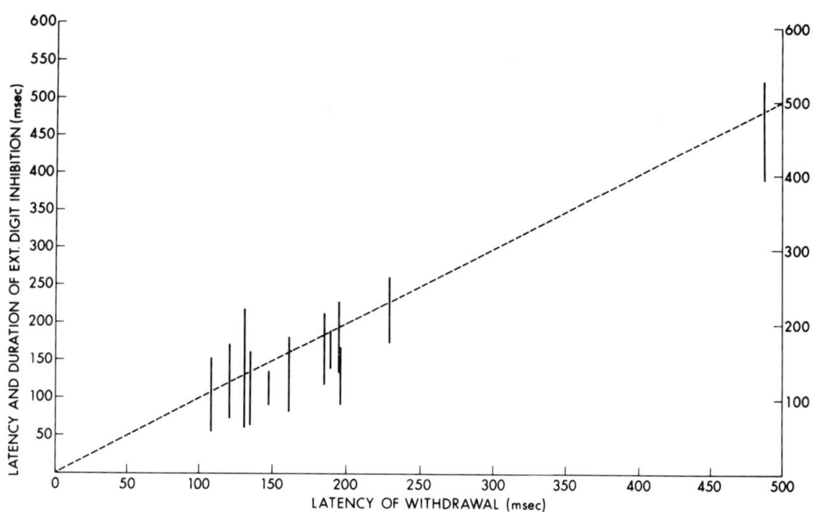

FIG. 6. Relationship of period of inhibition of extensor digitorum EMG activity to latency of withdrawal. Data from CPs of Fig. 5 where precontact extensor activity was prominent. Bottom and top of each vertical line show onset of reduction and abrupt increase in EMG activity, respectively. Broken diagonal facilitates comparison of occurrence of withdrawal and extensor activation.

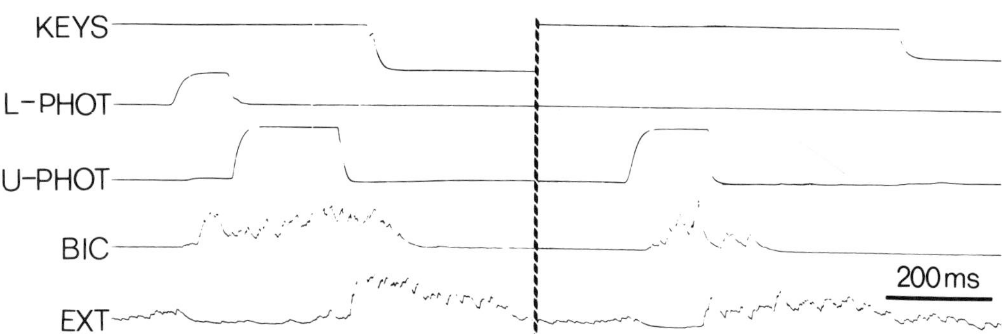

FIG. 7. Effect on EMG pattern in CP of changing the distance traversed to the top edge of the contacted surface. In addition to upper photocell assembly (U-Phot) situated at top end of vertical plate (Fig. 3), another (L-Phot) was attached 7.5 cm lower down on plate. Forepaw contacted low and high positions on vertical plate in left and right records, respectively. A larger downward deflection on 'keys' channel indicates a larger horizontal displacement on landing. Data are displayed by inkwriter. (This Figure is taken from (9)).

placing reaction and prepares the cat for landing on a support. Although not part of the tactile placing reaction, the prior increase in extensor tone provides a background against which inhibition occurring during withdrawal may be revealed. The latency and duration of extensor inhibition are evident in Fig. 6.

A profound change in EMG pattern occurs when the forepaw clears the top edge of the vertical plate. Biceps activity is reduced but that of extensor digitorum increases, usually quite abruptly. Triceps activity may increase concomitantly with that of the extensors (Fig. 23-2 and -8) or later. However, delicate CPs may occur without a detectable increase in triceps activity.

The increase in extensor digitorum activity usually occurs 20-50 msec after the start of the fast return of the photocell output. This implies that loss of contact at the top edge may be an important sensory cue determining the change in EMG activity. However, a few CPs show zero or even negative delays (Fig. 6); i.e., the extensors are switched on prior to the forepaw's having cleared the top edge. Such early activation is compatible with either a sensory cue derived from hairs proximal to the tips of the digits or a ballistic component. Significantly, when the initial contact occurred far from, compared with close to, the top edge, as in Fig. 7- left and right, respectively, the latency of abrupt extensor digitorum activation was markedly increased, a finding that is incompatible with a ballistic activation of extensors triggered by the initial contact. The association of extensor activation with restitution of the photocell output regardless of the distance through which the forepaw has travelled strongly supports the hypothesis that loss of contact at the top edge of hairs situated at or near the distal part of the forelimb is an important sensory cue that terminates withdrawal and precipitates the landing phase.

Searching movements also exhibit a sequence of biceps followed by extensor digitorum activation, but the interval between activations of these muscles in considerably

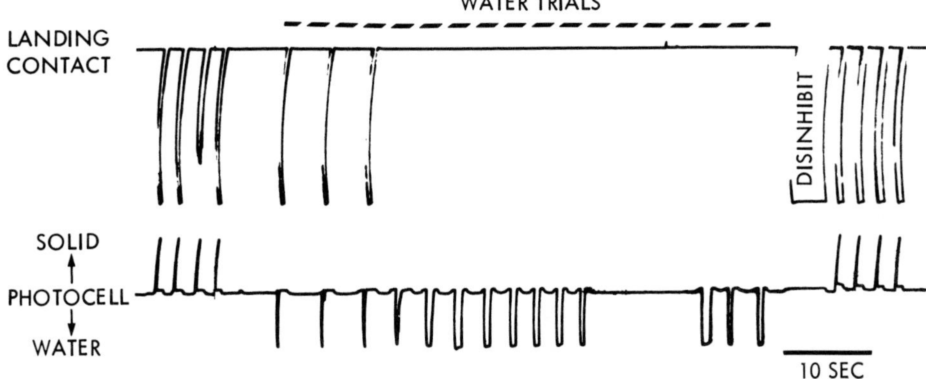

FIG. 8. Plasticity of CP. Upward and downward deflections on photocell record indicate tests with solid and water compartments, respectively. From left to right, 4 positive CPs occurred when the forepaw landed on a solid platform. Subsequently, the water compartment was substituted resulting in 3 CPs onto water, followed by 11 failures. After resting the forepaw on the solid platform for 3 1/2 sec, 4 positive CPs occurred onto the solid platform.

less than that observed during CP. The early onset of extensor activity may reflect the lack of inhibitory input from hairs when the paw is searching in the air, compared with moving vertically up a plate. Biceps activity during searching lasts longer and diminishes more gradually than in CP.

Plasticity of CP

The aversion exhibited by most cats to walking in puddles suggested the possibility of using water to condition CP. Substituting a water compartment for the solid surface on which the forepaw had previously landed modified CP in over one-half of the cats studied. Often, after 1-12 trials, most contacts result not in the forepaw's landing in the water (Fig. 8), but in one of the following: 1) Most commonly, flexion occurs at the wrist, with or without slight flexion at the elbow, and between trials the forepaw often adopts a flexed posture. 2) The forepaw lifts but hangs over the water. 3) A slight jerk of the forepaw occurs. 4) No movement is observed. 5) Movements occur that appear to search for a solid support. Immediate testing of the contralateral forepaw on the solid compartment results in positive CP.

Placing of the affected forepaw is restored by passively resting it on a solid surface for several seconds. Less commonly, "disinhibition" is incomplete until the affected paw has been rested several times. If, following disinhibition, a second set of trials into water is tested, the number required to inhibit CP is usually reduced, compared with the first set. Such occurrence of "savings" implied a "memory" system that resists disinhibition.

The Neural Circuits Subserving CP

The above description of CP implies the need for signalling 1) the steady state lack of support under one or more paws, and 2) the occurrence and location of contact with the limb. Lack of support is probably signalled by the reduction of discharge from touch and pressure receptors located on the ventral aspect of the paw rather than by proprioceptors, because CP can be elicited regardless of whether the limb is flexed or extended and when the digits are dorsiflexed. With gentle stimulation, CP is unambiguously elicited by contact with hairs alone. We have not studied the afferent spinal pathways subserving CP. Prior reports are conflicting; in the cat, CP was undisturbed by section of the dorsal columns but was abolished by a mediodorsal lesion of the lateral columns (29). In the monkey, section of the dorsal columns abolished CP for 10 days— 4 months (23).

The analysis of the neural circuitry subserving CP is dealt with in the sections below and is summarized in the diagram of Fig. 9.

N. Ventralis posterior

The evidence in the monkey (12) that the postcentral gyrus is essential for CP suggested that VP is the intermediary relay for the cutaneous input subserving CP. Lesions were made in VP in 12 cats, 5 of which were observed for 2—4 months. The lesions typically resulted in loss of CP to stimulation of specific contralateral skin areas, *without* the occurrence of cross-placing of the unaffected paw (cf. the effects of VL-VA lesions). During the first to third postoperative days following massive VP lesions, CP was either absent or rarely obtainable to stimulation of the contralateral forepaw and hindpaw. During the same period, CP was present to stimulation of the limbs ipsilateral to the lesion, visual placing was usually present bilaterally, and proprioceptive correction occurred to passive flexion of the wrist contralateral to the lesion. The subsequent clinical course depended on whether the lesion included

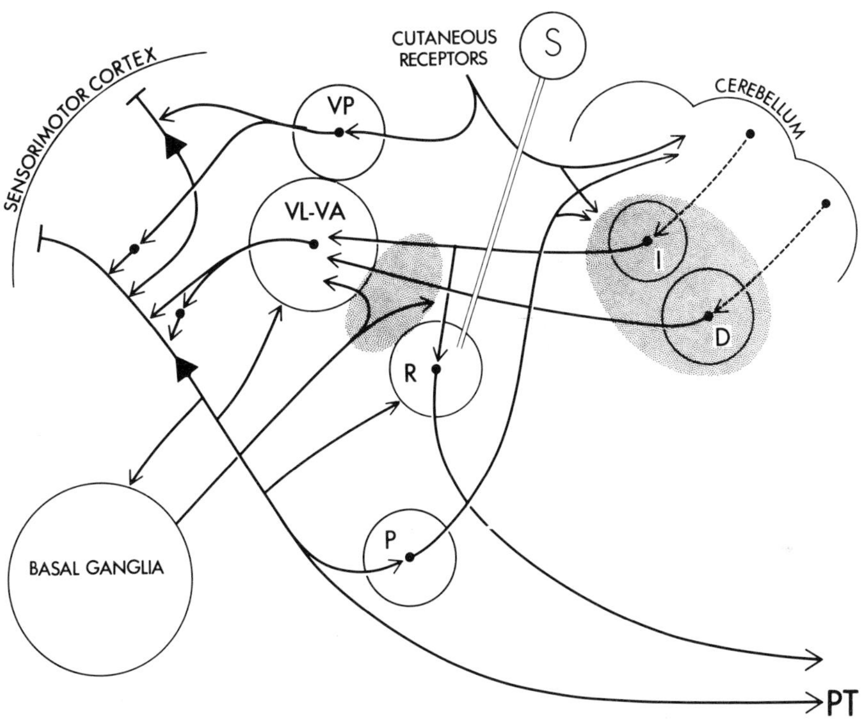

FIG. 9. Diagram of some neural structures with their interconnections, whose role in CP is discussed in this report. Abbreviations: VP(N. ventralis posterior), VL-VA-(N. ventralis lateralis and anterior), R - (red N.), P -(pontine N.), I -(N. interpositus), D -(N. dentatus) and PT (pyramidal tract). S-bipolar electrodes in red N. for delivering tonic 100/sec stimuli. Shading indicates two levels at which the cerebello-thalamo-cortical circuit was interrupted, with differing consequences to the red N. It is emphasized that not all portions of the motor control system believed to be important in CP are included in the diagram, nor are all the connections shown to the indicated structures; e.g., indirect afferent inputs to basal ganglia, VL-VA and red nucleus are omitted. Synaptology derived from (7, 16, 19, 26, 35, 46, 49).

cells ventrally placed in the nucleus. Where such cells were spared, CP could be elicited from the extremities of the affected paw, especially the dorsal and radial aspects, but was absent following stimulation at more proximal sites. In cat-39 (Fig. 10), from the fourth postoperative day until over 3 months later, CP was virtually absent to stimulation of the lateral aspect of the arm above the elbow, the anterior aspect from the elbow upwards, and the hindlimb. During the same period, CP was present to stimulation of the dorsal, radial and ulnar aspects of the digits, but was only variably present to testing between the wrist and elbow. After lesions that included ventral VP cells, CP to delicate stimulation of the digits was abolished. In addition, lowering the affected paw onto the surface of water at 30—32° C failed to result in the immediate withdrawal seen in cats either without lesions (30) or with VP lesions that spared ventral cells. A striking lack of motor impairment following a VP lesion was shown by the occurrence of cross-placing in the affected forepaw when the normal limb was stimulated peripherally but held proximally to stop it from placing.

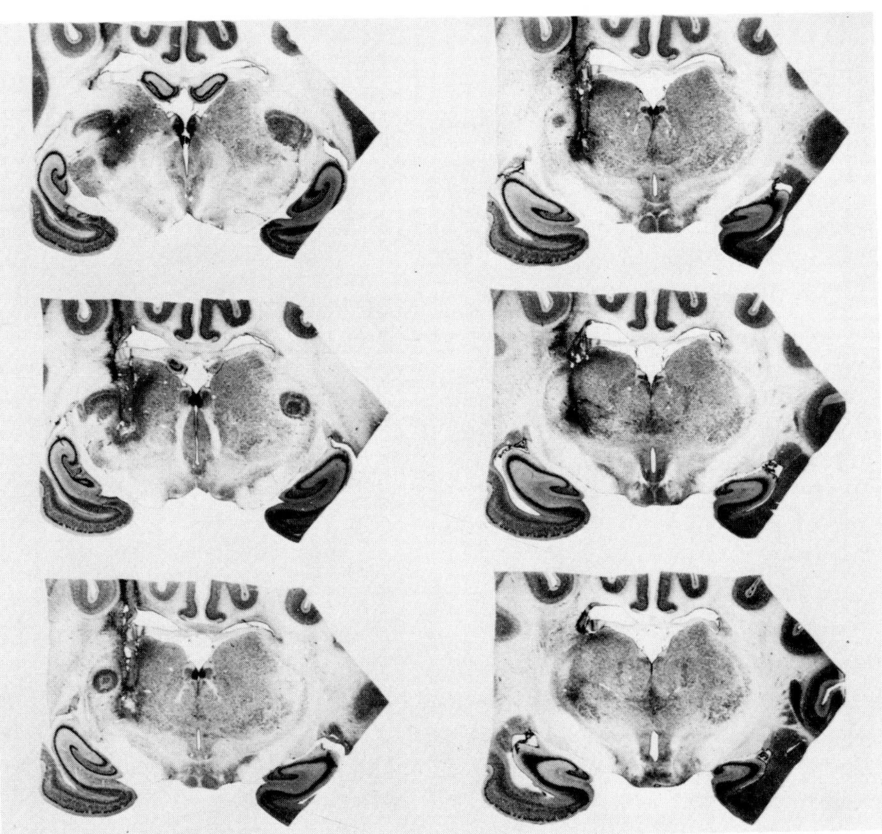

FIG. 10. Photomicrographs of representative sections through thalamic VP lesions cat-39.

Lesions such as those of Fig. 10 are too laterally placed to affect significantly the cerebellar input to VL (see below). A more medial lesion that was intended to sever the cerebellar input to VL was followed by the return of CP to stimulation of the dorsal and ulnar aspects of the paw within 6 days, but CP to stimulation of the radial aspect was absent for the subsequent 2 month period of observation. Radial stimulation was ineffective despite 'facilitation' (see methods) or injection of d-amphetamine, i.m. The inference that the lesion had extended laterally into medial VP was histologically confirmed.

Terminal exploration of somatosensory areas I and II under pentobarbital anesthesia disclosed in several cats unexpectedly large primary responses (20—60% of control side) to stimulation of contralateral peripheral sites that had previously failed to elicit CP. Clearly, additional recordings made at varying times after a VP lesion are required to analyze these findings.

CP was lost following a VP lesion even when anterior VPL was spared. The corollary, that destruction of anterior VPL alone would not abolish CP, was confirmed, in one cat by the return of CP on the fourth postoperative day. In summary, the effects of a VP lesion are what might be expected from the representation of the body surface mapped by evoked potentials (34). To a varying extent, all of the effective lesions encroached on the posterior nuclear group (37), but given the lack of topographical representation in these nuclei, it seems unlikely that loss of CP to stimulation of specific peripheral loci can thus be explained.

After a VP lesion, EMGs recorded from biceps showed absent, or delayed (68—234 msec) responses to contact with the paw; those recorded from the long extensors of the digits showed no inhibition. Similarly, a cat in which VPL was cooled showed both a reduction and a delay in the activation of biceps and a delayed inhibition of the extensor digitorum.

As previously described in acute preparations (40), individual VP neurons are powerfully activated after a short latency by peripheral stimulation. In the awake cat, increased firing of individual VP neurons commenced in the 0-10 msec bin following contact, as in FIG. 11. The simultaneously recorded biceps EMG started increasing in the 20-30 msec period. Taking minimum delays of 4 and 8 msec (see below) for transmission from VP→ PT neurons and from PT neurons → biceps EMG, there is no basis for rejecting the hypothesis that VP is part of the dynamic circuit initiating all phases of CP. Furthermore, VP neurons responding to stimulation of the dorsal aspect of the forepaw show reduced firing when the top edge is cleared, which suggests that VP may transmit the sensory cue causing a directed landing.

The Sensorimotor Cortex

Lesions of varying size and location were made in the sensorimotor cortex and SII of 7 cats. An example of an extensive lesion destroying the left sensorimotor cortex, adjoining medial cortex and virtually all of SII is shown in Fig. 12. This lesion is more extensive than that illustrated in Fig. 3 of Bard (11). On the first postoperative day, the cat could walk, feed and even shake food rapidly from the right forelimb. CP and visual placing were present in the left forelimb but, together with proprioceptive

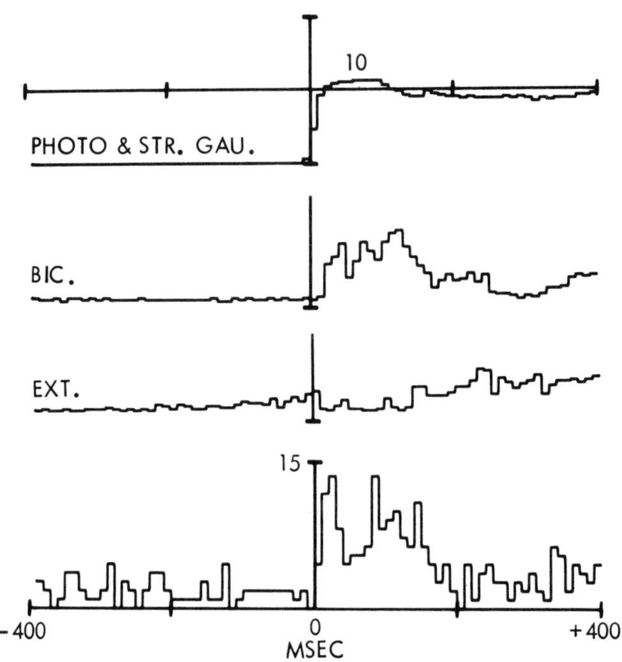

FIG. 11. Pre- and postcontact histograms of activity of a VP neuron (at bottom), integrated EMGs and CP transducer outputs. In top histogram, transducer channel initially recorded photocell output and then, during return of photocell output, switched to strain gauge output. (Transition between these outputs smeared by summing.) Pre- and postcontact histograms of this and all subsequent Figs. (except Fig. 27) displayed in 10 msec bins. Numerals at top are numbers of CPs summed. In bottom histogram, numerals on ordinate calibrate numbers of spikes/bin.

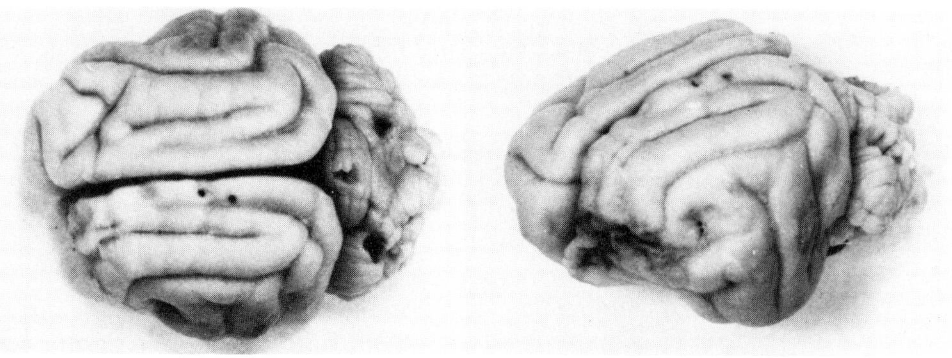

FIG. 12. Photograph of lesion of left sensorimotor cortex (cat N-15). Recording in Fig. 28-right obtained from right N. interpositus of this cat.

correction, were absent on the right side. The unsupported right forelimb had a markedly hyperextended posture, and made no searching movements. By 16 days, proprioceptive correction to ventroflexion of the wrist had returned, but correction at the digits was absent, and the cat stood on its 'fist'. Testing repeatedly failed to elicit either CP or early biceps activation on the affected side (Fig. 28-right), except on two occasions when rubbing the hairs on the dorsum of the affected paw elicited a long latency, "stiff-legged", hypermetric placing. In other cats, possibly because more of SII was spared, such stereotyped placings although still rare, were more often elicited. Such placings have been observed 3-37 days after cortical removal; they are usually best elicited by stimulation of the dorsal or radial aspects of the paw, more rarely by ulnar, and never by proximal stimulation of the limb. The movement is very poorly directed as compared with normal CP, usually resulting in a landing on the horizontal surface only after a dorsal contact. The possibility that such stereotyped placings were "spontaneous" movements was excluded by EMG recordings which revealed an increased latency (42-59 msec) for biceps activation. Extensor inhibition occurred later and was less prominent than normal; thus, although triggered by contact with hairs, stereotyped placing, because of the extended posture of the lower forepaw, may be completed through proprioceptive correction of the paw, which is passively ventroflexed during the lifting phase.

The likelihood of placing after sensorimotor cortical lesions was markedly increased 1-3 hours following the administration of d-amphetamine (1-2 mgm/kg, i.m.), an effect previously described after larger doses of dl-amphetamine (10 mg/kg, i.p.; note cat 26-left side (33)). Post-amphetamine placing was smoothly executed, but had a longer latency than normal; it was readily obtainable with dorsal stimulation, but was very rare with stimulation of the ulnar aspects of the digits. The latency of biceps activation in post-d-amphetamine placing was slightly increased, e.g., 25-50 msec. Tonic stimulation of the red N. at 100/sec also markedly increased the likelihood of placing, but the execution was less coordinated than with d-amphetamine. The effect of red N. stimulation was manifest as early as the first postoperative day and also long after the terminals of corticofugal axons would be expected to have ceased transmitting (e.g., at 14 days—4 1/2 months).

Four and one-half months after the lesion of sensorimotor cortex as shown in Fig. 12, the left forepaw was immediately withdrawn from water at 30.5 °C, but the right forepaw stood in water at this temperature. However, when tested with water at 11.5° C, the right forepaw immediately withdrew and gave a quick shake.

The possible dynamic role of sensorimotor cortex in CP was investigated by recording from individual bulbar PT axons. Most PT neurons responding during CP increased or decreased their firing rates too late to have initiated the earliest EMG activity, but could still have contributed to the regulation of later activity. However, the small fraction of hair field PT neurons that responded powerfully to contact with distal contralateral forepaw discharged prior to the earliest biceps activity. The PT neuron of Fig. 13 had a receptive field localized to hairs over digit II of the contralateral forepaw. Contact with the mediodorsal aspect of the paw (including the neuronal receptive field) resulted in an increase in discharge, starting in the 10-20 msec postcontact period. The integrated VP recording similarly showed an increase in the

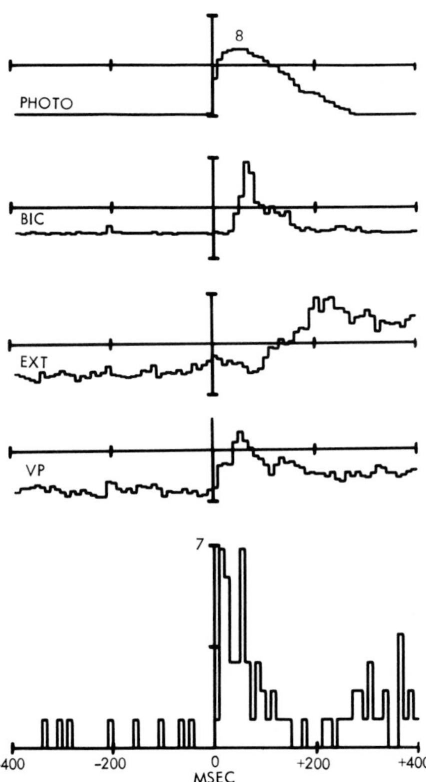

FIG. 13. Pre- and postcontact histograms of activity of a PT neuron (at bottom), integrated population recording from VP, EMGs and photocell outputs. Terminal stimulation through EXT electrodes produced ulnar deviation at wrist. Other details in legend of Fig. 11.

10–20 msec period. Histograms displayed in 4 msec bins showed latencies of 8–12 msec and 12–16 msec of VP population and PT unit responses, respectively. Measurements on individual CPs showed intervals of 3.5–7.5 msec between the earliest VP and earliest PT responses. The earliest biceps activity started in the 30–40 msec postcontact period (36–40 msec with 4 msec bins), implying that the earliest PT response led biceps activation by at least 20 msec. However, in cats with a stimulating electrode assembly implanted over sensorimotor cortex, biceps activation tends to occur later than in cats without such implants, implying that sensorimotor cortical function is slightly depressed. In normal cats, given that activation of biceps starts in the 20–30 msec period, and assuming that the earliest PT response could be earlier than that in Fig. 13 by no more than a few milliseconds, an interval of approximately 10 msec is estimated between early PT discharges and biceps activation.

A striking feature of large diameter, cutaneous field PT neurons is that powerful discharges can be elicited by contact stimuli that do not result in placing movements;

such dissociation occurs with cutaneous stimulation of the supported or held limb of an awake or a sleeping cat. Furthermore, high frequency driving of PT neurons by cutaneous stimulation is unimpaired following massive VL-VA lesions which impair CP (see section on VL-VA). Following a massive VP lesion that abolishes CP, the maintained driving of PT neurons normally observed during rubbing of forelimb skin is lost. PT responses to stimulating the face may be retained, possibly because VPM is partially spared by the lesion; dropping the cat or forward acceleration during CP testing may lead to increased PT discharge, presumably because vestibular input (32) is preserved. Less accountably, rubbing the lower back and hindquarters may also increase PT discharge, perhaps because of sensory input of a sexual character. After a VP lesion, pre- and postcontact histograms obtained on 10 individual PT neurons revealed either increased or decreased firing at latencies of 60-150 msec following stimulation of the contralateral paw. PT responses to stimulation of the unaffected (ipsilateral) forepaw started earlier than those to stimulation of the affected paw, e.g., at 20-30 msec. We conclude that early response by PT neurons to contact stimulation is mediated by VP, but is not a sufficient condition for placing movements; furthermore an alternative pathway may elicit a late PT response, but this alone is also insufficient for CP.

N. Ventralis Lateralis and Anterior

Lesions of varying size and location were made in VL-VA of 20 cats. Massive lesions of VL-VA that included ventral portions of these nuclei abolished contralateral CP for varying periods depending on the peripheral site of stimulation. Typically, CP and visual placing returned on the control side on the first postoperative day. When unsupported, the forelimb contralateral to the lesion usually adopted an extended posture, and did not show searching movements. CP was absent, but cross-placing of the unstimulated, unaffected forepaw occurred as early as the first postoperative day, implying that the function of VP was unimpaired. Visual placing and proprioceptive correction following ventroflexion of the wrist returned at various times from the first postoperative day onwards. Subsequently, during the first postoperative week, stimulation of dorsal or, less usually, radial aspects of the paw resulted occasionally in CP, but the paw was carried high, the reaction was slowed and usually fatigued after one or a few trials. Even when CP was absent, a prominent jerk due to transient flexion at the elbow, or a partial withdrawal, or repetitive withdrawals were often observed. The early component of biceps activation was prominent. Over the first three postoperative weeks, the probability of CP increased and both its latency and fatiguability were reduced. At this stage of recovery, stimulation of the affected paw often resulted in placing of both paws. CP to stimulation of the ulnar aspect occurred rarely at 2 weeks and was still highly improbable at one month. Searching movements were the last to return. In cat N-6 (Fig. 14), the extensive left sided VL-VA lesions spared only a small portion of VA dorsally and extended minimally into VP and lateralis posterior. One month postoperatively, CP was absent to stimulation of the ulnar aspect of the right forepaw but had returned to stimulation of the dorsal and radial aspects by the twelfth day. Terminal exploration under pentobarbital

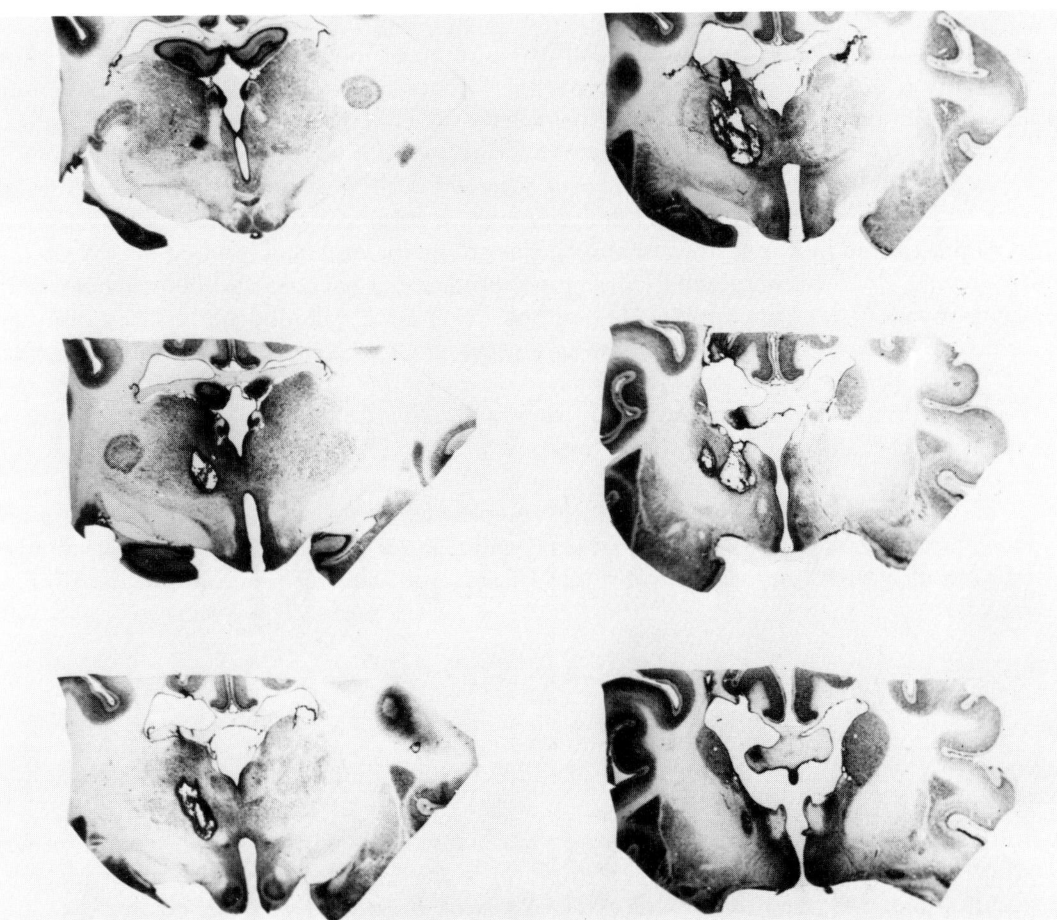

FIG. 14. Photomicrographs of representative sections through thalamic VL-VA lesions of cat-N6.

anesthesia disclosed a left cruciate response to stimulation of the right brachium conjunctivum with amplitude 3% of that of the control (right) side response. High-frequency trains of stimuli to each motor cortex elicited normal EMG responses in the corresponding limbs, confirming that the lesion had not damaged corticofugal pathways in the internal capsule; furthermore, there was no significant difference in the D and I waves in left and right bulbar pyramids. Electrocutaneous stimulation of the ulnar aspect of each forepaw yielded equal SI primary responses, confirming that the lesion had not impaired transmission through VP.

If cells are spared ventrally, even large VL-VA lesions have quite transient effects on CP. In cat-28 (Fig. 15-right lesion), CP to stimulation of the dorsal and radial aspects of the left forepaw returned on the second postoperative day and to stimu-

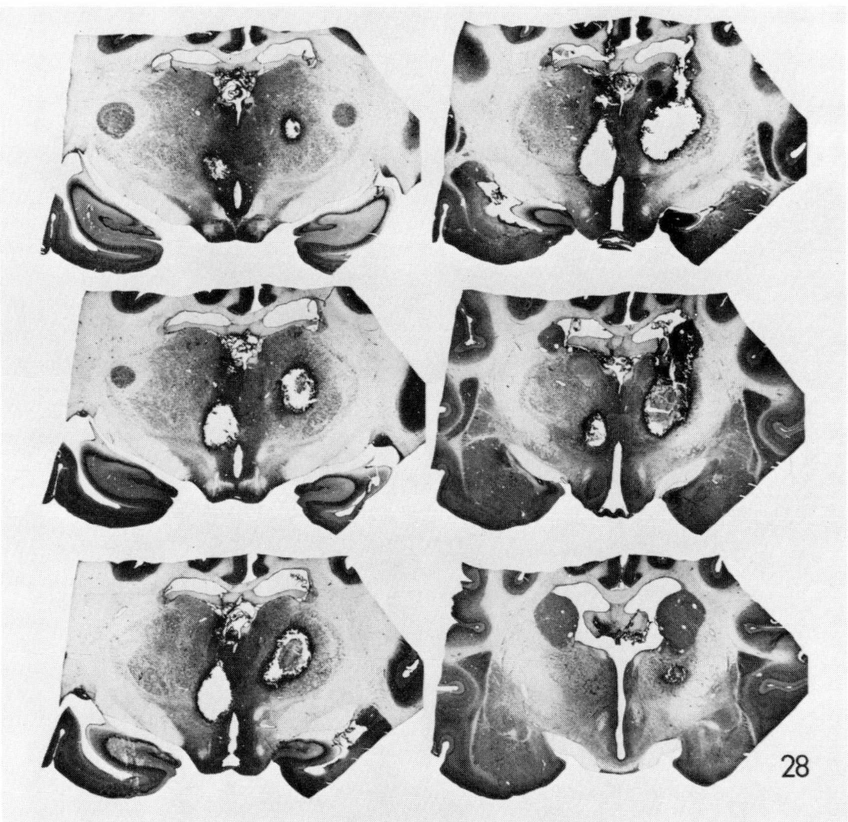

FIG. 15. Photomicrographs of representative sections through right VL-VA lesion and control left lesion of VM and mammillothalamic tract in cat -28.

lation of the ulnar aspect, upper arm and hindpaw on the fifth day. The cruciate response (recorded epidurally) to stimulation of N. interpositus was 64% of the 'control' response, which was 265 μV for an 8 mA pulse, i.e., it was probably unaffected by the left-sided lesion. The monosynaptic PT response to stimulation of VL-VA was reduced to 20% of the control value, indicating a severe loss of thalamocortical projection neu rons. By contrast with cat-28, CP to stimulation of the ulnar aspect of the forepaw in another cat was highly improbably for 3-4 weeks following a smaller but ventrally placed lesion that reduced the cruciate response to stimulation of N. interpositus-brachium conjunctivum to 25-30% of the control response.

With extensive lesions of VL-VA, the question arises as to whether the effects or CP are due to damage to nearby nuclei or tracts. An example of a control lesion is shown in Fig. 16; CP to stimulation of the dorsal, radial and ulnar aspects of the right forepaw returned on the first postoperative day. This implies that ventral and anterior portions of N. reticularis, anterior portions of VA, and the most medial portion of in-

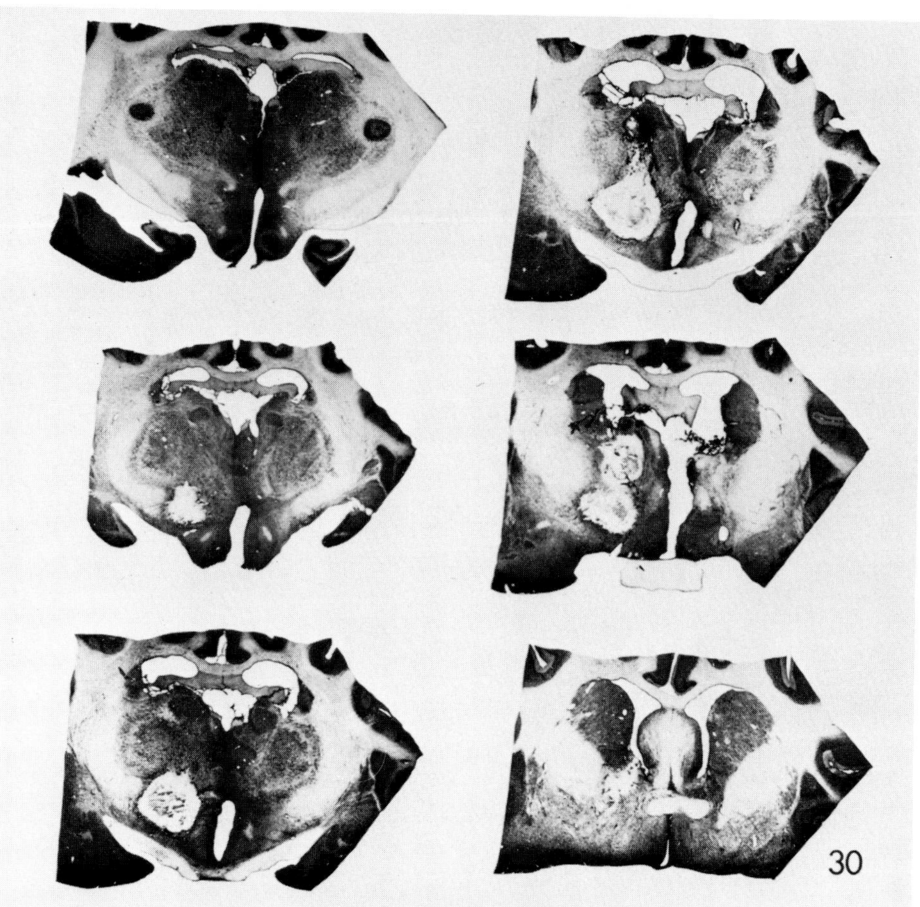

FIG. 16. Photomicrographs of representative sections through control lesion of ventral portion of reticular nucleus and adjoining capsule in cat-30.

ternal capsule are unimportant in CP. In Fig. 15-left, the control lesion destroyed much of ventralis medialis and severed the mamillothalamic tract; CP to stimulation of all three aspects of the right forepaw returned on the second postoperative day. Only transient reduction of CP followed lesions of N. centralis lateralis, the centre median N., N. prothalamicus and portions of the caudate N. adjoining VA. Destruction of N. lateralis posterior was followed by return of CP over a 3-7 day period. The lesion clearly encroached on dorsal VP; on terminal exploration, it was shown to have reduced the SI primary response to 60% of the control value. A temporary dysfunction of ventral VP may account for the delay in recovery.

Cooling VL-VA results in the reversible loss of contralateral CP (Fig. 17). The retention of short latency, e.g., 8 msec, EMG responses in forelimb muscles to interpolated stimuli to motor cortex is used as a physiological control for spread of the cold block to the internal capsule (cf. A and F). The release of cross-placing during cooling provides evidence that transmission through VP is unimpaired. Significantly, early bi-

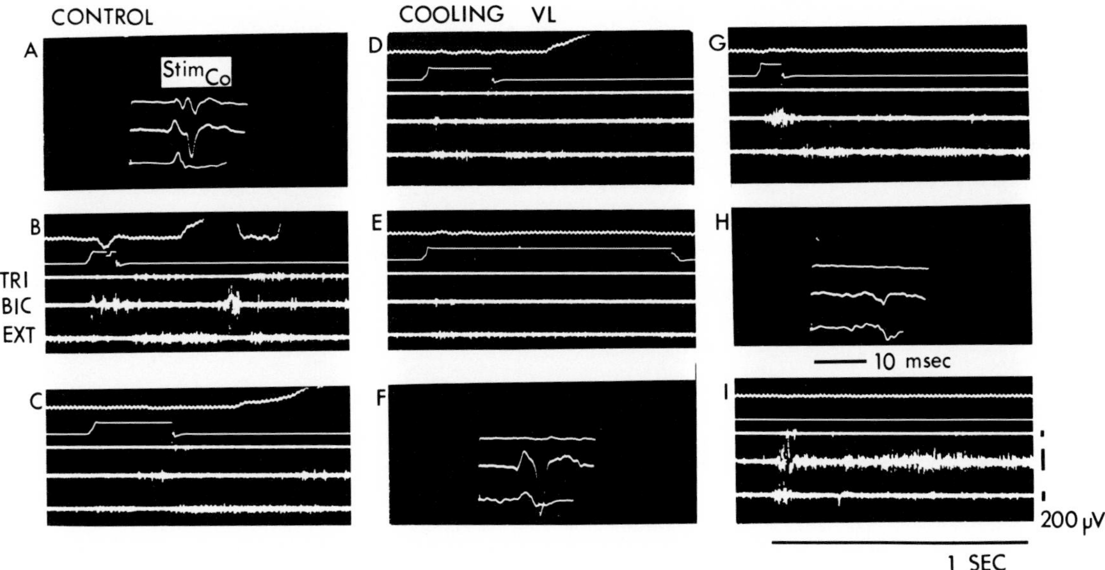

FIG. 17. The effect of cooling VL on contralateral CP. Sequence of records (A-I). Left column shows control EMG responses to (A) stimulus to motor cortex and (B, C) during CP. Transducer outputs and EMGs are shown in same order as in Fig. 4-left. Middle column shows CP present 11 sec after onset of cooling (D). From 17 sec onwards, CP was absent e.g., (E). Responses to cortical stimulus shown in (F). Subsequently, forepaw lifted once to contact stimulus (G), but did not place. Still later, responses to cortical stimulus were markedly reduced (H). Cooling discontinued after 70 sec. One min after cooling stopped, the forepaw could withdraw from cold water (I), but CP was still absent. (Nearly 9 min after cooling stopped, CP was occasionally present.)

ceps activity was not abolished by cooling, but inhibition of extensor digitorum was reduced.

The finding that CP is only temporarily abolished by VL-VA lesions raises the possibility that its loss, by analogy with spinal shock, is due to withdrawal of tonic facilitation by the main thalamic nucleus projecting to motor cortex. The following findings in cats 1-14 days after VL-VA lesions provide evidence against such a nonspecific effect: 1) High frequency driving of large PT neurons by cutaneous stimulation is unimpaired. 2) The ratio of the mean rates of discharge by PT neurons during waking/slow wave sleep is usually slightly above or below one (cf. monkeys (20)), while the ratio during activated sleep/slow wave sleep usually exceeds one, as described in normal monkeys by Evarts (20). 3) While the absolute level of activity in the population of PT neurons is not readily assessed, the bulbar PT shows much impulse traffic, with individual axons exhibiting high rates of discharge. In Fig. 19-legend, although the deprivation of synaptic drive to PT neurons was greater than interruption of the VL-VA input, in the awake cat high mean rates of discharge were encountered in the large PT axons that were recorded. (In normal awake cats, the largest PT axons, i.e., those with 0.5-1.0 msec corticobulbar conduction times, had mean rates of discharge as high as those with 1.0-1.5 msec conduction times, cf. in the monkey (21)). The interspike interval histograms of the partially 'deafferented' PT neurons in Fig. 19 are "dispersed" periodic in form and have fewer brief intervals than those of normal,

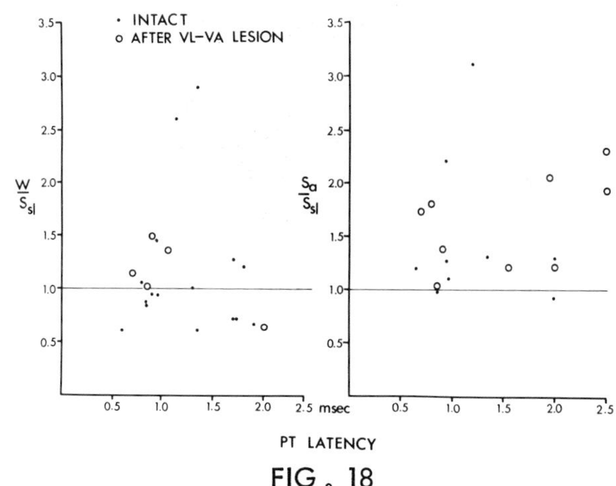

FIG. 18

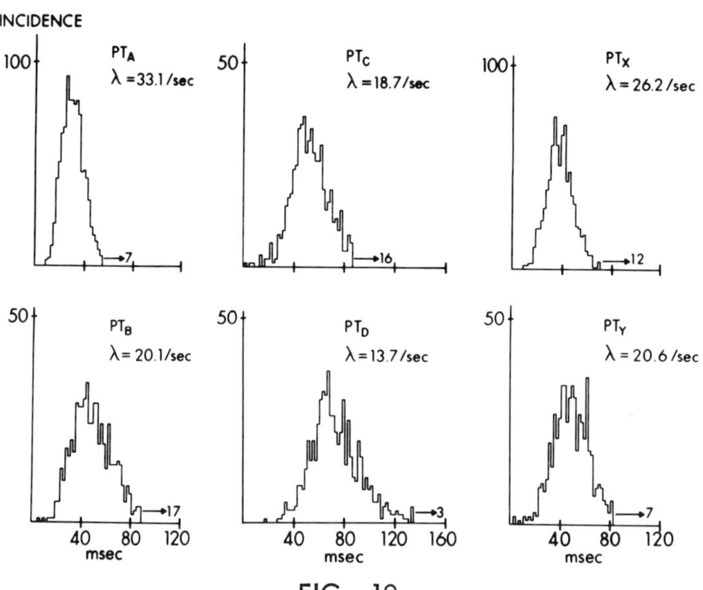

FIG. 19

awake cats where the percentage of intervals of 0–10 msec duration has a median of 4% (cf. PT neurons of monkey (20)).

The possible dynamic role of VL-VA in CP was assessed by recording from individual neurons in these nuclei. As a preliminary, the resting discharge was observed in quiet, awake cats (Fig. 20) and, in a few neurons, during sleep. In the awake state VL-VA neurons displayed a greater increase in mean rate with increasing alertness than did PT neurons. Mean rates of discharge for 3/4 of the neurons recorded were in the range of 0–30/sec. With rare exceptions (e.g., neuron AA-20-1), interspike interval distributions of resting activity in the awake state showed very few brief intervals and had a quasi-gamma shape. Semilog plots showed either a linear decrement of intervals longer than 20–30 msec, or skewing which was usually positive. The n-tuple distributions (Fig. 25 legend) usually showed marked convergence, i.e., the resting discharge is not well described by the random walk model (22).

VL-VA neurons responding during CP displayed either an increase in firing rate, usually followed by a reduction, or an initial reduction. Fig. 21 shows a neuron with an early phase of increased discharge starting during the 20–30 msec postcontact period and a second phase of increased discharge starting 300 msec later. Positive CPs (A–C) were accompanied by high frequency responses; when the cat became drowsy, the mean rate of precontact discharge was reduced, the neuronal response to contact was absent or reduced, and CP became negative (D, E). Subsequently, the neuron gave high frequency "spindling" discharges (F), which were desynchronized by peripheral stimulation (G), restoring both the evoked response and CP (H). Evidently, the occurrence of CP was contingent upon an early, high frequency response by the neuron

---

FIG. 18. Ratios of mean rates of discharge of individual PT neurons in awake and sleeping states compared in intact cats and 11–14 days following a VL-VA lesion. At left, ratio of rates during waking/slow wave sleep ($\frac{W}{S_{sl}}$) and at right, rates during activated/slow wave sleep ($\frac{Sa}{S_{sl}}$) are plotted as functions of orthodromic PT latency. Note that orthodromic PT latencies that exceed 1.5 msec are usually 'I' discharges in large PT axons rather than 'D' discharges in slow axons. In the cat with the VL-VA lesion, a PT axon responded at 1.95 and 0.45 msec to stimulating sensorimotor cortex and internal capsule respectively, and is plotted at the estimated 'D' latency, 0.7 msec. Another PT axon responding at 1.4 msec to stimulating internal capsule is plotted at 2.5 msec.

FIG. 19. Interspike interval histograms of resting discharge by 6 individual PT neurons recorded in a single penetration of bulbar PT of awake cat-11, 4 days after VL, dorsal VA, capsule laterally and most of VP destroyed. Partial contralateral sensorimotor cortex removal 1 week previously. Plot suppressed when every bin at increasing interspike intervals has counts of less than 3; arrow and numerals to right of histogram indicate total number of intervals not plotted. Orthodromic latencies for PT-A-Y were 1.05, 0.83, 0.80, 0.80, 0.95 and 0.90 msec, respectively. Axons A-D were recorded progressively more ventral in the bulbar PT, X and Y during withdrawal. Somatosensory stimulation was tested in B-Y and was ineffective.

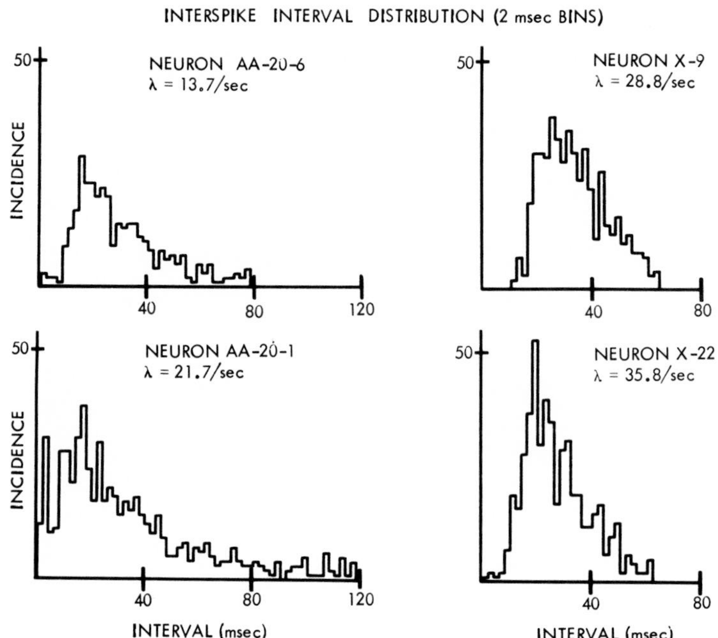

FIG. 20. Interspike interval histograms of resting discharge by 4 individual VL-VA neurons recorded in intact, awake cats. Neurons AA-20-6 and 20-1 were simultaneously recorded. Neurons X-9 and 22 responded to stimulation at level of red N. with latencies of 1.1-1.4 msec and 1.0-1.2 msec, respectively. X-22 responded to a stimulus to motor cortex with an antidromic latency of 0.6 msec, i.e., it is a projection neuron.

to contact (cf. hairfield PT neurons). The lack of a significant correlation between increased firing of this neuron and latency of withdrawal may be explained by the numerous synapses interposed between the recorded neuron and the effectors, each with independent sources of variability. The early increase in discharge by the neuron occurs too late to initiate the earliest phase of biceps activation; however, it could initiate later biceps activity and thus contribute dynamically to withdrawal. The occurrence of a second increase in activity when the muscles contributing to withdrawal had minimal activity suggests that this VL-VA neuron was related to the activity of more than one set of muscles.

N. Dentatus and Interpositus of Cerebellum

The possibility that the cerebellothalamic pathway (19, 31, 41) contributed to the VL-VA responses occurring during CP was evaluated in 7 cats by making extensive lesions in either N. interpositus or dentatus or both. (In two of these cats, a lesion of contralateral globus pallidus was subsequently made.) We confirmed neither the per-

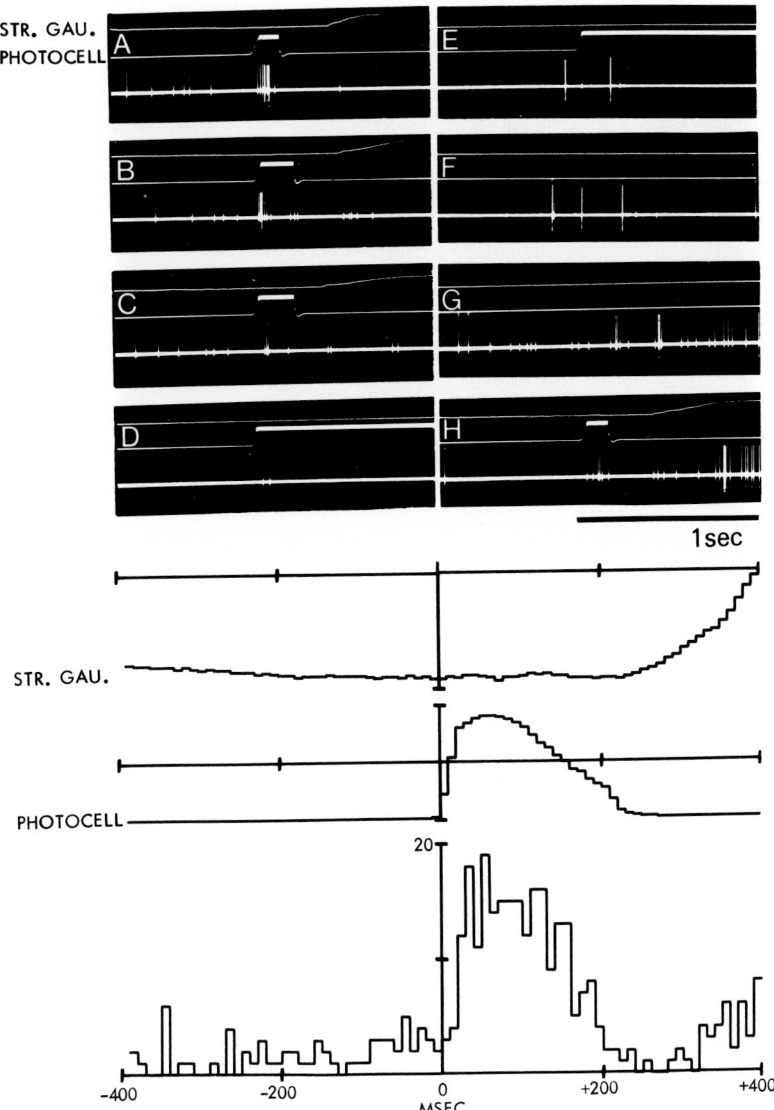

FIG. 21. Early responses by a VL-VA neuron during CP. Above, sequence of records (A-H). Positive CPs in (A-C) followed by failures (D-E). Pattern of spontaneous discharge in (F) altered by massaging a paw (G) followed by return of CP in (H). Upward deflection indicates positivity of microelectrode. Below, pre- and postcontact histograms of discharge by same neuron (at bottom) and CP transducer outputs. Rank order correlation between increased firing (postcontact bins 3 through 16) and latency of withdrawal (last precontact bin through postcontact bin 28) was -.14 (not significant) and between latency of withdrawal and latency of landing (postcontact bins 24 through 40) was -.40 ($p < .02$). (This Figure is taken from (9)).

manent loss of CP nor its temporary loss for 2-3 weeks following destruction of N. interpositus or dentatus (14, 15), respectively. CP of the ipsilateral forepaw usually returned on the first to the fourth postoperative day. In one cat, CP to stimulation of the dorsal and ulnar aspects of the forepaw returned on the eighth and twelfth postoperative days, respectively. The lesion of N. dentatus and interpositus was subsequently found to have extended into the lateral vestibular N. and the inferior cerebellar peduncle. The lesion in cat 32 (Fig. 22) spared a very few N. interpositus cells medially and a small ventral portion of N. dentatus ventrally; long latency, grossly hypermetric CP occurred to stimulation of the dorsal and ulnar aspects of the ipsilateral forepaw on the fourth postoperative day. Hypermetria is manifested during the withdrawal phase by lifting of the forepaw an excessive distance above the top edge, and during the landing phase by an excessive horizontal displacement. While "vertical" hypermetria is also prominent after other lesions of the motor control system, "horizontal" hypermetria is particularly pronounced after cerebellar roof nuclear lesions.

The increased latency of CP is related to the increased latency of biceps activation. The delay between clearing of the top edge and extensor digitorum activation is also increased. During recovery from roof nuclear lesions, e.g., 2 weeks later, the latency of withdrawal and of biceps activation are reduced towards normal, but hypermetria persists.

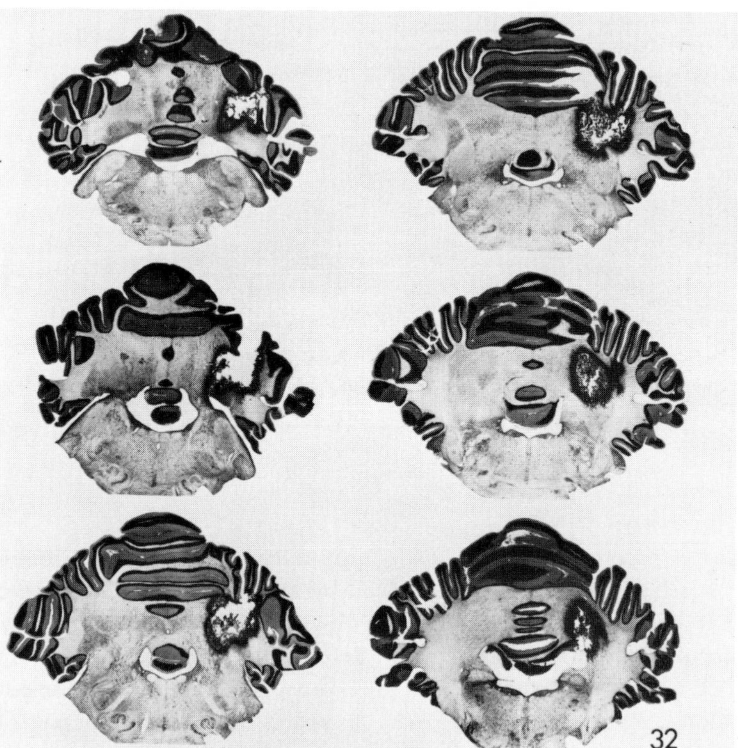

FIG. 22. Photomicrographs of representative sections through cerebellar roof nuclear lesion of cat-32.

Cross-placing occurred after lesions of N. dentatus and interpositus, but was not as consistent, nor did it appear as early as following VL-VA lesions.

Cooling N. dentatus and interpositus led temporarily to ipsilateral, hypermetric CP and greater cooling, to loss of CP and all searching movements. To reduce damage, the probe was implanted eccentrically at the periphery of the nuclei, lying partly in the white matter; despite this precaution, a careful examination usually disclosed a slight degree of hypermetria even before the cooling was started. Evidently, the two roof nuclei have few functionally redundant cells. Fig. 23 shows the loss of CP ipsilateral to the cooling (3, 4) with retention of contralateral CP (5). Biceps activation was unaccompanied by extensor digitorum depression. During tonic stimulation of the red N. (6, 7), CP was restored, with excellent timing of the reduction of biceps activity and activation of extensor digitorum and triceps.

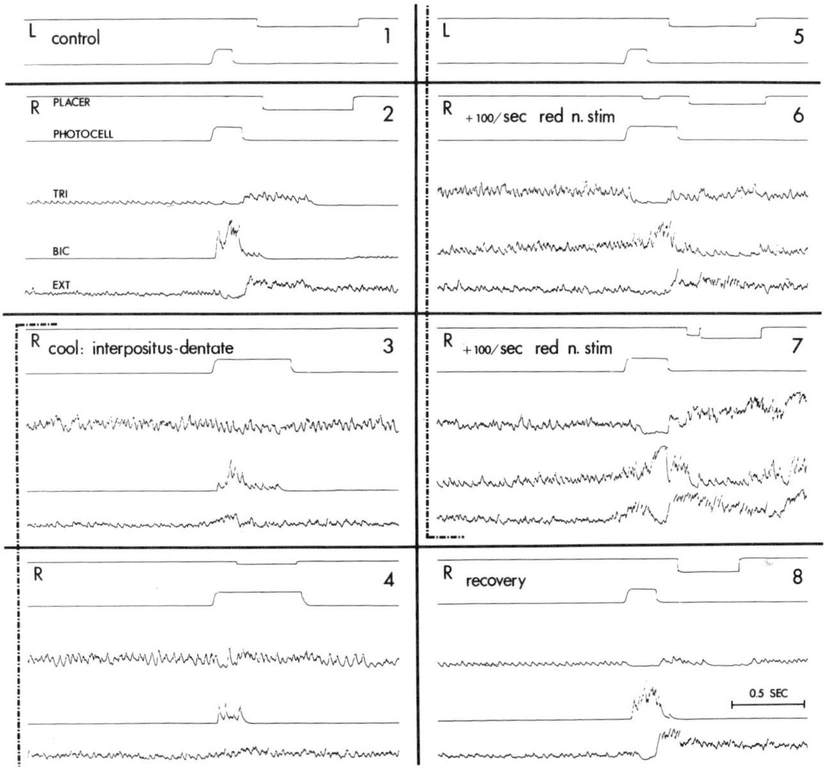

FIG. 23. Temporary loss of ipsilateral CP during cooling of N. interpositus and dentatus and its restoration by stimulation of the red N. Sequence of records 1-8. (L) and (R) identify the forepaw. Cooling started 19 sec before (3) and continued throughout (3-7). CP testing was ended in (3, 4) by removing the cat; placer key deflection in (4) is due to slight movement in holding the cat. Red N. stimulated throughout (6, 7). Record (8) taken approximately 9 min after cooling discontinued. (This Figure is taken from (9)).

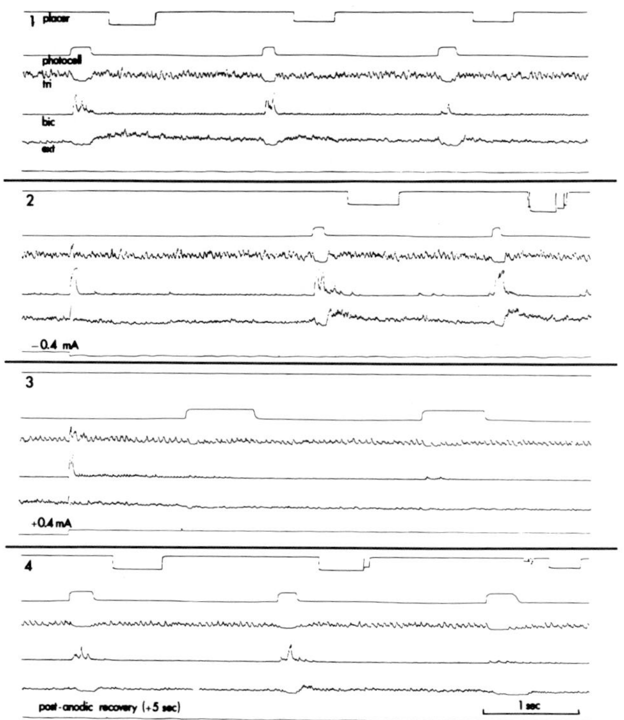
1 placer
photocell
tri
bic
ext
2
−0.4 mA
3
+0.4 mA
4
post-anodic recovery (+5 sec)
1 sec

FIG. 24

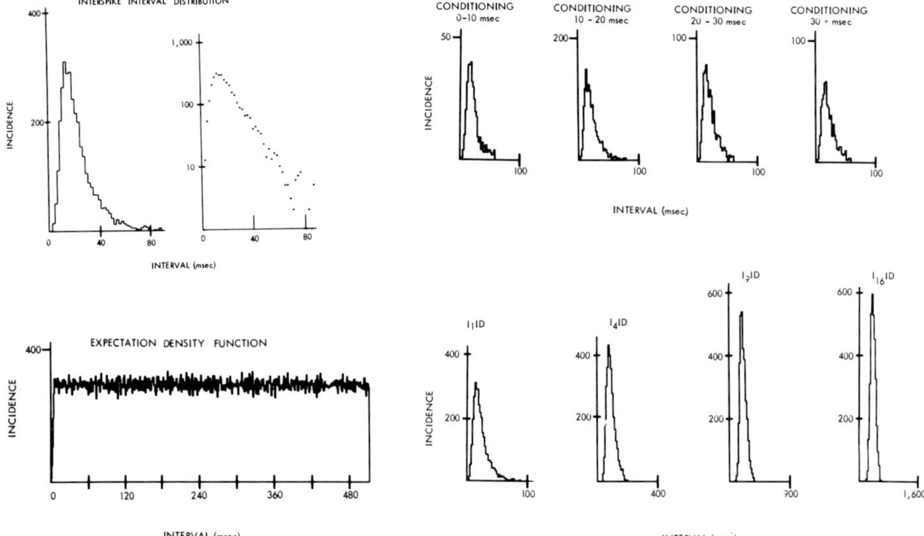
INTERSPIKE INTERVAL DISTRIBUTION
INCIDENCE
INTERVAL (msec)
CONDITIONING 0-10 msec
CONDITIONING 10 - 20 msec
CONDITIONING 20 - 30 msec
CONDITIONING 30 + msec
EXPECTATION DENSITY FUNCTION

FIG. 25

In 2 cats, we attempted to "block" the roof nuclei by passing current of either polarity through the cooling probe. In one cat (Fig. 24), CP and EMG activation could readily be 'switched off' by anodic current (3). With cathodal current (2), CP was made grossly hypermetric, with increased activation of both biceps and extensors. Applying an anodic pulse (lasting 550 msec) to the probe 10 msec after contact prevented CP from occurring; when the delay was 50 msec, CP was not prevented, implying that the essential roof nuclear contribution to CP had already occurred.

The dynamic role of N. interpositus in CP was assayed by recording the activities of individual interpositus neurons. As a preliminary, the resting discharge was analysed as indicated in Fig. 25. Out of a sample of 29 neurons, 26 were labelled as projection neurons, with antidromic conduction times from the level of caudal VL ranging from 0.5-1.3 msec. In the awake state, 3/4 of the projection neurons had high mean rates of discharge (40—90/sec), as previously reported for the monkey (44). However, a mean rate of resting discharge cannot readily be defined for some interpositus neurons which are virtually silent for many seconds and subsequently, without any obvious change in the behavioral state, 'turn on' at high frequency; such lengthy, silent periods are not included in the computations of mean rate given above. (Slight changes in orientation of the head or body may possibly account for this phenomenon.) For stable portions of the run, the interspike interval distribution usually had a quasi-gamma appearance, with a dead time of 1-8 msec. In a semilog plot, the incidence of intervals longer than 11-22 msec linearly decremented, resembling a Poisson process; less commonly, it showed positive skewing. The conditioned interval distribution (3) showed either a weak or no relationship between the duration of an interval and that of the immediately succeeding interval. The expectation density function revealed a periodic component in only one neuron and small inhomogeneities in 1/4 of the population. The n-tuple distribution showed convergence at the higher orders, i.e., the discharge pattern did not conform to the random walk model (22).

FIG. 24. Effect of anodal and cathodal polarization of N. interpositus and dentatus on CP. In (2,3) current at indicated intensity and direction passed through same cooling probe as was used in Fig. 23; at left, 'ON' transients occur approximately 1/2 sec after start of trace.

FIG. 25. Analysis of resting discharge of a N. interpositus projection neuron. N = 3,280 spikes; mean interval and standard deviation = 22.4 ± 13.8 msec. Antidromic latency with contralateral stimulation at level of caudal VL was 0.6 msec. Upper left, interspike interval distributions plotted with linear and semilog coordinates. Upper right, distribution of intervals immediately following each interval (conditioning) of duration between the indicated limits 0-10 msec, etc. (3). Mean interval and standard deviations: 21.9 ± 12.5, 22.4 ± 13.9, 22.2 ± 13.6 and 22.8 ± 14.4 msec, respectively. Lower right, distribution of n-tuples, i.e., interval between a given spike and the nth spike, with appropriate scaling of the time axis; n-tuple distribution is equivalent to scaled interval histogram (22).

Out of 20 individual neurons tested, 13 responded during CP. Most were initially activated and subsequently depressed (Fig. 26-left); others were initially depressed (Fig. 26-right) or, exceptionally, showed a cycle of initial activation, depression and final activation. In one-half of the responding neurons, activation commenced in the 20-30 msec period, or exceptionally, in the 10-20 msec period. During the period of increased firing, successive interspike intervals were very brief; e.g., the mean spike content/bin/CP=1 in Fig. 28-right and is increased to approximately 2 in several successive postcontact 10 msec periods, yielding a series of intervals of 5 msec mean duration.

In Fig. 26-left, biceps activation starts at 30-40 msec, i.e., the evoked discharge occurs prior to the EMG activity and therefore cannot be due to somatosensory feedback resulting from movement of the limb. Even when biceps activation starts at 20-30 msec (Fig. 26-right), there appears to be insufficient time for feedback from the movement. (In cats under chloralose anesthesia, the feedback latency for the initial negative field potential of N. interpositus to stimulation of the cut, peripheral end of a lower cervical root was 8.5 msec; calculated from the start of the EMGs, the feedback delay is estimated at 7 msec from proximal muscles and 9-10 msec from biceps and more distal muscles.)

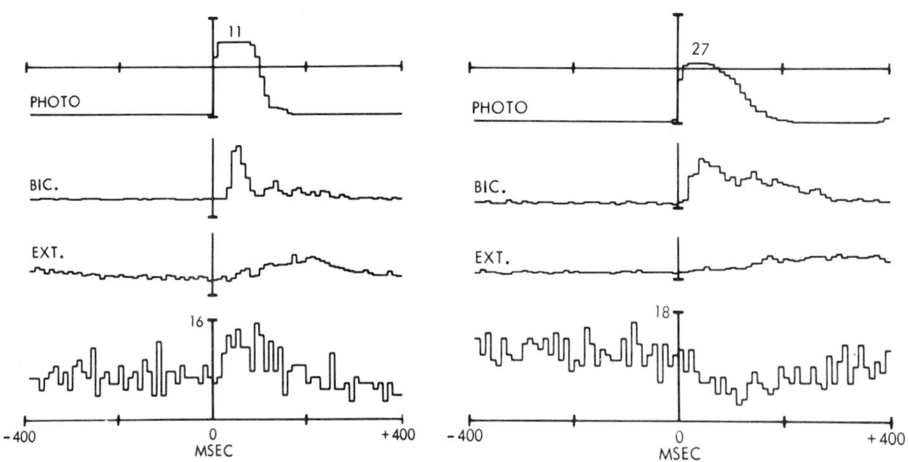

FIG. 26. Pre- and postcontact histograms of activities of two N. interpositus projection neurons (at bottom), EMGs and transducer outputs. Both neurons recorded in same cat. Antidromic latencies with caudal VL stimulation were 0.9 and 0.75 msec for neurons at left and right, respectively. At left, rank order correlation between increased firing (postcontact bins 3 through 14) and latency of withdrawal (postcontact bins 1 through 18) was -.88 ($p<.001$), between increased firing and area under BIC activation (postcontact bins 3 through 14) was + .80 ($p<.01$) and between increased firing and area under EXT activation (postcontact bins 7 through 18) was +.88 ($p<.001$). Correlation between early firing by neuron (postcontact bins 3 through 5) and early BIC activation (postcontact bins 4 through 6) was +.73 ($p<.02$). At right, correlations not significant. (This Figure is taken from (9)).

The increased neuronal discharge was strongly correlated with the latency of withdrawal (-.88) and with the amount of biceps (+.80) and extensor (+.88) activation. The correlation was less high (+.73) between the earliest phases of increased discharge and early biceps activation; this implies that the increased neuronal discharge was related more to the overall sequence of muscle activity in CP than to the initial biceps component.

Moving the cat to the placer often resulted in an increased discharge prior to contact (Fig. 27). This increase presumably was caused by vestibular input; its relationship to extensor digitorum activation prior to contact was not investigated.

A contingent relationship was demonstrated for late responses occurring during CP (Fig. 27). When the outcome of testing was a positive CP, the postcontact histogram revealed an increased discharge during the 200-400 msec period. This increase was absent when the limb only partially withdrew, implying that it was not directly related to the activity of muscles causing this component of CP; furthermore, the increased discharge preceded the landing on the placer keys, i.e., it did not result from sensory input from the ventral surface of the paw. By exclusion, the increased discharge reflects either the clearing of the top edge or the switching on of muscles subserving the landing phase.

The earliest phase of increased discharge by N. interpositus neurons occurred regardless of whether CP was positive or negative (Fig. 28-left); this does not necessarily

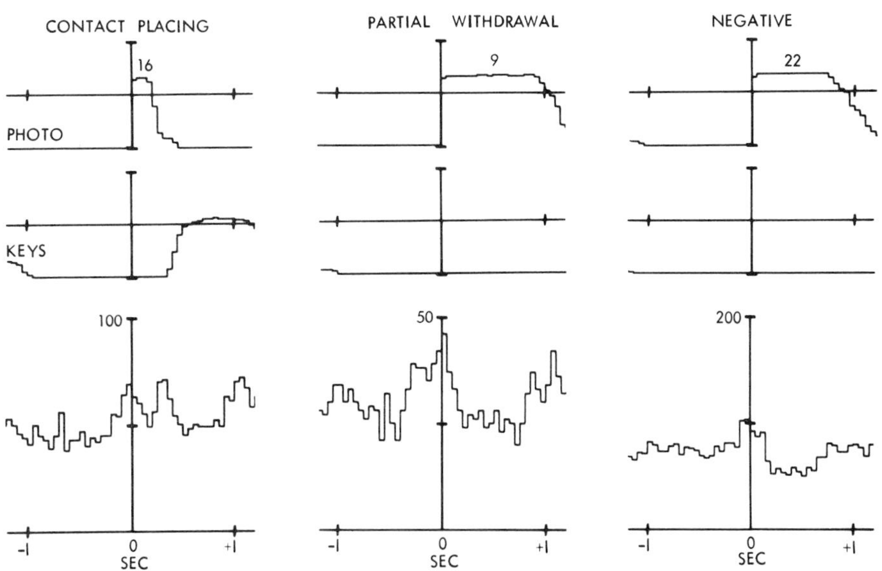

FIG. 27. Pre- and postcontact histograms of activity of a N. interpositus projection neuron (at bottom) and transducer outputs. Antidromic latency with caudal VL stimulation was 0.7 msec. Outcomes of 47 contact trials classified as 'contact placing' (note deflection on 'keys' channel), 'partial withdrawal' (note irregular plateau on photocell channel) and 'negative' (smooth plateau). Histograms displayed in 50 msec bins.

conflict with the correlation of increased discharge with EMG activity and with withdrawal reported above, but suggests other sources of variability or "decision points" in the intermediary pathway.

Recordings during the awake state from N. interpositus in Cat N-15 (Fig. 12), 4 months after removal of contralateral sensorimotor cortex yielded mean rates of discharge by 6 individual neurons in the range of 27-84/sec. (Antidromic conduction times from the contralateral red N. ranged between 0.55-0.75 msec). A semilog plot of the interspike interval distribution usually showed positive skewing. In 9 individual neurons tested, stimulation of the affected forepaw yielded either no alteration in activity or a small delayed increase with an even later reduction. Fig. 28-right shows a small increase in activity starting in the 50-60 msec period and is the most prominent example in the series. Although the size of the sample is small, the data suggest that an intact sensorimotor cortex contributes to early activation of interpositus neurons, but is unnecessary for a high resting discharge.

The Roles in CP of Red Nucleus and Inputs to VL-VA compared.

The upstream connections of N. dentatus are mainly with VL, but those of N. interpositus are with both VL and the red N. (19), which introduces an ambiguity in

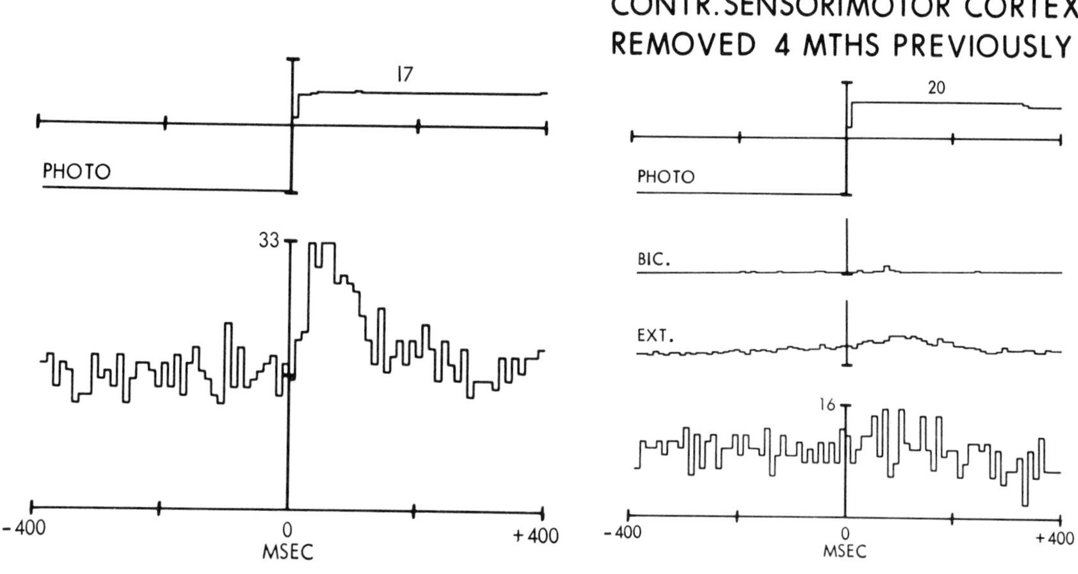

FIG. 28. Pre- and postcontact histograms of activities of two N. interpositus projection neurons (at bottom), EMGs and transducer outputs. Outcome of CP testing was negative. At left, antidromic latency with caudal VL stimulation was 0.7 msec. (In this cat, cooling probe previously implanted in capsule.) Recordings at right obtained from same cat as shown in Fig. 12. Antidromic latency with stimulation at level of contralateral red N. was 0.55 msec.

the interpretation of the effects of lesions of these roof nuclei. A massive lesion of the red N. caused a more profound deficit in CP than did a lesion either of N. interpositus-dentatus or of VL-VA. The lesion in Fig. 29 abolished CP to stimulation of the dorsal, radial and ulnar aspects of the contralateral forepaw for the entire period of observation—3 1/2 weeks. Cross-placing was prominent at the end of the second postoperative week, i.e., it appeared later than after a VL-VA lesion. Proprioceptive correction at the wrist and visual placing were virtually absent throughout, but the cat could walk during the third postoperative week. Torticollis was prominent. Terminal exploration under pentobarbital anesthesia revealed left cruciate responses to stimulation of the right brachium conjunctivum that were less than 5% in amplitude of the control (right) side responses. High frequency trains of stimuli delivered to each motor cortex elicited good contractions in either forelimb, confirming that the lesion had not damaged corticofugal pathways in the peduncle. Electrocutaneous stimulation of the distal forepaw disclosed only small differences in the amplitudes of the positive and negative components of the SI primary responses on the two sides, confirming that the lesion had not damaged the fast somatosensory projections.

A smaller lesion of the red N. was followed 1 1/2 weeks later by return of slow, easily fatiguable CP to stimulation of the dorsal and radial aspects of the forepaw, but a month after the lesion CP was still virtually absent to stimulation of the ulnar aspect; it was restored 3 hours after d-amphetamine was administered. Torticollis

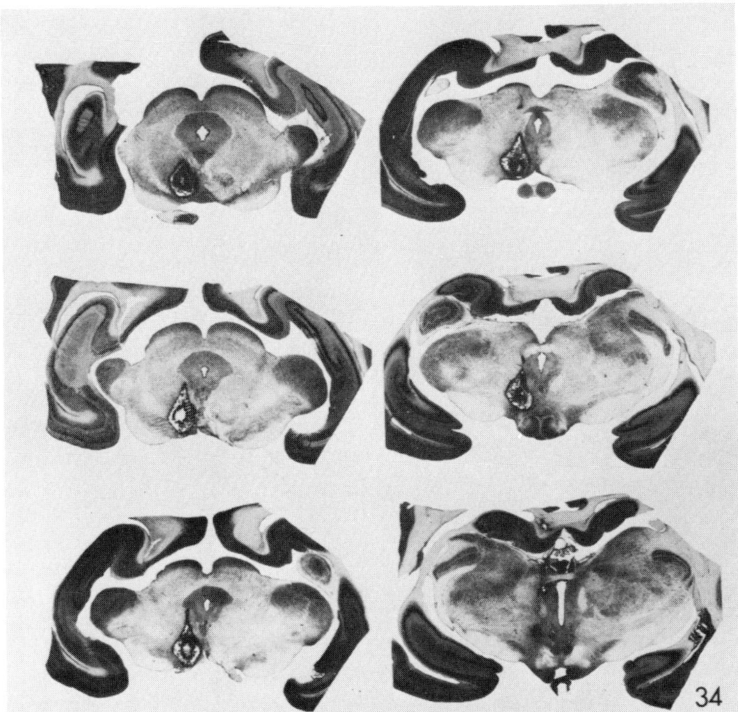

FIG. 29. Photomicrographs of representative sections through red N. lesions of cat-34.

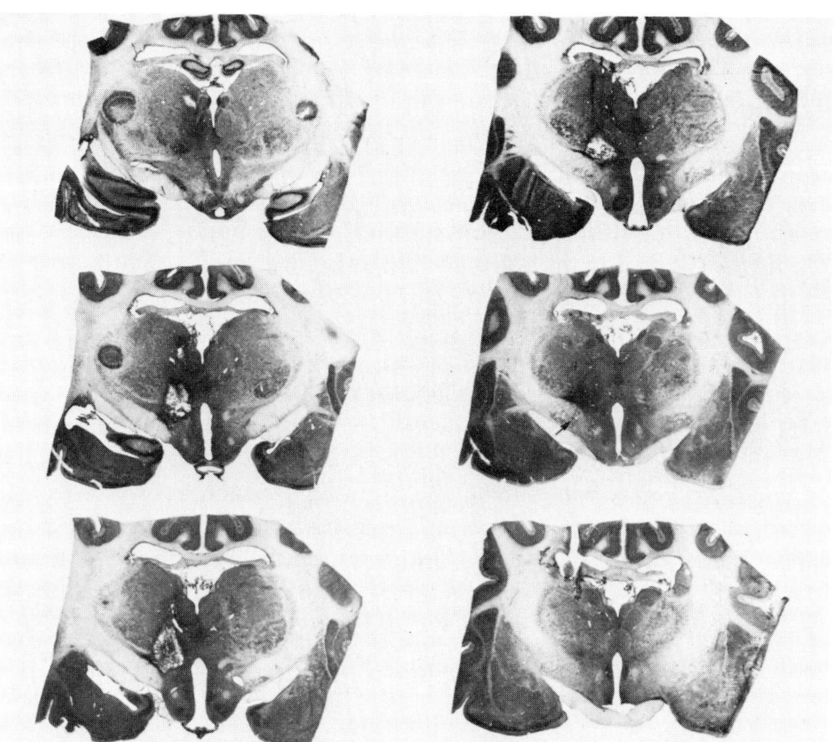

FIG. 30

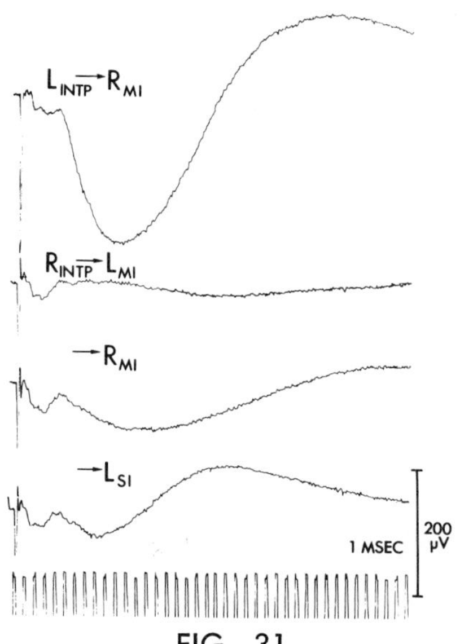

FIG. 31

and circling during walking were prominent. Cross-placing was absent while CP was absent, but became prominent at the end of 4 weeks. Terminal exploration disclosed a reduction in amplitude of the cruciate response to stimulation of N. interpositus to 8% of that on the control side. SI primary responses to mechanical stimulation of the affected forepaw were unimpaired.

The severe effect of a lesion of red N. implies that the role of the nucleus in CP is not restricted to processing the output of a cerebellar roof nucleus. Furthermore, the question is raised as to whether *any* of the effects of roof nuclear lesions depend on an upstream influence on VL; put another way, are all the effects of roof nuclear lesions described above attributable to the removal of a major input to, e.g., the red N.? We attempted to answer this question by interrupting the cerebellothalamic pathway between VL and the red N. Lesions were made in 12 cats at rostrocaudal levels ranging from A7-9. (The danger with rostral lesions is encroachment on caudal VL, while caudal lesions may damage the red N.). Typically, the lesions were located in Forel's field H_1 and the zona incerta, with variable amounts of encroachment on field H_2, ventromedial portions of caudal VL and VPM. Depending on the size and location of the lesion, the amplitude of the cruciate response to stimulation of contralateral N. interpositus and brachium conjunctivum was reduced to 42—less than 10% of that on the control side. Figure 30 shows a VL "deafferenting" lesion that terminally was shown to have reduced to a few percent of control amplitude the surface positive and negative components of the MI response to stimulation of contralateral N. interpositus. (Early components that were also recordable from SI were not reduced). This lesion was followed, on the second postoperative day, by occasional long-latency CP to stimulation of the dorsal, radial and ulnar aspects of the forepaw. Cross-placing was variably present. Visual placing was later initiated and more poorly coordinated than on the control side.

Both "vertical" and "horizontal" hypermetria of the forepaw were observed, especially to dorsal stimulation, after VL 'deafferenting' lesions, but the horizontal component was *less prominent than after cerebellar roof nuclear lesions*. The variability in occurrence and latency of CP following VL deafferenting lesions was remarkable. The mean latency of withdrawal was increased, but examples of individual withdrawals almost as rapid as on the control side were recorded, often when the cat appeared angry. Figure 32 shows both a rapid CP of the affected paw(3) and a slower, more typical CP (2). Cooling N. dentatus and interpositus was followed by reversible loss of ipsilateral CP, which was restored by tonic stimulation of substan-

---

FIG. 30. Photomicrographs of representative sections through VL 'deafferenting' lesions of cat-51. In right middle section, small arrow indicates marking lesion made with recording microelectrode in internal capsule.

FIG. 31. Summed cortical responses to stimulation of N. interpositus of cat-51. Terminal recordings from cat under pentobarbital anesthesia and immobilized with Flaxedil. (L) and (R) identify sides of brain. MI recording electrode at cruciate sulcus, SI recording electrode at ansate sulcus. Stimulus intensity 4 mA throughout.

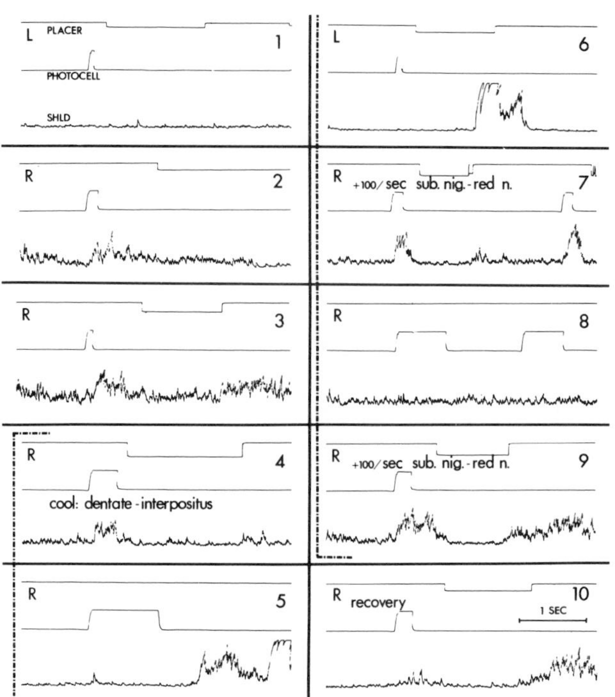

FIG. 32. Temporary loss of ipsilateral CP during cooling of N. dentatus and interpositus and its restoration by stimulation of substantia nigra—red N. despite 'deafferentation' of VL. Sequence of records (1-10). (L) and (R) identify the forepaw. EMG from anterior shoulder muscles. Cooling started 20 sec before (4) and continued throughout (4-9). Tonic stimulation throughout (7) and (9). CP returned 3 mins after cooling discontinued. Record (10) taken 121 min later.

tia nigra—red N. This result suggests that roof nuclear output is important in CP even when its influence through VL is prevented; presumably, such a component of the roof nuclear output is at least partly directed through the red N.

Some caution is required before the reduced probability and increased latency of CP following 'deafferenting' lesions can be attributed to loss of cerebellar input to VL. Numerous other pathways traverse the regions occupied by these lesions; among these is the pallidal outflow coursing rostrally to VL-VA and caudally to the midbrain. Massive lesions of globus pallidus abolish CP for only 1-3 days. Subsequently, the interval for landing is markedly increased. (Unfortunately, no electrophysiological observations were made to exclude the possibility that some or all of the above effects resulted from edema of the internal capsule.) It should be noted that the homologue of the medial segment of globus pallidus in carnivores is the entopeduncular nucleus (25) which is situated ventral to the internal capsule. Our attempts at destroying the nucleus without severely damaging the internal capsule have so far been unsuccessful. (The lesion in Fig. 16 destroyed a small rostral part of the entopeduncular N. and was unaccompanied by loss of CP.) Although evaluation of the role of the entopeduncular nucleus must await a more complete lesion, it seems unlikely that it is part of a dynamic circuit essential for CP, because globus pallidus—the most important input to the entopeduncular N.—was destroyed with only temporary loss of CP. Furthermore, a search for responses in VL-VA to stimulation of the entopeduncular N. disclosed only 3 out of 124 units that discharged at short latencies (17).

DISCUSSION

A sequentially ordered series of functions in CP may be distinguished as follows: 1) Signalling that one or more paws is unsupported. 2) Signalling the contact of a solid with part of the limb. 3) Processing the information provided by (2) leading to localization of the area contacted on the surface of the limb. 4) Transforming the spatiotemporal location code into a series of commands to the motor centers, producing a coordinated lifting-withdrawal movement. 5) Signalling the clearing of the top edge. 6) Replacing (4) by a series of commands to the motor centers producing a coordinated directed-landing movement. Finally, (1) is negated, thus completing CP. A nucleus may subserve any of the above functions either dynamically or by nonspecific or specific types of steady state action. "Dynamic" here means that the delay for change in nuclear activity equals, or is less than, that required for the particular function considered. The nonspecific type of steady state action is analogous to the classical concept of "tonic facilitation" of lower motor centers, withdrawal of such facilitation causing spinal shock. The above analysis of CP has attempted to avoid such nonspecific effects of lesions, the animals usually exhibiting walking, feeding, nociceptive reflexes, proprioceptive correction and visual placing. A specific steady state influence might be exemplified by the imposition on lower interneuron pools of a series of functional interconnections which permit the dynamic input from hair receptors to bypass the higher levels. Alternatively, local interneurons may be bypassed, wherever an afferent input bifurcates, monosynaptically exciting both the output neuron and interneurons which polysynaptically excite or inhibit the output neuron. Clearly, this type of steady state action functionally models a computer program which provides a set of instructions determining how future input will be processed. Regardless of whether the nuclear influence is dynamic or steady state, CP may be abolished permanently by a lesion (e.g. of VP), or it may recover (e.g. several weeks after a VL-VA lesion). A nuclear lesion (e.g. of N. interpositus) that fails to abolish CP may grossly impair the coordination either permanently or temporarily. Because of the numerous interconnections and hence the possibility of multiple loops in the higher motor control system, the recovery of CP several weeks, or less, after a nuclear lesion does not exclude the possibility that the nucleus had an important function in the intact organism. Either a dynamic or a specific steady state function should be considered when the centers that previously received input from the nucleus continue to exhibit neural activity (e.g. continued PT discharge after a VL-VA lesion).

Following removal of the sensorimotor cortex, CP is very rarely obtainable and biceps activation is virtually abolished, except after d-amphetamine. Although our data differ from those of Bard (11), we agree that CP is normally managed in the adult cat by the sensorimotor cortex (see later discussion). The question arises as to whether VP and sensorimotor cortex function *dynamically* in CP. Evidently the most difficult requirement for the establishment of such a dynamic circuit is to explain biceps activation occurring as early as 20-40 msec after contact. The circuit, skin→ VP→ large PT neuron→ biceps, can plausibly account for the shortest delays only if the 8 msec delay recorded between an electrical stimulus delivered to motor cortex and the EMG activation of biceps is of the same order as that obtaining with physiologically engendered corticofugal volleys. The forelimb EMG response to a high frequency train of electrical stimuli delivered to an individual motor cortical column, although shown to depend on the PT, has a much longer latency (e.g., 17 msec in Fig. 1 (10), 20 msec (42)). However, it may be argued that the many output columns activated by a contact stimulus lead to extensive spatial summation at the lower motor centers, thus reducing the delays consequent on temporal summation. Such an explanation is hypothetical, because our studies in the awake cat yield information about neither the *motor* effects of the PT neurons recorded, nor the total number activated by threshold contact.

In the acute preparation, PT neurons are polysynaptically activated by VP (7); at least two components are distinguishable, the latter of which is especially reduced by suction of posterior SI, cortex along the coronal sulcus, or SII (2). The reported sparing of CP in the cat after postcruciate but not precruciate lesions (1) suggests that the VP projection pathway subserving the earliest component of PT discharge is the most important in CP. However, in the study cited, SII, a source of powerful corticocortical excitation of PT neurons in motor cortex (2), remained intact and no electrophysiological controls were described for the amounts remaining of somatosensory cortex and cortex projecting to PT after the various lesions. Evidently, the relative contributions in CP of 'short' and 'long' cortical interneurons to excitation of PT neurons would be more easily weighed in the monkey.

It must be emphasized that the cutaneous 'input-output' column described in lightly anesthetized cats, because of its overall *positive* feedback action cannot account for the early EMG changes in CP, which initially entail an opposite overall action (cf. 10). However, a study in awake cats (42) disclosed in addition *aversive* motor responses such as flexion at the wrist and elbow to stimulation of zones containing units responding to light pressure or an air puff applied to the dorsum of the paw. The discrepancy between these two sets of observations could be resolved if cutaneous input were switched via interneurons either to 'flexor' or to 'extensor' output columns, depending on such factors as whether the paw is unsupported or the cat is awake. Alternatively, contingent 'switching' in interneuronal pools might occur downstream from the motor cortex; if switching occurs at any site, the lack of observed contingency in early cutaneous activation of PT axons favors a subcortical site.

Assuming that cortical input-output columns with an overall aversive action exist, is biceps activation a stimulus bound response to brushing of hairs during lifting? Allowing at least 8 msec for PT→ forelimb EMG and 14 msec for EMG→ movement→ PT, a minimum of 22 msec would be required to complete such a feedback loop. Significantly, we found that *transiently* bringing a one-inch thick platform in contact with an unsupported forelimb results in lifting of the paw to a height which is approximately a function of the distance up the forelimb that the contact occurred. Evidently, transient cutaneous stimulation of the forelimb results in an appropriately prolonged contraction of muscles producing lifting. The disparity between the number of afferent fibers activated with contact at different sites and the effector action implies a programmed, non-linear amplification of signals, rather than a simple input-output columnar representation. Furthermore, "skipping" during withdrawal (see Results) following contact with the dorsum of the paw again implies that excitation may be briefly maintained without requiring continuous input from the dorsum. We conclude that withdrawal, although triggered by cutaneous input, is probably maintained centrally by an iterative loop which is interrupted either by the change in cutaneous input when some part of the paw clears the top edge or, prematurely, by an internally generated signal. Iterative activity in cortical interneuron chains has long been inferred (28); most likely, the periodically incrementing PT response to a stimulus to VP depends on such local interneuronal circuits (7). However, such activity appears too brief to account for lifting-withdrawal; furthermore, lifting-withdrawal is initially absent or is replaced by a jerk following a VL-VA lesion that spares VP. The latter observation coupled with the finding that individual VL-VA neurons may discharge early enough to contribute to lifting-withdrawal and subsequent landing but not to the earliest biceps activity, implies that drive from VL-VA to sensorimotor cortex is normally required to complete lifting-withdrawal. VL-VA drive monosynaptically activates large PT neurons, certain cortical interneurons (7, 49) and doubtless other corticofugal neurons. In the awake state, disynaptic activation of large PT neurons by VL-VA via an excitatory cortical interneuron is slight (47); the "quenching" of PT discharge that results is well suited to permit the rapid following of changing VL-VA drive during movements. Furthermore, spatial focussing of VL-VA drive on the PT population would be enhanced. It may be noted that VL-VA and VP activate two populations of PT neurons that only partially overlap (2). In a sample of 54 individual bulbar PT axons responding to stimulation of the ventral nuclear group, 65% were fired by stimulation of VL-VA, 72% were fired by VP stimulation and 37% were fired by stimulation of either nuclear group (8). Whatever the role of the cutaneous field PT neurons in initiating biceps activity, they may also have an *informational* role; through collaterals widely distributed throughout the brainstem (16, 26, 35, 45, 46) they probably affect the motor response to subsequent discharge by the class of PT (and other corticofugal neurons) engaged by VL-VA.

Of the major inputs to VL-VA, the role in CP of that from the basal ganglia must await further evaluation; however, the preliminary evidence against the pallidal projection to VL-VA forming part of the dynamic circuit is given in the Results. By contrast, the evidence both from recording individual neurons and from lesions or reversible blocks suggests that discharge of N. interpositus could dynamically contribute both through VL and through another site (probably red N.) to lifting-withdrawal and subsequent landing, but not to the earliest biceps activity. N. interpositus is presently considered to receive excitatory collateral input from mossy and climbing fibers derived from ascending spinal pathways and descending corticofugal pathways (18, 19). Purkinje neurons contribute a direct inhibitory input and, if inhibited, could disinhibit interpositus neurons (19). The question arises whether corticofugal or ascending influences or both are required for early interpositus responses during CP. The finding that a VP lesion results in loss of CP, in absent or delayed BIC activation, and in the absence of early discharge of PT neurons to contralateral contact implies that any ascending somatosensory influence transmitted through N. interpositus (and perhaps dentatus) and VL-VA to the corticofugal systems is alone insufficient for CP. Our failure to record early responses by interpositus neurons in a cat whose contralateral sensorimotor cortex had been removed 4 months previously suggests an important role of corticofugal discharge in securing such early responses. However, our negative findings may reflect the sampling of a topographically inappropriate portion of the nucleus and, therefore, have not resolved this important question.

CP lost during cooling of N. interpositus and dentatus is restored during tonic stimulation of the red N., with good timing of extensor activation. This implies that roof nuclear output does not serve CP by transmitting a motor program uniquely stored in the cerebellum, nor does it uniquely signal to other nuclei e.g., that the top edge has been cleared. Roof nuclear action in the cruder aspects of CP appears to be a 'mass' facilitatory action, perhaps gated selectively in time through appropriate motor centers by signals generated elsewhere. The smoothness and economy of movement in normal CP is not restored by such tonic stimulation, evidencing an additional, more specific, coordinating function of the roof nuclear output.

Cerebellar output is sooner dispensed with, e.g., following roof nuclear lesions, than that of VL-VA. The inference that VL-VA has functions in CP additional to processing cerebellar output was supported by the finding that contralateral CP of the forepaw (but not cross-placing) was lost during cooling of VA-VL in a cat that had previously had massive lesions of globus pallidus, N. dentatus and interpositus, sparing only an anterior portion of the latter. Such findings are consistent with a contribution to CP by a short iterative loop between sensorimotor cortex and VL.

When analyzed by the procedures described, the resting discharge of individual interpositus neurons often approximates a Poisson process modified by a recovery function at short intervals. This finding is perhaps surprising considering the emphasis made of precise timing operations by the cerebellum (19). By analogy with sensation, it may be argued that the background state against which a change occurs is relatively unimportant, but it is hard to apply this view to the sphere of movement where the tensions required and the distances to be moved are all markedly influenced by the initial conditions. It is suggested that in the resting state, roof nuclear output is largely coded *spatially*, i.e., by combinatorial arrangements of active projection neurons, the mean rate of discharge in each providing the main temporal code. The slight, but definite hypermetria produced by the mere presence of a cooling probe suggests that, by comparison with VL-VA, there is very little redundancy in the spatial coding. The deficit in brief intervals during resting activity has the corollary that a series of brief intervals occurring after contact stimulation is a highly improbable event and therefore has a high information content. Recently, *brief* intervals in discharges by PT neurons were found to be well correlated with short latencies of movement (38).

A distinction was made earlier between a location code for the area on the limb contacted and the series of motor commands that result in placing. The information yielded by contact stimulation of a given forelimb has quite different consequences on the two sides; e.g., contact with the ulnar aspect of the right forepaw leads to *abduction* of a normal right forelimb, but leads to *adduction* of the left forelimb during cross-placing. Unless a representation of the site contacted is available bilaterally and is preserved separate from the motor consequences, the occurrence of such 'mirror reversal' in one type of behavior—CP—could lead to inappropriate movements in other types. By this hypothesis, an analysis of the mode of information transfer across the midline during cross-placing may promote an understanding of the coding employed in spatial localization.

Nothing is known of the intrinsic program that generates command signals in CP. However, considerable advantages would accrue if elements of the program peculiar to CP were stored in a higher level motor language; e.g., the initial representation at the highest order might be of "clear the top edge," translated successively into "lifting-withdrawal" and then commands, generated by iterative loops, issued to the individual muscle groups. The economy in space achieved by locally storing representations of "goals" or "set points" is offset by the neural activity expended elsewhere in translation to the lower order language. The latter might not be a disadvantage if the lower order language, in appropriate combinations, is shared by numerous inputs.

The question arises as to whether the neural connections that are required for CP in the adult are formed by learning, genetic specification or a combination of the two factors. On the day after birth, kittens usually exhibit CP, albeit of long latency (6), to stimulation of the dorsum of the paw. An underweight kitten, weighing 59 gm, exhibited CP on the day of birth. Although not conclusive, such findings suggest that CP is genetically determined rather than learnt (cf. 39). The striking increase in speed and coordination of CP during the next few weeks more likely results from maturation of the brain than from reinforcement. (Significantly, conditioned inhibition of CP by water with disinhibition was usually absent until the sixth week.) Removal, at various ages up to the end of the third week, of sensorimotor cortex, medial cortex and most or all of SII is followed within a few hours by return of CP, not differing significantly from that on the control side. (One to two months later, CP becomes depressed and is virtually abolished.) If the cortical removal is made after the fifth week, the deficit in CP begins to resemble that of the adult (6). Thus, CP can initially be controlled by a subcortical circuit whose connections are most likely genetically specified. Subsequently, the sensorimotor cortex plays a major role, but vestigial control by the subcortical circuit is perhaps revealed by the rare, stereotyped placing seen after sensorimotor cortical removal and by the more frequent placing during tonic stimulation of the red N. or after administration of d-amphetamine. The location of the subcortical circuit has not been determined; in particular, the role of the red N. remains to be elucidated.

Although CP is manifestly a response to sensory stimulation, the unsupported paw of an alert cat exhibits also searching movements whose timing is unpredictable by an external observer. Searching occurs only in a particular context—lack of support, but so also do human 'voluntary' movements. The neural substrate of such searching movements may provide a model system for studying volitional movement.

SUMMARY

Techniques for measuring the parameters of CP are described. During lifting-withdrawal, biceps and the flexor mass of the forearm are activated; the extensor digitorum and triceps are depressed. An initial phase of biceps activity (latency 20-40 msec) is often distinguishable from a later phase which completes the withdrawal. Regardless of the vertical distance traveled, the extensor digitorum is activated when the top edge is cleared, implying that loss of contact triggers the directed landing phase; other observations suggest an additional, ballistic component in withdrawal. CP is readily inhibited by placing into water and 'disinhibited' by resting the affected paw on a solid surface.

The neural circuits subserving CP were initially analyzed by making lesions in, or cooling parts of, the motor control system; subsequently, by unit recording, an attempt was made to distinguish dynamic and steady state functions of these areas. Lesions in VP resulted in the loss of CP, including any early biceps response, to stimulation of the corresponding skin area. Removal of sensorimotor cortex abolished normal CP and early biceps activation, but rare, stereotyped placings to stimulation of the dorsum of the paw persisted; their frequency was markedly increased by 100/sec stimulation of the red N. and by d-amphetamine. The temporary recovery of CP is attributed to control by a subcortical circuit, as evidenced also by return of CP within minutes or hours after removal of sensorimotor cortex in kittens younger than 3 weeks. (Subsequently, CP was lost at 1-2 months of age.) Based on an estimate of the delay for PT→forelimb EMG, the earliest discharge of individual VP and PT neurons precedes biceps activation by an interval sufficient for the dynamic circuit initiating CP to include the disynaptic pathway VP→ PT.

Massive lesions of VL-VA were followed by a temporary loss of CP and the appearance of cross-placing of the unaffected paw. Cutaneous driving and resting activity of PT neurons were still present. Placing to stimulation of the ulnar aspect of the paw and 'searching' movements were still depressed one month postoperatively, when placing to stimulation of the dorsal and medial aspects had substantially recovered. Prior to recovery, the response to stimulation of the dorsum tended to be 'jerky,' with sparing of the initial biceps component. Cooling VL-VA resulted in reversible loss of CP. The earliest responses by VL-VA neurons occurred in the 20-30 msec post-contact period; i.e., too late to initiate biceps activation, but early enough to contribute to withdrawal.

Following lesions of N. interpositus, dentatus or both, CP to stimulation of all three ipsilateral forepaw fields usually returned by the fourth postoperative day, but was markedly hypermetric. Cooling of these roof nuclei abolished CP, but it could be restored by tonic stimulation of the red N. The resting discharge of N. interpositus projection neurons had a high mean rate and approximated a Poisson process modified by a recovery function at brief interspike intervals. Two-thirds of the neurons responded during CP; one-half of these responded in the 20-30 msec postcontact period. Early responses in some neurons were highly correlated with latency of withdrawal and amount of EMG activity. Such early responses were absent in N. interpositus neurons recorded 4 months after removal of sensorimotor cortex.

Lesions of red N. resulted in a deficit in CP greater than that produced by a VL-VA lesion; therefore, lesions were made in Forel's fields H_1 and H_2, interrupting the cerebellar input to VL, but sparing that to the red N. Following such lesions, CP had a reduced probability and an increased latency. The horizontal component of hypermetria was less than after the roof nuclear lesions, suggesting that cerebellar input to red N. is important in control of CP. Such VL-VA 'deafferenting' lesions caused less deficit in CP than that resulting from massive VL-VA lesions, implying that VL-VA has a role in CP additional to processing cerebellar input.

The neural circuitry subserving CP is discussed and the roles of the VP and VL-VA thalamocortical projection systems are evaluated. We believe that the tactile placing reaction is a suitable model for the study of higher motor control in the adult, during development and during recovery following lesions; it may also provide a convenient system for studying plasticity.

ACKNOWLEDGMENTS

It is a pleasure to acknowledge the assistance given by Drs. M. Rosenblum and Norman White in many of the experiments.

This work was supported by grants from the USPHS, NS-03491, 01603 and NS-5304.

REFERENCES

1 ADKINS, R.J., CEGNAR, M.R. and RAFUSE, D.D. Differential effects of lesions of the anterior and posterior sigmoid gyri in cats, Brain Research, 30(1971) 411-414.

2 AMASSIAN, V.E. Discussion. In M.D. Yahr and D.P. Purpura (Eds.), Neurophysiological basis of normal and abnormal motor activities, Raven Press, New York, 1967, 288-292.

3 AMASSIAN, V.E., MACY, J. Jr., WALLER, H.J., LEADER, H.S., and SWIFT, M. Transformation of afferent activity at the cuneate nucleus. In: Information Processing in the Nervous System, Proc. International Union Physiol.Sci., 3 (1964) 235-254.

4 AMASSIAN, V.E., ROSENBLUM, M. and WEINER, H. Thalamocortical systems related to contact placing of forelimb of cat, Fed. Proc. 28 (1969) 455.

5 AMASSIAN, V.E., ROSENBLUM, M., and WEINER, H. Role of thalamic N. ventralis lateralis and its cerebellar input in contact placing, Fed. Proc., 29 (1970) 792.

6 AMASSIAN, V.E., ROSS, R. and DONAT, J. Development of contact placing and thalamocortical organization in kittens, Fed. Proc., 30 (1971) 434.

7 AMASSIAN, V.E., and WEINER, H. Monosynaptic and polysynaptic activation of pyramidal tract neurons by thalamic stimulation. In D.P. Purpura and M.D. Yahr (Eds.), The Thalamus, Columbia Univ. Press, New York, 1966, 255-282.

8 AMASSIAN, V.E. and WEINER, H., Unpublished observations.

9 AMASSIAN, V.E., WEINER, H., and ROSENBLUM, M. Neural systems sub-

serving the tactile placing reaction: a model for the study of higher level control of movement, Brain Research, 40(1972) 171-178.

10 ASANUMA, H., STONEY, S.D., Jr., and ABZUG, C. Relationship between afferent input and motor outflow in cat motorsensory cortex, J. Neurophysiol., 31 (1968) 670-681.

11 BARD, P. Localized control of placing and hopping reactions in the cat and their normal management by small cortical remnants, Arch. Neurol. & Psychiat. 30 (1933) 40-74.

12 BARD, P. Studies on the cortical representation of somatic sensibility, Harvey Lect., 33 (1938) 143-169.

13 CANNON, B.W., MAGOUN, H.W., and WINDLE, W.F. Paralysis with hypotonicity and hyperreflexia subsequent to section of basis pedunculi in monkeys, J. Neurophysiol., 7 (1944) 425-437.

14 CHAMBERS, W.W., and SPRAGUE, J.M. Functional localization in the cerebellum: I. Organization in longitudinal cortico-nuclear zones and their contribution to the control of posture, both extrapyramidal and pyramidal, J. comp. Neurol., 103 (1955) 105-129.

15 CHAMBERS, W.W., and SPRAGUE, J.M. Functional localization in the cerebellum: II. Somatotopic organization in cortex and nuclei, Arch. Neurol. & Psychiat. 74 (1955) 653-680.

16 CLARE, M.H., LANDAU, W.M., and BISHOP, G.H. Electrophysiological evidence of a collateral pathway from the pyramidal tract to the thalamus in cat, Exptl. Neurol., 9 (1964) 262-267.

17 DORMONT, J.F., OHYE, C., and ALBE-FESSARD, D. Comparison of the relationships of the nucleus entopeduncularis and brachium conjunctivum with the thalamic nucleus ventralis lateralis in the cat. In F.J. Gillingham and I.M.L. Donaldson (Eds.), Third Symposium on Parkinson's Disease, Livingstone, Edinburgh, 1969, 108-112.

18 ECCLES, J.C. Circuits in the cerebellar control of movement, Proc. Nat. Acad. Sci. (U.S.A.), 58 (1967) 336-343.

19 ECCLES, J.C., ITO, M., and SZENTAGOTHAI, J. The Cerebellum as a Neuronal Machine, Springer, New York, 1967.

20 EVARTS, E.V. Temporal patterns of discharge of pyramidal tract neurons during sleep and waking in the monkey, J. Neurophysiol., 27 (1964) 152-171.

21 EVARTS, E.V. Relation of discharge frequency to conduction velocity in pyramidal tract neurons, J. Neurophysiol., 28 (1965) 216-228.

22 GERSTEIN, G.L., and MANDELBROT, B. Random walk model for the spike activity of a single neuron, Biophys. J., 4 (1964) 41-68.

23 GILMAN, S., and DENNY-BROWN, D. Disorders of movement and behavior following dorsal column lesions, Brain, 89 (1966) 397-418.

24 HENNEMAN, E., COOKE, P.M., and SNIDER, R.S. Cerebellar projections to the cerebral cortex, Res. Publ. Ass. nerv. ment. Dis., 30 (1952) 317-333.

25 JUNG, R., and HASSLER, R. The extrapyramidal motor system. In J. Field, H.W. Magoun, and V.E. Hall (Eds.) Handbook of Physiology, Sec. 1, Vol. II, Neurophysiology. American Physiological Society, Washington, D.C., 1960,

863-927.
26 KLEE, M.R., and LUX, H.D. Intracelluläre Untersuchungen über den Einfluss hemmender Potentiale im motorischen Cortex. II Die Wirkung electrischer Reizung des Nucleus caudatus, Arch. Psychiat. Nervenkrankh., 203 (1962) 667-689.
27 LIDDELL, E.G.T., and PHILLIPS, C.G. Pyramidal section in the cat, Brain 67 (1944) 1-9.
28 LORENTE de NO, R. The cerebral cortex architecture, intracortical connections and motor projections. In J.F. Fulton, The Physiology of the Nervous System. Oxford Univ. Press, New York, 1938, 291-325.
29 LUNDBERG, A. and NORSELL, U. Spinal afferent pathway of the Tactile Placing Reaction, Experientia, 16 (1960) 123.
30 MACHT, M.B., and KUHN, R.A. Responses to thermal stimuli mediated through the isolated spinal cord, A.M.A. Arch. Neurol. & Psychiat., 59 (1948) 754-778.
31 MASSION, J., ANGAUT, P. and ALBE-FESSARD, D. Activités evoquées chez le chat dans la région du nucleus ventralis lateralis pars diverses stimulations sensorielles: I. Étude macro-physiologique, Electroenceph. clin Neurophysiol., 19 (1965) 433-451.
32 MEGIRIAN, D., and TROTH, R. Vestibular and muscle nerve connections to pyramidal tract neurons of cat, J. Neurophysiol., 27 (1964) 481-492.
33 MEYER, P.M., HOREL, J.A., and MEYER, D.R. Effects of dl-amphetamine upon placing responses in neodecorticate cats, J. comp. physiol. Psychol., 56 (1963) 402-404.
34 MOUNTCASTLE, V.B., and HENNEMAN, E. Pattern of tactile representation in thalamus of cat, J. Neurophysiol., 12 (1949) 85-100.
35 OSHIMA, T., PROVINI, L., TSUKAHARA, N., and KITAI, S.T. Cerebro-cerebellar connections mediated by fast and slow conducting pyramidal tract fibers, Proc. International Union Physiol. Sci., 7 (1968) 332.
36 PATTON, H.D., and AMASSIAN, V.E. The pyramidal tract: its excitation and functions. In J. Field, H.W. Magoun and V.E. Hall, (Eds.), Handbook of Physiology, Sec. 1, Vol. II, Neurophysiology, American Physiological Society, Washington, D.C., 1960, 837-861.
37 POGGIO, G.F., and MOUNTCASTLE, V.B. A study of the functional contributions of the lemniscal and spinothalamic systems to somatic sensibility, Bull. Johns Hopkins Hosp., 106 (1960) 266-316.
38 PORTER, R. Relationship of the discharges of cortical neurones to movement in free-to-move monkeys, Brain Research, 40(1972) 39-43.
39 RADEMAKER, G.G.J. Das Stehen, Springer, Berlin, 1931.
40 ROSE, J.E., and MOUNTCASTLE, V.B. Activity of single neurons in the tactile thalamic region of the cat in response to a transient peripheral stimulus, Bull. Johns Hopkins Hosp., 94 (1954) 238-282.
41 SAKATA, H., ISHIJIMA, T. and TOYODA, Y. Single unit studies on ventrolateral nucleus of the thalamus in cat: its relation to the cerebellum, motor cortex and basal ganglia, Jap. J. Physiol., 16 (1966) 42-60.

42 SAKATA, H., and MIYAMOTO, J. Topographic relationship between the receptive fields of neurons in the motor cortex and the movements elicited by focal stimulation in freely moving cats, Jap. J. Physiol., 18 (1968) 489-507.

43 STERIADE, M., APOSTOL, V., and OAKSON, G. Control of unitary activities in cerebello-thalamic pathway during wakefulness and synchronized sleep, J. Neurophysiol., 34 (1971) 389-413.

44 THACH, W.T. Discharge of Purkinje and cerebellar nuclear neurons during rapidly alternating arm movements in the monkey, J. Neurophysiol., 31 (1968) 785-797.

45 TOWER, S. Pyramidal lesion in the monkey, Brain, 63 (1940) 36-90.

46 TSUKAHARA, N., FULLER, D.R.G., and BROOKS, V.B. Collateral pyramidal influences on the corticorubrospinal system, J. Neurophysiol., 31 (1968) 467-484.

47 WEINER, H. and AMASSIAN, V.E. Monosynaptic and disynaptic discharge of pyramidal tract neurons during sleep and wakefulness. In Mario Bertini, (Ed.), Psicofisiologia Del Sonno E Del Sogno, Vita e Pensiero, Milan, 1970, 40-47.

48 WELT, C., ASCHOFF, J.C., KAMEDA, K. and BROOKS, V.B. Intracortical organization of cat's motorsensory neurons. In M.D. Yahr and D.P. Purpura (Eds.), Neurophysiological basis of normal and abnormal motor activities, Raven Press, New York, 1967, 255-293.

49 YOSHIDA, M., YAJIMA, K. and UNO, M. Different activation of the two types of the pyramidal tract neurons through the cerebello-thalamocortical pathway, Experientia, 22 (1966) 331-332.

Corticothalamic Projections and Sensorimotor Activities
T. Frigyesi, E. Rinvik, and M.D. Yahr, editors. © 1972
Raven Press, New York.

Alterations in Spinal Monosynaptic Reflex Produced by Stimulation of the Substantia Nigra

D. H. York

Descending extrapyramidal pathways from bulbar structures to spinal motorneurons and interneurons have been known since the early work of Lloyd (3) and Magoun and Rhines (4).

Involvement of the basal ganglia in descending spinal pathways was demonstrated by the observation that monosynaptic spinal reflexes were inhibited by caudate stimulation (5). It has also been demonstrated by Segundo and co-workers (6) that ventral root discharges in the L7 segment evoked by dorsal root stimulation are usually augmented, but occasionally reduced by repetitive stimulation of higher extrapyramidal centers (caudate and putamen as well as pallidum and claustrum). A depression of the reflex response was obtained only from the striatum (caudate and putamen).

The present experiments were undertaken to determine if stimulation of the substantia nigra (SN) could also modify spinal reflexes and might be involved in a descending pathway to the spinal cord.

Studies were undertaken in adult cats anesthetized initially with diethylether and ethylchloride followed by chloralose (60 mg/Kg, I.V.). An array of five bipolar stimulating electrodes was stereotaxically inserted into the SN. A lumbar laminectomy was performed exposing L6, L7 and S1 spinal roots. A spinal pool of warmed paraffin was maintained at 37°C. Spinal reflexes were recorded by stimulating the dorsal root and recording from the ventral root and from an adjacent dorsal root. The reflex amplitude was averaged in a Biomac 1000 computer. Electrode placements in SN were confirmed by histological sections of the mesencephalon.

The effect of SN stimulation on spinal reflexes was studied in 28 cats by initially applying a conditioning pulse (0.05 mA, 0.1 msec) or train of pulses (500-800/sec, 10 msec) to SN, which preceded the dorsal root stimulus by 10-60 msec. Both potentiation and depression of the monosynaptic reflex were observed. However, the most predominant effect was potentiation of the monosynaptic reflex with little or no effect on

---

* Medical Research Council of Canada Scholar

the polysynaptic response. Contralateral SN stimulation produced similar effects to ipsilateral activation. The potentiation of the monosynaptic reflex by SN was apparent at different intensities of dorsal root stimulation from 1-15X, group I threshold, with most measurements being performed at 10-15X, group I threshold, which is supramaximal for the monosynaptic pathway.

Stimulation of SN did not produce a measurable dorsal root potential, nor were any changes in primary afferent terminal excitability apparent upon SN stimulation when tested by Wall's technique (1, 2, 7). In order to rule out the possibility of involvement of other areas during SN stimulation, the following controls were undertaken. Bilateral section of the cerebral peduncles at the level of the pons did not alter the SN-induced potentiation of the spinal monosynaptic reflex. This result would suggest that the effects observed on spinal reflexes were not due to activation of the corticospinal system.

The possibility that the effects observed involved a pathway from SN projecting to anterior structures of the striatum or thalamus was ruled out, since an ipsilateral cross-section of the brain just anterior to the SN stimulating electrodes did not abolish the effect of SN on spinal reflexes.

Investigation of various adrenergic antagonists was also undertaken to further elucidate the pharmacological properties of this descending pathway. The SN induced potentiation of the monosynaptic reflex is consistently blocked by chlorpromazine (1-4 mg/Kg) and by haloperidol (0.5-1 mg/Kg). This blockade occurs without a change in amplitude of the control monosynaptic reflex. Atropine (0.5 mg/Kg) and methysergide (0.1-0.5 mg/Kg) do not effect the potentiation of reflexes by SN.

Further experiments are under way to determine the precise course of this pathway, the type of motorneurons affected and changes which occur in motorneuron conductance during SN activation.

ACKNOWLEDGMENT. This work was supported by the Medical Research Council of Canada.

REFERENCES

1 ANDERSEN, P., ECCLES, J.C. and SEARS, T.A., Presynaptic inhibitory action of cerebral cortex on the spinal cord. Nature 194 (1962) 740-741.

2 ANDERSEN, P., ECCLES, J.C. and SEARS, T.A., Cortically evoked depolarization of primary afferent fibers in the spinal cord. J. Neurophysiol., 27 (1964) 63-77.

3 LLOYD, D.P.C., Activity in neurons of the bulbospinal correlation system. J. Neurophysiol., 4 (1941) 115-134.

4 MAGOUN, H.W. and RHINES, R., An inhibitory mechanism in the bulbar reticular formation. J. Neurophysiol., 9 (1946) 165-171.

5 PEACOCK, S.M., Jr., and HODES, R., Influence of forebrain on somatomotor activity; facilitation. J. Comp. Neurol., 94 (1951) 409-426.

6 SEGUNDO, J.P. and LARRANAGA, W., Striatal influence upon units in posterior column nuclei. An. Fac. Med. Montevideo, 44, 424-431.

7 WALL, P.D., Excitability changes in afferent fiber terminations and their relation to slow potentials. J. Physiol. (Lond.) 142 (1958) 1-21.

Corticothalamic Projections and Sensorimotor Activities
T. Frigyesi, E. Rinvik, and M.D. Yahr, editors. © 1972
Raven Press, New York.

Pre- and Postcentral Neuronal Discharge in Relation to Learned Movement

Edward V. Evarts

Previous studies (2) have shown that neurons in the precentral motor cortex of the monkey become active prior to the performance of a learned hand movement. This finding is in accord with the classical view that neurons of the precentral motor cortex (area 4) have a role in initiating motor activity. In the studies which are described here, recording was restricted to the precentral motor cortex. It is well known, however, that movements can be elicited by electrical stimulation of postcentral as well as precentral motor cortex, and the entire concept of a "motor" as contrasted to a "sensory" cortex has often been questioned (c.f. Towe, 10). Thus the question arises as to whether discharge prior to movement may occur in the "sensory" as well as the "motor" division of the sensorimotor cortex.

In this connection, it should be recalled that, in addition to receiving powerful inputs from peripheral receptors, postcentral neurons receive inputs from nonsensory areas of the brain. A role for these nonsensory inputs to sensory areas is proposed in the theory of corollary discharge (6, 7). According to this theory, impulses pass from motor to sensory areas and activity in the sensory areas is elicited not only by feedback from the periphery but also by an input which is corollary with the motor output.

In the postcentral area, strong inputs do indeed exist from the adjacent precentral area (4). The increase in activity of precentral motor cortex neurons prior to movement provides one source of impulses entering the postcentral area prior to movement. In addition to these inputs from motor cortex, the postcentral gyrus receives inputs from cerebellar nuclei via the thalamus. The finding of Thach (8, 9) that neurons in the dentate nucleus become active prior to movement suggests another possible route whereby neurons in the postcentral gyrus might be impinged upon by impulses prior to any feedback from the periphery. This route, from dentate nucleus to nucleus ventralis posterolateralis of the thalamus and thence to cortex, provides a pathway for activating postcentral neurons which parallels the lemniscal pathway. Indeed, it has been shown that a single neuron in nucleus ventralis posterolateralis may be impinged upon by either a path from the dentate nucleus or by the classical lemniscal pathway (1, 5).

The preceding discussion suggests at least two pathways which may excite discharge in postcentral neurons prior to movement. However, these inputs may not be sufficiently strong to initiate all-or-none discharge; they may modify responses of postcentral neurons to sensory feedback rather than initiate all-or-none activity in and of themselves. In light of these uncertainties, it seemed worthwhile to observe the discharge of postcentral neurons in association with movement. The experiment which will be described presents the results of a study aimed at discovering whether modifications of discharge in postcentral neurons occur prior to movement (as a result of inputs from other parts of the central nervous system) or following movement (presumably as a result of sensory feedback from periphery).

METHODS

The major question here was one of timing; consequently the movement selected for study was one whose time of onset could be easily detected. A monkey was rewarded for a short reaction-time movement in response to a light stimulus whose time of occurrence was unpredictable. Under the stipulated conditions the monkey made a ballistic movement of abrupt onset. The results in this report are those of a monkey who grasped a handle and maintained steady wrist flexion until light onset, at which time he made a prompt extensor movement. Following the extensor movement, wrist extension was maintained until the light reappeared, at which time a prompt flexor movement was made. This was followed by maintained wrist flexion, etc. Following training, stimulating electrodes were permanently implanted in the medullary pyramid to identify pyramidal tract neurons by their antidromic responses to medullary stimulation, and a chamber was attached to the skull to allow single unit recording in both precentral and postcentral gyri. Knowledge of when postcentral and precentral neurons discharged with respect to the same stereotyped movement performed by the same monkey made it possible to infer when pre- and postcentral neurons discharged with respect to each other.

RESULTS

Since the aim of the present study was to discover the temporal relations between movement and the activity of neurons in sensorimotor cortex, it was necessary to obtain a measure of the onset of the movement. Recordings of arm muscle EMG and force applied to the handle provided this measure. Average responses of rectified EMG were obtained for each of a series of muscles. The first detected change of force exerted on the handle grasped by the monkey served as the temporal reference point for the EMG averaging. The force change associated with the movement, rather than the photic stimulus that triggered the movement, was selected as the reference point because the activity of muscles was time-locked to the force change, whereas the interval from stimulus to muscular response showed the wide variation characteristic of the type of reaction time task that monkeys performed.

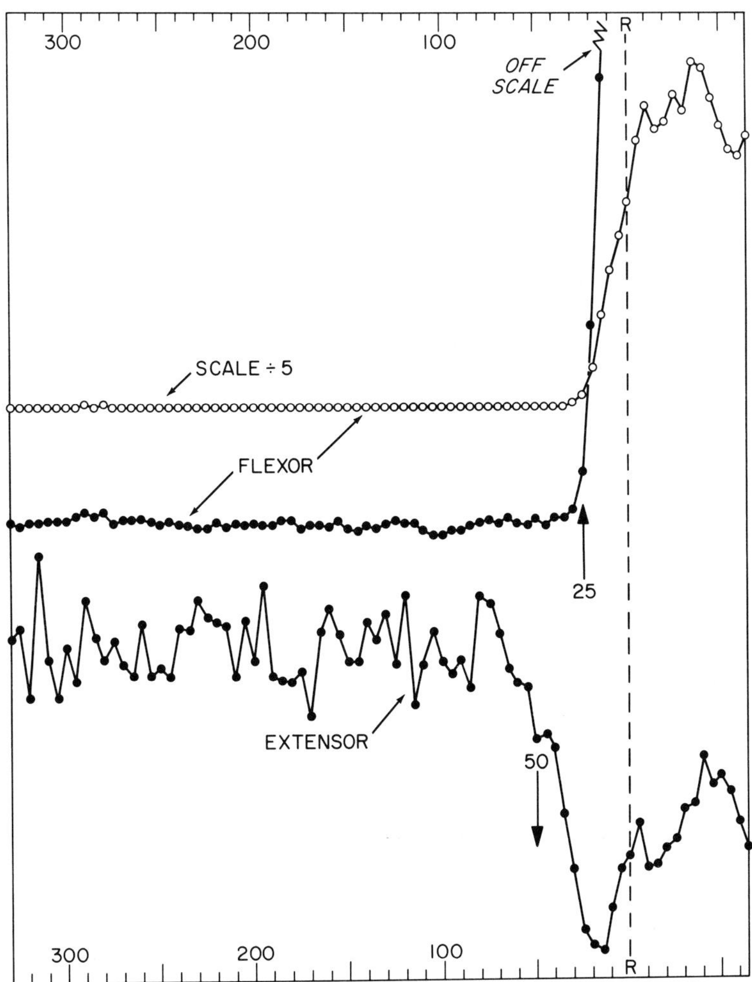

FIG. 1. Muscle Activity with Flexion. Electromyographic activity of flexor and extensor muscles was rectified and averaged with respect to the motor response (R), R being the time at which the first force change associated with movement was detected. The abscissa gives time in msec before and after R. For flexion, activity of flexor muscles started to increase 25 msec prior to R, whereas a decrease of activity in the antagonist extensor muscles began 50 msec prior to R.

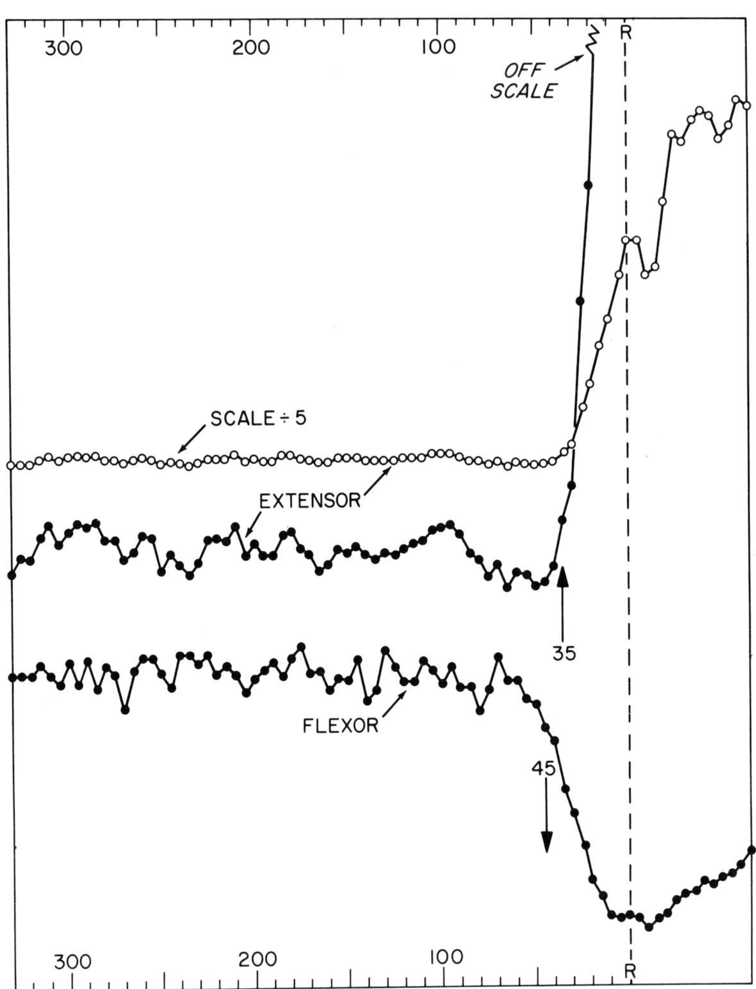

FIG. 2. Muscle Activity with Extension. For extension, a decrease of activity of wrist flexor began 45 msec prior to R, whereas the increase of activity in wrist extensors occurred 35 msec prior to R.

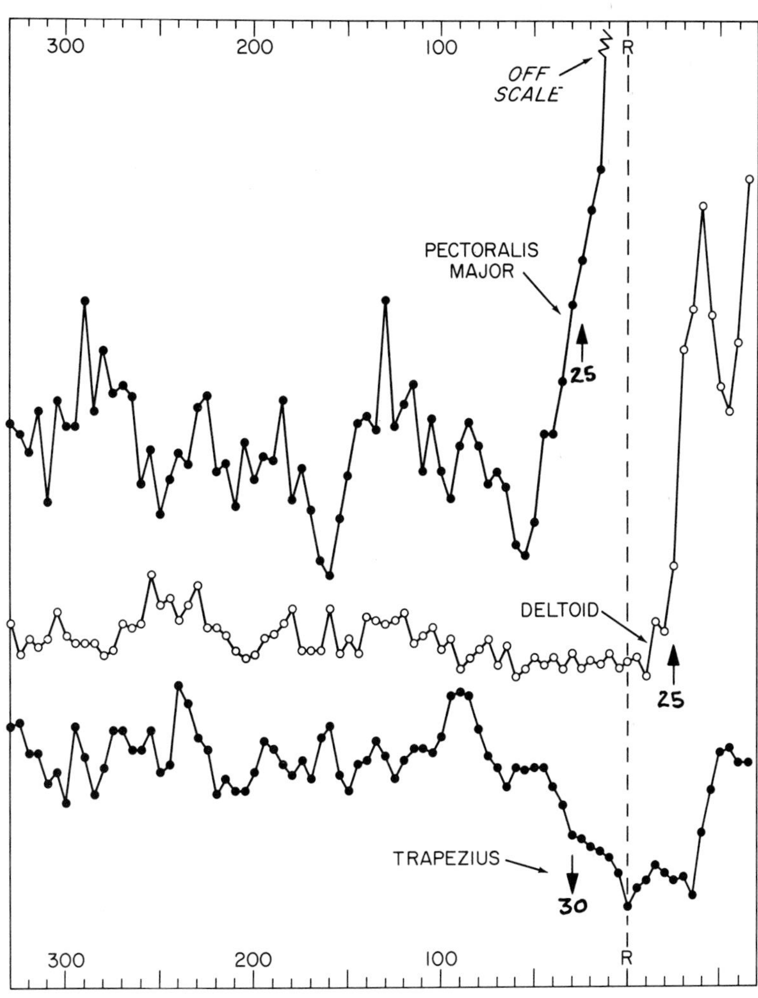

FIG. 3. Activity of Proximal Muscles. Average EMG records of three proximal muscles are shown for flexion. The changes in these muscles were less marked and tended to occur later than the changes occurring in distal prime movers of the wrist. The numbers next to the arrows show that trapezuis had a decrease of activity 30 msec prior to R, deltoid increased 25 msec following R, and pectoralis major increased 25 msec prior to R. The abscissa is in msec with respect to R.

Figure 1 shows average EMG responses of wrist flexors and extensors for the movement of flexion and Fig. 2 shows average responses of the same two muscle groups for the movement of extension. For both movements, decrease of activity in the antagonist precedes the increase of activity in the agonist, as already described by Hufschmidt and Hufschmidt (3). Figure 1 shows that for wrist flexion, the flexor muscles increase 25 msec prior to detection of the force change, whereas there is a decrease of extensor activity 50 msec prior to the detection of force change. For wrist extension (Fig. 2), the extensors increase 35 msec before detection of force change, while the flexors decrease 45 msec before detection of the force change. Recordings from more proximal muscles were also made, and the results for some of these muscles are shown in Fig. 3. It is clear that proximal muscles are also involved in this movement, but their changes occur somewhat later and are less marked than is the case for the prime movers of the wrist.

As mentioned above, the reference point for averaging muscle activity was the first detected change of force exerted on the handle; this first detected change of force will be referred to as the RESPONSE (R). Just as EMG activity can be averaged with respect to R, so the activity of a single cell can be averaged with respect to R. Figure 4 shows the activity of a single neuron in the postcentral gyrus with respect to R and with respect to the stimulus (S) as well. The peri-response histogram for this cell shows that it had an increase in activity during the first "bin"

FIG. 4. A Postcentral Neuron. Raster display of activity for a single postcentral neuron with respect to stimulus (left) and motor response (right). The large dot in each row of the left raster (the S-raster) shows the time of occurrence of the motor response (R). In this S-raster the stimulus occurs at the center line in the raster and activity is displayed for 500 msec before and after S. In the R-raster each row has been shifted to the left to bring R to the center of the raster, and here activity is displayed for 500 msec before and after R. Below each raster is a histogram which sums raster activity in 20 msec bins. In the left (peri-S) histogram the arrow indicates the time of occurrence of S, whereas in the right (peri-R) histogram the arrow indicates the time of occurrence of R. The R-histogram at the right has been scaled down by a factor of 2. The increase of activity in this postcentral neuron began in the first bin (0 to 20 msec) after R.

FIG. 5. Precentral and Postcentral Neuron Onset Times. Peri-response latencies were determined for several hundred precentral and postcentral neurons which showed a change (either increase or decrease) of activity in association with movement. This figure shows two distributions of peri-response latencies, one for precentral neurons and the other for postcentral neurons. The abscissa gives time in msec before and after R. Ordinate is number of units. For further details, see text.

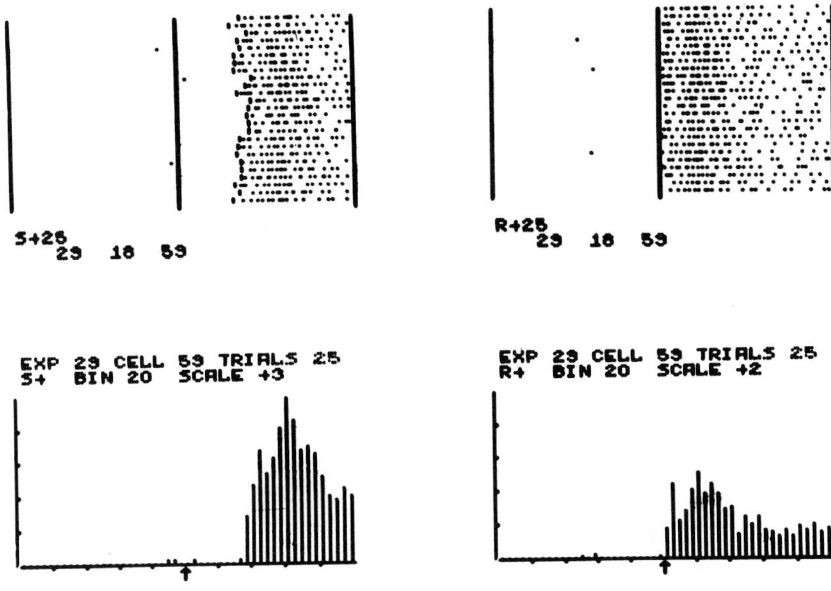
S+25
29 18 59
R+25
29 18 59
EXP 29 CELL 59 TRIALS 25
S+ BIN 20 SCALE +3
EXP 29 CELL 59 TRIALS 25
R+ BIN 20 SCALE +2

FIG. 4

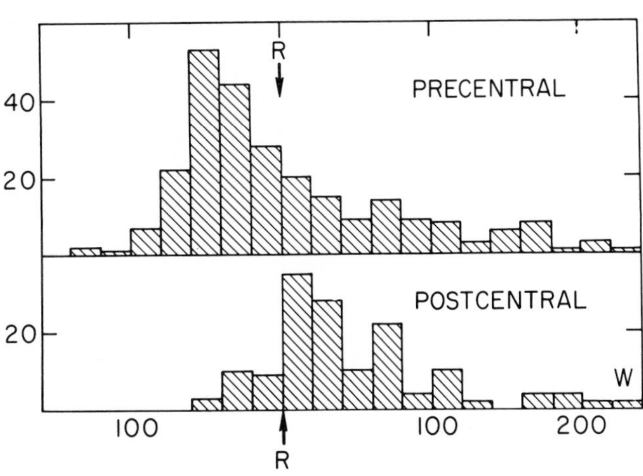
R
PRECENTRAL
40
20
POSTCENTRAL
20
W
100
100
200
R

FIG. 5

following R. Since the bin width for this peri-response histogram is 20 msec, this cell showed an increase in activity at some point between 0 and 20 msec following R.

For each of several hundred cells in pre- and postcentral gyrus showing a change of activity in relation to movement, the "bin" in which the change began was determined. These "peri-response latencies" are shown in Fig. 5. It can be seen that precentral neurons become active earlier than postcentral neurons. The most common time during which precentral neurons become active is between 60 and 40 msec before R whereas the most common time for postcentral cells to become active is between 0 and 20 msec after R. The earliest cells in precentral gyrus become active between 140 and 120 msec prior to R, whereas the earliest cells in postcentral gyrus become active between 60 and 40 msec prior to R.

DISCUSSION

These results demonstrate that, as a group, neurons in postcentral cortex discharge later than neurons in the precentral cortex in association with the learned motor response which was investigated in the present study. Granting this difference between pre- and postcentral neurons, several questions have not been answered by these experiments; two of these questions will be discussed in the following section.

The first question concerns the type of movement which was performed in the present experiment; it was a ballistic movement whose execution was not dependent upon sensory feedback from the periphery. Precision with respect to joint position, force of movement, or tactile feedback was not an important part of the motor performance. It was necessary merely that the animal propel his wrist as rapidly as possible from one position to another. The displacement was terminated by an external object; it was a movement that an animal might well perform after dorsal root section.

It is known that inputs to the postcentral gyrus provide precise information as to tactile, joint, and deep pressure modalities, and it might be argued that discharge of postcentral neurons prior to movement should not be expected under conditions in which inputs from these modalities are irrelevant to the task being performed. In contrast, it is possible that, were a movement carried out for the purpose of tactile exploration, postcentral neurons might become active prior to the movement if the purpose of this prior activity were to sharpen or focus the transmission of the sensory feedback from the movement. These considerations would suggest that, before concluding that postcentral neuron activity does not precede movement, it is necessary to investigate additional sorts of movement, especially movements which involve exploration and precise displacement.

The second point concerns the implications of the findings with respect to possible differences in neuronal activity in association with active compared to passive movement. The finding that most postcentral neurons discharge only following movement, presumably as a result of sensory feedback, does not imply that these discharges are the same as they would be following passive stimulation of receptors. It would, indeed, be interesting to examine the patterns of activity in postcentral neurons under conditions in which the animal's movements control receptor stimulation and contrast these patterns of activity with those generated when the experimenter produces the same inputs to receptors—but without the active participation by the animal.

SUMMARY

Activity of neurons in precentral and postcentral gyrus was recorded in monkeys during performance of learned flexion and extension movements of the wrist. The movements were triggered by a light stimulus, and the animal was rewarded for short reaction-time responses. Changes of activity in precentral neurons began 60-80 msec prior to changes of activity in postcentral neurons. Though there was a clear differentiation in onset times for pre- and postcentral neurons in association with this ballistic movement, these findings leave a number of questions unanswered. In particular, it would seem necessary to carry out additional experiments comparing pre- and postcentral neuronal activity during carefully controlled exploratory movements in which the feedback from sensory receptors is an important aspect of motor performance.

ACKNOWLEDGMENT

Much of this discussion was stimulated by P.D. Wall, who pointed out that observations made on "lurching" movements, such as those investigated in this study, should not be the basis for extrapolation to movement in general.

REFERENCES

1 BAVA, A., MANZONI, T., URBANO, A. Cerebellar influences on neuronal elements of thalamic somatosensory relay-nuclei. Arch. Sci. Biol.,(Bologna), 50 (1966) 181-204.

2 EVARTS, E.V. Pyramidal tract activity associated with a conditioned hand movement in the monkey. J. Neurophysiol.,29 (1966) 1011-1027.

3 HUFSCHMIDT, H.I. and HUFSCHMIDT, T. Antagonist inhibition as the earliest sign of a sensory motor reaction. Nature, 174 (1954) 607.

4 JONES, E.G and POWELL, T.P.S. Connexions of the somatic sensory cortex of the Rhesus monkey. I. Ipsilateral cortical connexions. Brain, 92 (1969) 477-502.

5 NAKAGOSHI, I. Certain influences of the cerebellum on impulses to and from the somato-sensory cortex in the cat. J. Kyoto Prefect. Med. Univ.,75 (1966) 1-14.

6 SPERRY, R.W. Neural basis of the spontaneous optokinetic response produced by visual inversion. J. Comp. Physiol. Psychol., 43 (1950) 483-489.

7 TEUBER, H.-L. Alterations of perception after brain injury. In: Brain and Conscious Experience, J.C.Eccles, (Ed.), New York, Springer-Verlag, 1966, pp. 182-216.

8 THACH, W.T. Discharge of cerebellar neurons related to two maintained postures and two prompt movements. I. Nuclear cell output. J. Neurophysiol., 33 (1970) 527-536.

9 THACH, W.T. Discharge of cerebellar neurons related to two maintained postures and two prompt movements. II. Purkinje cell output and input. J. Neurophysiol., 33 (1970) 537-547.

10 TOWE, A.L. Sensory-motor organization and movement. In: Central Control of Movement, E.V. Evarts, (Ed.) Cambridge, Mass., MIT Press, 1971, pp. 40-51.

DISCUSSION

ASANUMA:

Thank you very much Dr. Evarts. I am very much impressed with your elegant work and I am quite certain that you have thought about the following problem before planning the experiments. You have used visual stimulation and we know that there is a specific projection from the eye to the visual cortex. You were recording from the sensory cortex and not from the visual cortex. What I would like to ask is, for example, by using the same program, if there are neurons in the visual cortex which when responded to visual stimulation, the movement occurs. I think this kind of ques- is a natural one and since your experimental set-ups are so elaborate and such fine ones, this question could have been answered, but you choose the sensory cortex instead of the visual cortex in this experiment. Why did you?

EVARTS:

Well, the reason for investigating the sensory cortex of the post-central gyrus here was to see if there was clean functional differentiation between sensory and motor divisions of the sensorimotor cortex. In future studies I think it may be possible to obtain information along the lines that you have suggested. In our next experiment we are going to train monkeys to make a hand movement the stimulus for which comes directly into the sensory and the motor cortex. I think a point of considerable interest here is how information is processed between input and output if some of the input gets directly into the motor cortex. The situation we would look at is one in which the animal holds a particular position and then at a time which is unpredictable to him, the resistance against which he is pressing while he holds this position gives way and the animal's arm starts to move at time and speed which is unpredictable to the animal. The animal must sense how fast his arm is moving and must make a correction such that he will reach a certain preassigned end point at a basis for making a correction comes in through the moving arm and it is quite clear from many studies done in the past, by you and others, that this information will reach both the precentral and the postcentral gyrus. Most relevant to the studies that you have done would be to what extent information from the part which is to be moved goes to the output neurons in the precentral gyrus. I think that when we put the input into the sensorimotor area via the hand and look at the output from the same area we can get some of the points that you have raised in your question.

STERIADE:

Concerning your precentral neuron which was inhibited by the flexion movement and was facilitated in spontaneous firing by the extension movement, I was impressed by looking at your slide, that the background firing was strikingly different in these two cases. Perhaps you would like to comment if such an opposite effect was due to a certain function of this neuron or only reflects opposite states in the background firing of this particular cell in different movements.

EVARTS:

A difference in steady state activity depending upon which of the two forces the animal is exerting is very common, especially when the electrode is in the focal region for representation of wrist movement. This slide that Dr. Steriade referred to showed the same cell under conditions of steady state flexion and steady state extension. It is a very common finding that changes in the steady state force exerted by the animal is associated with changes in the discharge frequency of motor cortex units. I think that it is analogous to what's going on in the muscle. This is not surprising, since there is a rather tight coupling between neurons in the motor cortex and the activity of particular muscle groups.

PRIBRAM:

This isn't a question, it is a comment on Dr. Asanuma's question. We have used gross evoked potentials to study the question of what goes on in the visual cortex and similar situations and find that before the animal learns, the electrical activity in the visual cortex reflects only stimulus differences. However, after an animal learns a task such as this, potentials in the visual cortex do reflect response differences, provided one averages the record backward from the time of response not the time of stimulus presentation. Note that this is monkey primary visual cortex (area 17) on the lateral surface near the foveal region. Thus, motor activity becomes encoded in the striate visual cortex during learning.

EVARTS:

No, we have never looked in the visual cortex.

GILMAN:

I was fascinated by your statement that one of the first events peripherally is a relaxation of a tonically active muscle. I wonder if you think that relaxation is related to your discharging pyramidal of precentral neuron and if not to what is it related.

EVARTS:

I really don't know the answer to your question as to what underlies the early cessation of activity in tonically active muscle prior to movement. We have recorded activity from many different muscles in association with reaction time performance in monkeys and this phenomenon of antagonist relaxation is widespread. This phenomenon also has been described by a number of previous investigators, e.g., Hufschmidt and Hufschmidt in 1954. I tend to suspect that the decrease of muscle activity may be controlled by some structure other than the cerebral cortex, but I couldn't say what this structure is.

Corticothalamic Projections and Sensorimotor Activities
T. Frigyesi, E. Rinvik, and M.D. Yahr, editors. © 1972
Raven Press, New York.

The Effect of Local Cooling of the Motor Cortex upon Experimental Parkinson-like Tremor, Shivering, Voluntary Movements, and Thalamic Unit Activity in the Monkey

H. Jasper, Y. Lamarre and A. Joffroy

It has been known since the very first description of Parkinson's Disease that the characteristic tremor of this syndrome is abolished by lesions of the internal capsule associated with hemiplegia of the limbs involved in the tremor (3). This original observation was made possible by James Parkinson from his own personal experience. Since this time, there have been many neurosurgical interventions designed to arrest Parkinson tremor by ablations or sections involving the motor cortex or premotor regions or the pyramidal tract. Such operations have been successful with regard to the arrest of tremor but with unfortunate consequences for voluntary movement, because of varying degrees of hemiparesis.

In the course of previous experiments of the analysis of cortical function associated with experimental Parkinson-like tremor which follows local lesions in the tegmentum of the midbrain, we have published with Drs. Cordeau, Gybels, and Poirier an unexpected observation made in the course of studying the firing patterns of single cells in the sensory and motor cortex as related to tremor movements in the unanesthetized monkey (4). For purposes of these studies, we placed a plastic plug into the skull which held a micromanipulator by means of which we could insert microelectrodes into various depths in the cortex in the chronic animal preparations while recording tremor movements and the electromyogram. In a few of these animals, the plug which was screwed into the skull during anaesthesia resulted in an arrest of the experimental tremor localized to the contralateral muscles represented by the cerebral cortex over which the plug had been placed. It was soon discovered that the tremor would return to these muscles by simply unscrewing the plug to relieve the relatively light pressure upon the cortex which had resulted from it being inserted too far. This accidental observation demonstrated how sensitive this Parkinson-like tremor was to even rather minor interference with the blood supply of the motor cortex. We noted at that time that the arrest of tremor due to light pressure on the surface was not always accompanied by a comparable loss in voluntary movements in the limb.

In order to analyse this question further, we have undertaken to study the effect of motor cortex upon experimental Parkinson-like tremor in the monkey by means of a cooling chamber inserted in the skull over a local area of motor cortex (7). In this preparation, we also are able to insert microelectrodes into various regions of the thalamus and to study at the same time the change in firing patterns of thalamic cells which accompany the cooling of the motor cortex to the point of arrest of tremor. This makes possible also, by graded cooling, to study the relationship between the degree of cooling necessary for arrested tremor and that necessary for the arrest of finely coordinated voluntary movements of the extremities which characterize motor cortical function in the monkey.

Previous studies on thalamic unit discharge patterns in monkeys with experimental Parkinson-like tremor have shown that there are many cells in the rostral portion of nucleus ventralis lateralis which continue to fire in bursts at approximately the tremor frequency even though the tremor movements have been completely arrested by Flaxedil (11). Other cells located more posteriorly, including those in the ventro basal complex, stopped firing when the actual movements of tremor were arrested with Flaxedil. This observation is consistent with the previous studies in the sensory and motor cortex (4) showing that cells in the post-central gyrus fire with a rigid and precisely synchronized relationship with tremor movements and are arrested when the movements stop while cells in the motor cortex may not be so rigidly synchronized with movements and may burst at similar frequencies even though movements are not detectable.

METHODS

The cortical cooling chamber technique used in these studies has been described elsewhere (7). The cooling chamber consisted of a cylinder made of very thin stainless steel with an inlet and outlet for the circulation of cooled fluid at different velocities controlled by an automatic circulating pump. In the center of this chamber was an opened tube through which was inserted recording electrodes and a thermistor in order to monitor the temperature on the cortical surface at the center of the cooling chamber throughout the period of observation. There were, in addition, stimulating and recording electrodes attached to the undersurface of the chamber in order to make possible the recording of direct cortical electrical responses, evoked potentials and spontaneous electrical activity at different temperatures.

For purposes of microelectrode recording from the thalamus, there were 2 methods employed. The first was similar to that employed with Dr. Gilles Bertrand at the Montreal Neurological Institute during stereotaxic operations in man (5, 6). It consisted of a probe which could be inserted in the skull through which could be passed a Tungsten microelectrode attached to a micrometer drive. The probe could be either straight or curved like a stylet making possible exploration of large areas of the thalamus without changing the position of the guide which was permanently set into the skull in our chronic animal preparations.

In order to provide for greater stability of microelectrode recording in the unanaesthetized animal, the microelectrode technique has been revised by Dr. Lamarre (12) to fix the head more rigidly in by means of strong attachments to the skull and clamping of a plastic chamber into the top of a perspex table upon which is mounted a precise microdrive. This was installed according to stereotaxic coordinates accurately calibrated so that microelectrodes can then be placed according to known coordinates and various parts of the thalamus can be explored while at the same time cooling the motor cortex. In order to do this effectively, it was necessary to place the microelectrodes chamber posteriorly at an angle of 40° so that this chamber would not interfere with the cooling chamber installed over the motor cortex.

Histological controls were then carried out of the needle tracts to locate precisely the site in the thalamus from which unit recording was made. All of the data was prerecorded on an Ampex Tape Recorder which included electromyograms of antagonist muscles involving the tremor, tremor movements themselves by means of a transducer and the temperature of the surface of the cortex by means of the thermistor on the cortex in the centre of the cooling chamber. From these continuous tapes, analysis of relationships between units, muscle activity, tremor movements and temperature could be made subsequent to the experiment. Records were then selected for photography and for computer calculation on a PDP9 computer.

These experiments have to date been carried out successfully on 4 animals, the major portion of the results being taken from 3 animals. Cinematographic records of the effect of cooling on the tremor and voluntary movements have been made in two animals.

Experimental tremor was induced in these animals by the method developed with Dr. Poirier (4, 15, 16) and being used for many other experiments in our laboratories. It consists of inserting a coagulating electrode by stereotaxic control into the tegmentum of the brain stem at about the level of the substantia nigra, a technique modified from that originally described by Ward, McCulloch and Magoun (17). Lesions are made usually unilaterally near the midline at stereotaxic coordinates A 5-6, L 1-4 and H+1 to H-3. Some of the animals thus prepared show spontaneous Parkinson-like tremor movements in the opposite side of the body involving more or less of the musculature. In some instances, face, arm and leg were all involved while in others the tremor was more marked in the arm or the leg and more rarely in the face. In many of these animals, the tremor movements involved primarily the proximal musculature while in others, the distal musculature was also involved and pill rolling movements as seen in Parkinson patients were then observed. In all other respects, these movements corresponded to those seen in Parkinson patients, both with regard to tremor frequency and its arrest by anaesthesia or natural sleep. The tremor was also arrested by voluntary movement. The frequency is usually between 4 and 5/sec. The nature of the lesions and the tremor have been described elsewhere (16).

Only a portion of these animals show spontaneous tremor, about 1 in 3 in our series. In some, only a few tremor movements may be seen, not sufficient for adequate study. Consequently, we have used harmaline to produce the tremor in animals who did not show it spontaneously and also to exaggerate the tremor in those which showed only a minimal amount, inadequate for detailed study. Harmaline injected in the amount of 15-20 mg intramuscularly in a monkey with a tegmental lesion regularly produced a marked increase in the Parkinson-like tremor, localized only to the side of the body opposite to that of the lesion (2, 16). It developed gradually within about 15-20 min following the injection and lasted for at least 1 or 2 hours, and sometimes longer.

Harmaline injected into animals who have not had a tegmental lesion will not produce this form of tremor. With larger injections, especially given intravenously, the animal does develop a different sort of tremor at a much higher frequency. It appears more like shivering movements (10). These are accompanied by considerable agitation. It is quite easy to distinguish between harmaline-induced tremors and the effect of harmaline on increasing or revealing a latent tremor in an animal with a tegmental lesion.

In the animals used for the cooling experiments, there were 2 who showed spontaneous tremor and 2 who required harmaline. The effect of cooling was studied both on the tremor without harmaline and in the exaggerated tremor following harmaline administration. In one animal, shivering movements were also observed induced during cortical cooling so that we were able to study the microelectrode records of thalamic unit responses during shivering movements as well as during the Parkinson-like tremor in the same animal. They could easily be distinguished in frequency and cortical cooling produced opposite effects, arresting the Parkinson-like tremor while enhancing the shivering movements.

RESULTS

Effect of Cooling Motor Cortex Upon Tremor, Shivering, and Voluntary Movements

Cooling of the motor cortex to a surface temperature of 16-18° C in an animal with active spontaneous tremor, or even when reenforced with harmaline injection, caused complete cessation of tremor movements in the limb contralateral to the area of cortical motor representation. Tremor movements persisted in the face and leg areas when only the arm area was cooled. Arrest of tremor was remarkably rapid, requiring only 5-10 seconds once the cortical surface temperature had reached the vicinity of 18° C. It did not reappear as long as this temperature was maintained (up to 15 min in these experiments). Upon cessation of cooling, tremor returned promptly (within 10-15 secs) when cortical surface temperature had reached the vicinity of 25-30° C providing the cortex had not been cooled below 16° C for more than about 1 minute. With longer periods of cooling at lower temperatures (down to 10° C) recovery was delayed and sometimes required several minutes even after cortical surface temperature had returned to normal (38° C).

Voluntary movements of the affected limb, even fine coordinated movements of the fingers, were preserved after complete arrest of tremor providing surface cortical temperature was reduced just sufficient for tremor arrest. Cooling below this temperature (to about 12° C) resulted in loss of voluntary finger movements as well, even though gross movements of limb persisted. It was possible, therefore, to dissociate motor cortical function controlling the expression of Parkinson-like tremor in these experimental animals with tegmental lesions from those functions making possible fine finger movements.

In the one animal in whom shivering movements were induced by cortical cooling, these movements persisted even when surface cortical temperature was reduced sufficiently for arrest of both voluntary finger movements and Parkinson-like tremor in the affected limb. The shivering movements in this animal consisted of a tremor at 13/sec as compared to 4.3/sec for the Parkinson-like tremor. There were, in addition, occasional tonic spasms of the limbs. Both the tremor and tonic spasms were increased by cortical cooling to temperatures which caused complete arrest of the 4.3/sec tremor as well as arrest of fine finger movements. Shivering movements persisted for several minutes even after the cortex was rewarmed to normal temperature and voluntary finger movements and the 4.3/sec tremor had returned. These observations would suggest that the motor cortex is not required for the expression of shivering as it is for Parkinson-like tremor and for finely coordinated finger movements.

Effect of Cooling of Motor Cortex Upon Thalamic Units Discharging Synchronous with Parkinson-like Tremor and Shivering Movements

As in previous studies in experimental animals (9, 11) and in man (5), exploration of the ventral thalamus with a stereotaxically controlled microelectrode, a variety of units were encountered, only some of which showed precise temporal relationships with tremor movements. Only those showing such relationships were selected for detailed study during cortical cooling in these experiments.

In the more caudal portion of the ventral thalamus, units were encountered which fired in bursts precisely timed with the tremor frequency. They also fired in response to passive movements of the affected limb. These "sensory" units ceased firing in bursts at regular intervals when the tremor movements were arrested by cortical cooling, as might be expected.

In more rostral portions of the ventral thalamus, in n. Ventralis Lateralis, units were found which fired in bursts at the tremor frequency, but failed to fire with passive movements of the affected limb. Nevertheless, the firing pattern of many of these cells was altered during cortical cooling sufficient to arrest tremor movements. These units continued to fire in bursts, but at a lower frequency and with less regularity than before. A typical example is illustrated in Fig. 1 in which a unit showed a burst pattern at 4.3/sec clearly associated with the tremor movements prior to cooling, but continued to fire in irregular bursts at 1.5 to 2.5/sec when tremor movements were arrested by cortical cooling. It returned to a more rapid and regular burst frequency when the cortex was allowed to return to a surface temperature of 35° C with return of tremor movements, though synchronization with tremor movements was less precise at this time. Even though we were unable to demonstrate that these cells would respond to passive movements, and consequently were probably not simple "sensory" units, cortical cooling did produce a definite effect upon the frequency and regularity of their firing pattern.

There were a few apparently "non-sensory" cells recorded also from n. Ventralis Lateralis which fired in regular bursts at the tremor frequency, but which continued to fire in equally regular bursts at the same frequency even when tremor was arrested by local cortical cooling. These were relatively rare as compared to those described

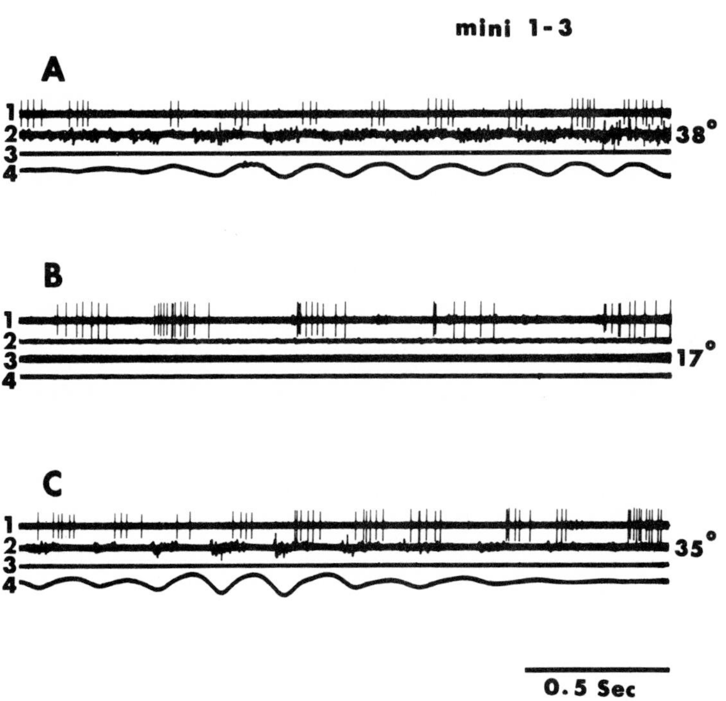

FIG. 1. Thalamic unit firing in bursts (first line) at the tremor frequency in the contralateral arm, as indicated in the needle EMG from the biceps muscle (second line) and by the strain-gauge transducer record of arm movements (fourth line in each strip). (A) Records taken before cooling of the motor cortex. The cortical temperature is 38° C and is indicated by the line superimposed on the biceps EMG (line 2). (B) Records taken during arrest of tremor after cooling of the motor cortex to 17° C (temperature line now displaced downward over line 3). The thalamic cell fires in burst but irregularly and at a lower frequency when tremor is arrested. (C) Records obtained after cortex has rewarmed to 35° C and tremor reappeared. The cell resumes its rhythmic firing synchronous with the muscle tremor.

above. One of these cells is illustrated in Fig. 2, firing with tremor in the arm at a frequency of about 4/sec. In this animal spontaneous tremor occurred only in the arm, and almost exclusively in the arm even when reenforced with harmaline. However at the height of harmaline reenforcement occasional tremor movements of the leg were also observed.

One might assume that thalamic units which continued to burst at the tremor frequency even when tremor in one limb was arrested by cortical cooling merely represented those which were functionally related to muscles of the other limb or face not af-

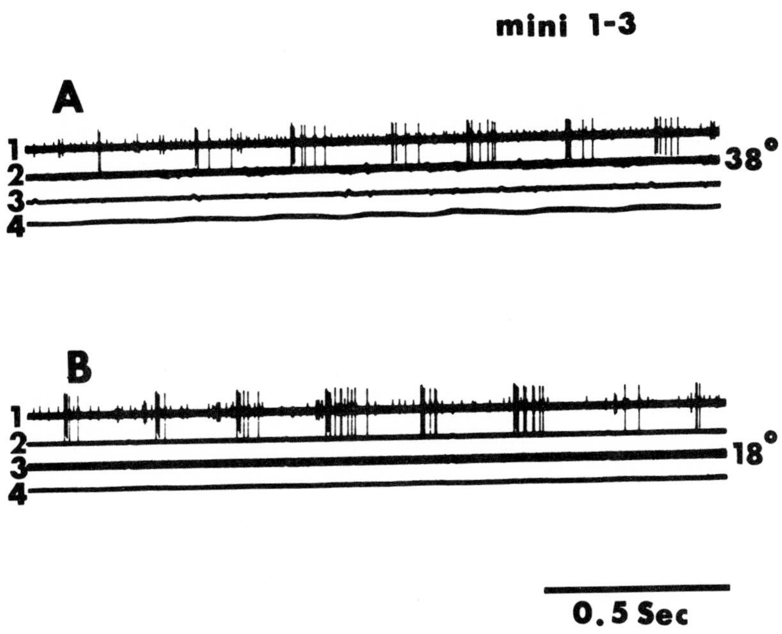

FIG. 2. Thalamic unit firing in bursts at 4/sec during 4/sec tremor in the contralateral arm (A). This firing pattern is undisturbed when tremor is arrested after cooling of the motor cortex to 18° C (B). (Lines 1 to 4: same identification as in Fig. 1.).

fected by local cortical cooling. In some instances in the present experiments, these units continued to burst at the tremor frequency even though no tremor movements of any part of the body could be observed. However, the possibility that there might have been minimal tremor movements in some part of the body which escaped our notice still remains, so that interpretation of these findings remains uncertain.

In the animal exhibiting generalized shivering consisting of tremor at 13/sec occasionally interrupted by tonic spasms, we were also able to record thalamic units firing in bursts synchronous with the 13/sec tremor, and firing continuously during the tonic spasms. However, these were not the same cells which fired in bursts with the 4-5/sec tremor in the same animal. In Fig. 3 is shown an example of a cell firing in bursts at the tremor frequency of 4.8/sec in A during tremor movements at the same frequency. In B the same muscles became involved in shivering movements with arrest of the 4.8/sec tremor and the same unit ceased firing in bursts, and did not follow the 13/sec shivering movements. In C there was a combination of shivering and Parkinson-like tremor and this unit began again to fire in bursts with the latter tremor, but not with the shivering movements of the same muscles.

In Fig. 4 (A and B) is shown a typical small spike firing in rapid bursts at 13/sec

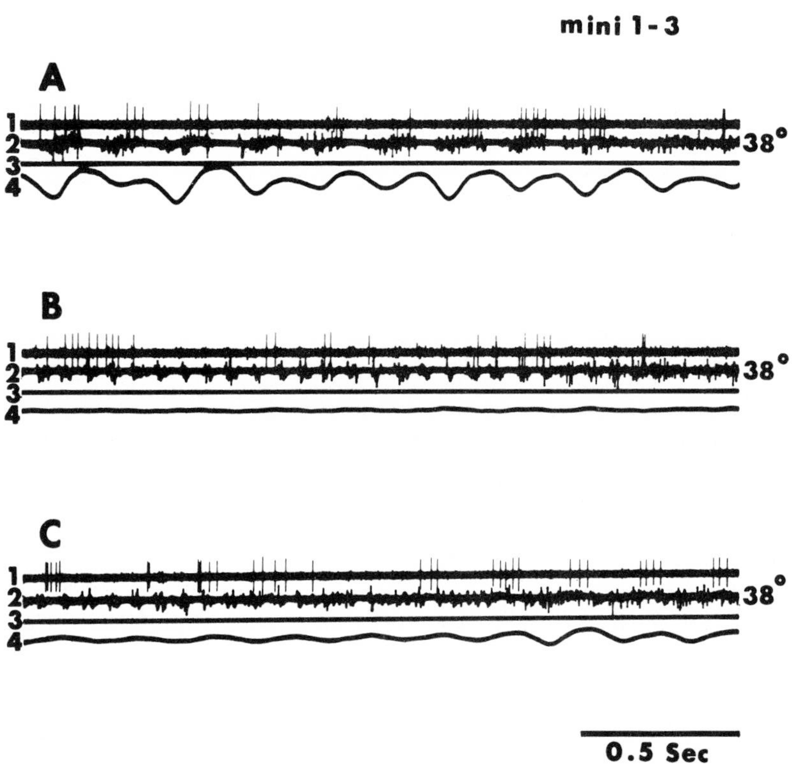

FIG. 3. Thalamic unit firing in bursts in relation with the Parkinson-like tremor in the contralateral arm (A) but not with the faster 13/sec tremor recorded in the same muscle (B). Records C show the behaviour of the same unit during consecutive episodes of fast tremor (first half of the record) and slow, Parkinson-like tremor (second half of the record). The unit fires only in relation with the slow 4/sec tremor. The cortical temperature was normal during all these recordings. (Lines 1 to 4; same identification as for Fig. 1.).

during tremorous shivering movements at the same frequency, with continuous tonic discharge during sustained spasms of the same muscles (Fig. 4A). This cell did not follow the Parkinson-like tremor in these same muscles. In Fig. 4 C and D is shown another cell which fired infrequently without relation to Parkinson-like tremor (C) but which began to fire in burst at the frequency of shivering movements when they appeared (D). In other examples it was found possible to record from the same microelectrode position and at the same time, cells firing in bursts at 13/sec and others firing in bursts at about 4/sec. The cells firing at 13/sec burst frequency continued to fire at this frequency during cooling of the motor cortex sufficient to arrest 4/sec tremor movements, but

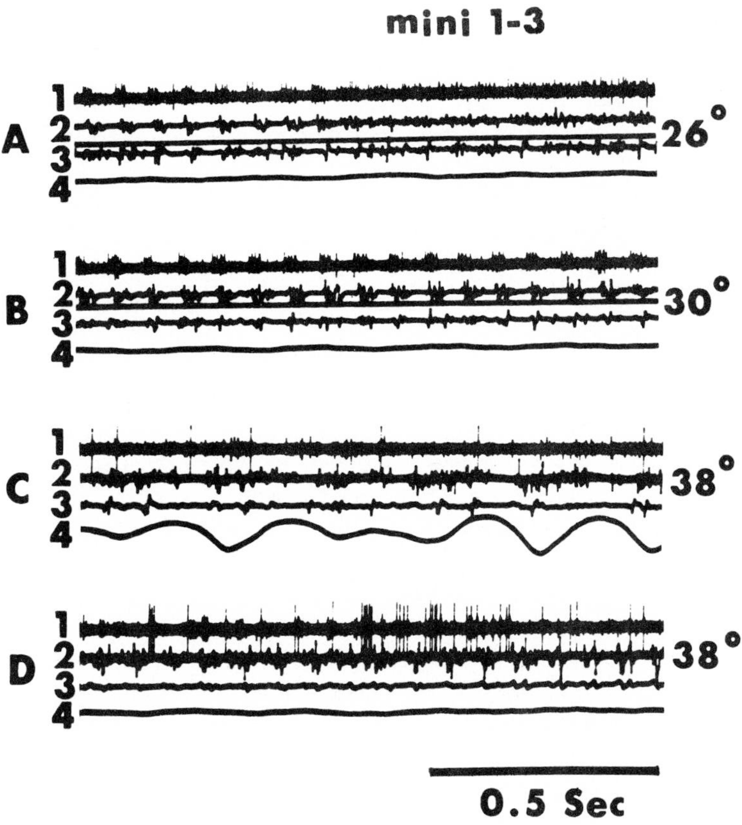

FIG. 4. Thalamic units firing in bursts at the frequency of the 13/sec tremor in the contralateral arm. Lines 2 and 3 are the biceps and triceps EMG and line 4, the strain-gauge transducer record of the arm movements. The cortical temperature is indicated by a line which overlies the biceps EMG records (line 2) when the temperature is 38° C (C and D). The cell in A and B is firing in relation with the fast tremor movements and also during episodes of spasm (second half of record A). Records C and D show another unit which fires infrequently during Parkinson-like tremor (C) but which engages into rhythmic bursting synchronous with the 13/sec tremor (D).

which had no effect or even enhanced the shivering movements with 13/sec tremor.

This showed that thalamic units participating in shivering movements consisted of, at least in part, a different population of neurones than those involved in Parkinson-like tremor and were differently affected by cooling of the motor cortex. Likewise the tremor movements were differently affected; the shivering movements persisting at surface cortical temperatures well below those required to arrest both the Parkinson-like tremor and voluntary finger movements of the hand.

DISCUSSION

These experiments demonstrate clearly, once again, that the motor cortex plays an important and essential role in neuronal mechanisms involved in Parkinson-like tremor movements. Furthermore they suggest that the nature of this role may not be simply that the cortico-spinal pyramidal tract is the efferent pathway necessary for the conduction of tremorogenic volleys of impulses of subcortical origin as has been sometimes assumed in the past. The fact that, with graded cooling, tremor is rapidly arrested at temperatures which do not interfere with finely coordinated voluntary finger movements proves that the two functions of the same motor cortex may be dissociated.

This suggests that it may be the cortico-fugal extrapyramidal projections of the motor cortex to thalamus, striatum, or to other subcortical structures rather than direct pyramidal projections which are most important in the mechanisms whereby the motor cortex exerts such an important control over tremor movements.

Direct recording from the pyramidal tract and the effect of its interruption has not been carried out as yet in these experiments. Such studies will be necessary before concluding that the pyramidal tract may not also be involved in the modulation or mediation of Parkinson-like tremor movements.

Interpretation of results from microelectrode studies of thalamic cells which fire in bursts at the tremor frequency is not certain at this preliminary stage of our experiments. The fact that certain cells which do not respond to passive movements are found to be firing in bursts at the tremor frequency would suggest that they are not being controlled by simple afferent feed-back from the tremor movements. Why then was their burst frequency slower and less regular when the tremor was arrested by cortical cooling? It is possible that cortico-fugal fibers terminating directly in the thalamus, or via the striatum, may be involved. If so, a thalamo-cortico-thalamic reverberating circuit may be of importance in the genesis of Parkinson-like tremor.

Interpretation of the fact that other cells continue to fire in bursts at the tremor frequency even after the tremor in a given limb is arrested by cortical cooling, and tremor in other muscles was not visible, may mean simply that these units were not related to the area of cortex being subjected to cooling, and that tremor movements in other muscles may have escaped our notice. It does seem quite clear from the present experiments that motor cortical functions necessary for the preservation of finely coordinated movements of the fingers are distinct from those responsible for Parkinson-like tremor movements and it is likely that the more direct corticospinal (pyramidal) pathways are those in the control of fine finger movements.

The fact that shivering movements were induced or triggered reflexly by cortical cooling in an animal predisposed by harmaline, and that thalamic cells firing in bursts at the frequency of the trembling of shivering (13/sec) were not the same as those taking part in the Parkinson-like tremor at 4/sec shows that the two forms of tremor have a different neuronal mechanism, at least in part, and that shivering movements are not dependent upon intact cortical function as is the Parkinson-like tremor.

These results are consistent with the findings of Battista et al. (2) who were able to show that lesions of the n. Ventralis Lateralis of the thalamus, and in Globus Pallidus in the monkey served to arrest the Parkinson-like tremor in animals with tegmental lesions, but failed to affect the more rapid tremor induced by harmaline alone. The harmaline tremor has been shown to depend primarily on structures lower in the brain stem and cerebellum, and it can be induced in cats or in monkeys after decerebration at the intercollicular level (10, 13).

The fact that many VL thalamic cells continued to fire in bursts at or near the tremor frequency even following the arrest of tremor movements by neuromuscular blocking agents (gallamine triethiodide) has previously shown their lack of dependence upon sensory feedback from tremor movements. Parkinson-like tremor in these animals has been shown to continue, relatively unaltered, or even to increase in amplitude and regularity following complete deafferentation by dorsal root section (8, 14). Arrest of tremor by cortical cooling has been shown to have a marked effect on the firing pattern of nearly all cells of thalamic VL even though they were firing in bursts well timed with tremor movements prior to cooling of the motor cortex with its associated arrest of tremor movements. This is clearly different from the effect of tremor arrest by neuromuscular blocking agents. The change in the pattern of VL unit firing with arrest of tremor by cortical cooling is not due, therefore, to the absence of sensory feedback from the tremor movements, but implies a more active participation of the motor cortex in direct or indirect cortico-thalamo-cortical pathways which seem apparently necessary for the development of the Parkinson-like tremor in these experimental animals, and probably also in man.

It has been demonstrated by many previous studies of thalamic unit discharge recorded during stereotaxic surgery of Parkinson patients (1, 6) that there are cells in VL which fire in bursts at the tremor frequency even in the absence of tremor movements. This is consistent with the observation in experimental animals showing that in these cells the tremor movements cannot be the origin of the rhythmic bursting of thalamic cells at this frequency. The fact that the firing pattern of these cells is altered when tremor is arrested by cortical cooling implies a more direct participation of the motor cortex in tremorogenesis and in the control of VL unit discharge independent of the tremor movements themselves. The fact that tremor can be arrested by thalamic lesions involving these cells (and others in their vicinity) as well as by lesions or cooling of motor cortex implies that thalamo-cortical interrelationships are of major importance in neuronal mechanisms essential to Parkinsonian tremor in man as well as in experimental animals.

SUMMARY

Local cooling of the surface of the motor cortex to 16-18° C produced rapid arrest of the experimental Parkinson-like tremor at 4-5/sec in animals with local tegmental lesions without paralysis of fine finger movements which were lost only at lower temperatures. Microelectrode recording of the firing patterns of single cells in the ventral thalamus show cells firing in burst at the tremor frequency which did not respond to passive movements. Nevertheless, these "non-sensory" cells changed their pattern to much slower irregular bursts during arrest of tremor by cortical cooling. It is concluded that the motor cortex plays an important role in Parkinson-like tremor mechanisms independent of its mediation of voluntary fine finger movements, possibly due to extrapyramidal cortico-fugal projections or a thalamo-cortico-thalamic reverberating circuit including perhaps the striatum.

REFERENCES

1 ALBE-FESSARD, D., GUIOT, G., LAMARRE, Y. and ARFEL, G. Activation of thalamocortical projections related to tremorogenic processes. In D.P. Purpura and M.D. Yahr (Eds.), The Thalamus, Columbia University Press, New York, 1966, pp. 237-253.

2 BATTISTA, A.F., NAKATANI, S., GOLDSTEIN, M. and ANAGNOSTE, B. Effect of harmaline in monkeys with central nervous system lesions. Exp. Neurol., 28 (1970) 513-524.

3 BUCY, P.C. The corticospinal tract and tremor. In W.S. Fields (Ed.), Pathogenesis and Treatment of Parkinsonism, Charles C. Thomas, Springfield, Ill., 1958, pp. 271-293.

4 CORDEAU, J.P., GYBELS, J., JASPER, H. and POIRIER, L.J. Microelectrode studies of unit discharges in the sensorimotor cortex. Investigations in monkeys with experimental tremor, Neurology, 10 (1960) 591-600.

5 JASPER, H.H. and BERTRAND, G. Thalamic units involved in somatic sensation and voluntary and involuntary movements in man. In D.P. Purpura and M.D. Yahr (Eds.), The Thalamus, Columbia University Press, New York, 1966, pp. 365-390.

6 JASPER, H.H. and BERTRAND, G. Recording from microelectrode in stereotaxic surgery for Parkinson's disease, J. Neurosurg., 24 (1966) 219-221.

7 JASPER, H.H., SHACTER, D.G. and MONTPLAISIR, J. The effect of local cooling upon spontaneous and evoked electrical activity of cerebral cortex, Can. J. Physiol. Pharmacol., 48 (1970) 640-652.

8 JOFFROY, A.J. and LAMARRE, Y. Rhythmic unit firing in the precentral cortex in relation with postural tremor in a deafferented limb, Brain Research, 27 (1971) 386-389.

9 LAMARRE, Y. and CORDEAU, J.P. Étude du mécanisme physiopathologique responsable, chez le singe, d'un tremblement experimental de type Parkinsonien, Actualites Neurophysiologiques, 7 (1967) 141-166.

10 LAMARRE, Y., De MONTIGNY, C., DUMONT, M. and WEISS, M. Harmaline-induced rhythmic activity of cerebellar and lower brain stem neurons. Brain Research, 32 (1971) 246-250.

11 LAMARRE, Y. and JOFFROY, A.J. Thalamic unit activity in monkey with experimental tremor. In A. Barbeau and F.J. McDowell (Eds.), L-Dopa and Parkinsonism, F.A. Davis Co., Philadelphia, 1970, pp. 163-170.

12 LAMARRE, Y., JOFFROY, A.J., FILION, M. and BOUCHOUX, R. A stereotaxic method for repeated sessions of central unit recording in the paralyzed or moving animal, Rev. Can. Biol., 29 (1970) 371-376.

13 LAMARRE, Y. and MERCIER, L-A. Neurophysiological studies of harmaline-induced tremor in the cat. Can. J. Physiol. Pharmacol., 49 (1971) 1049-1058.

14 OHYE, C., BOUCHARD, R., LAROCHELLE, L., BEDARD, P., BOUCHER, R., RAPHY, B. and POIRIER, L.J. Effect of dorsal rhizotomy on postural tremor in the monkey, Exp. Brain Res. 10 (1970) 140-150.

15 POIRIER, L.J., LAMARRE, Y. and CORDEAU, J.P. Neuroanatomical study of an experimental postural tremor in monkeys. Second Symposium of Parkinson's Disease, J. Neurosurg., (Suppl.) 24 (1966) 191-193.

16 POIRIER, L.J., SOURKES, T.L., BOUVIER, G., BOUCHER, R. and CARABIN, S. Striatal amines, experimental tremor and the effect of harmaline in the monkey, Brain 89 (1966) 37-52.

17 WARD, A.A. Jr., McCULLOCH, W.S. and MAGOUN, H.W. Production of an alternating tremor at rest in monkeys. J. Neurophysiol., 11 (1948) 317.

Corticothalamic Projections and Sensorimotor Activities
T. Frigyesi, E. Rinvik, and M.D. Yahr, editors. © 1972
Raven Press, New York.

Projection of the Visual Cortex to the Lateral Geniculate Nucleus in the Cat

Horstmar Holländer

Extensive anatomical and physiological studies of the cat's visual system have revealed that there is a strong projection from the retinae to the lateral geniculate nucleus (LGN) (5, 7, 13, 18, 19, 21, 28, 30, 37, 40) and from the lateral geniculate nucleus to the visual cortex (8, 12, 14, 22, 23, 29, 30, 33, 43, 46). Both projections, which together form the afferent visual pathway to the cortex, are strictly retinotopically organized. The cortex, in turn, sends fibres back to the LGN (3, 10, 11, 16, 20, 27, 32, 35). This corticogeniculate fibre system provides the anatomical basis for transmission of corticofugal influences to the lateral geniculate nucleus (1, 2, 24, 26, 38, 41, 44, 45). There is general agreement on the existence of a corticogeniculate projection. Most likely the corticogeniculate fibres are identical with the type I axons in Golgi preparations (15, 16). Electron microscopic degeneration studies have shown that terminals of Guillery's RSD type (17) undergo degeneration after cortical lesions (25). Details of the organization of the corticogeniculate pathway, especially concerning its site of origin, are still a matter of controversy.

First, a short description of the geniculo fibre system will be given to provide a better understanding of the organization of the corticofugal system.

GENICULOCORTICAL PROJECTION

This projection has recently been studied by Garey and Powell (12), Wilson and Cragg (46), and Niimi and Sprague (33). The main route of the geniculocortical projection originates in the layered part of LGN and terminates in the striate area or area 17. The periphery of the visual field is represented near the splenial sulcus and the vertical meridian at the border between area 17 and 18 (4). Besides the projection to area 17, the LGN in the cat projects to area 18 and area 19. Area 18 receives fibres from the layers of LGN and possibly also from the medial interlaminar nucleus (MIN). In this geniculocortical projection to area 18 the vertical meridian again is represented at the 17/18 border; the periphery, however, is represented laterally near the border to area 19. Area 19 receives a projection from MIN

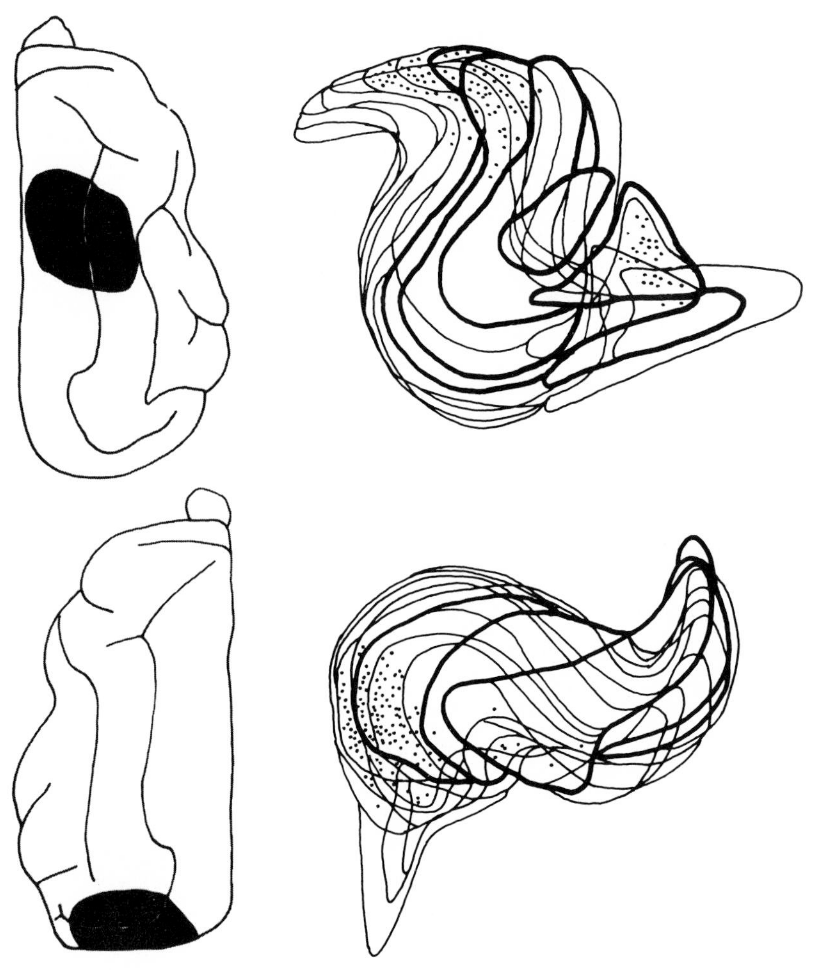

FIG. 1. Two experiments with a large rostral lesion (upper half) and a large caudal lesion (lower half) of the visual cortex. The lesions are represented by the black areas and the terminal degeneration in the degeneration reconstructions are indicated by dotting.

Upper left: Extent of the rostral lesion. x 19

Upper right: Degeneration reconstruction of the LGN (medial aspect) corresponding to the rostral lesion. x 13

Lower left: Extent of the caudal lesion. x 19

Lower right: Degeneration reconstruction of the LGN (lateral aspect) corresponding to the caudal lesion. x 10

and possibly also from the layers. In addition, there is evidence that the layers of LGN also project to the suprasylvian gyrus. All of the geniculocortical projections are organized rostrocaudally in the same manner. The lower visual field is represented rostrally and the upper, caudally in the visual cortex. The ventral nucleus of LGN, which also receives direct retinal fibres, seems not to project to the visual cortex.

CORTICOGENICULATE PROJECTION

Lesions of the visual cortex produce localized fibre degeneration in the LGN. This has been repeatedly demonstrated with the Marchi technique (35) and also with the Nauta technique and its modifications (10, 16, 27, 32). It is not quite clear, however, which of the areas of the visual cortex give rise to the corticogeniculate fibres. Kusama et al. (27) observed degeneration in the LGN only after lesions of area 17. On the other hand Szentagothai (42) mentioned that fibre degeneration in the LGN is produced only by lesions of the peristriate cortex which supports the finding of Widen and Ajmone-Marsan (45) that inhibitory effects in LGN can be most readily produced by stimulating visual II which corresponds to area 18, and not visual I, which corresponds to area 17. Most of the authors, however, obtained results indicating that area 17 as well as area 18 project back to the LGN (3, 10, 11, 16, 32). These discrepancies led us to reinvestigate the corticogeniculate pathway (20).

MATERIALS AND METHODS

Small thermal lesions were made in the visual cortex of cats. In most of the experiments the postoperative survival time was 4 days. The cortex including the lesion was embedded in paraffin and cut in series. The extent of the lesion was determined with respect to the borders between the different cortical architectonic areas (34, 36). The degeneration in the lateral geniculate nucleus was studied with the Nauta-Laidlaw (31) and the Fink-Heimer (22) techniques. Serial drawings of the LGN with the sites of degeneration were plotted with an electronic pantograph (6) at a magnification of 30 on translucent sheets. The sheets were stacked over each other in register between plexiglas plates. The resulting three dimensional degeneration reconstructions were photographed in transmitted light.

RESULTS

1. LARGE LESIONS INCLUDING AREA 17, 18, AND 19.

Two experiments with large cortical lesions are presented in Fig. 1. The location and the extent of the lesions are drawn as black areas in the upper and lower left drawing. The photographs on the right side show the corresponding degeneration reconstructions of the LGN; the outlines of the nucleus in the different sections are drawn as lines. The terminal degeneration is represented by the dots. The experiments show that the rostral visual cortex projects to rostral parts of the LGN and that the caudal visual cortex projects to caudal parts of the LGN. This indicates that the corticogeniculate projection and the geniculocortical projections have the same rostro-caudal organization. The degenerating fibres in the LGN are very thin. The degeneration is densest in layer A, diminishes rapidly in A_1 and C, and in C_1 only occasional fragments of degenerating fibres are found.

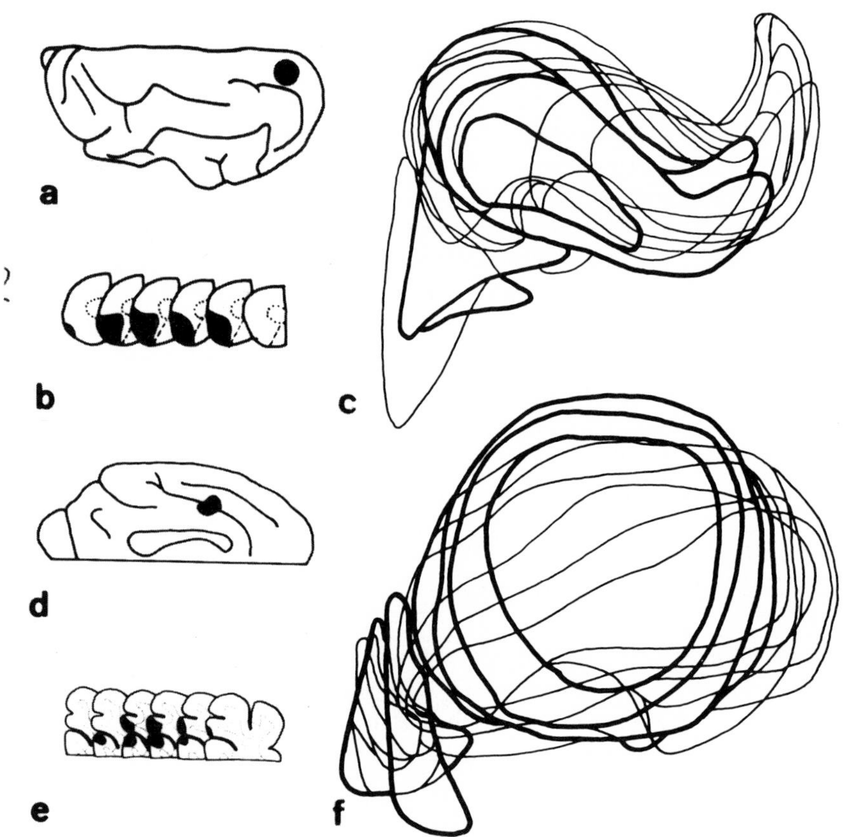

FIG. 2. Two experiments with lesions restricted to area 17. Same symbols as in Fig. 1.

a. Extent of the lesion which is situated at the cortical representation of the central area. x 1.25

b. Histological series through the lesion. The border between area 17 and 18 is indicated by the broken line.

c. Corresponding degeneration reconstruction of the LGN (lateral aspect). x 10

d. Extent of the lesion which is situated at the medial aspect of the hemisphere. x 1.25

e. Histological series through the lesion.

f. Corresponding degeneration reconstruction of the LGN (rostral aspect). x 13

2. LESIONS RESTRICTED TO AREA 17.

Figure 2 shows two examples of area 17 lesions. In Figure 2b and e, serial sections through the lesions are shown to demonstrate the position of the lesion with respect to the areas 17/18, their borders and their depths. In both cases the lesions are restricted to area 17 and do not involve the white matter. In the first experiment, the lesion is situated in the region of the central area representation, and the second,

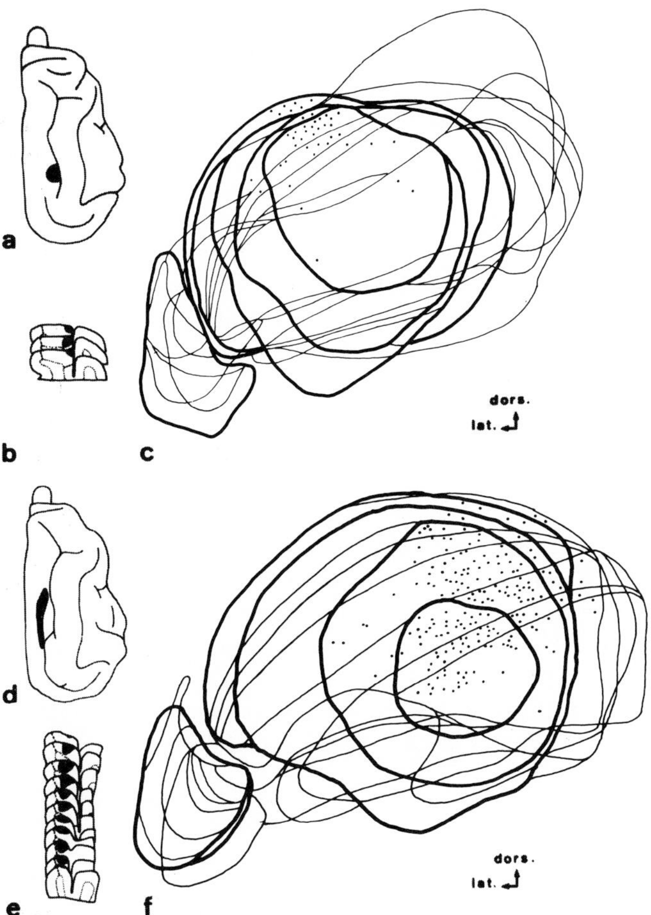

FIG. 3. Two experiments with lesions restricted to area 18. Same symbols as in Fig. 1.

a. Extent of the lesion which is situated in the lateral area 18. x 0.9
b. Histological series through the lesion. The broken lines indicate the 17/18 and the 18/19 border.
c. Corresponding degeneration reconstruction of the LGN (rostral aspect). x 12
d. Extent of the lesion which is situated in the medial area 18. x 0.9
e. Histological series through the lesion.
f. Corresponding degeneration reconstruction of the LGN (rostral aspect). x 12

at the medial surface of the hemisphere. The degeneration reconstruction shows that there was no terminal degeneration in the dorsal or ventral LGN. These negative results were observed in 5 additional cases with area 17 lesions. In all of these cases, however, there were distinct degenerations in the lateral posterior nucleus of the thalamus indicating that the lack of degeneration in LGN is not due to a technical deficiency. In one case, the lesion was placed in the most caudal part of area 17 and degeneration was observed in the caudal part of LGN. In this case an involvement of area 18 was doubtful.

3. LESIONS RESTRICTED TO AREA 18.

Lesions restricted to area 18 produce distinct degeneration in the LGN. Figure 3 shows two examples of area 18 lesions. The first is a small lateral lesion near area 19. The second has a lesion which is much larger and is situated near the border of area 17. The degeneration reconstructions show clear degeneration in both cases. The degeneration is restricted to the layered part of LGN. The extent of the degeneration corresponds clearly to the size of the lesion and its location. The lesion in the second case extends further rostrally and is situated more medially than the lesion in the first case. Correspondingly, the degeneration extends further rostrally in the second case and is situated more medially than the degeneration in the first case. That indicates that the mediolateral organization of the projection from area 18 is the same as in the afferent fiber system which projects to area 18.

4. LESIONS OF AREA 19 AND THE SUPRASYLVIAN GYRUS.

It has not been possible to produce lesions restricted to area 19 because of the hidden location of that area. In all our lesions which included parts of area 19, however, degeneration was observed in the medial interlaminar nucleus, which indicated that this part of LGN also receives cortical fibres from the same area to which it projects.

Lesions of the suprasylvian gyrus produce degeneration in the ventral nucleus of LGN and weak, diffuse degeneration in the dorsal part.

DISCUSSION

Our finding that lesions restricted to area 17 do not produce terminal degeneration in the LGN is supported by a recent study in the squirrel monkey by Spatz, Tigges and Tigges (39). These authors report that in their material there was no evidence of a projection from area 17 to the LGN. However, the results of Garey et al. (11) and Niimi et al. (32) who found degeneration in the LGN after lesions in area 17 require an explanation.

One critical factor was the depth of the lesion. Fibres coming from the medial part of area 18 traverse the white matter immediately underlying lateral parts of area 17. Thus lesions which are situated in this region of area 17 and include little of the white matter produce degeneration in the LGN by destruction of fibres coming from area 18 (20). In the squirrel monkey lesions in area 17 including the underlying white matter produce degeneration in the LGN, although it is difficult to determine how such lesions would damage fibers arising in area 18. A second factor which might explain the different findings after area 17 lesions is the survival time. LGN undergoes rapid and severe retrograde degeneration after lesions of the visual cortex (30). Lesions of area 17 may produce Nauta degeneration in the LGN after 7 days survival. However, in these cases, the degeneration is in the typical wedge shaped area of retrograde nerve cell degeneration. It is difficult to prove beyond doubt that the Nauta degeneration in these cases is orthograde in nature and independent of the process of retrograde degeneration (for a discussion of the problem see Guillery (16) and Garey (11). We have chosen short survival times in our material to avoid severe retrograde degeneration in LGN. Therefore our experiments do not exclude a projection from area 17 which requires a longer survival time to degenerate than the projection from area 18 does. A possible way of solving the problem would be to inject a small amount of a labelled amino acid into area 17. If the projection to the LGN exists it should be possible to trace the corticofugal fibres autoradiographically without producing retrograde degeneration in the LGN.

The finding that all cases in which area 19 is included in the lesion show degeneration in MIN is in agreement with the results of Garey et al. (11) who made the same observation.

SUMMARY

There is a distinct projection from area 18 to the layered part of the LGN organized in the same manner as the geniculocortical projection to area 18. This fibre system degenerates already 4 days after the cortical lesion and seems to represent the main corticogeniculate route in the cat. Lesions confined to area 17 did not produce degeneration in the LGN after 4 days' survival. A projection from the most caudal part of area 17, however, could not be excluded.

Area 19 projects most likely to the MIN and possibly also to the ventral nucleus. The suprasylvian gyrus projects to the ventral nucleus and also weakly to the dorsal part of LGN.

ACKNOWLEDGMENTS

The encouraging discussions and helpful criticism of Professor R. W. Guillery are gratefully acknowledged. Thanks are due also to Mrs. E. Langer and Miss Bonnie Wallace for assistance in the preparation of the manuscript.

REFERENCES

1 AJMONE MARSAN, C., and MORRILLO, A. Cortical control and callosal mechanisms in the visual system of cat, E.E.G. clin. Neurophysiol., 13 (1961) 553-563.

2 ANGEL, A., MAGNI, F., and STRATA, P. The excitability of optic nerve terminals in the lateral geniculate nucleus after stimulation of visual cortex, Arch. Ital. Biol., 105 (1967) 104-117.

3 BERESFORD, W.A. Fibre degeneration following lesions of the visual cortex of the cat. In R. Jung and H. Kornhuber (Eds.), Neurophysiologie und Psychophysik des visuellen Systems, Springer, Berlin-Göttingen-Heidelberg, 1961, p. 247-255.

4 BILGE, M., BINGLE, A., SENEVIRATNE, K.N., and WHITTERIDGE, D.W. A map of the visual cortex in the cat, J. Physiol., (Lond.) 191 (1967) 116.

5 BISHOP, P.O., KOZAK, W., LEVICK, W.R. and VAKKUR, G.J. The determination of the projection of the visual field on to the lateral geniculate nucleus in the cat, J. Physiol. (Lond.), 163 (1962) 503-539.

6 BOIVIE, J., GRANT, G., and ULFENDAHL, H. The X-Y recorder used for mapping under the microscope, Acta Physiol. Scand., 74 (1968) 1A-2A.

7 COHN, R. Laminar electrical responses in the lateral geniculate body of cats, J. Neurophysiol., 19 (1956) 317-324.

8 DOTY, R.W. Potentials evoked in cat cerebral cortex by diffuse and by punctiform photic stimuli, J. Neurophysiol., 21 (1958) 437-464.

9 FINK, R.P., and HEIMER, L. Two methods for selective silver impregnation of degenerating axons and their synaptic endings in the central nervous system, Brain Res., 4 (1967) 369-374.

10 GAREY, L.J. Interrelationships of the visual cortex and superior colliculus in the cat, Nature 207 (1965) 1410-1411.

11 GAREY, L.J., JONES, E.G., and POWELL, T.P.S. Interrelationships of striate and extrastriate cortex with the primary relay sites of the visual pathway, J. Neurol. Neurosurg. Psychiat., 31 (1968) 135-157.

12 GAREY, L.J., and POWELL, T.P.S. The projection of the lateral geniculate nucleus upon the cortex in the cat, Proc. Roy. Soc. B., 169 (1967) 107-126.

13 GAREY, L.J.,and POWELL, T.P.S. The projection of the retina in the cat, J. Anat. (Lond.) 102 (1968) 189-222.

14 GLICKSTEIN, M., KING, R.A., MILLER, J., and BERKELEY, M. Cortical projections from the dorsal lateral geniculate nucleus of cats, J. Comp. Neurol., 130 (1967) 55-76.

15 GUILLERY, R.W. A study of golgi preparations from the dorsal lateral geniculate nucleus of the adult cat, J. Comp. Neurol., 128 (1966) 21-50.

16 GUILLERY, R.W. Patterns of fibre degeneration in the dorsal lateral geniculate nucleus of the cat following lesions in the visual cortex, J. Comp. Neurol., 130 (1967) 197-222.

17 GUILLERY, R.W. The organization of synaptic interconnections in the laminae of the dorsal lateral geniculate nucleus of the cat, Z. Zellforsch. Mikroskop. Anat., 96 (1969) 1-38.

18 GUILLERY, R.W. The laminar distribution of retinal fibers in the dorsal lateral geniculate nucleus of the cat: A new interpretation, J. Comp. Neurol., 138 (1970) 339-368.

19 HAYHOW, W.R The cytoarchitecture of the lateral geniculate body in the cat in relation to the distribution of crossed and uncrossed optic fibres, J. Comp. Neurol., 110 (1958) 1-64.

20 HOLLÄNDER, H. The projection from the visual cortex to the lateral genicu-

late body (LGB) in experimental study with silver impregnation methods in the cat, Exp. Brain. Res., 10 (1970) 219-235.
21 HUBEL, D.H., and WIESEL, T.N. Integrative action in the cat's lateral geniculate body, J. Physiol. (Lond.), 155 (1961) 385-398.
22 HUBEL, D.H., and WIESEL, T.N. Receptive fields, binocular interaction and functional architecture in the cat's visual cortex, J. Physiol., 160 (1962) 106-154.
23 HUBEL, D.H., and WIESEL, T.N. Receptive fields and functional architecture of two non-striate visual areas (18 and 19) of the cat, J. Neurophysiol., 28 (1965) 229-289.
24 IWAMA, K., SAKAKURA, H., and KASAMATSU, T. Presynaptic inhibition in the lateral geniculate body induced by stimulation of the cerebral cortex, Jap. J. Physiol., 15 (1965) 310-322.
25 JONES, E.G., and POWELL, T.P.S. An electron microscopic study of the mode of termination of cortico-thalamic fibres within the sensory relay nuclei of the thalamus, Proc. Roy. Soc., B. 172 (1969) 173-185.
26 KALIL, R.E., and CHASE, R. Corticofugal influence on activity of lateral geniculate neurons in the cat, J. Neurophysiol., 33 (1970) 459-474.
27 KUSAMA, T., OTANI, K., and KAWANA, E. Projections of the motor, somatic sensory, auditory and visual cortices in cats. In: Progress in Brain Research, M. Singer and J.P. Schade (Eds.), Volume 21A, Elsevier, Amsterdam, 1966, p. 292-322.
28 LATIES, A.M., and SPRAGUE, J.M. The projection of optic fibers to the visual centers in the cat, J. Comp. Neurol., 127 (1966) 35-70.
29 MARSHALL, W.H., TALBOT, S.A., and ADES, H.W. Cortical responses to gross photic and electrical afferent stimulation, J. Neurophysiol., 6 (1943) 1-15.
30 MINKOWSKI, M. Über den Verlauf, die Endigung und die zentrale Reprasentation von gekreuzten und ungekreuzten Sehnervenfasern bei einigen Saugetieren und beim Menschen, Schweiz. Arch. Neurol. Psychiat., 6 (1920) 201-252.
31 NAUTA, W.J.H. Silver impregnation of degenerating axons. In: New Research Techniques of Neuroanatomy, W.F. Windle (Ed.) Charles C. Thomas, Springfield, 1957, p. 17-26.
32 NIIMI, K., KAWAMURA, S., and ISHIMARU, S. Anatomical organization of corticogeniculate projections in the cat, Proc. Japan Acad., 46 (1970) 878-883.
33 NIIMI, K., and SPRAGUE, J.M. Thalamo-cortical organization of the visual system in the cat. J. Comp. Neurol., 138 (1970) 219-250.
34 OTSUKA, R., and HASSLER, R. Über Aufbau und Gliederung der corticalen Sehophare bei der Katzer, Arch. Psychiat. Neurol., 203 (1962) 213-234.
35 PROBST, M. Über den Verlauf der centralen Sehfasern (Rinden-Sehhugelfasern) und deren Endigung im Zwischen und Mittelhirne und über die Associations— und Commissurenfasern der Sehsphare, Arch. Psychiat., 35 (1902) 22-43.
36 SANIDES, F., and HOFFMANN, J. Cyto- and mycloarchitecture of the visual cortex of the cat and of the surrounding integration cortices, J. Hirnforsch.,

11 (1969) 79-104.
37 SANDERSON, K.J. The projection of the visual field to the lateral geniculate and medial interlaminar nuclei in the cat, J. Comp. Neurol., 143 (1971) 101-118.
38 SINGER, W., and CREUTZFELDT, O.D. Reciprocal lateral inhibition of on- and off-center neurones in the lateral geniculate body of the cat, Exp. Brain Res., 10 (1970) 311-330.
39 SPATZ, W.B., TIGGES, J., and TIGGES, M. Subcortical projections, cortical associations, and some intrinsic interlaminar connections of the striate cortex in the squirrel monkey (Saimiri), J. Comp. Neurol., 140 (1970) 155-174.
40 STONE, J., and HANSEN, S.M. The projection of the cat's retina on the lateral geniculate nucleus, J. Comp. Neurol., 126 (1966) 601-624.
41 SUZUKI, H., and KATO, E. Cortically induced presynaptic inhibition in cat's lateral geniculate body, Tohoku J. Exptl. Med., 86 (1965) 277-289.
42 SZENTAGOTHAI, J. The structure of the synapse in the lateral geniculate body, Acta Anat., 55 (1963) 166-185.
43 VASTOLA, E.F. A direct pathway from lateral geniculate body to association cortex, J. Neurophysiol., 24 (1961) 469-487.
44 VASTOLA, E.F. Steady-state effects of visual cortex on geniculate cells, Vision Res., 7 (1966) 599-601.
45 WIDEN, L., and AJMONE MARSAN, C. Effects of corticipetal and corticifugal impulses upon single elements of the dorsolateral geniculate nucleus, Exptl. Neurol., 2 (1960) 468-502.
46 WILSON, M.E, and CRAGG, B.G. Projections from the lateral geniculate nucleus in the cat and monkey, J. Anat., 101 (1967) 677-692.

Corticothalamic Projections and Sensorimotor Activities
T. Frigyesi, E. Rinvik, and M.D. Yahr, editors. © 1972
Raven Press, New York.

Comments on the Visual Pathways

Charles R. Noback

COMMENTS ON THE VISUAL PATHWAYS

These critical morphological studies that we have just heard are an emphatic reminder that, to establish the presence or absence of direct reciprocal connections between a thalamic nucleus and the cerebral cortex with silver or electron microscopic techniques to identify degenerating fibers, special attention must be directed to distinguish anterograde from retrograde axonal degeneration. The observations of Dr. Holländer suggest three related topics: (1) the diverse types of degeneration expressed by the neurons of the visual pathways and some aspects of the valuable neuroanatomical silver techniques which reveal the products of axonal degeneration; (2) the differences in the connections of the retino-dorsal lateral geniculate body (DLGB)—cerebral cortex pathways among representatives of different orders of mammals, and (3) the relation of these differences to the concepts of parallel evolution and convergent evolution.

Degeneration.

In response to a variety of etiological factors, the neurons of the visual system may degenerate in several ways. These include orthograde(anterograde) degeneration, retrograde degeneration, transneuronal (transsynaptic) degeneration and retrograde transneuronal (transsynaptic) degeneration. The well-known orthograde degeneration and retrograde degeneration in a neuron are the degenerative changes exhibited distal to and proximal to (relative to the cell body) the site of the lesion, respectively. Anterograde transneuronal degeneration refers to the degeneration or degenerative changes of neurons which are postsynaptic to other degenerating neurons. This degeneration is considered to be the consequence of a major deafferentation of the postsynaptic degenerating neurons. For example, following eye enucleation, the neurons of the DLGB exhibit anterograde transneuronal degeneration as a response to the degeneration of the ganglionic neurons of the retina. Retrograde transneuronal degeneration refers to the degeneration or degenerative changes in neurons which are presynaptic to other degenerating neurons. It is probably the consequence of a major deafferentation of the presynaptic neuron that degenerates. For example, following lesions of the visual cortex the ganglion neurons of the retina degenerate as a response to the retrograde degeneration of the presynapticDLGB neurons (neurons projecting to the DLGB and synapsing with DLGB neurons projecting to the cortex) projecting to the cerebral cortex. These types of degeneration are comprehensively discussed by Cowan (3).

Another aspect of degeneration relates to the time course of degenerative changes observed with light microscopy. These vary widely from a few days(orthograde axonal fragmentation may be observed in some neurons at 4 days following the injury) to many months for some atrophic changes in transneuronal degeneration. These variations depend upon the specific neurons involved, age of the animal and the histological methods used to demonstrate the degeneration or atrophy. The degenerative phenomena may include fragmentation of axons or myelin sheaths, chromatolytic changes in the cell body and atrophic changes. These different expressions and rates of neuronal degeneration are both advantageous and disadvantageous for obtaining data depending upon the experimental design of the problem. One disadvantage, as Dr. Holländer's results show, is the problem of determining whether direct reciprocal point-to-point interconnections exist between the DLGB and visual cortex—especially if both anterograde degeneration and retrograde degeneration occur following a cortical lesion. Hence the modern Glees technique, Nauta suppressive technique and its modifications, and Fink-Heimer methods and its modifications must be used with care and adroitly interpreted to obtain meaningful data. These methods are discussed in detail in the book edited by Nauta and Ebbesson (13). Following a lesion in the visual cortex in the cat, Guillery (7) notes evidence of both anterograde and retrograde axonal degeneration by 4 to 5 days in the lateral geniculate body.

Also following a cortical lesion in a cat, Jones and Powell (10) demonstrate that corticothalamic fibers (to the lateral geniculate body, medial geniculate body and ventral posterior nucleus) exhibit intense terminal degeneration by 4 days and degeneration of main axonal processes at 8 to 10 days. In his studies on corticofugal fibers in the rhesus monkey, Dr. Petras informed us that axonal degeneration, as revealed by silver techniques, is not noted until about 18 days. In critical problems, it may be essential to get further evidence to clarify the observations made, comparing the silver degeneration techniques with those obtained from electron microscopy (EM) and autoradiography. Following a lesion, details of synaptic connectivity can be clarified by the observation of degenerating fibers with EM. The use of tritiated proline or leucine may yield decisive evidence; These amino acids, after being incorporated into protein within the cell bodies of neurons, migrate distally within axons by axoplasmatic flow where they can be revealed in the terminals by autoradiographic techniques (18).

Pathway involving the retina, dorsal lateral geniculate body and visual cortex.

Many similarities and differences in the neuroanatomy and neurophysiology of many neural structures have been noted among species of mammals (and among the other classes of vertebrates). Previous speakers in this conference have referred to some differences in certain thalamic nuclei and their connections in the cat, a carnivore, and in the rhesus monkey, a primate. The recognition of these points is imperative in order to establish meaningful correlates.

Although the visual pathway involving the retina, DLGB and visual cortex in the cat and in the rhesus monkey exhibits many similarities, e.g., retinotopic and center-surround organizations, the following comments will stress several differences which have been reported, but not all necessarily firmly established, in the retinogeniculate, geniculocortical, and corticogeniculate projections. (1) The retinogeniculate fibers in (a) the cat, project from the contralateral eye to laminae A and B of the DLGB, from the ipsilateral eye to lamina A, and from both eyes to the intralaminar zone (11, 17); a modification of projections to lamina B is noted by Guillery (8), and in (b) the rhesus monkey, in common with the simians, apes and man, project from the contralateral eye to laminae 1, 4 and 6 of LGB and from the ipsilateral eye to laminae 2, 3 and 5. The retinofugal projections that decussate in the optic chiasma are expressions of a long phylogenetic history as compared to the nondecussating projections passing through the chiasma. All retinofugal fibers are said to decussate in the optic chiasma of living, non-mammalian vertebrates, whereas both decussating and nondecussating retinofugal fibers pass through the chiasma in the living mammals. (2) The geniculocortical fibers in (a) the cat, project to cortical areas 17, 18 and possibly 19 (1, 4, 5, 15) and (b) the rhesus monkey, project to the striate area 17 but not to areas 18 and 19. (3) The corticogeniculate fibers in (a) the cat, project from cortical area 18 and not from area 17 (9 and also the preceding chapter) and in (b) the rhesus monkey are not demonstrable from areas 17, 18 and 19 (2). These latter investigators base their conclusions of the absence of corticogeniculate projections in the rhesus monkey on their interpretation of the nature of the axonal degeneration following cortical lesions. This axonal degeneration within the DLGB revealed by EM and such degeneration silver methods as the Glees, Nauta-Gygax and Fink-Heimer—is stated to be due to retrograde degeneration of geniculate neurons projecting to the cortex.

Until all aspects of the geniculocalcarine and corticocalcarine projections are resolved, definitive statements concerning these connections are not possible. For example, on the basis of degeneration studies in the cat, Niimi, Kawamura and Ishimaru (14) maintain that fibers from area 17 do project in a topical manner to DLGB. They suggest that the inability of Dr. Hollander to observe this degeneration may be due to the short survival time of his animals.

Other differences in the visual pathways from those noted in the cat and rhesus monkey are found in such mammals as the tree shrew *Tupaia* (classified either as an insectivore or primate) and such prosimians as *Galago*, *Nycticebus* and *Tarsius* (6, 16)(reviewed by Giolli and Tigges, 1970, and Noback and Laemle, 1970).

Parallel evolution and convergent evolution.

The differences in the organization of the visual pathways between the cat—as a representative of the carnivores, and the rhesus monkey—as a representative of the primates (exclusive of the prosimians) are probably independently derived; they are probably expressions of an independent parallel evolution for a period of over 60 million years following the origin of these two orders of mammals in the late cretaceous era (12). The same principle applies to the evolutionary history of the differences observed in these pathways in other groups of mammals. As a corollary, the organization of the visual pathways in the cat is not primitive or ancestral to the organization of this pathway in the rhesus monkey.

On the other hand, the similarities in the organization of the pathways in two species in different orders may be expressions of features with a long phylogenetic history from common ancestors. Alternatively, they may be independently derived patterns, which would indicate convergent evolution.

REFERENCES

1 BURROWS, G.R., and HAYHOW, W.R. The organization of the thalamo-cortical visual pathways in the cat. Brain, Behavior and Evolution, 4 (1971) 220-270.

2 CAMPOS-ORTEGA, J.A., HAYHOW, W.R. and CLUVER, P.F. The descending projections from the cortical visual fields of Macaca mulatta with particular reference to the question of a cortico-lateral geniculate pathway. Brain, Behavior and Evolution 3 (1970) 368-414.

3 COWAN, W.M. Anterograde and retrograde transneuronal degeneration in the central and peripheral nervous system. In: W.J.H. Nauta and S.O.E. Ebbesson, eds., Contemporary Research Methods in Neuroanatomy, Springer Verlag, New York, 1970, pp. 217-251.

4 GAREY, L.J., and POWELL, T.P.S. The projection of the lateral geniculate nucleus upon the cortex in the cat. Proc. Roy. Soc. Lond. Ser. B, 169 (1967) 107-126.

5 GLICKSTEIN, M., KING, R.A., MILLER, J. and BERKLEY, M. Cortical projections from the dorsal lateral geniculate nucleus of cats. J. Comp. Neurol. 130 (1967) 55-76.

6 GIOLLI, R.A., and TIGGES, J. The primary optic pathways and nuclei of primates. In: C.R. Noback and W. Montagna, eds., The Primate Brain. Advances in Primatology, Appleton-Century-Crofts, New York 1 (1970) 29-54.

7 GUILLERY, R.W. Patterns of fiber degeneration in the dorsal lateral geniculate nucleus of the cat following lesions in the visual cortex. J. Comp. Neurol., 130 (1967) 197-222.

8 GUILLERY, R.W. The laminar distribution of retinal fibers in the dorsal lateral geniculate nucleus of the cat: a new interpretation. J. Comp. Neurol., 138 (1970) 339-368.

9 HOLLÄNDER, H. The projection from the visual cortex to the lateral geniculate

body (LGB). An experimental study with silver impregnation methods in the cat. Exptl. Brain Res. 10 (1970) 219-235.

10 JONES, E.G., and POWELL, T.P.S. An electron microscopic study of the mode of termination of cortico-thalamic fibres within the sensory relay nuclei of the thalamus. Proc. Roy. Soc. Lond. Ser. B, 172 (1969) 173-185.

11 LATIES, A.M., and SPRAGUE, J.M. The projection of optic fibers to the visual centers in the cat. J. Comp. Neurol., 127 (1966) 35-70.

12 McKENNA, M.G. The origin and early differentiation of therian mammals. In: J.M. Petras and C.R. Noback, eds., Comparative and Evolutionary Aspects of the Vertebrate Central Nervous System. Annals of the New York Academy of Sciences 167 (1969) 217-240.

13 NAUTA, W.J. H., and EBBESSON, S.O.E. Contemporary Research Methods in Neuroanatomy, Springer Verlag, New York. 1970 386 pp.

14 NIIMI, K., KAWAMURA, S. and ISHIMARU, S. Projections of the visual cortex to the lateral geniculate and posterior thalamic nuclei in the cat. J. Comp. Neurol., 143 (1971) 279-311.

15 NIIMI, K., and SPRAGUE, J.M. Thalamo-cortical organization of the visual system in the cat. J. Comp. Neurol., 138 (1970) 219-250.

16 NOBACK, C.R., and LAEMLE, L.K. Structural and functional aspects of the visual pathways of primates. In: C.R. Noback and W. Montagna, eds., The Primate Brain. Advances in Primatology. Appleton-Century-Crofts, New York, 1 (1970) 55-81.

17 SANDERSON, K.J. The projection of the visual field to the lateral geniculate and medial interlaminar nuclei in the cat. J. Comp. Neurol., 143 (1971) 101-118.

18 COWAN, W.M., GOTTLIEB, D.I., HENDRICKSON, A.E. and PRICE, J.L. The autoradiographic demonstration of axonal connections in the central nervous system. Brain Res. 37 (1972) 21-51.

DISCUSSION

PURPURA:

Dr. Hassler, would you care to comment?

HASSLER:

I can confirm the results of Tigges and Spatz drawn from experiments with a survival time of 4, maximum 5 days. We obtained the same results. The problem is very interesting because, you know perhaps that Broun and Wallenberg connected these recurrent fibers from cortex to thalamic nuclei with the problem of direction of attention. It would, thus, be very interesting that the visual system is an exception in that it does not have these recurrent fibers that do have a role in "mediating attention" to subcortical centers. So my question is: Is it not perhaps that the projections from the lateral geniculate to area 18 and 19 are collateral projections? I believe that most of the cells of the lateral geniculate project first to area 17; the other ones are collateral projections, so, for me, this is not a real problem.

PURPURA:

Dr. Holländer, would you answer that question. I think it is an important one.

HOLLÄNDER:

The projection to area 18 originates in the same part of the lateral geniculate nucleus as the projection to area 17; thus it may represent a collateral projection. However, the projection to area 19 seems to originate in the medial interlaminar nucleus and is therefore independent from the projection to area 17 and 18. Dr. Noback mentioned that the problem whether or not area 17 projects on the lateral geniculate nucleus could be solved by electron microscopy. I do not think that this is possible. Degenerating terminals occurring in the lateral geniculate nucleus after a cortical lesion may belong to axon collaterals of cells which have undergone retrograde degeneration. It is not possible to eliminate this uncertainty by degeneration experiments either by silver impregnation techniques or by electron microscopy. The only way to solve the problem, seems to me, to use autoradiographic techniques.

Corticothalamic Projections and Sensorimotor Activities
T. Frigyesi, E. Rinvik, and M.D. Yahr, editors. © 1972
Raven Press, New York.

Corticotectal Systems in the Cat: Their Structure and Function

Larry A. Palmer, Alan C. Rosenquist and James M. Sprague

The superior colliculus of mammals is not a unitary structure either anatomically or functionally, but is a compound neural center composed of several laminae of cells whose inputs arise from different origins and whose outputs travel to different terminations. The neocortex has an extensive projection to the superior colliculus. Of the two species thoroughly studied, every cortical area so far explored in the cat gives rise to efferent fibers terminating in the colliculi (23, 95); in the macaque only pre- and postcentral gyri are known to lack a corticotectal projection (56). In addition to the extensive and heterogeneous corticotectal system, the superior colliculus receives afferent information from the optic tract, inferior colliculus, spinotectal tract, trigeminal lemniscus, reticular formation and central gray matter (62). The intrinsic collicular neurons are organized in at least seven concentric laminae which are related to both afferent and efferent systems. For example, in the cat the superficial laminae are often called "visual", and receive fibers and terminals of the retinotectal tract and the corticotectal paths from visual areas 17, 18 and 19. By contrast, the lemniscal systems from spinal cord and medulla, and the corticotectal tract from somatic sensorimotor cortices terminate in intermediate and deep laminae. Thus, there is primary laminar matching of modalities from peripheral and cortical origins. Of major importance to this paper is the demonstration that many of the cytoarchitectural and functional divisions of the neocortical mantle project to the colliculus, and these have different patterns of termination in both cat (23, 95) and macaque (55, 56, 67). It is likely that this principle holds for other species as well.

Also of great interest is the recent finding that in tree shrews (59) the superficial ("visual") laminae give rise to an efferent pathway projecting to pretectum, dorsal lateral geniculate nucleus and to the LP-pulvinar, which in turn project to primary visual cortex and to cortex bordering the classical visual areas. This efferent path can be distinguished clearly from those originating in deeper laminae, which form the tectospinal, tectopontine, tectoreticular and interneurons in the path between tectum and oculomotor nuclei, as well as ascending projections terminating in subthalamus, intralaminar and posterior nuclei. This finding leads to two important conclusions: 1) that fibers from cells in the superficial and deep collicular laminae have different sites of termination, and 2) that visual information from the superficial layers reaches primary and association visual cortex. This latter finding suggests that visual corticotectal interactions are in both directions.

These anatomical findings provide the framework for certain functional generalizations which have guided the direction of our experiments: 1) there is extensive cortical modulation of collicular activity, 2) the characteristics of this modulation are determined by the cortical area of origin and the collicular laminae of termination, 3) there is marked interaction in visual information processing between cortical and collicular levels, and 4) many complex visual functions and behaviors depend on this interaction.

Despite the potential significance of these hypotheses our present state of knowledge about the functions of these many and diverse corticotectal systems is rudimentary. The present paper will examine in detail the structure and function of one such system in the cat, which originates in cortical areas 17-18 and terminates in the superficial strata of the superior colliculus.

I. ANATOMY

The anatomical and functional organization of the visual corticotectal pathways cannot be discussed logically without reference to the afferent sensory systems serving vision; we will therefore first summarize the anatomy of these. There is broad agreement that the optic tract of mammals terminates in at least five subcortical sites: 1) dorsal lateral geniculate (LGNd), 2) ventral lateral geniculate (LGNv), 3) pretectum (chiefly nucleus of the optic tract), 4) tectum (S. Coll.) and 5) accessory optic nuclei (24, 57). After much controversy there now appears to be clear evidence of a sixth system, the retinohypothalamic tract, terminating bilaterally in the suprachiasmatic nucleus in the cat and presumably other species (65). There is considerable anatomical evidence of the direct cortical projection of site 1 (LGNd); that site 4 (S. Coll) projects to the cortex via thalamic relays is now clear although some important details are lacking. These two systems form two afferent visual projections, largely, but not entirely, separated anatomically. Site 3 (Pretectum) also appears to project to the visual association cortex via the thalamus but few details are now available; whether it should be considered separate from, or a part of, the tectothalamic cortical system is not yet clear.*

A. Afferent Visual Pathways

The anatomical relationships of these two afferent visual projection systems in the

----

* Solution of this problem is complicated by the fact that many fibers ascending from the colliculus pass through the pretectum. Pretectal lesions apparently result in degeneration in most of the areas to which the colliculus projects (28, 73); in addition, however, degenerating fibers and terminals are present in large numbers in the pulvinar (28).

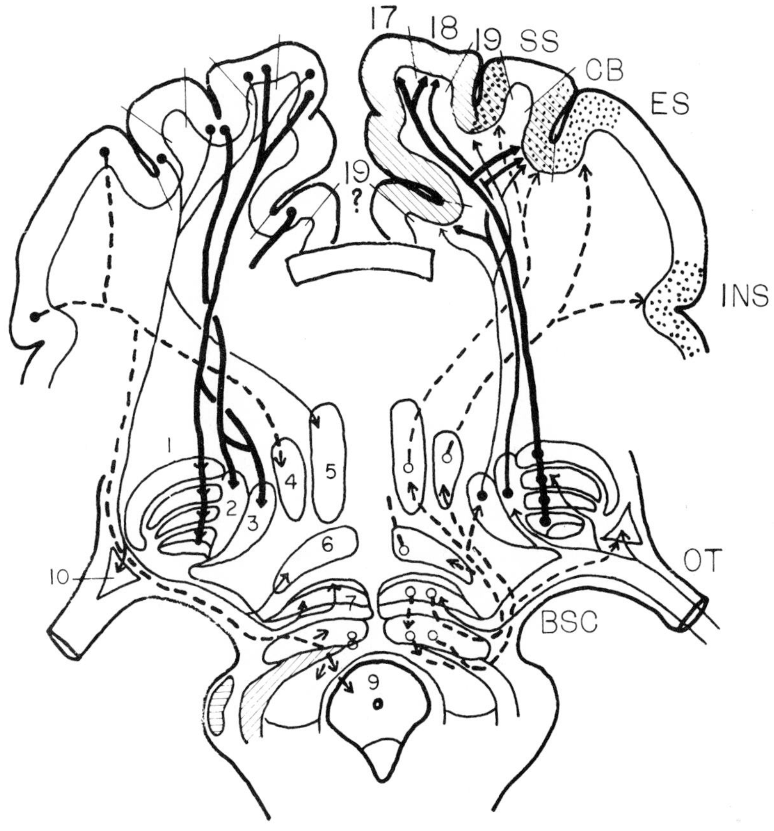

FIG. 1. Schematic drawing to show ascending paths of the tectal visual system (dashed lines) and the geniculate visual system (solid lines) on the right side, and descending paths on the left side. BSC = brachium of superior colliculus, CB = Clare-Bishop cortex, ES = ectosylvian cortex, INS = insular cortex, OT = optic tract. 1 = laminar part of lateral geniculate nucleus (LGNd), 2 = medial interlaminar part of LGNd, 3 = inferior pulvinar or posterior nucleus (NPI), 4 = caudal part of posterior nuclear group including suprageniculate + magnocellular medial geniculate nuclei, 5 = lateral posterior nucleus, 6 = pretectum, 7 = superior laminae of superior colliculus (SC), 8 = deep laminae of SC, 9 = central gray matter, 10 = ventral lateral geniculate, 17, 18, 19 = visual cortical areas.

cat are summarized schematically on the right side of Figure 1.* The ascending paths arising in superior colliculus are shown in dashed lines; these terminate in ventral lateral geniculate, in LGNd (laminae C1 and C2), pretectum (nucleus of optic tract, medial and lateral pretectal nuclei), in the lateral posterior nucleus and adjacent parts of pulvinar, and in the posterior nuclear group (suprageniculate, magnocellular part of medial geniculate and adjacent nuclear mass, Poi,Pol and Pom). Not shown are other tectal terminations in the subthalamus, parafascicular nucleus and intralaminar nuclei; these nuclei will not be considered further and we will limit our discussion to those thalamic termini with known cortical projections. The ascending tectal projection, or part of it, is bilateral, crossing in tectal and posterior commissures, and in the ventral supraoptic commissure (28, 62, 66, 73). The cortical targets of these tectothalamic sites, shown in stipple, are seen to be largely in the banks of the lateral (under 19), suprasylvian (under CB) and pseudosylvian sulci (under INS). The projection from the lateral pulvinar nucleus to the convexity of the suprasylvian gyrus (SS) is not shown (16, 27, 36), but it is probably closely related functionally.

The geniculocortical system is represented in Figure 1 by solid lines, the heaviest line indicating the projection of the laminar part of LGNd (A, A1, C,C1) to cortical areas 17, 18 and Clare-Bishop (CB). The pathway from the medial interlaminar (MIN) part of LGNd to area 18 (and perhaps adjacent parts of 19) and C-B is represented by a somewhat thinner line.** The thinnest line extends from the so-called posterior nucleus (NPI) to cortical areas 19 and C-B. Although N. posterior *** (inferior pulvinar) does not receive direct optic fibers, electrophysiological evidence indicates a retinotopic organization comparable to that of LGNd (54) and to the cortex to which it projects (45).**** Anatomically this thalamic nucleus appears to be a specialized part of the LP-pulvinar group which belongs functionally with the dorsal lat-

----

* Anatomical details of the projection of the retinal ganglion cells to the subcortical optic centers in the cat will be found in Hayhow (34) , Singleton and Peele (92), Laties and Sprague (57), Garey and Powell (24) and Guillery (29). For the ascending projection of the superior colliculus see Altman and Carpenter (1), Niimi, et al. (73), Graybiel (28), and for the cortical projections of the tectal system see Graybiel (27), and Heath and Jones (36). Details of the geniculocortical projection will be found in Glickstein, et al. (26), Wilson and Cragg (113), Garey and Powell (22), Niimi and Sprague (74) and Burrows and Hayhow (10).

** There is some evidence using silver stains (27, 28, 37) and autoradiographic techniques (20) which suggests that degeneration in area C-B after lesions in LGNd is due to severance of fibers of passage in LGNd which originate in the lateral posterior nucleus.

*** This terminology is a misnomer because of the confusion with that of the posterior nuclear group of Rose and Woolsey (85), Poggio and Mountcastle (80), Moore and Goldberg (64), Rinvik (81), Heath and Jones (36, 37). The posterior nucleus is probably part of the pulvinar (84) and is better designated inferior pulvinar nucleus according to Niimi et al. (72).

****The visual afferents to the inferior pulvinar (posterior nucleus) are not completely

eral geniculate complex.

The cortical targets of the geniculate complex are indicated by hatching in Figure 1 and are topographically separated from the collicular cortical targets except for the overlaps in the lateral and suprasylvian sulci.

In a paper of great significance to recent thinking in this field, Diamond and Hall (17) have discussed some hypothetical trends of evolutionary development of the central visual pathways. Their concept is that two visual systems developed in early mammals: A. The retinotectal system was the first to appear phylogenetically, and its cortical projection was mediated by the lateral posterior nucleus of the thalamus; B. The second system established a thalamic relay known as the lateral geniculate. The thalamic component of each system projected to a different but adjacent area of cortex, and in the more primitive living species, such as the hedgehog, these thalamocortical projections overlap extensively and the cortical cytoarchitecture is also rather poorly differentiated. Diamond and Hall visualize a second stage of development, exemplified by the tree shrew in which both thalamic nuclei and cortical targets of these two systems are clearly separated and well differentiated. They also postulated a third stage, seen in monkeys, apes and man in which the thalamic relay nucleus in the tectal system is further differentiated into parts; the older one receives tectal afferents directly and there is a newer, intrinsic part, the cortical projection of which becomes differentiated to form the association cortex.

The organization of visual pathways found in the cat appears to be somewhere between the second and third stage in the scheme of Diamond and Hall.

B. Efferent Visual Pathways

We shall now summarize the anatomical organization of the efferent projections from the cortices of these two components of the visual system, with emphasis on the corticotectal portion, shown on the left side of Figure 1.* Again the solid lines represent the efferent paths from geniculocortical system. Area 17 projects to A, A1 and C of the laminar part of LGNd** to LGNv, to the inferior pulvinar (posterior nucleus (NPI)), to lateral posterior nucleus (LP), to the pretectum (nucleus of the optic tract,

----

known. Because of the electrophysiological characteristics already referred to, Kinston, et al.(54) suggest that it is supplied from LGNd. Fibers from the superior colliculus are known to end in the inferior pulvinar in the cat (27,73), and in the macaque(63).

* Details of corticotectal projections in the cat can be found in Sprague (95), Meikle and Sprague (62), Garey, Jones and Powell (23), and of corticothalamic terminations in Meikle and Sprague (62), Garey, Jones and Powell (23), Diamond, Jones and Powell (18), Niimi, Kawamura and Ishimaru (71), Heath and Jones (35, 37), Jones and Powell (52).

** When reciprocal connections exist between a thalamic nucleus and a specific cortical area, such as LGNd and area 17, difficulty in distinguishing between orthograde and retrograde degeneration following lesions may result (11, 30). Thus, in contrast to others using silver degeneration methods, Hollander (43) believes that area 17 does not project to LGNd in the cat, because no degeneration is found in LGNd after short

NOT), and to the superior colliculus (S. Coll.); area 18 projects to laminar LGNd (chiefly lamina C) and to NIM, with few or no fibers to LGNv. Area 19 also sends fibers to NIM and a few to lamina C1, to LGNv, NPI, NOT, LP and S. Coll. The Clare-Bishop cortex sends no fibers to LGNd, but projects to LGNv, NPI, NOT, LP and S. Coll. Thus those cortices which receive fibers from the geniculate complex project back to these nuclei as well as to subcortical parts of the tectal visual system.

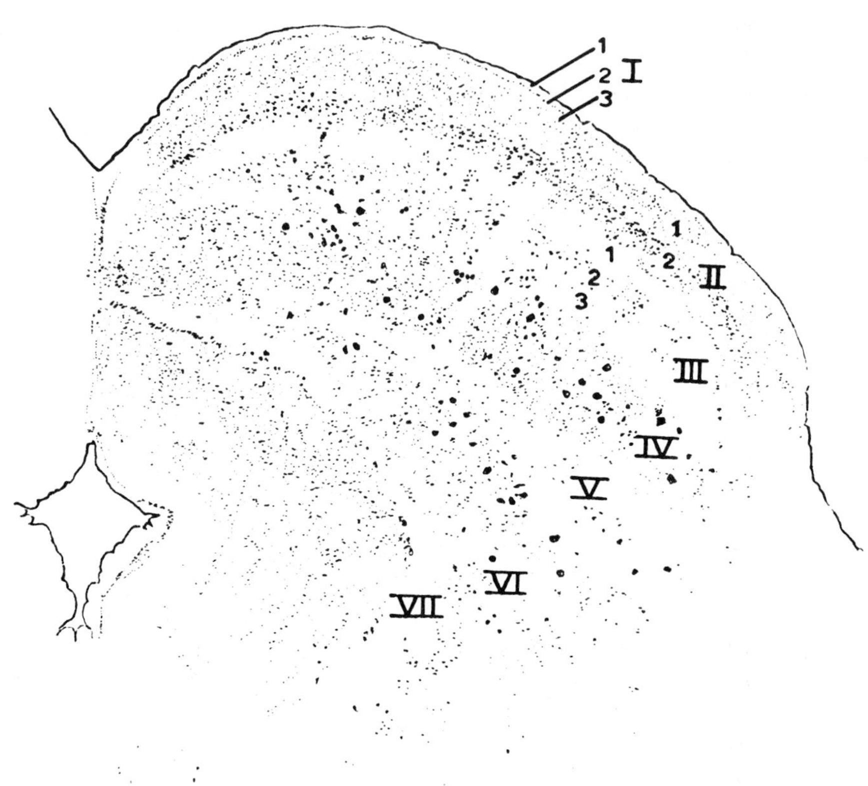

FIG. 2. Projection drawing of a coronal section (80μ, cresyl violet stain) of the right superior colliculus of the cat showing major (I–VII) and minor (1, 2, 3) laminae. I = Stratum zonale, II = S. griseum superficiale, III = S. opticum, IV = S. griseum intermediale, V = S. album intermediale or S. lemniscum, VI = S. griseum profundum, VII = S. album profundum. Taken from Kanaseki and Sprague, unpublished.

----

survival periods (3 days) which are thought to rule out retrograde effects. A clear answer to this question however has been obtained in this species using electron microscopy which demonstrates anterograde degeneration in LGNd after visual cortical lesions (51).

Although the corticofugal projections of the tectal visual system are not worked out in such detail, the pattern is clear for most areas. Area 19 and Clare-Bishop, the zones of overlap of the two systems, are described above. Insular cortex projects to suprageniculate (SG), the magnocellular part of medial geniculate (MGNm), caudal part of the posterior nuclear group (Poi), parts of the principal division of medial geniculate (MGNp) and S. Coll.; the dorsal corner of the posterior ectosylvian gyrus and the upper part of the anterior ectosylvian gyrus project to SG and MGNp (50, 52). The thalamic projections of the sulcal cortex are unknown. Thus, from present evidence, it appears that the cortex of the tectal visual system does not project either to LGNd or NPI.

There is an extensive projection from the cortical targets of both visual systems onto the superior colliculus (Figure 2) but the laminar distribution of the terminals from these cortical areas differ (23, 53, 95).

The parts of anterior and posterior ectosylvian gyri which receive from the tectal system project to the deeper collicular laminae-intermediate (IV), deep gray (VI) and to adjacent central gray matter; insular cortex projects to deep gray lamina and especially to the central gray matter (50). The association cortex in the convexity of the middle and anterior suprasylvian gyri which receives from the pulvinar (lateral pulvinar of Niimi et al., 72) has the most extensive collicular projection, terminating in laminae II, III, IV, V and VI, particularly in IV (intermediate gray)(23, 95). This is in contrast to the pattern of degeneration resulting from lesions in that part of the posterior suprasylvian gyrus corresponding to area 19 (Figure 3).

Foci of terminal degeneration in the colliculus after small lesions in areas 17 (CT7), 18 (CT2, 8) and 19 (CT4) are shown in Figure 3. In each case, most of the degeneration lies in the superficial layer of the superficial gray stratum (II_1), with only small amounts in the deep layer II_2, and in the stratum zonale (I2). Comparing the four animals the focus of degeneration is clearly more superficial in the cat with the 17 lesion. This animal also has more terminals in the zonal stratum (I), and the cat with lesion in area 19 has a sparse terminal degeneration in the upper part of stratum opticum (III_1). The fibers of these projections enter the colliculus via its brachium.* The C-B cortex terminates somewhat deeper, in the deep layer of SGS, in SO and into the intermediate gray stratum (SG_1), according to Heath and Jones (35) and Jones (50).

The corticotectal paths originating in areas 17 and 18 maintain the retinotopic organization present in the cortex, and terminate in retinotopic register with terminals of the incoming optic tract (23). As seen in Fink-Heimer stained material (38), terminals of the retinotectal fibers overlap extensively with these corticotectal terminations but differ in that they form a dense layer in SZ and most superficial part of SGS, in that area which is relatively clear in cat CT7 (Figure 3). The study by Sterling (100) using the electron microscope also indicates that cortical terminals reach their

----

* These areas of terminal degeneration using the Fink-Heimer technique are somewhat different than described in those studies using Nauta-Laidlaw (95) and Nauta-Gygax (23). Both of these methods demonstrate primarily the stem fibers and preterminal arborization and stain incompletely the actual terminal fields.

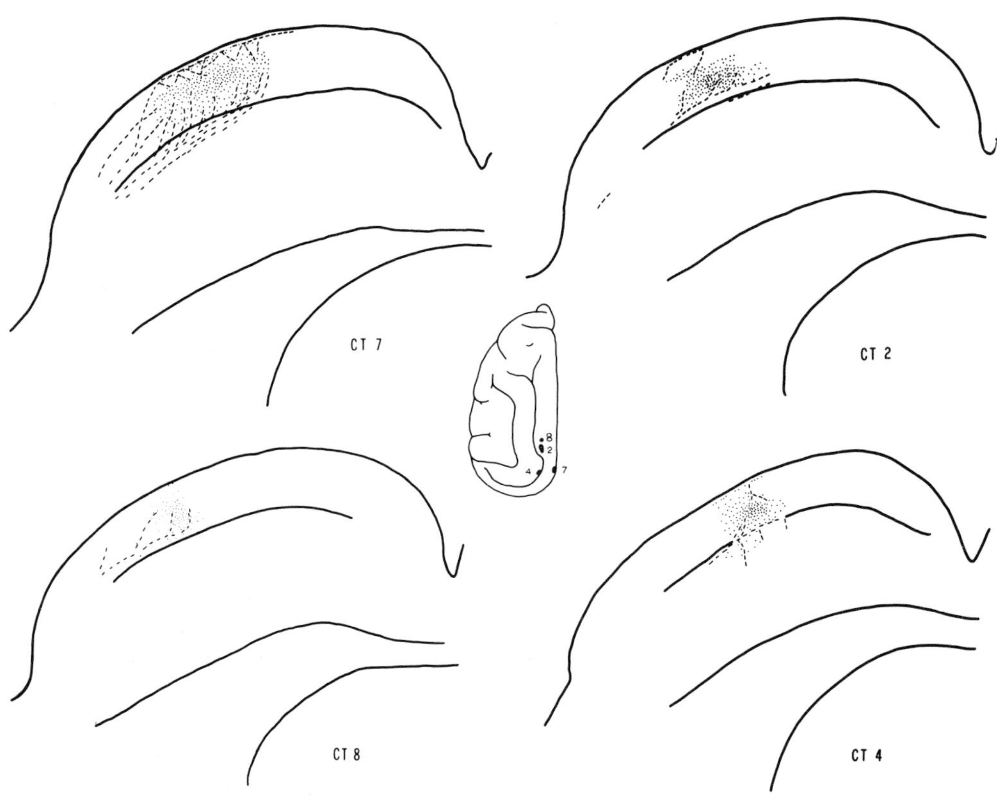

FIG. 3. Projection drawings of terminal field degeneration in the superficial gray (II of Figure 2) of the colliculi of four cats, 6 days after discrete cortical lesions in areas 17, 18 and 19 (see insert). Material stained according to the Fink-Heimer method; dots indicate fine particulate degeneration, dashed lines represent fibers. The border between superficial gray and optic strata was drawn from superimposed, adjacent cresyl violet stained sections. Taken from Lund and Sprague, unpublished.

maximum number somewhat deeper in SGS than do those from the retina. Details of the synaptic organization of retinotectal and corticotectal tracts are described by Sterling (100).

There is evidence that the corticotectal projections from area 19 (23) and C-B (50) are also retinotopically organized.

II. ELECTROPHYSIOLOGY-SUPERIOR COLLICULUS NEURONS

The above description outlines the anatomical organization of the extensive reciprocal connections which exist between two of the primary optic receiving sites: the visual cortex and the superior colliculus. The remainder of this paper will focus on the physiological interactions that occur in one tract of this system: the corticotectal tract which originates from cells in areas 17 and 18 of the cortex and terminates upon cells in the superficial laminae of the ipsilateral superior colliculus. We shall first describe receptive field properties of cells in the superficial laminae of the colliculus in normal cats and then characterize the changes seen in such cells following cortical removal. Finally, we shall describe the receptive field properties of corticotectal cells themselves and suggest how they may help to account for certain receptive field properties of the collicular cells to which they project.

We, as well as others (7, 31, 32, 40, 60, 82, 86, 87, 98, 102, 104, 106), have studied the receptive field properties of cells in laminae SGS and SO of the cat superior colliculus. To some extent techniques and results have varied among authors, and here we describe only our own procedures, results and conclusions regarding functional properties of these tectal neurons.

Cats were initially anesthetized with sodium pentothal and maintained with gaseous nitrous oxide and oxygen anesthesia. Animals were paralyzed with neuromuscular blocking agents (mixture of Flaxedil and d-tubocurarine) and standard procedures for refraction of the eyes were carried out. Natural light stimuli were projected onto a 6 foot-diameter white Plexiglas hemisphere which enabled us to study even the largest visual fields seen in the colliculus. Details of the techniques have been described by us previously (87).

In agreement with other authors, we found that movement was the single most important property of the visual stimulus in driving collicular cells. Because of this moving stimuli were used to locate cells and plot their receptive field borders. Receptive fields were circular or elliptical in shape and ranged in diameter from 2° near the center of gaze (rostral in the colliculus) to 60° in the periphery of the visual field (posterior in the superior colliculus).

Over 70% of all cells showed surround inhibition so that when the size of the stimulus extended beyond the excitatory receptive field there was a decrease in responsiveness. So long as the stimulus did not extend over the field borders, its size was not critical in affecting the responses in 60% of all cells tested. The remaining 40% of the cells showed either internal summation (more responses as the size of the stimulus was increased within the field) or internal inhibition (fewer responses as the size of the stimulus was increased within the field). We saw no evidence of any effect of shape or orientation of the stimulus in affecting tectal cells. In only one quarter of all cells tested was the response obtained from stationary spot stimuli turned on and off adequate for plotting receptive fields. Such responses at best were always far poorer than when the same spot was put in motion. We found that most cells had optimal velocities of stimulus movement, but most of them responded within a wide range.

In addition to responding best to moving stimuli, three-fourths of all cells showed a greater response to movements in one or more directions than to others. Such cells—

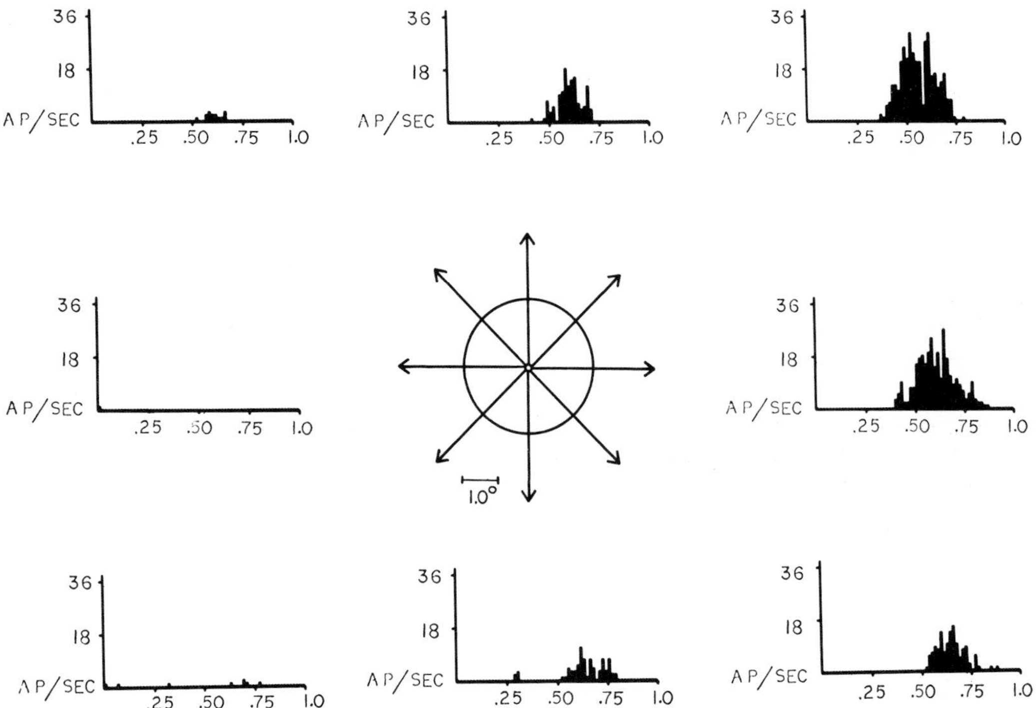

FIG. 4. An example of collicular direction selectivity. Cell recorded 100 μ below pial surface. Field 4° in diameter centered on the horizontal meridian, 7° to the right of the area centralis. 16 passes each with a 1/4° spot moving at 17°/sec through an excursion of 17°. 64 bins at 32 msecs each.

those which showed asymmetries in directional responses—were called direction selective (DS). An example of one such cell is shown in Figure 4. It is clear from the records that this cell responded best when the stimulus was moved in the up-right direction, and that the cell responded not at all to movements in a null direction 180° opposite to the preferred. A preferred direction lying 180° from the null direction was characteristic of all DS collicular cells studied.

Although the retinal input to the superior colliculus is 80–90% from the contralateral eye (57), virtually all collicular cells can be driven by either eye and 80% of them are driven about equally by either eye (Hubel and Wiesel's (44) ocular dominance groups 3–5). This reflects either a greater effectiveness of the small number of fibers from the ipsilateral eye or an additional ipsilateral eye input from elsewhere in the visual system.

The above characterization of cells in laminae SGS and SO of the cat colliculus agrees closely with the results of Sterling and Wickelgren (101), and Berman and Cynader (7) who followed similar procedures.

Wickelgren and Sterling (111) have added to our understanding of the cortical contribution to collicular function by showing certain changes in the properties of collicular cells after removal of the overlying ipsilateral visual cortex. Because of the importance of their results and because others have failed to confirm them (42, 58, 82) we undertook to repeat and extend their experiments.

In our initial study we first made large unilateral lesions of the visual cortex which included all of areas 17, 18, 19 as well as other cortical areas medial to the rhinal fissure. After 3 to 4 weeks postoperative survival we recorded from cells in the superior colliculus ipsilateral to the cortical lesion, using exactly the same procedures described previously for normal cats. We found no change in general responsiveness or spontaneous activity of these cells compared with those in normal animals, but we did see, as did Wickelgren and Sterling, clear and unequivocal changes in receptive field properties of such cells. First, the number of cells showing direction selectivity was reduced from the 75% seen in normal animals to about 12% in lesioned animals. This result shows that although cells still responded best to moving stimuli the mechanism of direction selectivity was greatly diminished after lesions. Second, the number of cells that could be driven by the ipsilateral eye was also greatly reduced: after these cortical lesions only 17% of the cells were about equally driven by either eye. The majority of cells (71%) were now driven exclusively by the contralateral eye, a percentage reflecting more closely the proportion of retinal fibers entering the colliculus from the contralateral eye (Figure 5). Third, we also saw an increase in the effectiveness in driving cells of stationary light stimuli turned on or off. Using such stimuli in these lesioned animals we were able to plot the receptive fields of about half of all cells isolated. However, even after cortical lesions stationary stimuli always elicited a much poorer response than moving stimuli.

The changes seen in these three properties,direction selectivity, eye dominance and response to transient stationary stimuli, after cortical lesions stand in marked contrast to the spatial properties of these same cells. We found no change in the percentage of cells showing surround inhibition, internal inhibition, or internal summation after cortical lesions.

From these experiments and those of Wickelgren and Sterling (111) and from recent work by Berman and Cynader (7), we conclude that the ipsilateral occipito-temporal cortex is largely responsible for providing the mechanism of direction selectivity to collicular cells, and that it is largely responsible for the ability of the ipsilateral eye to affect collicular cells and, lastly, that the cortex normally exerts some inhibitory influence over the responses of collicular cells to transient stationary stimuli. We conclude also that this cortex is probably not involved with the organization of the spatial receptive field properties of collicular cells.

In order to extend these results an additional series of experiments was undertaken in which the lesions were limited to cytoarchitectonically defined areas of the cortex (77, 88) to determine which of these areas are responsible for producing the changes reported above. Lesions limited to the Clare-Bishop area (13, 48, 115), to areas 18 and 19, to large amounts of cortex lateral to but sparing area 17 were ineffective in producing the changes. When the lesions included area 17 or were limited to 17, the full phenomenon appeared (see Fig. 6). Complete anatomical reconstruction of the cortical lesion based upon Nissl and myelin stained sections together with an analysis of the retrograde changes in the thalamus confirmed the extent of our lesion in each case.

We conclude that area 17 of the visual cortex is capable of maintaining normal collicular function with respect to the properties examined, and that only when area 17 is removed are the changes found. It should be cautioned, however, that whereas lesions anatomically limited to area 17 are effective, we cannot at present eliminate the possibility that such lesions might also functionally impair other cortical areas which receive projections from 17 and which project to the superficial colliculus (i.e., areas 18, 19, CB). This functional impairment might also be mediated by retrograde effects on the laminar part of the dorsal lateral geniculate body which projects to both areas 17 and 18 in the cat.

Our next question was whether the survival time after placement of a lesion in area 17 is a crucial factor in these changes. We allowed one animal with bilateral area 17 lesions to survive for 16 months before recording from the colliculi. We saw in this animal the same changes in the colliculus that we had seen after one month postoperative survival in other animals. There appears to be no compensation for these effects with time. We also wanted to know whether the changes seen in the colliculus after cortical lesions could be observed acutely—shortly after the lesion—or whether some period of reorganization was required. We removed area 17 in three animals and recorded one hour later in two of them and 3 days later in the third. We saw the same shift in the distributions of direction selectivity and eye dominance of the cells. Thus, we conclude that the changes reported above are the reflection of a cortical modulation of collicular activity, and are not due to a compensatory change which occurs over a period of time.

Further evidence for the role of the visual cortex in the organization of eye dominance of collicular cells comes from experiments using visual deprivation. In cats with one eye closed at birth most cells in area 17 of the adult animal, instead of being driven by both eyes as in the normally reared cat, are now driven solely by the nondeprived eye (112). Sterling and Wickelgren (102) reasoned that this change in eye dominance of cortical cells might be passed on to the superior colliculus. They found in cats similarly monocularly deprived for a period after birth, that both superior colliculi were driven exclusively by the nondeprived eye— just like those in the visual cortex. However, when the visual cortex was removed contralateral to the deprived eye, the ocular dominance of cells of the underlying colliculus underwent a dramatic shift, i.e., these cells were then driven by the deprived eye. In other words, cortical removal had not only removed the previously dominant ipsilateral eye input but also released the ability of the contralateral eye to excite cells. Figure 7 shows schematically the re-

---

FIG. 5. A comparison of the proportion of cells showing direction selectivity and binocular convergence in the superior colliculus for normal cats (A) and cats with cortical lesions (B). Combined results from 8 cats. (Reprinted by permission of Academic Press).

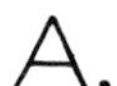
A.

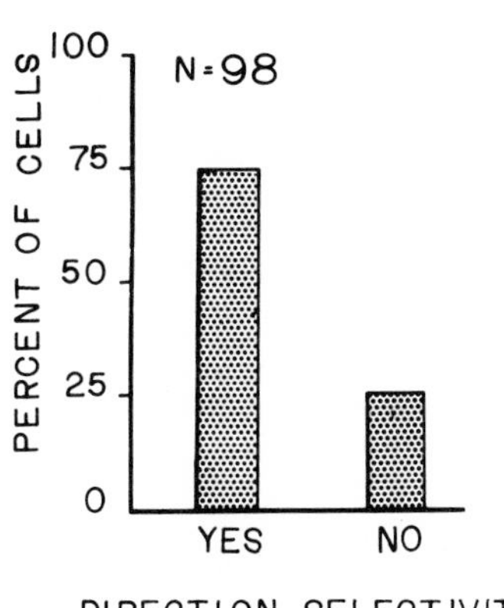
N=98
PERCENT OF CELLS
100
75
50
25
0
YES
NO
DIRECTION SELECTIVITY

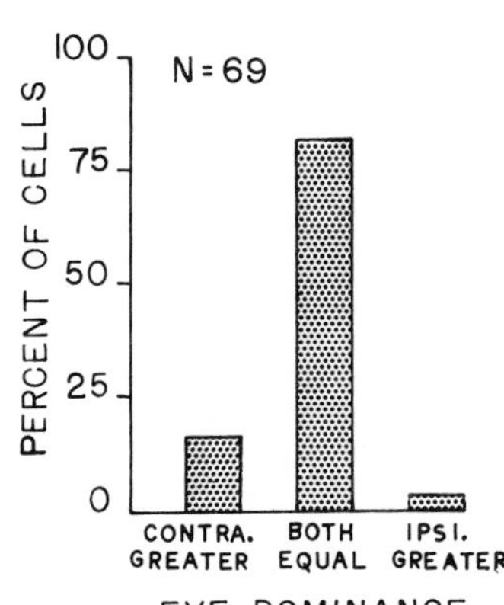
N=69
PERCENT OF CELLS
100
75
50
25
0
CONTRA. GREATER
BOTH EQUAL
IPSI. GREATER
EYE DOMINANCE

B.

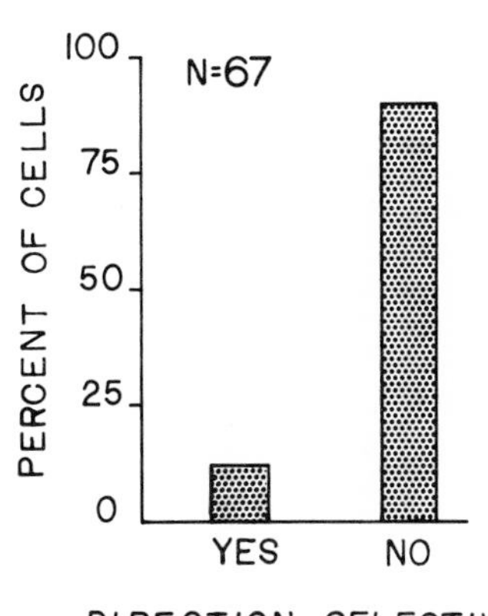
N=67
PERCENT OF CELLS
100
75
50
25
0
YES
NO
DIRECTION SELECTIVITY

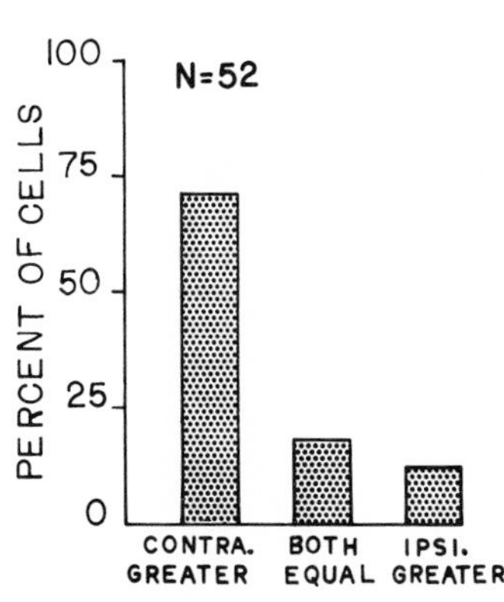
N=52
PERCENT OF CELLS
100
75
50
25
0
CONTRA. GREATER
BOTH EQUAL
IPSI. GREATER
EYE DOMINANCE

FIG. 5

sults from the eye closure experiments.

III. ELECTROPHYSIOLOGY—CORTICAL AND CORTICOTECTAL NEURONS

As shown above, the normal distributions of ocular dominance and direction selectivity for collicular cells in lamina SGS and SO are dependent on cortical area 17 and its corticotectal tract. In this section we shall compare the receptive field properties of the total population of visual cortical cells with those of corticotectal neurons.

The properties of cells in this and other cortical areas (17, 18, 19, CB) projecting to the superficial laminae have been described in some detail in the last decade. Two of the most striking attributes of most of these visual cortical neurons are again related to ocular dominance and direction selectivity. A high percentage of visual cortical neurons are driven strongly by both eyes, a property not present in retinal and lateral geniculate cells. Nearly all cortical cells are much more responsive to moving than to stationary stimuli and a high percentage are also direction selective.

A unique feature of visual cortical neurons is, however, their selectivity for elongated stimuli moving in space in a particular orientation. Cortical cells vary somewhat

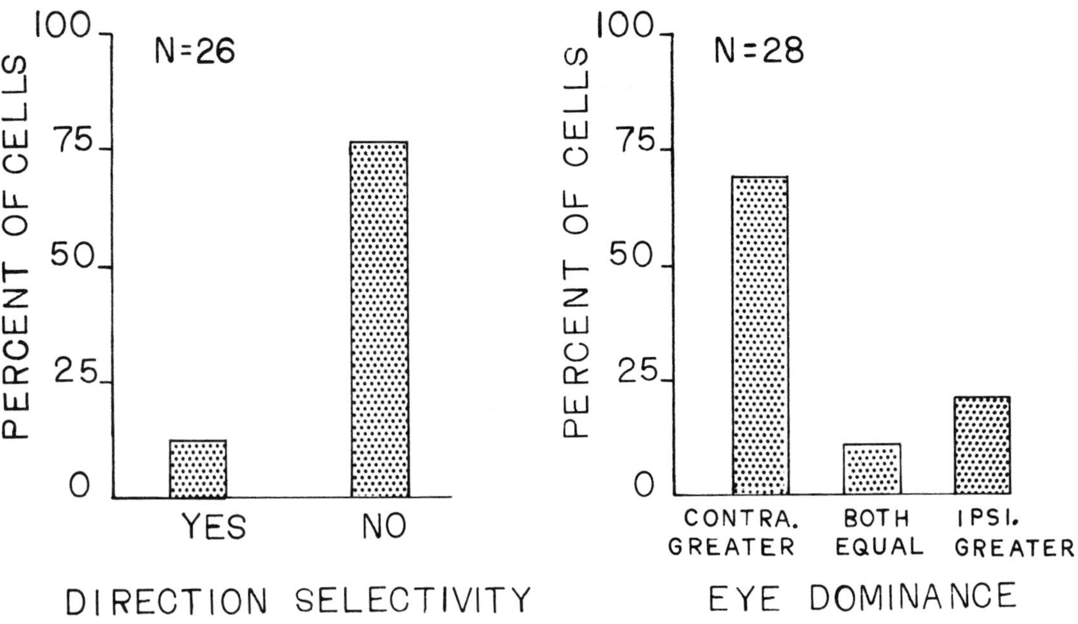

FIG. 6. The effects of chronic lesions limited primarily to cortical area 17 on direction selectivity and eye dominance of cells recorded in the colliculi ipsilateral to the lesions. Combined results from 3 cats. (Reprinted by permission of Academic Press).

in their sensitivity to orientation of stimulus edges but in general, a tilt of ± 20–30° from the optimal orientation will severely attenuate or abolish the response. Hubel and Wiesel (44, 45, 47) have described three classes of cells in the cat (and monkey) striate cortex. The receptive fields of *simple cells* can be plotted with small spots of light turned on or off, and are divided into specific on-regions and off-regions. There is summation of the response as the stimulus size is increased within each region and the two or more regions present are mutually antagonistic. Thus, a whole field flash generally elicits no response whatever. These cells are called simple because their responses to more complex moving stimuli could be roughly predicted from a stationary field plot. *Complex cells* on the other hand, have no obvious subregions within their receptive fields. Responses to small flashing spots are either absent or not organized into recognizable units. Such fields must be plotted with a moving stimulus.

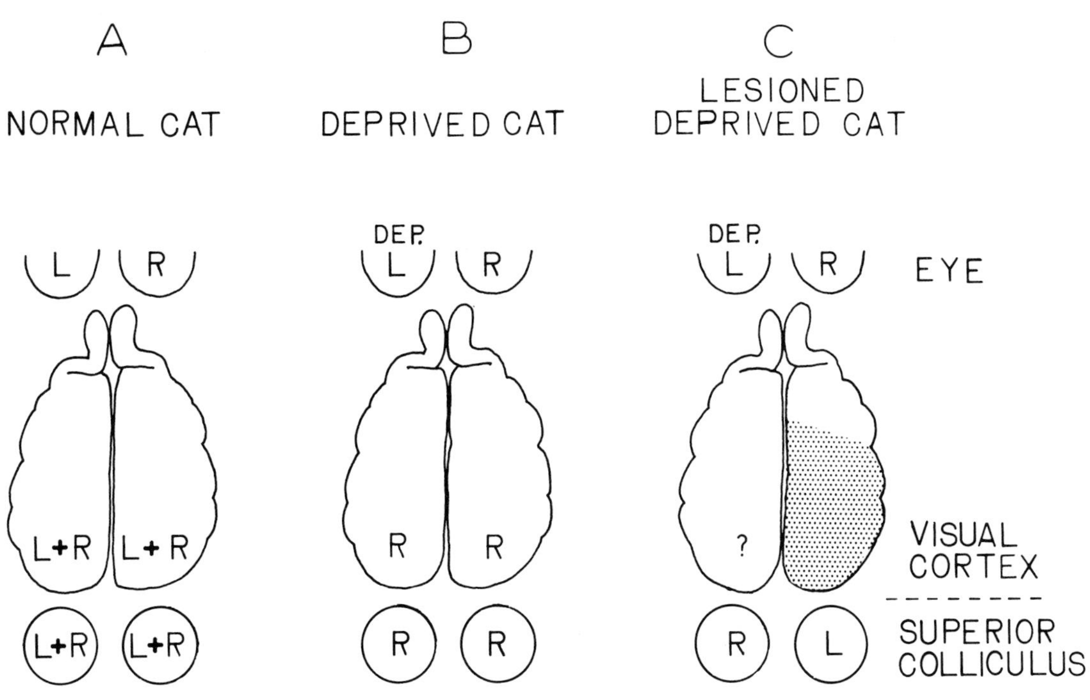

FIG. 7. Schema summarizing the results of Wiesel and Hubel (112) and Wickelgren and Sterling (102, 111). A. Most cortical and collicular cells are driven by both eyes in the normal cat. B. In the monocularly deprived cat cells in both visual cortices and superior colliculi are driven only by the previously non-deprived eye. C. When the visual cortex is removed on the side opposite to the deprived eye, the cells in the ipsilateral superior colliculus are no longer driven by the ipsilateral (non-deprived) eye, and the contralateral eye becomes effective in driving cells.

Whereas simple cells respond to stimuli moved over a very small retinal region with a short, low frequency burst, complex cells respond with a high frequency, fairly continuous discharge over a relatively large retinal area. Simple and complex cells show greater responses with increased stimulus length up to the length of the receptive field. Hypercomplex cells closely resemble complex cells, but they respond only when the stimulus length is restricted. The suppression of response for stimuli that are too long may be accomplished in several ways, most simply by means of inhibitory flanks at one or both ends of the field. All of these cells are orientation selective; many are binocular and direction selective as well. Simple, complex and hypercomplex cells are found in area 17, complex and hypercomplex in different proportions lie in 18, 19 and CB in the cat (44, 45, 48, 115).

Bishop and his associates (8, 79) have also classified cells as simple or complex but on rather different grounds. They classify a cell as simple if it responds with a low frequency burst (<100/sec) as an edge or slit moves over a very small retinal region ($< 1^\circ$) at a low stimulus velocity (generally 2°/sec or less). Whereas simple cells generally lack spontaneous activity, complex cells are usually active without any overt stimulation. Complex cells respond to much higher stimulus velocities over a wider retinal region ($> 3^\circ$) with a high frequency, maintained discharge. In our own experiments, we analyzed data in such a way that both sets of criteria were employed, and in most cases, the two systems have agreed on the classification of a given cell. Bishop et al. have not explicitly defined hypercomplex cells but it is clear from their descriptions that they find such cells in the striate cortex. In addition, they have mentioned cortical units which show no orientation selectivity of any kind.

In view of the effects of cortical lesions on the properties of tectal units, we undertook a series of experiments to determine directly what information is sent from cortical areas 17 and 18 to the colliculus. All procedures were standard and are described in detail elsewhere (78, 87). The experiment consisted of recording single unit activity from these cortical areas in paralyzed cats anesthetized initially with sodium pentothal (I.P.) and maintained for 2 or 3 days on N_2O and O_2. In addition, an array of stimulating electrodes was placed stereotaxically in the ipsilateral superior colliculus for identification of visual cortical cells projecting to the colliculus by means of antidromic stimulation. Placement of these electrodes was facilitated by recording a visual evoked response in the colliculus to a stroboscopic, whole field flash, and by recording an antidromic field potential over the lateral gyrus in response to collicular stimulation. Most cortical cells were in no way affected by electrical stimulation of the colliculus; a few were driven orthodromically perhaps through recurrent collaterals (33), and a small percentage were driven antidromically (9, 33). A small number of those cells driven antidromically had sufficiently large potentials to be isolated when studied using visual stimulation. These cells were then studied by first plotting the fields and then systematically varying the stimulus parameters to determine the sensitivity of the cell to various aspects of the stimuli. Data were stored on tape and PST histograms generated off-line on a PDP 12 laboratory computer (25). At present, 43 cells have been so isolated and examined.

Our primary interest was to determine the ocular dominance and direction selectivity of corticotectal cells. In addition, we were anxious to know if the corticotectal cells constitute a homogeneous population with respect to these and other properties. The homogeneity of properties in this projection system is demonstrated in Figure 8 and contrasts sharply with another visual cortical efferent system known to project through the corpus callosum. All three cortical cell types are found in the callosal tract and what appears to be approximately a uniforn cross section of cortical properties have been found there. This commissural fiber system is known to arrise in part from layers II and III of area 18 (110) and is evidently specialized only in the location of its receptive fields, all of which were found on or near the vertical meridian (5, 46).

The corticotectal cells we have studied have all shown the orientation selectivity of cortical cells. Nearly all were classified as complex cells; a few, as hypercomplex. We have also studied in detail about 100 cells not driven from tectal stimulation including a large number of simple cells in area 17. While it is clear on several grounds that simple and complex cells are truly separate cell types, in our opinion it is not clear that complex and hypercomplex cells are. Although some cells are clearly hypercomplex as defined above and some are clearly complex, many cells lie somewhere between with weaker or stronger inhibitory flanks reducing the response to a stimulus that is too long. Many cells were classed as complex during an experiment and these were found to have weak but definite inhibitory flanks when the data were subsequently analyzed off-line. Therefore, we would like to emphasize the fact that no simple cells were found to project to the tectum rather than the fact that a few hypercomplex cells did. These corticotectal cells were found exclusively in layer V of areas 17 and 18. This was determined by histological reconstruction of electrode tracks and localization of electrolytic lesions made at the time of recording.

Figure 8 also summarizes the ocular dominance distribution of the corticotectal population and presents for comparison the distribution obtained from other complex cells (not driven by collicular stimulation) recorded in areas 17 and 18. Our sample of complex cells *not* projecting to the colliculus agrees well with the distribution given by Hubel and Wiesel for area 17 of the cat (44). Whereas only about half of all complex cells are binocular (driven well by either eye, Hubel and Wiesel's groups 3, 4, 5), 90% of the corticotectal population falls into this class. Comparison of Figs. 5 and 8 will reveal a marked similarity between corticotectal and collicular distributions of ocular dominance.

Figure 8 also suggests that a higher percentage of corticotectal cells are direction selective than of the complex cell population as a whole. Preferred-null ratios of peak mean frequency (spikes/sec calculated from the average of the 5 bins centered on the maximum response, 79) in response to stimuli moving back and forth across the field were determined from PST histograms. The characteristics of the stimuli (orientation, velocity, length, width) were selected to give an optimal response before such measurements were taken. Cells whose preferred-null ratios exceeded 2.0 were classified as direction selective; 70% of the corticotectal cells fell into this class compared with 30% of the complex cells not projecting to the superior colliculus. The cut-off point at a P:N ratio of 2.0 was chosen mainly because subsequent quantitative studies of collicular cells suggested that the minimal P:N ratio we had called direction selective in our earlier work was between 1.8 and 2.0.

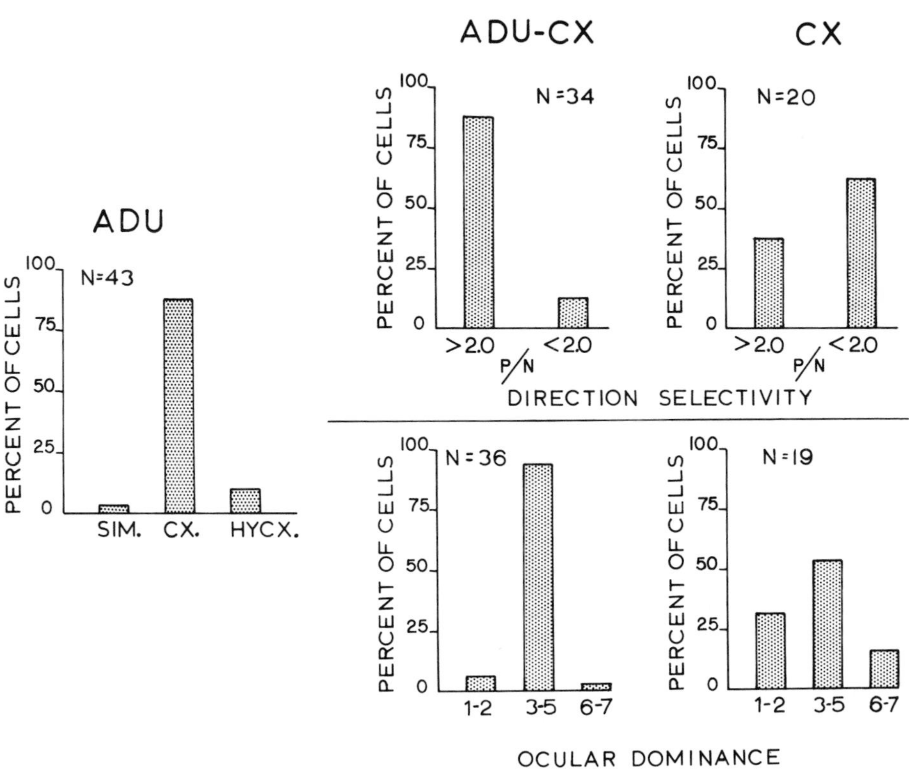

FIG. 8. Some properties of the corticotectal population (ADU), and comparison with complex cells not driven by the collicular stimulation (CX). See text for details.

The next problem which concerned us was the presence of orientation selective behavior in corticotectal cells and the lack of this property in the colliculus. One simple way to explain this masking out of orientation selectivity would be simply to assume the convergence of many cortical cells with different optimal orientations onto a given collicular cell. This may ultimately be found to provide a large part of the explanation but on closer examination, the situation appears more complex. Because direction selectivity of cells in the superficial colliculus depends in large part on cortical inputs, the question we really want to ask is, how can information about the direction of motion be preserved while information about the orientation of edges is lost?

At the present time, we cannot answer this question completely but we can approach a solution more closely by considering other differences between cortical and collicular cells. The available descriptions of cortical cells using slit stimuli indicate that the preferred and null directions of stimulus motion are separated by 90°, rather than by 180° as in the colliculus (44). We agree with this observation for corticotectal cells as long as the stimulus edges are maintained perpendicular to the direction of motion. But under these circumstances, orientation as well as direction of motion vary with respect to the receptive field. Since no response is ever obtained with edge stimuli oriented 90° to the optimal, this is the null direction for such elongated stimuli.

A further inconsistency between our understanding of cortical and collicular cells concerns sensitivity to small stimuli. Although the spatial properties of collicular cells do not depend on the cortex, in the intact animal a direction selective response is obtained from a large proportion of collicular units using a stimulus much smaller than the receptive field. Even for cells with very large fields, a 1/4° spot is usually an effective stimulus. Simple and complex cells, on the other hand, are described as showing spatial summation with stimulus length up to the length of the field (44, 45). There must be direction selective cortical cells which respond in some way to small, moving spot stimuli if they influence the firing of collicular cells to such stimuli.

We therefore examined the corticotectal and other adjacent cortical cells for their sensitivity to small moving spots and to variations in stimulus length. The results were somewhat surprising and are exemplified by the responses of a corticotectal cell to stimuli of various lengths, as shown in Fig. 9. This cell, found to be typical of 75% of the corticotectal population, did not show summation with increasing slit length, and was in fact strikingly insensitive to this stimulus parameter. In contrast, nearly all complex cells not driven by tectal stimulation showed clear summation with stimulus length, and simple cells always summate in such a way that the response is approximately a linear function of the stimulus length from some threshold up to the full field length. However, a few of the corticotectal cells did show pure summation and the remainder fell somewhere between this and complete insensitivity to stimulus length. The cell of Fig. 9 was also typical of most corticotectal cells in that the response was halved by a deviation of ± 35° from the optimal orientation when a field length slit was used.

When, however, the small spot so effective for this cell and others like it was moved across the receptive field in various directions, a response profile very similar to that of a collicular cell was obtained; as in Fig. 4. Thus, when the direction of stimulus motion alone is varied by using a small spot, the preferred and null directions are truly separated by 180° just as for most tectal units. The preferred direction for slit or spot movement was always the same.

The exact details of how groups of corticotectal cells interact with the retinal input to produce collicular receptive fields remains unknown. It is evident, however, that the corticotectal population carries to the colliculus the very information required to produce the properties lost there following lesions of this same cortex. The corticotectal cells are nearly all binocular, direction selective, complex or hypercomplex cells. Furthermore, most of these cells show less than pure summation with stimulus length and many show no summation at all. Therefore, these cells respond in a direction selective manner to any stimulus configuration known to be effective for cells in the colliculus. Thus far we have seen no differences between corticotectal cells from areas 17 or 18 although a functional difference has been implied from the cortical stimulation studies of McIlwain and Fields (61) and our own lesion studies (86, 87) reviewed above.

The best direction of stimulus movement for corticotectal cells was always perpen-

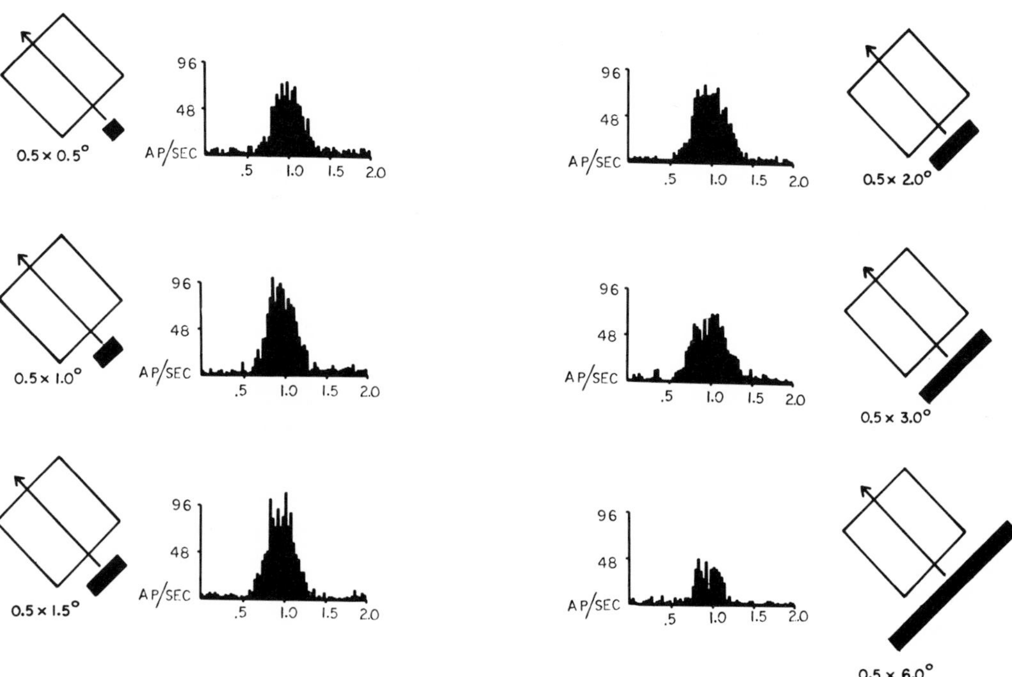

FIG. 9. Corticotectal cell showing relative insensitivity to variations in stimulus length. Field is 3.0 x 3.2° located 2.0° below and 3.5 ° to the right of the area centralis. Stimulus velocity is 4.5°/sec over 9.0°. Bin width is 32 msecs; 16 passes with each stimulus. Note the suppressive flanks apparent with the 6.0° slit. Latency from collicular stimulation was 1.0 msecs.

dicular to the long axis of their receptive fields even when small spot stimuli were presented. This finding suggested that the best direction of stimulus movement for a given collicular cell might be related to the orientations of the corticotectal cells converging upon it. Since a population of collicular units whose receptive fields fell in that portion of the visual field from which the corticotectal cell population was obtained did show a tendency for their best directions of stimulus movement to be away from the vertical meridian and into the contralateral visual field (7, 40, 87, 98, 101, 104), we might have expected a prevalence of vertical field orientations in the corticotectal population. The present experiments revealed no such prevalence; the field orientations of corticotectal cells were distributed randomly. This lack of correlation between the distributions of collicular best directions and corticotectal field orientations may be accounted for by supposing that there must be convergence of many corticotectal cells with a wide range of optimal orientations onto any given collicular cell in order to account for the lack of orientation selectivity in the latter.

The logic of this corticotectal projection system can be emphasized by comparing the properties of collicular cells with simple and complex cortical cells. In several ways, complex and collicular cells are similar but both are different from simple cells. 1) The latter are for example responsive only to slowly moving stimuli, few responding at all to velocities in excess of 10 deg/sec. In contrast, collicular and complex cortical cells respond generally to a wide range of velocities often including very slow movements and nearly always including much higher velocities in the neighborhood of 30-60 deg/sec. Thus, complex and collicular cells both respond at velocities of stimulus movement greater than the maximal velocity to which most simple cells respond. 2) Simple cells also tend to have very small receptive fields with centers often less than 1.0 deg. across. Complex cells have much larger fields, sometimes greater than 10 deg. across and nearly always greater than 2 deg., even for fields located on or near the area centralis. Collicular units recorded in the superficial lamina have fields ranging in size from 2 to 60 deg. along the major axis. 3) Collicular and complex cells have similar binocular interaction properties; they are both relatively insensitive to the exact position of objects in three dimensional space, when compared with simple cells (8). Thus, when comparing the discharge elicited by stimulation of either eye alone with that of both eyes when the fields are in correspondence, some complex and collicular units show facilitation for exact field super-position, although it is less marked than that characteristic of simple cells, and they lack the powerful inhibitory trough on either side of exact super-position typical of certain simple cells. 4) Whereas complex cells vary considerably in their sensitivity to stimulus length, all simple cells summate with machine-like precision from some threshold up to the full-field length. The corticotectal cells in particular seem to be largely insensitive to variations in stimulus length and respond well to any stimulus configuration known to be effective in the colliculus. 5) We have alluded previously to the subregions found in the receptive fields of simple cells which can be mapped by using small flashing spots. One consequence of this is that the "spontaneous" activity of many simple cells can be affected, often dramatically, by a stationary edge or slit positioned within one of these regions. Usually a greater discharge rate is produced by slowly moving the same stimulus over the field, although occasionally a simple cell is found which is not at all selective for movement. The discharge of complex and most superficial collicular cells is never significantly modified with stationary stimuli. These cells are completely selective for movement.

The response properties of both simple and complex cells are possibly dependent on selective innervation by specific types of lateral geniculate neurons, as recently described by Cleveland et al. (15, see also 21). The latter authors have shown that there is a dual projection system from retina to cortex. The transient (or Y) system mediated by fast conducting fibers from retina to lateral geniculate and from geniculate to cortex responds to stimulus movement of high velocities and changes in flux within the field, whereas the slowly conducting sustained (or X) system responds to sustained contrast. In another series of experiments, Hoffmann and Stone (41, 103) have shown that complex cells are activated with shorter latencies than other cell types following stimulation of optic chiasm or optic radiation. This implication that complex cells are innervated by the transient system (although perhaps not exclusively) is well correlated with the observed movement selectivity of complex cells and with the fact that only complex cells project to the tectum which itself is predominantly responsive to moving stimuli. That both sustained and transient systems project directly to the colliculus from the retina, either as stem fibers or collaterals, is suggested by anatomical (76) and physiological (14) evidence.

Hubel and Wiesel's (44, 45) scheme of an hierarchical organization of visual cortical cell types proposed that complex cells are formed by the convergence of several simple cells. Some difficulties presented by this theory regarding velocity information and latency to optic radiation stimulation are cited above, but such an organization would provide the basis for the observation that lesions of area 17 alone abolish direction selectivity and binocular convergence in the colliculus since no simple cells are known to exist outside of area 17.

Simple cells then seem to be primarily concerned with the precise position and orientation of edges in three dimensional space whereas complex cells may be more concerned with the movement of such stimuli. Both systems project through the callosum to the opposite hemisphere but only complex cells project onto the tectum, a structure known to be involved in the control of eye movements.

DISCUSSION

We have described a corticotectal system whose cell bodies lie in layer V of visual cortical areas 17 and 18, and whose axons enter the colliculus via its brachium and superficial part of the stratum opticum. They terminate on dendrites of cells in the superficial gray stratum, chiefly its upper part, and sparsely in the zonal stratum.

Study of the receptive fields of these corticotectal neurons indicates that they form a rather homogeneous group of complex cells, different in several ways from other, non-corticotectal complex cells in the same cortex. In fact the corticotectal neurons are similar to cells in the superficial laminae of the superior colliculus, except for the cortical property of orientation specificity. These corticotectal neurons carry to the colliculus the information required to produce the properties of binocular activation and direction selectivity which are lost in most tectal units after lesion of this same cortex. Thus these cortical and collicular neurons form a functional unit, whose behavioral potentialities we will explore.

I. Visual Attention and Orientation

Classically, the colliculus has been recognized as a center controlling reflexive eye movements involved in target acquisition and maintenance, the visual grasp reflex (39). Incoming information to the colliculus from auditory, tactile or visual channels may elicit complex orienting movements involving the eyes, head and whole body so organized as to bring the source of stimulation into the central visual field.

In support of this classical notion of collicular function is the fact that bilateral collicular lesions after a period of apparent blindness result in persistent deficits in head and eye movements; visual following is slow and the animal easily loses moving targets. In addition, however, a clear deficit is also seen in attention, orientation to, and localization of visual acoustic or tactile stimuli. When tectal lesions are placed unilaterally (99) head and eye movements are normal in the ipsiversive direction only; after transitory, contralateral hemianopia, moving stimuli in the contralateral visual field evoke attention but orientation to and localization of such objects remains poor. When stimuli are presented simultaneously in both fields the contralateral stimulus is ineffective and the animal responds to the ipsilateral side only. The motor deficit with little visual neglect can be produced by lesions of the tectospinal tract. Contralateral visual neglect without the motor deficit arises after lesions of the brachium of the superior colliculus and parts of the tectothalamic system (99). We shall return later to a discussion of other sensory deficits seen after collicular lesions.

Although the colliculus is unquestionably implicated in visual attention and orientation, we consider it unlikely that the corticotectal tract from area 17 is involved in these functions in the cat. Thus lesions of area 17, or 17 + 18, greatly reduce the incidence of binocular driving and direction selectivity in the colliculus, yet such animals show no obvious deficits in eye and head movements, or in attending to or localizing objects in space (6, 19, 97). Furthermore, in the developing kitten visual attention and gross orientation appear before the superficial collicular units show direction selectivity and binocularity (75).

II. Eye Movements

It does seem likely, however, that the fine control of saccadic and smooth pursuit eye movements necessary to foveate and track objects moving in various directions and at varying velocities in 3-dimensional space is dependent on the presence of direction selective and velocity sensitive binocular neurons somewhere in the visual system. In the cat such neurons are present in cortical areas 17 and 18 and in the superficial layers of the superior colliculi; the tectal properties of direction selectivity and binocularity are supplied primarily by the striate corticotectal path. Electrical stimulation of the superior colliculus in cat (39, 49, 94, 107) and macaque (83, 90) elicits eye movements of a variety of amplitudes and directions determined by the locus of stimulation. Similar effects are obtained by stimulation of the visual cortex, and are lost following destruction of the colliculus (90, 94), although eye movements elicited by stimulation of the frontal eye fields remain. Thus, the visual cortex is linked to the oculomotor system through the tectum. Wurtz and Goldberg (116) and Schiller and Koerner (90) have elegantly demonstrated that cells in intermediate and deep laminae of the macaque colliculus fire in a highly organized and specific way before saccadic eye movements appear. These units have weakly responding receptive fields; their discharge specifically precedes those eye movements which move the fovea in certain directions from its initial position onto objects which had previously been in that receptive field. Other work suggests that such cells are also found in the colliculi of rabbits (89) and cats (105). The likely significance of such units in the mechanisms controlling the precision of saccadic and smooth pursuit movements is reinforced by the finding of Schiller and Koerner (90) that after collicular ablation macaques are permanently unable to acquire and maintain foveation of visual targets.

The organization of the striate corticotectal system is such that collicular units having receptive fields within the central 60-70° of the visual field are driven by both eyes in the cat. In keeping with the indicated role of the tectum in guiding eye movements for foveation and following, and with the deficits in spatial localization produced by tectal lesions, it is logical to propose that localization in depth and the vergence eye movements associated with it are dependent on the activity of this corticotectal path. This system probably has little to do with fine stereoscopic depth perception (which is presumably mediated by simple cortical cells) except for its dependency on convergence of the eyes on appropriate planes as objects are sought in space.

III. Complex Behaviors

That the superior colliculus is involved in perception and discrimination is clearly established in the tree shrew (form, 12), rat (spatial, 4), hamster (spatial, 91), cat (form, 6, 96), and macaque (movement, 2).* Although the deficits in these particular tests appear not to be due to visuomotor deficiencies, the responsible lesions in all studies but one destroyed most or all of the colliculi. In the tree shrew, however, the lesions were both superficial and total; those with deep lesions appeared blind and lacked visual orientation and following; in contrast, those with superficial lesions retained the normal, brisk, visually guided behavior characteristic of this species. Both groups of animals, however, were unable to discriminate upright from inverted triangles, a task easily achieved by tree shrews lacking striate cortex.

Following total or near total lesions of superior colliculus and part of the pretectum, cats had no deficit in a light-dark discrimination, but showed prolonged learning of upright versus inverted triangles (solid or outline), upright versus horizontal bars, and were unable to learn to discriminate cross from circle of same area and flux.

Accompanying anatomical studies in the tree shrew (59) show that the superficial collicular laminae receive afferents from retina and area 17 of the cortex (like the cat and many other species); the efferent projection from the superficial laminae ends in pretectum, dorsal and ventral lateral geniculates and in LP-pulvinar. The second and fourth of these terminal sites project to visual "sensory" and visual "association" cortices respectively (it is likely that this tectal pathway is present in cat and most mammals). In contrast, the deep collicular laminae give rise to the classical "motor" systems to reticular formation, pons and spinal cord, as well as ascending tracts to the posterior thalamic nuclei, subthalamus and intralaminar nuclei.

These results in the tree shrew indicate that the deficits in form perception and discrimination which are known to follow total collicular lesions in this species are related primarily to the superficial laminae in which retinotectal and striate corticotectal tracts terminate. Furthermore, these deficits are clearly independent of mechanisms controlling visual orientation and tracking. Whether a comparable function for the superficial laminae exists in the cat is not now known, but is under investigation in this laboratory.

Cortical lesions in the cat limited to area 17 (6, 19) or to areas 17 and 18 (3, 97) result in no loss in preoperatively learned light-dark discrimination nor in retention or original learning of several form discriminations (upright vs. inverted solid triangles, cross versus circle, horizontal versus vertical stripes). The unpublished results of

----

* When the lesions involve the pretectum in addition to the colliculus the deficit in form discrimination is more marked in the cat (6, 68); such deficits are also present after damage to pretectum alone in rats (108) and macaques (109).

Sprague et al. (97) indicate that cats without areas 17 and 18 also have normal ability to perform repeated reversal of these patterns. Such animals, as well as cats with only area 17 removed, did show prolonged learning of outline triangles embedded in circles. Both of these tests, particularly the last, are difficult for normal cats.

Tree shrews, like cats, show normal tracking and following and gross depth perception after striate lesions. There is no loss in a preoperatively learned light-dark discrimination. Black-white, color, vertical-horizontal lines and triangle discriminations are not retained after striate lesions in the tree shrew, but relearning is at the preoperative rate or faster. When the vertical-horizontal discrimination was retested using reflected, rather than transmitted light the animals showed prolonged learning. No relearning was possible in tests which introduced an irrelevant (distracting) cue, i.e., triangles embedded in a circle, and vertical-horizontal stripes with irrelevant hue.

The similarities seen in these tests in cats and tree shrews after bilateral removal of area 17 are rather striking. We cannot carry the parallel further vis-a-vis the function of the striate corticotectal tract, because comparable data from single unit recording are not available in the tree shrew. On behavioral grounds alone, however, it appears clear that the described deficits in form discrimination following tectal lesions are not caused by interruption of this corticotectal tract. This discussion does not account for the possible role of the corticotectal tracts coming from areas 19 and Clare-Bishop and terminating in the superficial laminae. When 19 is included with 17 and 18 in cortical lesions (19, 93, 114), or when 19 is involved with the suprasylvian gyrus leaving 17 and 18 intact (6, 96), form discrimination is prolonged or absent.

SUMMARY

This paper presents anatomical, physiological and behavioral data on the organization of certain corticotectal systems in the cat. Anatomically, separate pathways arise in cytologically defined cortical areas 17, 18 and 19. All of these paths reach the colliculus via its brachia and the fibers traverse the tectum in the superficial part of the optic stratum (SO). All of these fibers terminate in the superficial gray stratum (SGS), especially its upper part, with a few in the stratum zonale. There appear to be differences in the foci of greatest density of terminals: those from area 17 are more superficial and those from 19 are deeper, with a few spilling into the upper layer of stratum opticum. The focus of retinotectal terminals is even more superficial, although these also show considerable overlap with all three corticotectal systems.

Removal of area 17 is followed by at least three unequivocal changes in the responses of neurons lying in collicular laminae SGS and SO. There is a marked decrease in the number of cells which are binocularly driven with a resulting dominance of the contralateral eye; there is an equally marked diminishment in the percentage of neurons showing direction selectivity to moving stimuli; there is an increase in the responsiveness of many neurons to stationary, punctate light stimuli turned on or off. These alterations in the receptive field organization of superficial collicular neurons did not follow ablation of any occipitotemporal cortex other than area 17. Such changes are interpreted as clear evidence of a naturally occurring cortical modulation of their activity, since the same changes follow acute lesions of 1 hour as well as chronic lesions of up to 16 months duration.

Isolation of the responsible corticotectal neurons and study of their receptive fields revealed a rather homogeneous group of complex-hypercomplex cells lying in layer V of cortical areas 17 and 18 (19 is yet to be studied). When the field properties were compared with other adjacent complex cells not projecting to the colliculus, a higher percentage of corticotectal cells were found to be a) binocular, b) direction selective and c) driven by small spots of light as well as by slits and edges. Using spots as stimuli, the direction selective properties and the low incidence of spatial summation also resembled the receptive fields of collicular cells. Thus, this corticotectal system carries that neural information to the superior colliculus which is lost in tectal cells after lesions of this cortex.

From the evidence reviewed here, we believe it is unlikely that the corticotectal system in the cat is critical in visual attention and orientation, or in the ability of the animal to perceive and discriminate differences in flux or visual forms. Rather the evidence suggests that this pathway is involved in the elaboration of the known collicular mechanism which controls precise foveation and tracking of moving objects. In addition this corticotectal system may provide binocular information to the mechanism of vergence eye movements required for depth perception.

ACKNOWLEDGMENTS

This research was supported in part by National Institutes of Health research grant EY00577 and training grant GM01994.

We wish to express our appreciation to Mrs. J. Levy and Miss A. DiBerardino for their technical assistance and to Mr. Lawrie Winning for the photography. It is also our pleasure to thank M. Fujita and E. Shalna and their associates at the Instrumentation Lab and Machine Shop of the Institute of Neurological Sciences. Lastly, we are indebted to Dr. George Gerstein for the use of his computer facility and to John Stevens for valuable assistance in programming.

REFERENCES

1 ALTMAN, J. and CARPENTER, M.B. Fiber projections of the superior colliculus in the cat. J. Comp. Neurol. 116 (1961) 157-178.

2 ANDERSON, K.V. and SYMMES, D. The superior colliculus and higher visual functions in the monkey. Brain Research, 13 (1969) 37-52.

3 BADEN, J.P. and URBAITIS, J.C. and MEIKLE, T.H., Jr. Effects of serial bilateral neocortical ablations on a visual discrimination by cats. Exp. Neurol., 13 (1965) 233-251.

4 BARNES, P.J., SMITH, L.M. and LATTO, R.M. Orientation to visual stimuli and the superior colliculus in the rat. Quart. J. Exp. Psychol., 22 (1970) 239-247.

5 BERLUCCHI, G., GAZZANIGA, M.S., and RIZZOLATTI, G. Microelectrode analysis of transfer of visual information by the corpus callosum. Arch. ital.

Biol., 105 (1967) 583-596.
6 BERLUCCHI, G., SPRAGUE, J.M., LEVY, J. and DiBERARDINO, A.C. Pretectum and superior colliculus in visually guided behavior and in flux and form discrimination in the cat. J. Comp. Physiol. Psychol., 1972. Monogr. Suppl., 78 (1972) 123-172.
7 BERMAN, N. and CYNADER, M. Comparison of receptive field organization of the superior colliculus in Siamese and normal cats. 1972. In preparation.
8 BISHOP, P.O. Beginning of form vision and binocular depth discrimination in cortex. In: The Neurosciences Second Study Program, Ed. by F.O. Schmitt, Rockefeller University Press, 1970, New York.
9 BISHOP, P.O., BURKE, W., and DAVIS, R. Single unit recording from antidromically activated optic radiation neurons. J. Physiol., 162 (1962) 432-450.
10 BURROWS, G.R. and HAYHOW, W.R. The organization of the thalamo-cortical visual pathways in the cat. Brain Behav. Evol., 4 (1971) 220-272.
11 CAMPOS-ORTEGA, J.A., HAYHOW, W.R. and DE V. CLUVER, P.F. The descending projections from the cortical visual fields of Macaca mulatta with particular reference to the question of a cortico-lateral geniculate pathway. Brain, Behav. Evol., 3 (1970) 368-414.
12 CASAGRANDE, V.A., HARTING, J.K., MARTIN, G.F. and DIAMOND, I.T. Superior colliculus of the tree shrew (Tupaia glis): Evidence for a structural and functional subdivision into superficial and deep layers. 1972, In preparation.
13 CLARE, M.H. and BISHOP, G.H. Responses from an assiciation area secondarily activated from optic cortex. J. Neurophysiol., 17 (1954) 270-277.
14 CLARE, M.H., LANDAU, W.M. and BISHOP, G.H. The relationship of optic nerve fiber groups activated by electrical stimulation to the consequent central postsynaptic events. Exp. Neurol., 24 (1969) 400-420.
15 CLELAND, B.G., DUBIN, M.W. and LEVICK, W.R. Sustained and transient neurons in the cat retina and lateral geniculate nucleus. J. Physiol., 217 (1971) 473-496.
16 DE V. CLUVER, P.F. and CAMPOS-ORTEGA, J.A. The cortical projection of the pulvinar in the cat. J. Comp. Neurol., 137 (1969) 295-308.
17 DIAMOND, I.T. and HALL, W.C. Evolution of neocortex. Science, 164 (1969) 251-262.
18 DIAMOND, I.T., JONES, E.G. and POWELL, T.P.S. The projection of the auditory cortex upon the diencephalon and brain stem in the cat. Brain Research, 15 (1969) 305-340.
19 DOTY, R.W. Survival of pattern vision after removal of striate cortex in the adult cat. J. Comp. Neurol., 143 (1971) 341-369.
20 EDWARDS, S.B., ROSENQUIST, A.C., and PALMER, L.A. 1972. In preparation.
21 ENROTH-CUGELL, C. and ROBSON, J.G. The contrast sensitivity of retinal ganglion cells of the cat. J. Physiol., 187 (1966) 517-552.
22 GAREY, L.J. and POWELL, T.P.S. The projection of the lateral geniculate nucleus upon the cortex in the cat. Proc. Roy. Soc. B., 169 (1967) 107-126.
23 GAREY, L.J., JONES, E.G. and POWELL, T.P.S. Interrelationships of striate and extrastriate cortex with the primary relay sites of the visual pathway. J.

Neurol. Neurosurg. Psychiat. 31 (1968) 135-157.

24 GAREY, L.J. and POWELL, T.P.S. The projection of the retina in the cat. J. Anat., 102 (1968) 189-222.

25 GERSTEIN, G.L. and KIANG, N.T. An approach to the quantitative analysis of electrophysiological data from single neurons. Biophysical Journal 1 (1960) 15-28.

26 GLICKSTEIN, M., KING, R.A., MILLER, J. and BERKLEY, M. Cortical projections from the dorsal lateral geniculate nucleus of cats. J. Comp. Neurol., 130 (1967) 55-76.

27 GRAYBIEL, A.M. Some thalamocortical projections of the pulvinar-posterior system of the thalamus in the cat. Brain Research, 22 (1970) 131-136.

28 GRAYBIEL, A.M. Some fiber pathways related to the posterior thalamic region in the cat. Brain, Behav. Evol. 1972. In press.

29 GUILLERY, R.W. The laminar distribution of retinal fibers in the dorsal lateral geniculate nucleus of the cat: a new interpretation. J. Comp. Neurol., 138 (1970) 339-368.

30 GUILLERY, R.W. Patterns of fiber degeneration in the dorsal lateral geniculate nucleus of the cat following lesions in the visual cortex. J. Comp. Neurol., 130 (1967) 197-213.

31 HARUTIUNIAN-KOZAK, B., KOZAK, W. , DEC, K. and BALCER, E. Responses of single cells in the superior colliculus of the cat to diffuse light and moving stimuli. Acta Biol. Exp., 28 (1968) 317-331.

32 HARUTIUNIAN-KOZAK, B., KOZAK, W. and DEC, K . Visually evoked potentials and single unit activity in the superior colliculus of the cat. Acta Neurobiol. Exp., 30 (1970) 211-232.

33 HAYASHI, Y. Recurrent collateral inhibition of visual cortical cells projecting to superior colliculus in cats. Vision Res., 9 (1969) 1367-1380.

34 HAYHOW, W.R. The cytoarchitecture of the lateral geniculate body in the cat in relation to the distribution of crossed and uncrossed optic fibers. J. Comp. Neurol., 110 (1958) 1-48.

35 HEATH, C.J. and JONES, E.G. Connections of area 19 and the lateral suprasylvian area of the visual cortex of the cat. Brain Research, 19 (1970) 302-305.

36 HEATH, C.J. and JONES, E.G. An experimental study of ascending connections from the posterior group of thalamic nuclei in the cat. J. Comp. Neurol., 141 (1971) 397-426.

37 HEATH, C.J. and JONES, E.G. The anatomical organization of the suprasylvian gyrus of the cat. Erg. Anat. Entwickls., 45 (1972) 6-64.

38 HEDREEN, J. Patterns of axon terminal degeneration seen after optic nerve section in cats. Anat. Rec., 163 (1969) 198.

39 HESS, W.R., BURGI, S. and BUCHER, V. Motorische Functionen des Zektal— und Tegmentalsgebietes. Mschr. Psychiat. Neurol., 112 (1946) 1-52.

40 HOFFMANN, K.-P. Retinotopische Beziehungen und Struktur rezeptiver Felder im Tectum opticum und Praetectum der Katze. Z. vergl. Physiologie, 67 (1970) 26-57.

41 HOFFMANN, K.-P. and STONE, J. Conduction velocity of afferents to cat

visual cortex: a correlation with cortical receptive field properties. Brain Res., 32 (1971) 460-466.

42 HOFFMANN, K.-P and STRASCHILL, M. Influences of cortico-tectal and intertectal connections on visual responses in the cat's superior colliculus. Exp. Brain Res., 12 (1971) 120-131.

43 HOLLANDER, H. The projection from the visual cortex to the lateral geniculate body (LGB). An experimental study with silver impregnation methods in the cat. Exp. Brain Res., 10 (1970) 219-235.

44 HUBEL, D. and WIESEL, T.N. Receptive fields, binouclar interaction and functional architecture in the cat's visual cortex. J. Physiol., 160 (1962) 106-154.

45 HUBEL, D.H. and WIESEL, T.N. Receptive fields and functional architecture in two nonstriate visual areas (18 and 19) of the cat. J. Neurophysiol. 28 (1965) 229-289.

46 HUBEL, D.H. and WIESEL, T.N. Cortical and callosal connections concerned with the vertical meridian of visual fields in the cat. J. Neurophysiol., 30 (1967) 1561-1573.

47 HUBEL, D. H. and WIESEL, T.N. Receptive fields and functional architecture of monkey striate cortex. J. Physiol., 195 (1968) 215-243.

48 HUBEL, D.H. and WIESEL, T.N. Visual area of the lateral suprasylvian gyrus (Clare-Bishop area) of the cat. J. Physiol., 202 (1969) 251-260.

49 HYDE, J.E. and ELIASSON, S.G. Brainstem induced eye movements in cats. J. Comp. Neurol., 108 (1957) 139-171.

50 JONES, E.G. Personal communication.

51 JONES, E.G. and POWELL, T.P.S. An electronmicroscopic study of the mode of termination of corticothalamic fibres within the sensory relay nuclei of the thalamus. Proc. Roy. Soc. B., 172 (1969) 173-185.

52 JONES, E.G. and POWELL, T.P.S. An analysis of the posterior group of thalamic nuclei on the basis of its afferent connections. J. Comp. Neurol., 143 (1971) 185-216.

53 KAWAMURA, S., NIIMI, K. and SPRAGUE, J.M. Projection of the visual cortices to posterior thalamus, pretectum and superior colliculus in the cat. 1972. In preparation.

54 KINSTON, W.J., VADAS, M.A and BISHOP, P.O. Multiple projection of the visual field to the medial portion of the dorsal lateral geniculate nucleus and the adjacent nuclei of the thalamus of the cat. J. Comp. Neurol., 136 (1969) 295-316.

55 KUYPERS, H.G.J.M. In: Interhemispheric relations and cerebral dominance, Ed. V.B. Mountcastle. Johns Hopkins Pres , Baltimore, 1962, pp. 114-116.

56 KUYPERS, H.G.J.M. and LAWRENCE, D.G. Cortical projections to the red nucleus and brainstem in the Rhesus monkey. Brain Res., 4 (1967) 151-188.

57 LATIES, A.M. and SPRAGUE, J.M. The projection of optic fibers to the visual centers in the cat. J. Comp. Neurol., 127 (1966) 35-70.

58 MARCHIAFAVA, P.L. and PEPEU, G. The responses of units in the superior colliculus of the cat to a moving visual stimulus. Experientia, 22 (1966) 51-55.

59 MARTIN, G.F., HARTING, J.K., HALL, W.C. and DIAMOND, I.T. Efferent

projections of the superior colliculus in the tree shrew (T u p a i a g l i s): An analysis of the projections of individual strata. Anat. Rec., 1972, In press.
60 McILWAIN, J. and BUSER, P. Receptive fields of single cells in the cat's superior colliculus. Exp. Brain Res., 5 (1968) 314-325.
61 McILWAIN, J.T. and FIELDS, H.L. Superior Colliculus: Single unit responses to stimulation of visual cortex in the cat. Science, 170 (1970) 1426-1428.
62 MEIKLE, T.H., Jr. and SPRAGUE, J.M. The neural organization of the visual pathways in the cat. Intern. Rev. Neurobiol., 6 (1964) 149-189.
63 MISHKIN, M. Cortical visual areas and their interactions. In: The Brain and Human Behavior, Ed. A.G. Karczmar, Springer-Verlag, 1972, In press.
64 MOORE, R.Y. and GOLDBERG, J.M. Ascending projections of the inferior colliculus in the cat. J. Comp. Neurol., 121 (1963) 109-136.
65 MOORE, R.Y., KARAPAS, F. and LENN, N.J. A retinohypothalamic projection in the rat. Anat. Rec., 169 (1971) 382-383.
66 MYERS, R.E. Projections of superior colliculus in monkey. Anat. Rec., 145 (1963) 264.
67 MYERS, R.E. Cortical projections to midbrain in monkey. Anat. Rec., 145 (1963) 337-338.
68 MYERS, R.E. Visual deficits after lesions of brain stem tegmentum in cats. Arch. Neurol., 11 (1964) 73-90.
69 NIIMI, K. Personal communication.
70 NIIMI, K. and INOSHITA, H. Cortical projections of the lateral thalamic nuclei in the cat. Proc. Japan Acad., 47 (1971) 664-669.
71 NIIMI, K., KAWAMURA, S. and ISHIMARU, S. Projections of the visual cortex to the lateral geniculate and posterior thalamic nuclei in the cat. J. Comp. Neurol., 143 (1971) 279-312.
72 NIIMI, K. and KUWAHARA, E. The dorsal thalamus of the cat and comparison with monkey and man. J. Comp. Neurol., 1972, In press.
73 NIIMI, K. , MIKI, M. and KAWAMURA, S. Ascending projections of the superior colliculus in the cat. Okajimas Fol. Anat. Jap., 47 (1970) 269-287.
74 NIIMI, K. and SPRAGUE, J.M. Thalamo-cortical organization of the visual system in the cat. J. Comp. Neurol., 138 (1970) 219-250.
75 NORTON, T.T. The development of receptive field properties in the superior colliculus of kittens. Anat. Rec., 1972, In press.
76 O'LEARY, J.L. A structural analysis of the lateral geniculate nucleus of the cat. J. Comp. Neurol., 73 (1940) 405-430.
77 OTSUKA, R. and HASSLER, R. Uber Aufbau und Gliederung der corticalen Sehsphare bei der Katze. Arch. Psychiat. Nervenkr., 203 (1962) 212-234.
78 PALMER, L.A. 1972. In preparation.
79 PETTIGREW, J.D., NIKARA, T. and BISHOP, P.O. Responses to moving slits by single units in cat striate cortex. Exp. Brain Res., 6 (1968) 373-390.
80 POGGIO, G.F. and MOUNTCASTLE, V.B. A study of the functional contributions of the lemniscal and spinothalamic systems to somatic sensibility. Bull. Johns Hopkins Hosp., 106 (1960) 266-316.
81 RINVIK, E. A re-evaluation of the cytoarchitecture of the ventral nuclear com-

plex of the cat's thalamus on the basis of corticothalamic connections. Brain Research, 8 (1968) 237-254.

82 RIZZOIATTI, G., TRADARDI, V. and CAMARDA, R. Unit responses to visual stimuli in the cat's superior colliculus after removal of the visual cortex. Brain Research, 24 (1970) 336-339.

83 ROBINSON, D.A. Eye movements evoked by superior colliculus stimulation in the alert monkey. Vision Res., In press. 1972.

84 ROSE, J.E. The thalamus of the sheep: cellular and fibrous structure and comparison with pig, rabbit and cat. J. Comp. Neurol., 77 (1942) 469-523.

85 ROSE, J.E. and WOOLSEY, C.N. Cortical connections and functional organization of the thalamic auditory system of the cat. In: Biological and Biochemical Bases of Behavior, Eds., H.F. Harlow and C.N. Woolsey, Univ. of Wisconsin Press, Madison. 1958, pp. 127-150.

86 ROSENQUIST, A.C. and PALMER, L.A. Responses of single cells in the cat superior colliculus after cortical lesions. Anat. Rec., 169 (1971) 414-415.

87 ROSENQUIST, A.C. and PALMER, L.A. Visual receptive field properties of cells of the superior colliculus after cortical lesions in the cat. Exp. Neurol., 33 (1971) 629-652.

88 SANIDES, F. and HOFFMAN, J. Cyto- and myeloarchitecture of the visual cortex of the cat and of the surrounding integration cortices. J. Hirnforschung, 11 (1969) 79-104.

89 SCHAEFER, K.P. Microableitungen im Tectum opticum des frei beweglichen Kaninchens. Arch. Psychiat. Ztschr. Neurol., 208 (1966) 120-146.

90 SCHILLER, P.H. and KOERNER, F. Discharge characteristics of single units in superior colliculus of the alert Rhesus monkey. J. Neurophysiol., 34 (1971) 920-936.

91 SCHNEIDER, G.E. Contrasting visumotor functions of tectum and cortex in the golden hamster. Psychologische Forschung., 31 (1967) 52-62.

92 SINGLETON, M.C. and PEELE, T.L. Distribution of optic fibers in the cat. J. Comp. Neurol., 125 (1965) 303-328.

93 SPEAR, P.D. and BRAUN, J.J. Pattern discrimination following removal of visual neocortex in the cat. Exp. Neurol., 25 (1969) 331-348.

94 SPIEGEL, E.A. and SCALA, N.P. Ocular disturbances associated with experimental lesions of the mesencephalic central gray matter. Arch. Ophthal., 18 (1937) 614-632.

95 SPRAGUE, J.M. Corticofugal projections to the superior colliculus in the cat. Anat. Rec., 145 (1963) 288.

96 SPRAGUE, J.M., BERLUCCHI, G. and DiBERARDINO, A. The superior colliculus and pretectum in visually guided behavior and visual discrimination in the cat. Brain Behav. Evol., 3 (1970) 285-294.

97 SPRAGUE, J.M., LEVY, J., Di BERARDINO, A.C. and CONOMY, J. Perceptual deficits following cortical and tectal lesions in cats. 1972. In preparation.

98 SPRAGUE, J.M., MARCHIAFAVA, P.L. and RIZZOLATTI, G. Unit responses to visual stimuli in the superior colliculus of the unanesthetized, mid-pontine cat. Arch. ital. Biol., 106 (1968) 169-193.

99 SPRAGUE, J.M. and MEIKLE, T.H., Jr. The role of the superior colliculus in visually guided behavior. Exp. Neurol., 11 (1965) 115-146.

100 STERLING, P. Receptive fields and synaptic organization of the superficial gray layer of the cat superior colliculus. Vision Res. Supplement 3 (1971) 309-328.

101 STERLING, P. and WICKELGREN, B.G. Visual receptive fields in the superior colliculus of the cat. J. Neurophysiol., 32 (1969) 1-15.

102 STERLING, P. and WICKELGREN, B.G. Function of the projection from the visual cortex to the superior colliculus. Brain Behav. Evol., 3 (1970) 210-218.

103 STONE, J. and HOFFMANN, K.P. Conduction velocity as a parameter in the organization of the afferent relay in the cat's lateral geniculate nucleus. Brain Research, 32 (1971) 454-459.

104 STRASCHILL, H. and HOFFMAN, K.P. Functional aspects of localization in the cat's tectum opticum. Brain Research, 13 (1969) 274-283.

105 STRASCHILL, M. and HOFFMANN, K.P. Activity of movement sensitive neurons of the cat's tectum opticum during spontaneous eye movements. Exp. Brain Res., 11 (1970) 318-326.

106 STRASCHILL, M. and TAGHAVY, A. Neuronale Reaktionem im Tectum opticum der Katze auf bewegte und stationare Lichtreize. Exp. Brain Res., 33 (1967) 353-367.

107 SYKA, J. and RADIL-WEISS, T. Electrical stimulation of the tectum in freely moving cats. Brain Research, 28 (1971) 567-572.

108 THOMPSON, R. Localization of the "visual memory system" in the white rat. J. Comp. Physiol. Psychol., Monogr. Suppl., 69 (4, pt. 2) 1969.

109 THOMPSON, R. and MYERS, R.E. Brainstem mechanisms underlying visually guided responses in the Rhesus monkey. J. Comp. Physiol. Psychol., 74 (1971) 479-512.

110 TOYAMA, K., MATSUNAMI, K. and OHNO, T. Antidromic identification of association, commissural and corticofugal efferent cells in cat visual cortex. Brain Research, 14 (1969) 513-517.

111 WICKELGREN, B.G. and STERLING, P. Influence of visual cortex on receptive fields in the superior colliculus of the cat. J. Neurophysiol., 32 (1969) 16-23.

112 WIESEL, T.N. and HUBEL, D.H. Comparison of the effects of unilateral and bilateral eye closure on cortical unit responses in kittens. J. Neurophysiol., 28 (1965) 1029-1040.

113 WILSON, M.E. and CRAGG, B.G. Projections from the lateral geniculate nucleus in the cat and monkey. J. Anat. 101 (1967) 677-692.

114 WINANS, S.S. Visual form discrimination after removal of the visual cortex in cats. Science, 158 (1967) 944-946.

115 WRIGHT, M.J. Visual receptive fields of cells in a cortical area remote from the striate cortex in the cat. Nature, 223 (1969) 973-975.

116 WURTZ, R.H. and GOLDBERG, M.E. Superior colliculus cell responses related to eye movements in awake monkeys. Science, 171 (1971) 82-84.

DISCUSSION

KUYPERS:

Dr. Sprague mentioned the difference between his findings in the cat and ours in the monkey. For the record, we found (Kuypers and Lawrence, Brain Research, 4: 151, 1967) that in the monkey the areas adjoining the central sulcus do not project to the tectum. This may correlate with physiological data which indicate that electrical stimulation of these pericentral areas in the monkey do not elicit eye movements (cf. I.H. Wagman, In: The Oculomotor System, Harper and Row, New York, 1964). In our material the fibers from the caudal part of the precentral gyrus do not project heavily to the superior colliculus but the projection is directed to a more lateral area at the foot of the colliculus. This area we called the dorsolateral mesencephalic tegmentum, which also receives lemniscal fibers. We tend to think that one is dealing here with a somatosensory mesencephalic area intervening between the visual and the auditory mesencephalic areas.

PURPURA:

I suppose the basic question here is do we really have to think about two separate visual systems, one system for exploring space and the other for examining the details of patterned space. As I hear your message I believe you are saying that attempts to separate these two systems physiologically will be difficult and perhaps of little heuristic value in view of the close behavioral coupling between the two "systems."

SPRAGUE:

Thank you Dr. Kuypers for your point of clarification on the anatomy.

In response to Dr. Purpura's comment, there is good anatomical evidence for at least two separate visual systems in mammals, which we have already summarized in this paper. Evidence from signle unit studies and from deficits in visually guided behavior and in perception and discrimination indicate that these two systems process the visual input differently, and mediate different aspects of visual behavior. Having said this however, it is important to stress the interaction of the two systems at many levels in mediating many complex visual behaviors. We feel that formulations of visual functions which emphasize exclusive properties of cortex or midbrain are misleading. Our study in the cat has defined the anatomy and physiology of one corticotectal system at both cortical and collicular levels; in the intact animal, the responses of cells at both levels of this system are remarkably similar. Cortical modulation of the tectal cells is shown by the changes in receptive field properties after removal of area 17.

Corticothalamic Projections and Sensorimotor Activities
T. Frigyesi, E. Rinvik, and M.D. Yahr, editors. © 1972
Raven Press, New York.

Association: Cortico-cortical and/or Cortico-subcortical

Karl H. Pribram

I accepted the challenge presented by this Symposium because a body of work on the functional connections of the non-human primate association cortex is coming to fruition. The results of a long series of neuroanatomical, neurophysiological and neurobehavioral experiments have led me to revise the classical views on the functions of the association cortex which I had been taught. What are these views and what are the data that led to revision?

Webster's dictionary defines "association" as "the process of forming...connections or bonds between sensations, perceptions, ideas or feelings." The classical view of the functions of association cortex therefore implies that input from several primary sensory systems converges onto the association areas. And, in fact, a large number of electrophysiological studies on cats has delineated several cortical areas characterized by cells that can be stimulated through two or more sensory channels (45). These polysensory cortical areas are not the topic of the present paper. They have as yet been inadequately studied in primates although one fact relevant to this discussion has emerged. When the same techniques were used to delineate the polysensory cortical systems in cat and monkey, it became apparent that the primate precentral motor cortex is one of the major such polysensory areas (1). More of this later.

In primates, including man, an entirely different set of areas has been identified as "association cortex." Both clinical and experimental evidence shows these areas to be sensory specific rather than polysensory. It is this evidence, and that for the functions in behavior of this sensory specific association cortex and even what we have discovered about the anatomical substrate for these functions that have shaken my faith in the classical view.

THE CLINICAL EVIDENCE

In patients, damage to certain parts of the brain has been correlated with a loss of the ability to identify objects. This disability can be manifest in any one of the major sensory modes. For instance, when a visual deficit occurs, the subdominant hemisphere is especially involved (24) approximately at the inferior junction of the occipital and temporal lobes. According to Henry Head (17), Sigmund Freud is responsible for the usage of the term agnosia to describe this syndrome, a term which epitomizes the problems posed by its occurrence.

Von Monakov (26) called attention to these problems in a thorough review of relevant data. The issues can be summarized in two related questions: 1. Is agnosia dependent on the occurrence of primary sensory difficulties? 2. Can agnosia occur in the absence of involvement of the primary sensory projection systems? Von Monakov's answer to the first question was an unequivocal "no", an opinion shared on the basis of more recently acquired and very carefully obtained data by Bay (5). With the negative answer to the behavioral question in mind, Von Monakov reviewed the anatomical data and also gave a tentative "no" in answer to the possible exclusion of sensory systems in agnosia. However, he was by no means completely convinced or convincing on this point.

THE NON-HUMAN PRIMATE

Because of the difficulty of obtaining evidence on precise and limited brain injury in man, I decided some years ago to attempt to produce animal models of the agnosias (and other disorders of psychological processes) produced by brain damage. Such animal models would allow long-term behavioral analysis and relatively complete specification of the brain locus and perhaps even of the brain mechanisms involved in cognition. The ensuing program of research has proved effective, and I wish today to share some of its critical experimental results with you.

The immediate problem in making animal models was to identify areas in the brain cortex of monkeys that were homologous to those of man in producing behavioral disturbances. To this end a series of anatomical (8, 11, 29-31), chemical, viz., neuronography (22, 32, 33), and electrophysiological (12, 18, 20, 23, 37, 46) studies were undertaken. The results of these experiments were then used as a guide to making resections of cortex in a series of experiments in which a battery of behavioral tests was administered (visual, auditory, somatosensory and gustatory discriminations; delayed response and alternation; locomotor activity; conditioned avoidance of foot shock).

But often the subsystems of forebrain determined by one technique did not match exactly those determined by another. Further, there was no guarantee that the dissection wrought by a particular anatomical or physiological technique would accord with the neurobehavioral classification I sought. Resections for testing behavioral effects were therefore made in any one experiment on the most logical basis of what was known at the time so that each experiment could stand on its own. However, when approximately half a hundred rhesus monkey models had been produced the results were collated by a method called "the intercept of sums technique" (27). Briefly, by this method, one adds together on a standardized brain diagram all of the areas of the resections that produced a particular behavioral deficit, then in a separate diagram adds together all of the areas of the resections that produced no deficit on that test; and overlays the two summations. The extent of summed lesions producing deficit that lies beyond the margins of the non-deficit-producing sum is the area critically involved in producing the behavioral difficulty. That this area and only this area is so involved was then tested by limiting resections to the "intercept" area and reproducing the behavioral difficulty in its entirety.

MONKEY BEHAVIOR

What is the nature of this behavioral difficulty? First and critically, there is a correlation between locus of lesion in the posterior association cortex and agnosia in one or another sensory mode. (Frontal or limbic lesions do not produce sensory discrimination deficits.) Figures 1 and 2 summarize the results of these "intercept-of-sums" studies.

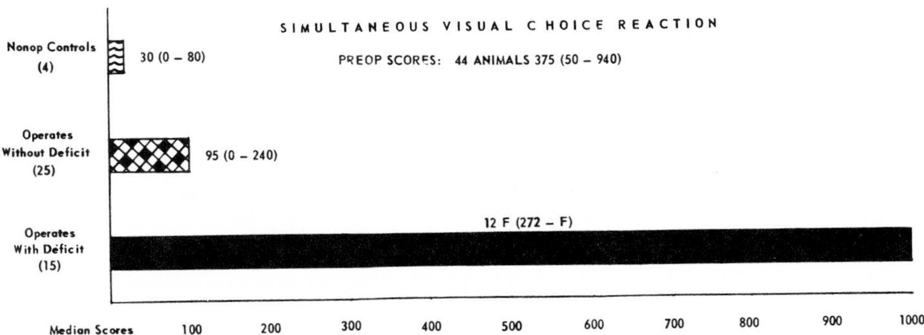

FIG. 1. Bar graph of median scores taken by monkeys to perform a visual discrimination task (the printed patterns + vs □). The number of animals per group is indicated below group name; the range from which median scores are taken appears in parentheses next to the median.

Second, a lesion producing a sensory specific deficit does not affect all behaviors in that mode equally. For instance, after resections of the inferior temporal gyrus, visual tracking was unaffected—monkeys could, despite severe visual discrimination deficits, catch gnats in midair with alacrity. But whenever a visually guided choice had to be made, monkeys with inferotemporal cortex resections showed impairment and this impairment was roughly proportional to the difficulty experienced by normal monkeys in learning the discrimination.

I want to limit discussion here to the brain area found to be homologous to that producing visual agnosia in man and to report only a few of a long series of experiments undertaken to determine the nature of this visual discrimination deficit. One

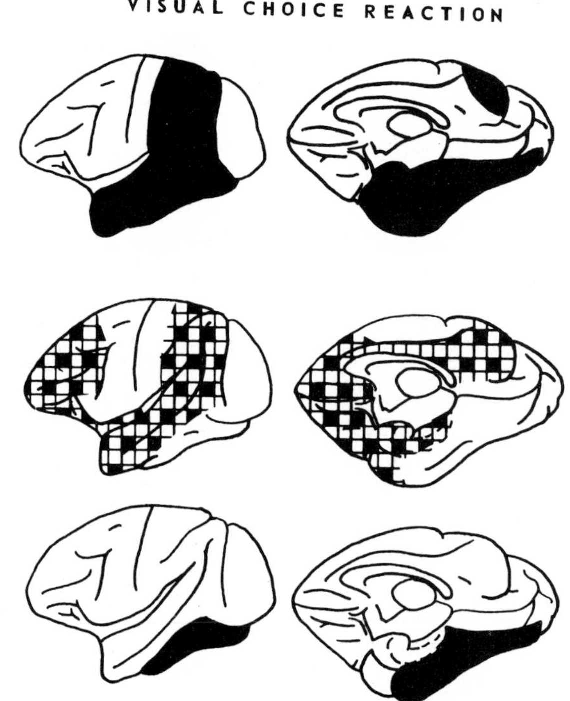

FIG. 2. The upper diagram A represents the sum of the areas of resection of all of the animals grouped as showing a deficit on the visual discrimination task noted in Figure 1. The middle diagram B represents the sum of the areas of resection of all of the animals grouped as showing no-deficit in Figure 1. The lower diagram C represents the intersect of the area shown in black in the upper diagram and that not checkerboarded in the middle diagram. This intersect represents the area invariably implicated in visual choice behavior in these experiments.

of the critical experiments asked the question whether the monkeys with inferotemporal cortex resections had difficulty in distinguishing among visual cues or whether some other difficulty was responsible for their discrimination deficit (34). The monkeys were taught a very easy discrimination: to choose between a simultaneously presented ash tray and tobacco tin. Though the lesioned monkeys took significantly longer to acquire the discrimination than did the controls, the task was mastered by all monkeys. Then a change was made in the way in which the ash tray and tobacco tin were presented. Instead of a simultaneous discrimination, two forms of a successive discrimination task were instituted. In one—the go-no/go procedure—the monkey found a

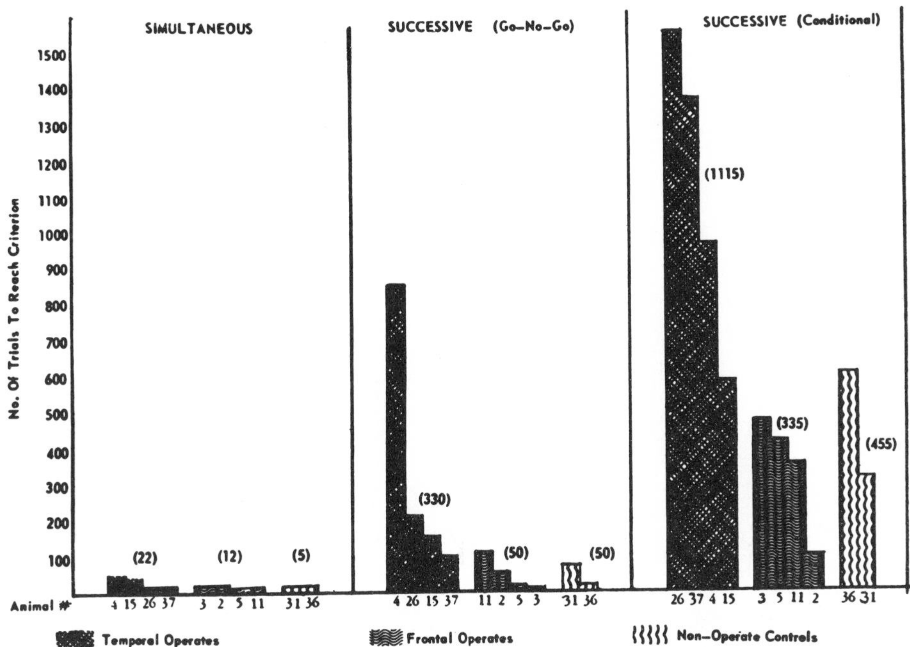

FIG. 3. Comparison of learning scores of three groups of animals (inferotemporal operates, anterofrontal operates, and non-operate controls) in a simultaneous task and two types of successive tasks in which the same cues were used. The increment of impairment of the inferotemporal group, as compared with controls, appears roughly proportional to the increasing difficulty of the task for controls.

peanut in a single box when the ash tray was present but no peanut when the tobacco tin adorned the top of the box. In the other, two boxes were present as in the simultaneous procedure but at this time the ash tray placed between them indicated that a peanut was located in the right hand box and the tobacco tin placed in the same position indicated that the peanut could be found in the left hand box. Compared with their controls, monkeys with inferotemporal cortex lesions showed severe difficulties in adjusting to the successive procedures. This, despite the fact that they could be shown on the same day in the simultaneous task to readily distinguish between ash tray and tobacco tin.

If the difficulty experienced by monkeys with inferotemporal resections—one is tempted to say, their agnosia—is not due to an inability to distinguish among objects, to what then is it attributable? Another change in the discrimination procedure provided a first clue to an answer to this question. In this modification several, rather than just two, cues were used (38). In this experiment the lesioned

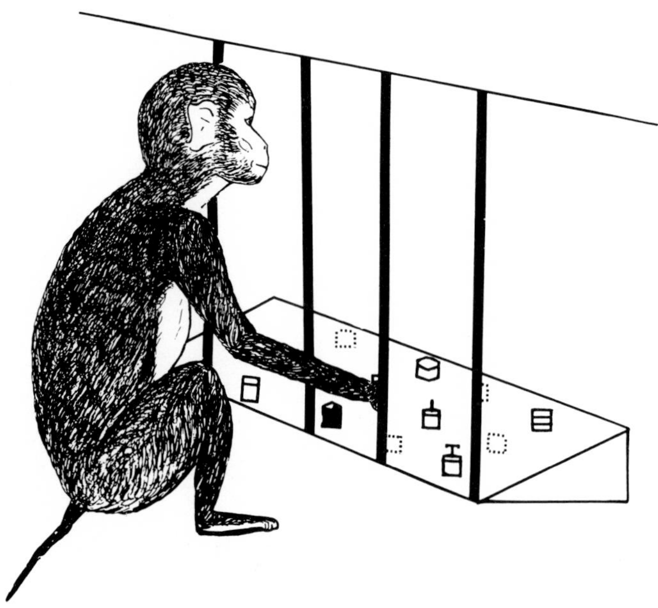

FIG. 4. Diagram of the multiple object problem showing an example of the seven object situation. Food wells are indicated by dashed circles, each of which is assigned a number. The placement of each object over a food well was shifted from trial to trial according to a random number table. A record was kept of the object moved by the monkey on each trial; only one move was allowed per trial. Trials were separated by lowering an opaque screen to hide from the monkey the objects as they were repositioned.

monkeys were shown to choose among fewer of the alternatives than their controls, suggesting a limitation on their ability to sample from an array of stimuli.

In another experiment Butter (7) showed that this limitation in sampling also occurred with respect to features within a particular cue. He taught monkeys to discriminate between two complex geometric designs and then dropped first one then another of the lines making up the designs. Normal subjects retained the ability to discriminate over a wide variety of such transformations of the cues. Monkeys with inferotemporal cortex resections began to fail after the initial transformations were undertaken.

These three experiments suggest that *selective* attention becomes impaired by the lesion, i.e., the number of alternative stimulus features which can be attended

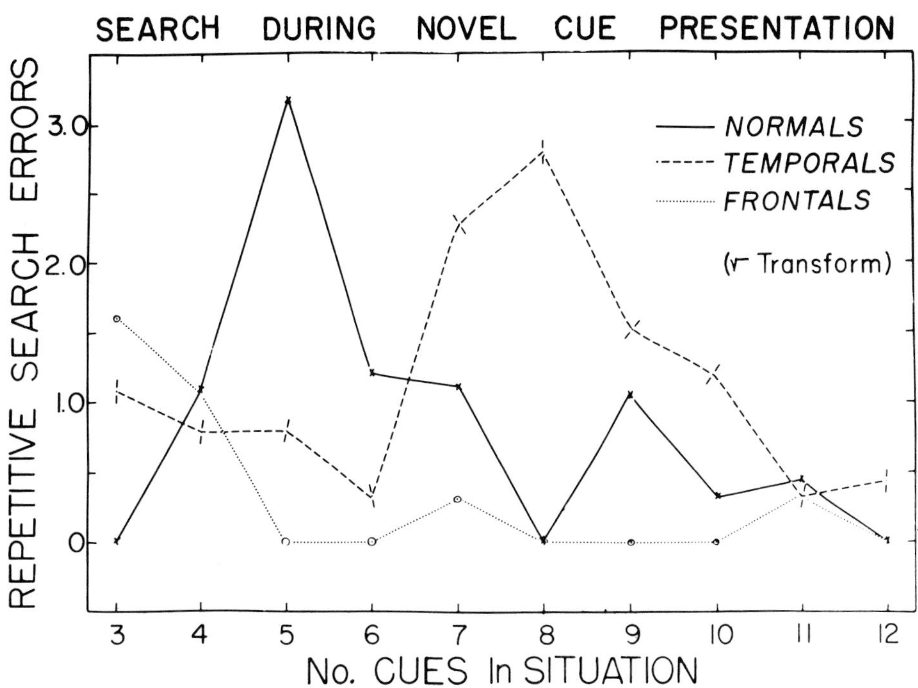

FIG. 5. Graph of the average of the number of repetitive errors made in the multiple object experiment during those search trials in each situation when the additional, i.e., the novel, cue is first added.

becomes restricted; the physiological studies suggest that the mechanism in this restriction is altered channel redundancy.

Confirmation of these hypotheses comes from an additional set of experiments. In this series the question was asked whether perhaps the difficulty in selective attention was due to a change in the way in which the lesioned monkeys observe cues. A Mackworth eye camera (21) was used to record the eye movements of monkeys (2) while they oriented to a change in one of a number of displayed cues. The course of habituation was also recorded and the distribution of eye movements was shown (4) to be indistinguishable from that of control subjects. (However, the monkeys with inferotemporal resections moved their eyes more often than did their controls.) When, on the other hand, I tried to train the monkeys to observe one of two cues by differentially reinforcing their looking at it, I failed with the lesioned group though their unoperated controls responded readily (3). These results point up another aspect of the nature of the involvement of the inferotemporal cortex in selective attention. One of the ways attention can become selective is through differential reinforcement, and the inferotemporal cortex appears to be critically involved in this process.

THE EFFERENT HYPOTHESIS

The next questions to be answered concern the neural mechanism involved in selective attention and the relationship between selective attention and agnosia. As already noted, the classical view of the agnosias posits some association between "sensations, perceptions, ideas or feelings." These associations are assumed to occur via cortico-cortical connections between primary sensory receiving areas, connections which converge onto the association areas of the cortex. This hypothesis of the critical importance of cortico-cortical associations in the production of agnosias (and aphasias) is being actively pursued in man (14). But in monkey, a series of experimental results has led to an alternate view. The monkey brain appears not to be critically connected by its cortico-cortical pathways. In one experiment a comparison was made between the effects on visual discrimination of cross-hatching and undercutting the inferotemporal cortex. Cross-hatching, i.e., interrupting transcortical connections failed to impair visual discrimination learning. Undercutting the inferotemporal cortex on the other hand produced as much difficulty as does resection of this cortex (Figs. 6 and 7 and Table 1).

TABLE 1

	Animal	3 vs. 8	R vs. G	3 vs. 8
Crosshatch	158	380	82	0
	159	180	100	0
	161	580	50	0
	166	130	0	0
Undercut	163	(1014)	100	300
	164	(1030)	200	(500)
	167	704	50	0
	168	(1030)	150	(500)
Normal	160	280	100	0
	162	180	100	0
	165	280	100	0
	170	350	100	0

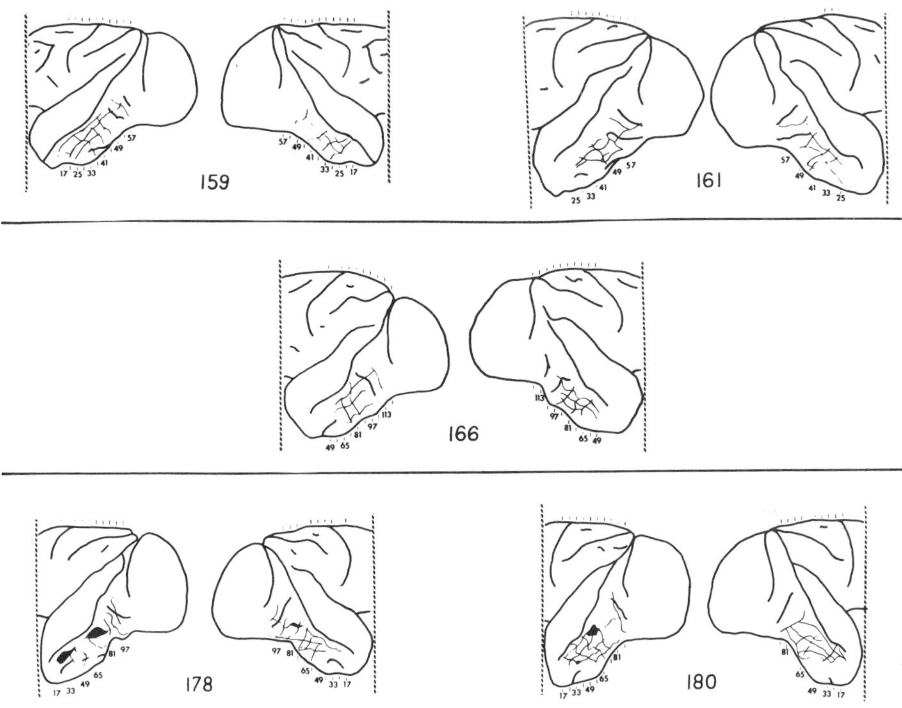

FIG. 6. Reconstructions of the cross-hatch lesions of Ss 159, 161, 166 (original learning), and 178 (retention). (Fine lines indicate the lesions.)

The question arises as to where the undercut fibers of the inferotemporal cortex connect. One possibility that must be considered is that the undercutting has severed U fibers originating in the striate area, the primary visual cortex. This possibility is ruled out by the fact that all known cortico-cortical connections of the striate area are with the peristriate cortex. There remains, of course, the possibility of a two-step indirect connection between visual projection and inferotemporal cortex via the peristriate area. To test this possibility, the striate and temporal cortex were radically disconnected from one another by making essentially complete resections of peristriate cortex and testing the effects on visual discrimination behavior. The results of this experiment confirmed those of earlier ones (9) in that monkeys could readily perform visual discriminations despite the radical disconnections (Fig. 8), (36).

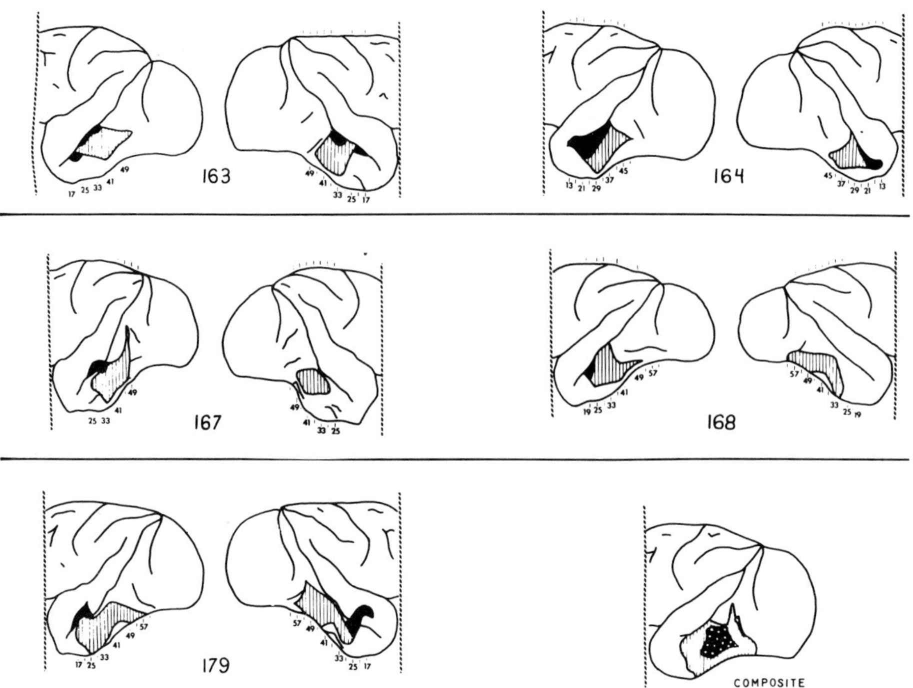

FIG. 7. Reconstructions of the undercut lesions of Ss 163, 164, 167, 168 (original learning), and 179 (retention). (Black indicates superficial cortical damage; stripes indicate the deep lesion.)

Where else could the undercut temporal lobe fibers critical to visual discrimination connect? A second possibility is that a second visual input system, in parallel with the primary projection system, has been interrupted. Such a second system has been described to exist in lower primates (16, 42), and there is a thalamic input to the inferotemporal cortex of the rhesus monkey from the pulvinar (6, 8) which could be the homologue of the second system of lower primates. However, experiments in which the pulvinar was destroyed failed to influence visual discrimination (10); in an as yet unpublished study (25), some 35 such lesions which destroyed the entire extent of the pulvinar and more, have left visual discrimination intact.

Because of results such as these, which have become ever more persuasive in recent years, I suggested some fifteen years ago yet a third alternative for the criti-

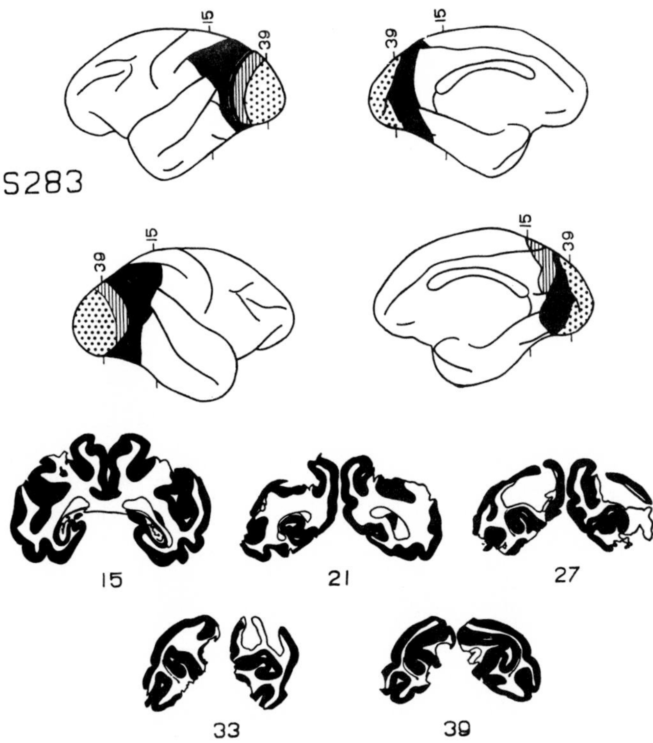

FIG. 8. Reconstruction of bilateral prestriate lesions after which monkey could still perform a visual discrimination (the numerals 3 vs. 8).

cal connections of the inferotemporal cortex: viz., that corticofugal, efferent fibers leave the temporal lobe to connect downstream with visual structures such as the superior colliculus to alter the functions of the primary visual projections. I specified the tegmental region of the brain stem rather than the thalamic because preliminary anatomical studies had shown no direct connections from the temporal cortex to the lateral geniculate nucleus (47). I want now to report a series of electrophysiological studies undertaken to test the hypothesis that the inferotemporal cortex exerts control over visual input and to determine the pathways by which this control may be effected.

The clearest evidence that the temporal cortex can control the activity of visual input system comes from studies of the effects of electrical stimulation of the inferotemporal cortex on unit activity recorded from cells in the visual input system by microelectrodes. The results of a series of experiments demonstrating this corticofugal effect is shown in Figure 9 (43, 44).

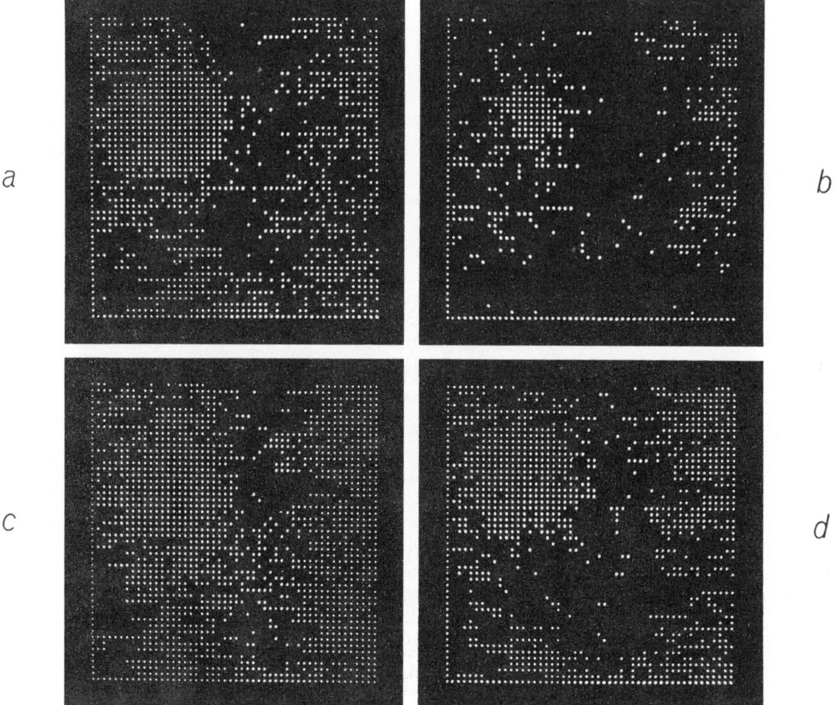

FIG. 9. Visual-receptive field maps show how information flowing through the primary visual pathway is altered by stimulation elsewhere in the brain. Map a is the normal response of a cell in the geniculate nucleus when a light source is moved through a raster-like pattern. Map b shows how the field is contracted by stimulation of the inferior temporal cortex. Map c shows the expansion produced by stimulation of the frontal cortex. Map d is a final control taken 55 minutes after recording a.

Two questions are immediately raised by this demonstration: 1. What are the efferent pathways to the visual input system from the temporal cortex, and 2. What is the functional significance of these pathways? The anatomical question had already been posed in the studies (of Whitlock and Nauta) referred to above and was reinvestigated by electrophysiological methods (38). Essentially four major corticofugal pathways have been shown to exist. 1. The connection from the temporal cortex to the superior colliculus, already mentioned, turns out to originate only in the posterior part of the inferotemporal cortex (and in the peristriate cortex). Therefore this connection by itself cannot account for the role of the inferotemporal cortex in vision. 2. A connection between inferotemporal cortex and amygdala which, however, arises only from the most anterior extremity of the cortex involved in vision. In view of the close connection between temporal pole and amygdala and the fact that resections of neither the pole nor amygdala produce visual impairment, I feel that these connections represent an overlap between inferotemporal and polar areas. These considerations plus the facts that there are no direct connections between inferotemporal cortex and other limbic structures (such as the hippocampus) and that resections of limbic structures do not lead to visual discrimination deficits tends to disconfirm hypotheses (14) which explain the functions of the association cortex of monkeys on the assumption that such connections are critical. 3. A connection between inferotemporal cortex and pulvinar. Interestingly, this connection is not with that part of the pulvinar (posterior inferior) which projects to the inferotemporal cortex but with a portion somewhat anterior and lateral. Thus a simple direct feedback loop appears precluded. The possible functional role of these connections therefore remains unexplained. 4. A connection between inferotemporal cortex and the basal ganglia: tail of the caudate nucleus and ventral putamen. The vast extent of this connection and the large size of the potentials evoked in the basal ganglia by inferotemporal stimulation came as a surprise in the electrophysiological experiments. Anatomical studies, however, have confirmed the stimulation data (Fig. 10) (19) and, in my opinion, these connections account fully for the results obtained by Rosvold and Szwarcbart (39) that stereotaxic lesions in the region of the tail of the caudate nucleus and ventral putamen drastically disrupt visual discriminations. What remains to be uncovered is the pathway by which the basal ganglia control visual input. Experiments to do this are now under way.

In summary, neuroanatomical, neurophysiological and neurobehavioral experiments indicate that it is likely that the visual functions of the inferotemporal cortex depend on corticofugal efferents to the basal ganglia which influence the primary visual projection system by an as yet unspecified pathway.

CHANNEL REDUNDANCY AND ATTENTION

Given the probability that the brain's association areas work by way of corticofugal efferents that alter the functions of the primary projection system, the question arises as to how that efferent control is manifest. A clue toward an answer to this question has come from a series of electrophysiological experiments on the effects of

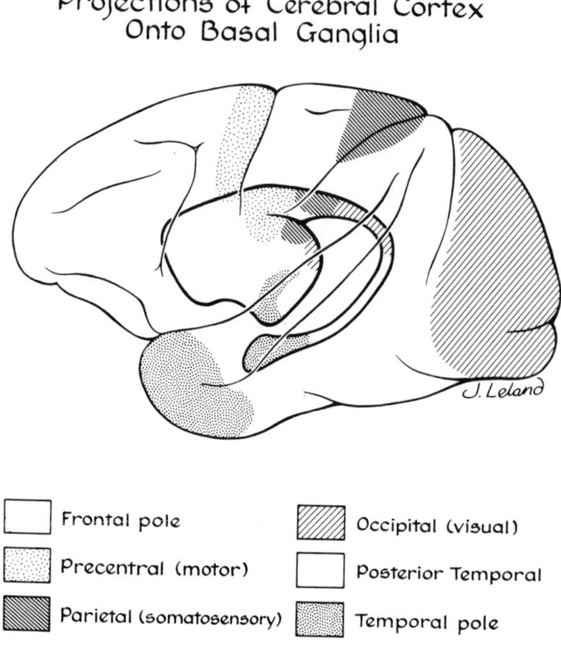

FIG. 10. Diagram of the projections of cerebral cortex onto the caudate nucleus and putamen. There is considerable overlap not shown in diagram.

electrical stimulation of the inferotemporal cortex on recovery cycles in the visual input system (43). In fully awake monkeys such recovery cycles were initiated by presenting double flashes separated by a varying interval of between 25 and 250 msec. The amplitude of the two responses evoked at the visual cortex was measured and the ratio of second to first plotted as a function of the interflash interval. The plot gave the recovery function of the system for a particular monkey and this remained stable over weeks of testing. Continuous electrical stimulation of the inferotemporal cortex was then begun and the recovery function obtained under the new condition. Figure 11 shows the effect of such stimulation: the recovery is slowed by stimulation of the inferotemporal cortex.

An interpretation of these results can be made in information processing terms: slowing of recovery indicates that a greater number of fibers of the input channel remain "busy" for longer during the stimulation condition. This effectively reduces

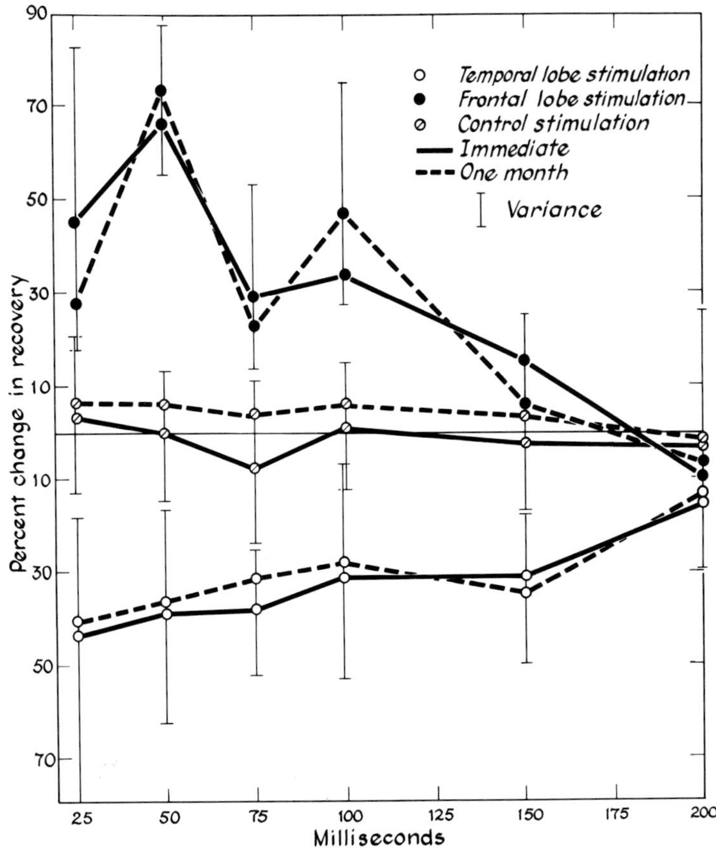

FIG. 11. The change produced by cortical stimulation in recovery of a response in an afferent channel. Cortical stimulation of 8 Hertz was maintained continuously for several months. Control stimulations were performed on the parietal cortex. Records were made immediately after the onset of stimulation and weekly thereafter. The initial recovery functions and those obtained after 1 month are shown. Vertical bars represent actual variability of the records obtained in each group of four monkeys.

the number of fibers carrying the signal evoked by the second flash and thus reduces redundancy in the channel whenever more than a single brief signal is processed. Redundancy reduction implies an enhanced information density in the channel, i.e., at any moment, the channel capacity for processing information becomes increased.

Because of the importance of these results to an understanding of the functions of the inferotemporal cortex, additional studies were undertaken. Very quickly we found that we had not specified all of the variables necessary for replication. Sometimes the effect on recovery function was seen clearly; in other experiments it was lacking. Finally a fortuitous accident pointed the direction our research must take. Because of the crowded condition of the laboratory, Lauren Gerbrandt, then a post-doctoral fellow, began to perform the recovery cycle experiments at night. His wife was pressed into service to help catch and place the monkey in a restraining chair. One evening, after good results had been pouring in nightly, she brought a friend along to help pass the waiting time while her husband was testing. She told her friend of the experiment and the usual wifely chatter continued for a time in the large room in which the experiment was conducted. And lo! the slowing of recovery previously obtained whenever the inferotemporal cortex had been stimulated now ceased. Gerbrandt called me and we quickly put his serendipitous observation to test. We took a record under normal quiet conditions and then opened the testing cage so the monkey could see me and took another record. The recovery function became slowed while the monkey attended me and this slowing was comparable to that produced by inferotemporal cortex stimulation in the inattentive condition. While the monkey was visually or auditorily attending, the temporal lobe stimulation had no further slowing effect. In short, behavioral attention and electrical stimulation of the inferotemporal cortex converged to produce the same effect on input channel redundancy.

A direct test of the importance of the attention variable in the recovery function experiment was then made. Other research (41) had shown that the potential evoked in the visual cortex of awake monkeys by an electrical pulse delivered to the lateral geniculate nucleus was sensitive to attentiveness. Using such a probe stimulus we first checked and confirmed the earlier observation and then used this phenomenon as a probe to gauge attentiveness in a recovery cycle experiment run during the day. Recovery functions obtained during periods of attention (e.g., when someone in high heels came down the hall) as gauged by the probe were separated by computer from those obtained during periods of inattention. Now beautiful records of slowing were again recorded consistently—but only during the periods when the monkeys were inattentive (13). Our initial experiments had taken much longer to perform than subsequent ones since we were still groping and so tested the monkeys daily with a large number of stimuli (e.g., single flash, double flash, single click, double click, click-flash and flash-click) repeated over and over. Not only the monkeys but the experimenters became inattentive; I remember many occasions when the monkey had to be prodded from time to time to keep him from falling asleep—a procedure which helped keep me from doing the same.

The results of these experiments suggest that the inferotemporal cortex is somehow involved in the process of visual attention, a suggestion supported by the findings of Gross et al.(15) that unit recordings from cells in this cortex register when the monkey is visually attending. The nature of this attentive process and its relation to recognition becomes evident from the results of yet another series of experiments,

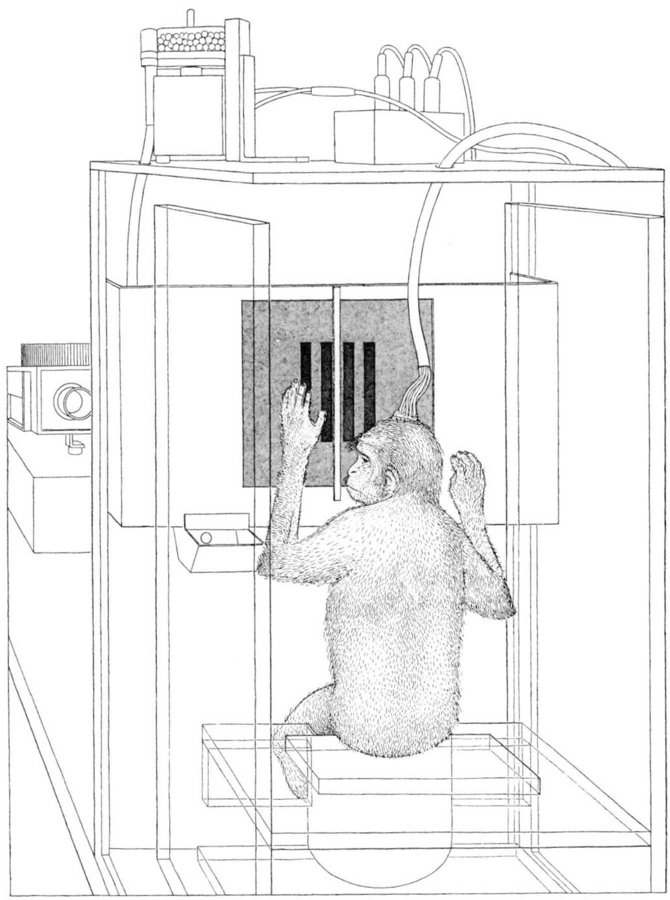

FIG. 12. On the translucent panel in front of him, the monkey sees either a circle or a series of vertical stripes, which have been projected from the rear. He is rewarded with a peanut, which drops into the receptable at his left elbow, if he presses the right half of the panel when he sees the circle or the left half when he sees the stripes. Electrodes record the wave forms that appear in the monkey's visual cortex as he develops skill at this task. Early in the experiments the wave forms show whether the monkey sees the circle or stripes. Eventually they reveal in advance which half of the panel the monkey will press.

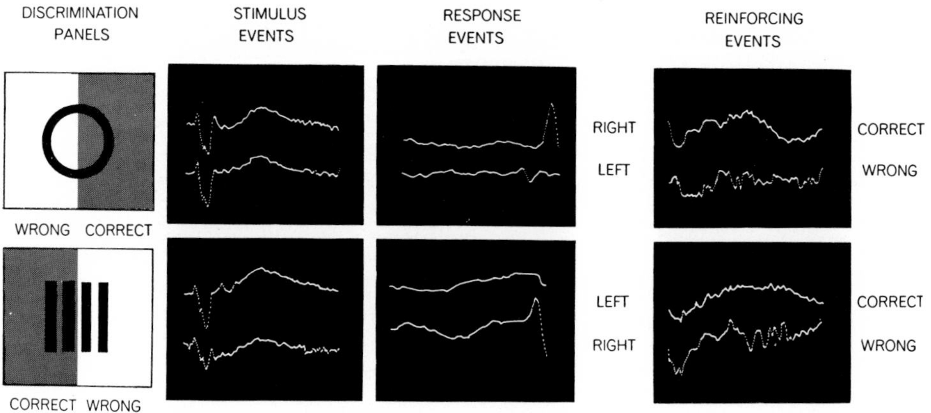

FIG. 13. Results of visual-discrimination experiment are shown in the wave forms recorded from the striate (visual) cortex of a monkey. The waves are those after he has learned the task illustrated in Figure 12. The records under "Stimulus events" are wave forms that appear immediately after the monkey has been shown a circle or stripes. The records under "Response events" were generated just prior to the moment when the monkey actually responded by pressing either the left or the right half of the panel. The records under "Reinforcing events" were produced when the monkey was rewarded with a peanut if he was correct or not rewarded if he was wrong. The correct response was to press the right half of the panel on seeing a circle, the left half on seeing stripes. A difference in the "stimulus" wave forms indicates whether the monkey has seen stripes or a circle. After he has learned his task well, sharp differences appear in the response and reinforcing records. The response wave forms, which are actually "intention" waves, show one pattern (the one with the sharp peak) whenever the monkey is about to press the right half of the panel, regardless of whether he has seen a circle or stripes. If he has actually seen stripes, of course, pressing the right half of the panel is the wrong response. Thus the wave forms reflect his intention to press a particular half of the panel. They could hardly reveal whether his response is going to be right or wrong because at this point he still "thinks" he is about to make the correct response.

described below.

The most recent set of experiments performed in my laboratories demonstrates this relationship directly. Electrical recordings were made from the primary visual (35) and inferotemporal (40) cortices during visual discrimination performances. In order to generate analyzable transients in the brain, the cues were flashed briefly (1 microsec.) onto a translucent divided panel each side of which could be pressed in order to obtain reinforcement (Fig. 12). In the primary visual cortex, wave forms could be distinguished that reflected the differences between the cues presented to the monkey's retina (Fig. 13). In the inferotemporal cortex no such distinction could be made out. When, however, a somewhat more complicated task was presented—cues that differed in two dimensions, i.e., both in color and shape—the electrical activity recorded from the inferotemporal cortex correlated with the dimension responded to by the monkey. Specifically (but somewhat oversimply) monkeys were trained to discriminate color (e.g., green was rewarded, reinforced) until stable criterion performance was reached when recordings were made. Then they were taught the shape dimension (e.g., circle was reinforced), and again when stable performance was reached, recordings were made (Figs. 14 and 15). The records were then compared by computer analysis and differences were demonstrated. Note that the stimulus configuration displayed to the monkey's retina is identical in the two situations: only the reinforcing contingencies and therefore the responses generated are different. This is demonstrated by the fact that in this situation the brain electrical records anchored to the time of stimulus presentation do not reflect the dimension attended—only when the records are analyzed using the moment of response (panel pressing) do these differences in brain record show up.

CONCLUSION

These penultimate experiments demonstrate once again that the inferotemporal cortex is primarily involved in the "motor" function of responding to, rather than the "sensory" process of distinguishing between, visual cues. Thus if association does take place by virtue of the association cortex, it is not association between cues but between cue and the outcome of response, i.e., between cue and reinforcer. The system of which association cortex is a part and which apparently includes the basal ganglia is involved in establishing a m o t o r set which reinforces discrimination learning through enhancing the process of selective attention. This is accomplished in part at least by increasing the capability of input channels to simultaneously transmit and select among different signals. Recognition, making identifications in the sensory world, depends on this m o t o r process. When lesions of the association cortex of the brain impair identification, agnosias result.

Thus, an answer to Von Monakov's questions has been obtained, at least for the monkey. Agnosia does involve sensory (channel) capacity. Lesions of the association cortex affect sensory processing because the critical connections of the association cortex are the efferents to the input systems, not the afferents from them. But the input systems per se need not be anatomically disrupted in order that agnosia

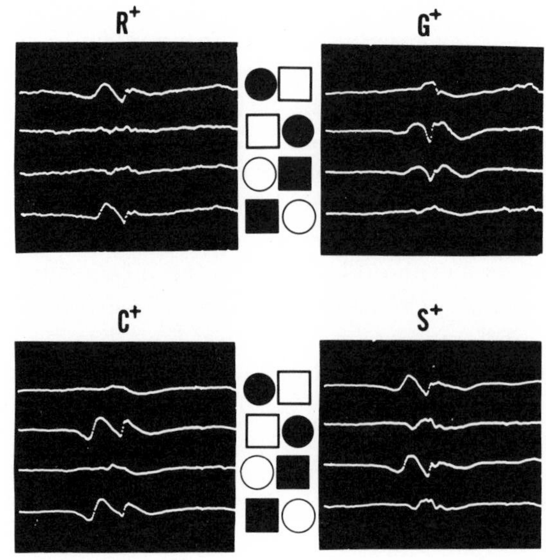

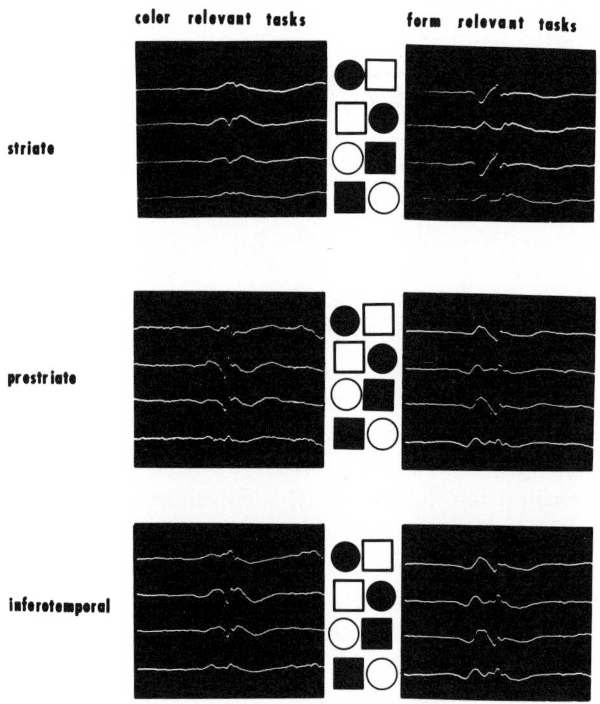

Figures 14 and 15

FIGS. 14 and 15. Results of an experiment demonstrating the functions of the inferotemporal cortex by behavioral electrophysiological techniques. The experiment is similar to the one described in Figs. 12 and 13. A monkey initiates a flashed stimulus display and responds by pressing either the right or left half of the display panel to receive a reward while electrical brain recordings are made on line with a small general purpose computer (PDP-8). In this experiment the flashed stimulus consisted of colored (red and green) stripes and circles. Reinforcing contingencies determined whether the monkeys were to attend and respond to the pattern (circle vs stripes) or color (red vs green) dimension of the stimulus. As in the earlier experiment, stimulus, response, and reinforcement variables were found to be encoded in the primary visual cortex. In addition, this experiment showed that the association between stimulus dimension (pattern or color and the outcome of the response occurs first in the inferotemporal cortex. This is presented in recording 3 of Fig. 14 where the electrophysiological data averaged from the time of response (forward for 250 msec and backward 250 msec from center of record) show clear differences in waveform depending on whether pattern or color is being reinforced. Note that this difference occurs despite the fact that the retinal image formed by the flashed stimulus is identical in the pattern and color problems. Once the monkeys have been overtrained, this reinforcement produced attentional association between a stimulus dimension and response and also becomes encoded in the primary visual cortex as shown in Fig. 15.

be produced. The inability to recognize, to selectively attend to and identify the objective world, can be the result of lesions restricted to the association cortex. This cortex is not involved in association among inputs, nor in distinguishing between them, but in establishing, on the basis of reinforcement, a motor set that determines attentive selection among alternatives.

REFERENCES

1 ALBE-FESSARD, D. Activites de projection et d'association du neocortex cerebral des mammiferes. Extrait du Journal de Physiologie, 49 (1957) 521-588.

2 BAGSHAW, M.H., MACKWORTH, N.H. and PRIBRAM, K.H. Method for recording and analyzing visual fixations in the unrestrained monkey. Perceptual and Motor Skills, 31 (1970) 219-222.

3 BAGSHAW, M.H., MACKWORTH, N.H. and PRIBRAM, K.H. The effect of inferotemporal cortex ablations on eye movements of monkeys during discrimination training. Int. J. Neuroscience, 1 (1970) 153-158.

4 BAGSHAW, M.H., MACKWORTH, N.H. and PRIBRAM, K.H. The effect of resections of inferotemporal cortex on the amygdala on visual orienting and habituation (in preparation).

5 BAY, E. Principles of classification and their influence on our concepts of aphasia. In: Disorders of Language, edited by A.V.S. de Reuck and M. O'Connor. Little Brown and Company, Boston, 1964, pp. 122-142.

6 BLUM, J.S., CHOW, K.L.,and PRIBRAM, K.H. A behavioral analysis of the organization of the parieto-temporo-preoccipital cortex. J. comp. Neurol., 93 (1950) 53-100.

7 BUTTER, C.M. The effect of discrimination training on pattern equivalence in monkeys with inferotemporal and lateral striate lesions. Neuropsychologia, 6 (1968) 27-40.

8 CHOW, K.L. A retrograde cell degeneration study of the cortical projection field of the pulvinar in the monkey. J. comp. Neurol., 93 (1950) 313-339.

9 CHOW, K.L. Further studies on selective ablation of associative cortex in relation to visually mediated behavior. J. comp. physiol. Psychol., 45 (1952) 109-118.

10 CHOW, K.L. Lack of behavioral effects following destruction of some thalamic association nuclei in monkey. Arch. Neurol. Psychiat., 71 (1954) 762-771.

11 CHOW, K.L., and PRIBRAM, K.H. Cortical projection of the thalamic ventrolateral nuclear group in monkeys. J. comp. Neurol., 104 (1956) 57-75.

12 FULTON, J.F., PRIBRAM, K.H., STEVENSON, J.A.F., and WALL, P.D. Interrelations between orbital gyrus, insula, temporal tip and anterior cingulate. Trans. Amer. Neurol. Assoc., 175 (149).

13 GERBRANDT, L.K., SPINELLI, D.N., and PRIBRAM, K.H. The interaction of visual attention and temporal cortex stimulation on electrical activity evoked in the striate cortex. Electroenceph. clin. Neurophysiol., 29 (1970) 146-155.

14 GESCHWIND, N. Disconnexion syndromes in animals and man: Part I. Brain, 88 (1965) 237-294.

15 GROSS, C.G., BENDER, D.B., and ROCHA-MIRANDA, C.E. Visual receptive fields of neurons in inferotemporal cortex of the monkey. Science, 166 (1969) 1303-1305.

16 HALL, W.C., and DIAMOND, I.T. Organization and function of the visual cortex in hedgehog. I. Cortical cytoarchitecture and thalamic retrograde degeneration. Brain, Behav. Evol. I (1968) 181-214.

17 HEAD, H. Studies in Neurology. Medical Publications, Oxford, 1920.

18 KAADA, B.R., PRIBRAM, K.H., and EPSTEIN, J.A. Respiratory and vascular responses in monkeys from temporal pole, insula, orbital surface and cingulate gyrus. A preliminary report. J. Neurophysiol., 12 (1949) 347-356.

19 KEMP, J.M., and POWELL, T.P.S. The cortico-striate projection in the monkey. Brain, 93 (1970) 525-546.

20 LENNOX, M.A., DUNSMORE, R.H., EPSTEIN, J.A., and PRIBRAM, K.H. Electrocorticographic effects of stimulation of posterior orbital, temporal and cingulate areas of Macaca mulatta. J. Neurophysiol., 13 (1950) 383-388.

21 MACKWORTH, N.H. A stand camera for line-of-sight recording. Perception & Psychophysics, 2 (1967) 119-127.

22 MACLEAN, P.D., and PRIBRAM, K.H. A neuronographic analysis of the medial and basal cerebral cortex. I. cat. J. Neurophysiol., 16 (1953) 312-323.

23 MALIS, L.I., PRIBRAM, K.H., and KRUGER, L. Action potentials in "motor" cortex evoked by peripheral nerve stimulation. J. Neurophysiol., 16, (1953) 161-167.

24 MILNER, B. Psychological defects produced by temporal lobe excision. In: The Brain and Human Behavior (Proc. Assoc. for Res. in Nerv. & Ment. Dis., Vol XXXVI), Williams & Wilkins Co., Baltimore, 1958, pp. 244-257.

25 MISHKIN, M., and ROSVOLD, H.E. (unpublished study).

26 MONAKOV, C. VON. Die Lokalisation im Grosshien und der Abbau der Funktion Durch Korticale Herde. J.F. Bergmann, Wiesbaden, 1914.

27 PRIBRAM, K.H. Toward a science of neuropsychology: (Method and data). In: Current Trends in Psychology and the Behavioral Sciences, Ed. R.A. Patton, University of Pittsburgh Press, Pittsburgh, 1954, pp. 115-142.

28 PRIBRAM, K.H. On the neurology of thinking. Behav. Sci., 4 (1959) 265-287.

29 PRIBRAM, K.H., and BAGSHAW, M.H. Further analysis of the temporal lobe syndrome utilizing frontotemporal ablations in monkeys. J. comp. Neurol., 99 (1953) 347-375.

30 PRIBRAM, K.H., CHOW, K.L., and SEMMES, J. Limit and organization of the cortical projection from the medial thalamic nucleus in monkeys. J. comp. Neurol., 95 (1953) 433-448.

31 PRIBRAM, K.H., and FULTON, J.F. An experimental critique of the effects of anterior cingulate ablations in monkeys. Brain, 77 (1954) 34-44.

32 PRIBRAM, K.H., LENNOX, M.A., and DUNSMORE, R.H. Some connections of the orbito-fronto-temporal, limbic and hippocampal areas of Macaca mulatta. J. Neurophysiol., 13 (1950) 127-135.

33 PRIBRAM, K.H., and MACLEAN, P.D. A neuronographic analysis of the medial and basal cerebral cortex: II. Monkey. J. Neurophysiol., 16 (1953) 324-340.

34 PRIBRAM, K.H., and MISHKIN, M. Simultaneous and successive visual discrimination by monkeys with inferotemporal lesions. J. comp. physiol. Psychol., 48 (1955) 198-202.

35 PRIBRAM, K.H., SPINELLI, D.N., and KAMBACK, M.C. Electrocortical correlates of stimulus response and reinforcement. Science, 157 (1967) 94-96.

36 PRIBRAM, K.H., SPINELLI, D.N., and REITZ, S.L. Effects of radical disconnexion of occipital and temporal cortex on visual behavior of monkeys. Brain, 92 (1969) 301-312.

37 PRIBRAM, K.H., ROSNER, B.S., and ROSENBLITH, W.A. Electrical responses to acoustic clicks in monkey: extent of neocortex activated. J. Neurophysiol., 17 (1954) 336-344.

38 REITZ, S.L., and PRIBRAM, K.H. Some subcortical connections of the inferotemporal gyrus of monkey. Exp. Neurol., 25 (1969) 632-645.

39 ROSVOLD, H.E., and SZWARCBART, M.K. Neural structures involved in delayed-response performance. In: The Frontal Granular Cortex and Behavior. Eds. J.M. Warren and K. Akert, McGraw Hill, New York, 1964, pp. 1-15.

40 ROTHBLAT, L., and PRIBRAM, K.H. Selective attention: an electrophysiological analysis of monkey (submitted to Brain Research).

41 SCHOOLMAN, A., and EVARTS, E.V. Responses to lateral geniculate radiation stimulation in cats with implanted electrodes. J. Neurophysiol., 22 (1959) 112-129.

42 SNYDER, M., and DIAMOND, I.T. The organization and function of the visual cortex in the tree shrew. Brain, Behav. Evol. 1 (1968) 244-288.

43 SPINELLI, D.N., and PRIBRAM, K.H. Changes in visual recovery functions produced by temporal lobe stimulation in monkeys. Electroenceph. clin. Neurophysiol., 20 (1966) 44-49.

44 SPINELLI, D.N., and PRIBRAM, K.H. Changes in visual recovery function and unit activity produced by frontal cortex stimulation. Electroenceph. clin. Neurophysiol., 22 (1967) 143-149.

45 THOMPSON, R.F., JOHNSON, R.H., and HOOPES, J.J. Organization of auditory somatic sensory, and visual projection to association fields of cerebral cortex in the cat. J. Neurophysiol., 26 (1963) 343-364.

46 WALL, P.D., and PRIBRAM, K.H. Trigeminal neurotomy and blood pressure responses from stimulation of lateral cerebral cortex of Macaca mulatta. J. Neurophysiol., 13 (1950) 409-412.

47 WHITLOCK, D.G., and NAUTA, W.J. Subcortical projections from the temporal neocortex in Macaca mulatta. J. comp. Neurol., 106 (1956) 183-212.

DISCUSSION

METTLER: I don't think we should be deluded by the rather casual way that Karl presented this material. This is an elegant display of experimental techniques in an area which is extremely difficult to handle, and I congratulate you, Karl. What he has just shown you throws into relief the importance of two systems concerning which we have so far had only a few hints during the presentations of the last two days. He has opened the way to a new symposium, dealing with the interconnections of the cortex and striatum and pallidum, on the one hand, and between the striatum and pallidum with the thalamus, on the other. What is the difference between the functions of the cortex and extrapyramidal systems insofar as peak performance in sensory, motor and associative functions are concerned? The difference he has shown you is one of power, from the point of view of what we may call the associational handling of sensory experience. Without the striatum the animal is quite unable to relate itself to its environment at a satisfactory level of self-maintenance. Without its cortex it is unable to relate itself accurately to its environment but it still can do it. The cat, maligned feline though it may be, is able to get along reasonably well without much cortex but if you add a sizeable striatal deficit to this, the animal looks at you with vacuous eyes and, in an uncomprehending manner, will walk out of a third floor window with complete unconcern.

Corticothalamic Projections and Sensorimotor Activities
T. Frigyesi, E. Rinvik, and M.D. Yahr, editors. © 1972
Raven Press, New York.

Hexapartition of Inputs as a Primary Role of the Thalamus

Rolf Hassler

In the history of brain research, there have been many attempts to understand the functional role of the great subcortical ganglion, the thalamus.* The question should properly be asked as to why the 120 nerve cell complexes which form the thalamus according to the author (12, 13, 15) are inserted in all the sensory systems, except the olfactory, on the way to their analyzing cortical fields. At first, the answer seems easy—not all of the distinct thalamic nuclei project to cortical fields; only 60 (i.e., half) do so, while the other half of the nuclei project to subcortical centers exclusively or in addition to a collateral cortical projection.

A more explicit interpretation of the thalamus function is offered by determining the number of terminal nuclei of each sensory system in the thalamus. A thalamic nucleus is characterized by the site where its terminals exert action and by the afferents which it receives. Particularly in the thalamus each nucleus has its own peculiar cytoarchitecture with a special but variable type of interneuron (Fig. 1) and its own peculiar fiber arrangement or myeloarchitecture.

The thalamus is comprised of nine regions: anterior, medial, intralaminar, lateral, geniculate bodies, pulvinar, ganglion habenulae (or pedunculi conarii), all distinguished by BURDACH (1819-1826) (5); and the periventricular gray and the reticulate regions (or Gitterschicht). Because of their phylogenetic age, the central gray of the third ventricle and the habenula are excluded from the present discussion. These regions are also exceptions in that they do not have the special thalamic type of small

----

* The expression thalamus, θαλαμος, was first used by GALEN (8) when he stated: "The optic nerves originate sidewards on the end of the front ventricles: these ventricles (!) form, so to say, a closet for them," (Greek "thalame"). Referring to the upper parts of the diencephalon, the term, thalamus nervorum opticorum, was first used by WILLIS (1676) (42). As early as 1724, SANTORINI (37) found this name inapt, because the origin of optic nerves is only near to them. In fact, the supplementary adjective, opticus, is misleading and should be omitted, because all sensory and even the motor and coordinating systems are represented in the thalamus.

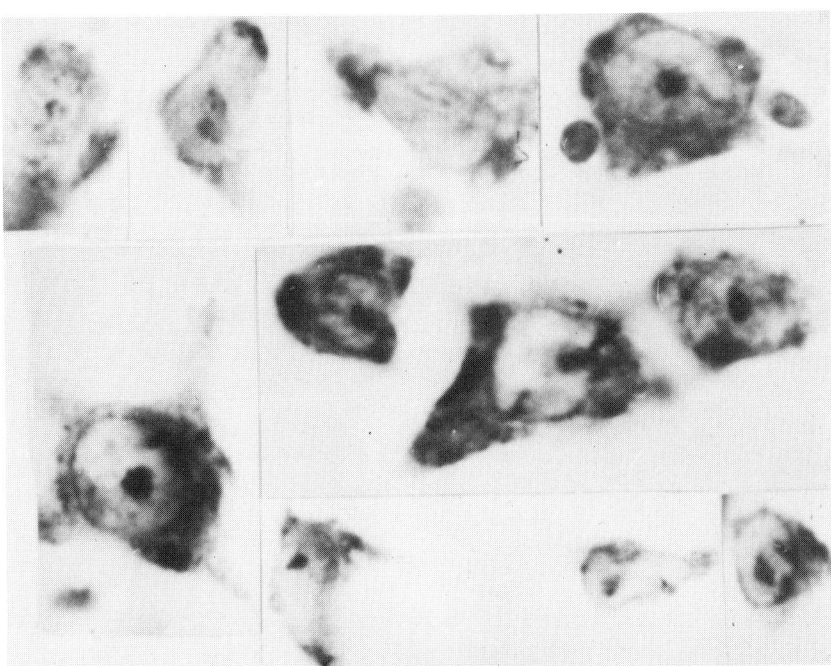

FIG. 1. Examples (a,b,c,g,h) of small interneurons of specific thalamic nuclei. Characteristic are the small but not clear nucleus with a small and especially pale nucleolus bordered by a dark marginal body and the centrally light cytoplasm with marginally accumulated Nissl bodies. A proposed name therefore was parvonucleolar cells. In d, e and the middle of f: three typical nerve cells of the medial nuclei of the thalamus.

interneuron which otherwise seems to be thalamospecific.

The lateral thalamic region comprises all the ventral nuclei for special sensory systems. Above these ventral nuclei two sets of nuclei extend, supplied by 1) only some collateral terminals (zentrolateral nuclei), or by 2) a few or none at all (dorsal nuclei). The geniculate bodies are derivatives of the ventral nuclei for teleceptive senses; the parts of the pulvinar are derivatives of the dorsal or zentrolateral segments of the lateral thalamic region. Each of the different portions of the reticulate zone of the thalamus is allied with a special portion of the lateral region. The same applies to the nuclei of the envelope of the medial nucleus. Thus the predominant mass of thalamic nuclei can be considered together, excluding the two phylogenetically old structures and the "intrinsic" anterior and medial nuclei.

There are at least 12 different afferent systems of projections to the ventral and corresponding thalamic nuclei:

1. visual
2. auditory
3. taste tract

4. spinothalamic (somatotopic including quintothalamic fibers from subnucleus caudalis tractus spinalis trigemini)
5. cervicothalamic (somatotopic including quinto-thalamic fibers from subnucleus oralis tractus spinalis trigemini)
6. medial lemniscus (somatotopic including lemniscus trigemini from the main sensory nucleus)
7. spindle afferents (somatotopic: tractus spinocerebellaris dorsalis, nucleus cuneatus externus and radix mesencephalica trigemini)
8. vestibular (ipsiversive) system
9. efferent cerebellar systems
10. non-horizontal directional systems from the nuclei of posterior commissure
11. internal pallidar (contraversive) system
12. external pallidar system.

I will first try to explain the terminal nuclei of the spinothalamic tract. 1. Its relay nucleus in the parvocellular ventrocaudal nucleus (V.c.pc) projects to the area 3b of postcentral gyrus in man (16) as well as in higher primates including baboon; 2. its integrative nucleus of the first level, the Z.c (caudal zentrolateral nucleus), also receives spinothalamic terminals (Fig. 2); 3. its integrative nucleus of the second level is probably represented in the caudal dorsal nucleus (D.c) without direct spinothalamic input; 4. it participates with the limitans and intralaminar nuclei in the truncothalamic or unspecific projection system (Fig. 2); 5. it contributes many terminals to the magnocellular nucleus of the medial geniculate body (G.m.mc), as do all the somatosensory systems of different modalities and other sensory systems. That may be called a composite or, better, multisensory nucleus, as the cortical area to which this nucleus projects was first called by Mickle and Ades (30). 6. The last termination of spinothalamic fibers belongs to the reticulate nucleus of the thalamus (Rt.v.c) which borders on the ventrocaudalis posterior and parvocellularis.

If we consider the spinothalamic input to the reticulate nucleus,* it must be pointed out that the reticulate zone or zone grillagée, is divided into 6 segments with 18 subnuclei since each ventral, zentrolateral or dorsal nucleus (Fig. 3) is laterally bordered by a reticulate nucleus with a special structure. Until recently, the different parts of the reticulate nucleus were regarded as cortex-dependent nuclei with a more extensive projection region in the cortex than the particular thalamic nucleus (1, 15, 35). The Scheibels (39) and Minderhoud (31), however, found that neurons of the reticulate nucleus also have thalamic projections and degenerate to a more marked extent after thalamic than after cortical lesions. On the basis of my studies of hemitrophia cerebri and complete capsular degeneration, I can confirm that the reticulate nucleus in the human always degenerates less than the neighboring ventral nucleus after destruction of the corticothalamic fibers (Fig. 4A+B+C+D). What is the peculiarity of

----

* "Reticulate nucleus" is used in this chapter as a synonym for "thalamic reticular nucleus." (Eds.)

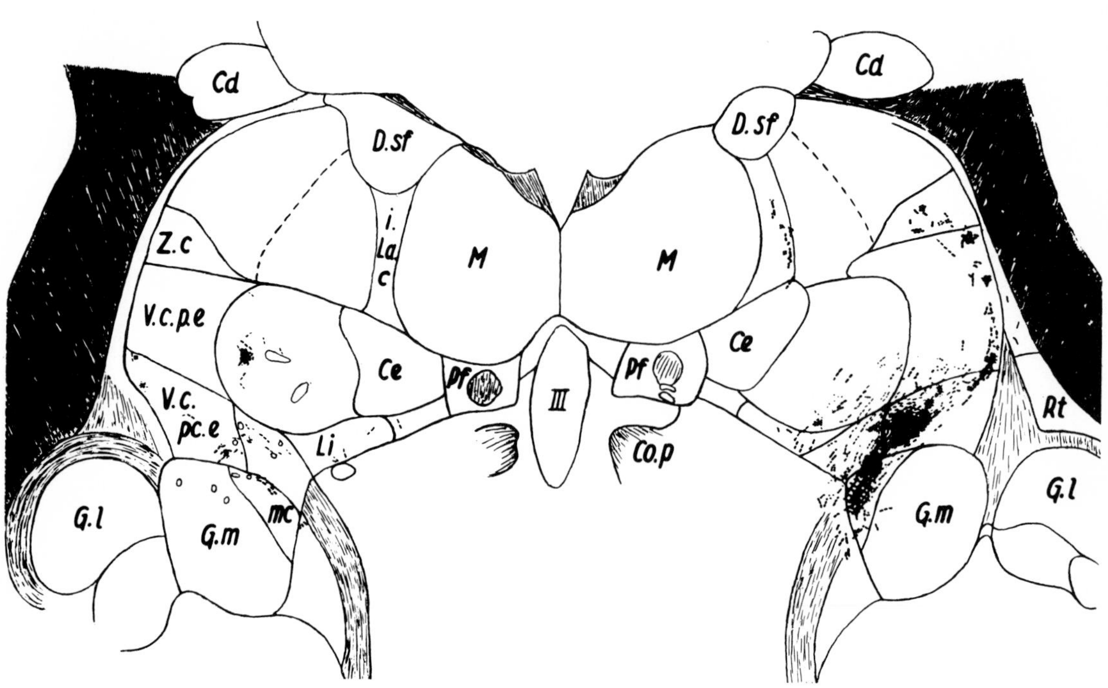

FIG. 2. Diagram of different nuclei containing terminal degenerations, in the spinothalamic tract in the baboon using Nauta-Gygax-technique after anterolateral chordotomy at level C4. The main pool of degenerated fibers turn laterally after entering the thalamus to terminate in 1. the magnocellular nucleus of medial geniculate body (G.m.mc) (polysensory); 2. the (basal) parvocellular part of the ventro-caudal nucleus (V.c.pc.e) (specific relay); 3. the caudal zentrolateral nucleus (Z.c) above the lemniscal nucleus (V.c.p.e) which also seems to receive some spinothalamic terminals (first integrative level). 4. A few terminal degenerations are found in the ventro-caudal reticulate (Rt.v.c) which is the feedback nucleus. A smaller portion of degenerated fibers turns medially in the door of the thalamus. Their terminations are unspecific (protopathic) and involve 5. the limitans nucleus (Li) and the intralaminar nuclei (i.La). (After Hassler, Imai, Kusama, and Wagner, unpublished).

FIG. 3. In a horizontal section, each ventral nucleus bordering the internal capsule (Ca.i) is laterally accompanied by a special structurally differentiated portion of the reticulate nucleus of the thalamus. Each portion receives the same afferents as the pertinent special ventral nucleus: The ventro-caudal nuclei (V.c.p and V.c.a) by the nucleus reticulatus ventro-caudalis (Rt.v.c); the ventro-intermediate nucleus (V.im.e) by the reticulate ventro-intermediate (Rt.v.im); the zentrolateral nucleus (Z.o) by the reticulate zentrolateral oral nucleus (Rt. z. o.); the ventro-oral anterior nucleus (V. o. a.) by the reticulate ventro-oral (Rt. v. o.) and the lateropolar nucleus (L. p. o.) by the reticulate polar nucleus (Rt. po.)

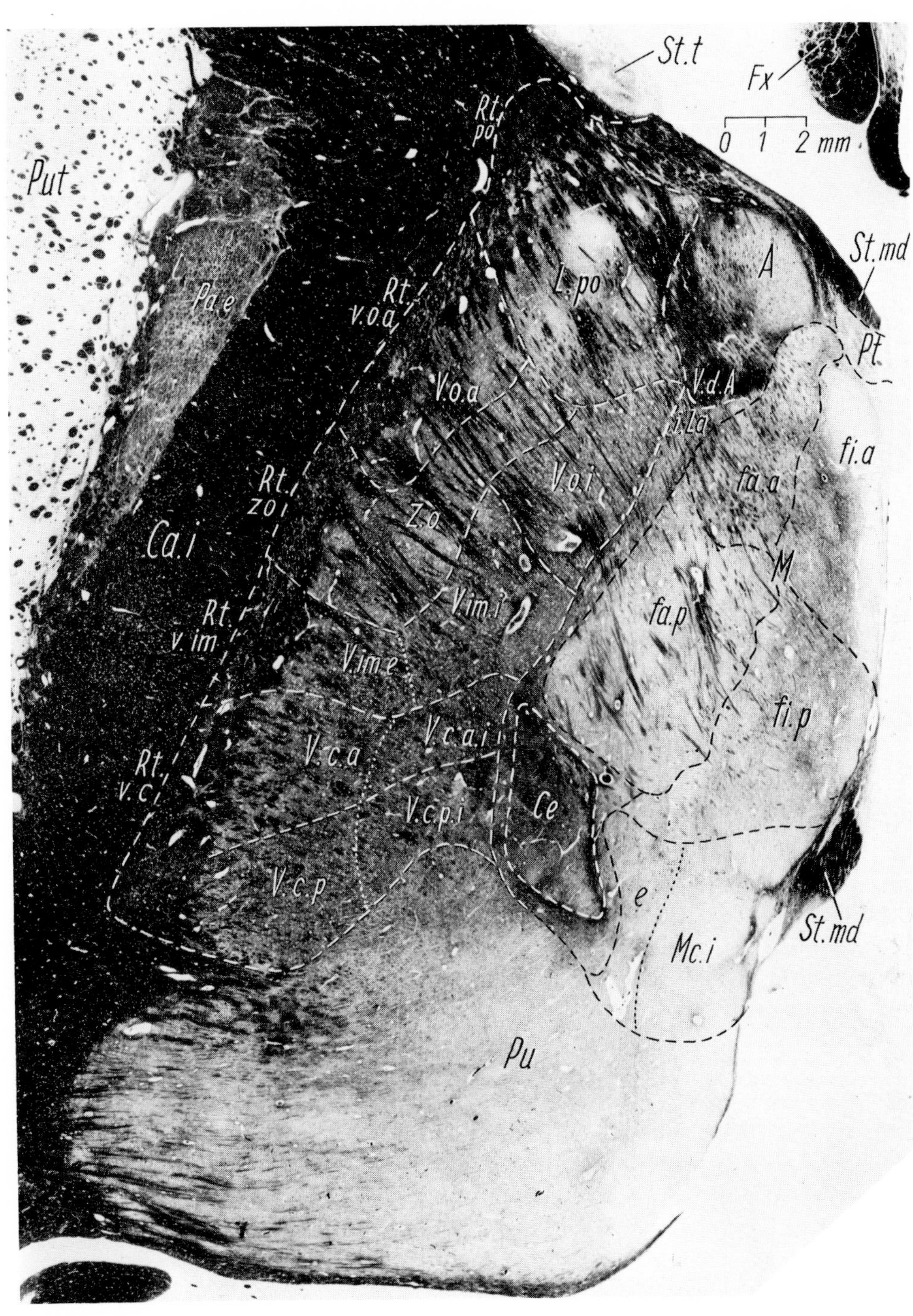
St.t
Fx
0 1 2 mm
Put
Rt. po
Pa.e
Rt. v.o.a
L.po
A
St.md
Pt
V.o.a
V.d.A
i.La
fi.a
fa.a
V.o.i
Rt. zo
Z.o
Ca.i
M
V.im.i
fa.p
Rt. v.im
V.im.e
fi.p
V.c.a.i
V.c.a
Rt. v.c
V.c.p.i
Ce
V.c.p
e
St.md
Mc.i
Pu

FIG. 3

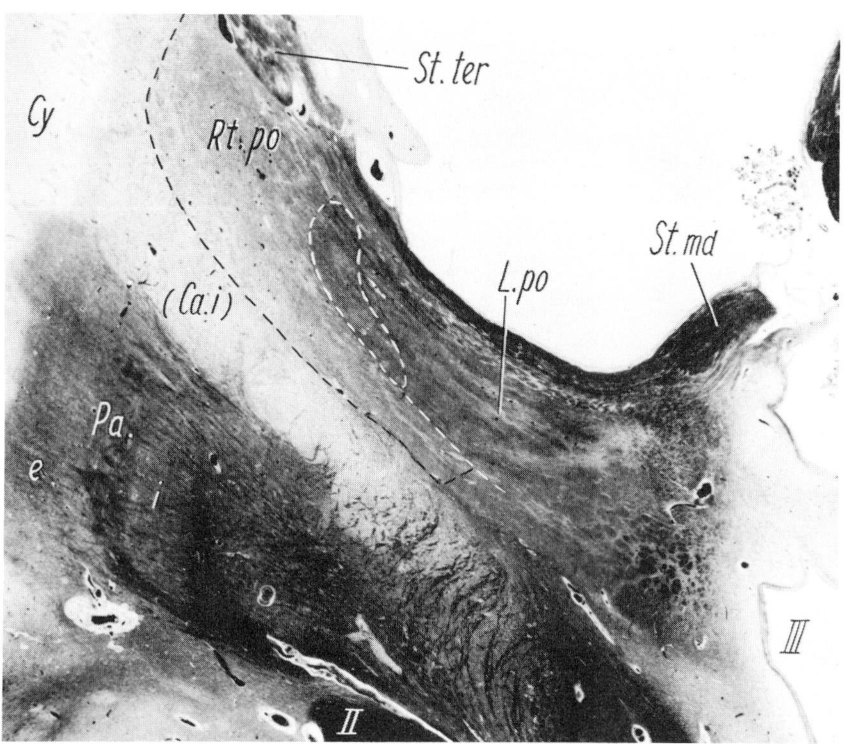

FIG. 4A. Except for its most medial portion, the internal capsule (Ca.i) of this human is almost completely degenerated due to a hemorrhage in the putamen and the rostral internal capsule. The black dots and small black curves in the capsule below L.po are direct pallidothalamic fibers connecting the dark pallidum with the lateropolar nucleus (L.po) which has lost most of its efferent fiber bundles. The reticulate nucleus lateral to L.po (Rt.po), is deprived of all fiber bundles and some of its single fibers. The corresponding Nissl picture (4B) shows the nerve cell degeneration and disintegration in L.po whereas in Rt.po most of the nerve cells are merely somewhat shrunken but preserved and the glia is proliferated.

these reticulate nuclei? Each receives special afferent inputs from one of the great sensory systems (15), which also supply the neighboring ventral nucleus. According to the Scheibels (39) and Minderhoud (31), these reticulate nuclei conduct back to the palliothalamic as well as to the truncothalamic nuclei. They are excited by feedback messages (efference copy) and may operate as thalamic equivalents of the recurrent inhibition best represented by the Renshaw cells of the anterior horn (7).

Another example of the set of six different thalamic nuclei of one functional system is the vestibular input to the thalamus, which we have investigated with Grippo (10) in the cat. 1. The main relay nucleus is the internal part of the intermediate ventral nucleus (V.im.i) as described by the Marchi- (14) and fiber degeneration

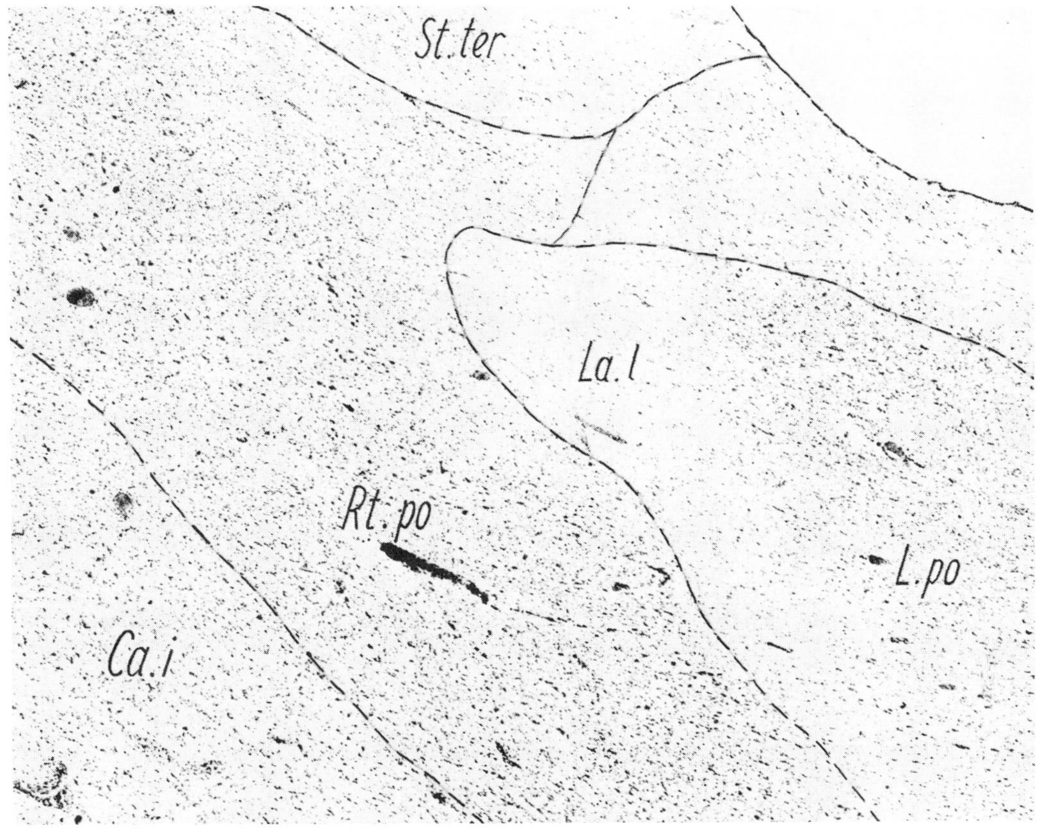

FIG. 4B

methods (11) now confirmed by the Nauta-Gygax method (Fig. 5A). It may project to the area 6a γ of the motor cortex. The stimulation of the whole vestibulo-thalamo-cortical pathway results in an ipsiversive turning of the head and foretrunk (14, 16). 2. The narrow integrative nucleus above the V.im.i, called intermediate zentrolateral (Z.im.i) is supplied by some small collateral degeneration of vestibular fibers (Fig. 6). 3. The larger second integrative level above the Z.im.i, called intermediate dorsal nucleus (D.im.i) does not directly receive terminals or collaterals from the vestibular system. 4. The vestibulothalamic pathway also includes a multisensory thalamic nucleus, namely the magnocellular medial geniculate (G.m.mc). It receives somatosensory, acoustic, visual and vestibular impulses, and projects to the "composite" multisensory area in the anterior ectosylvian gyrus (30), architectonically characterized as area 2 preinsular (2 pr. I) in the cat by Hassler and Muhs (24). This "composite area" should no longer be regarded as a special vestibular area, but as a multisensory convergent thalamocortical system. 5. The parafascicular nucleus (Pf) and magnocellular centrum medianum are the truncothalamic or unspecific nuclei of the vestibular pathway (Fig. 5B), whereas vestibular connections to reticulate nuclei have not

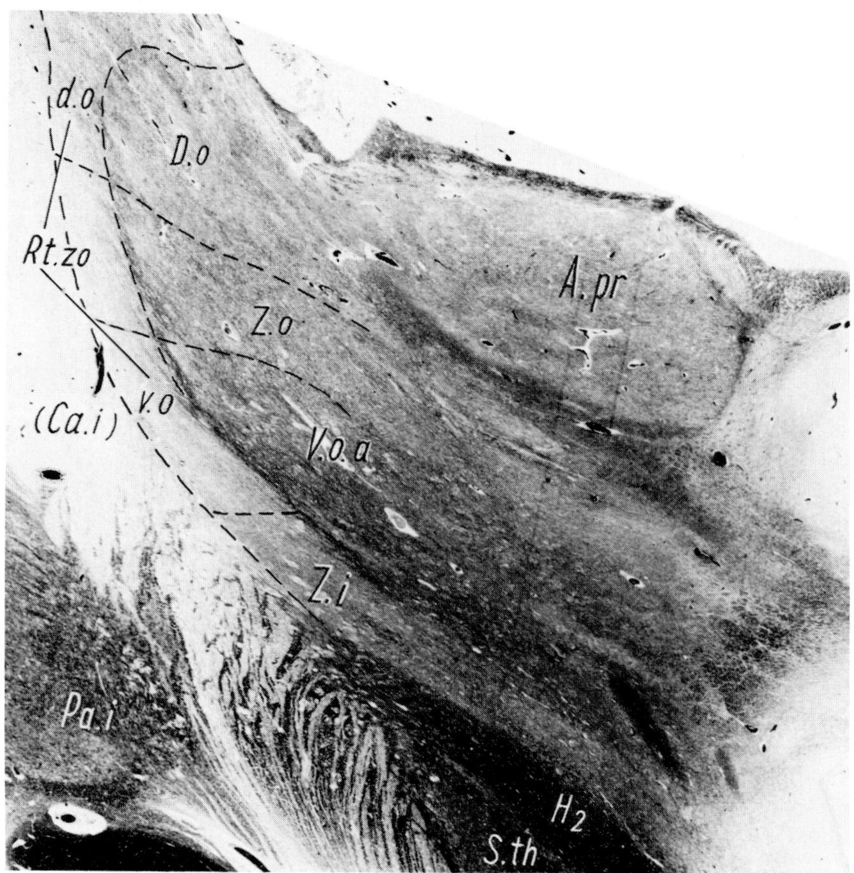

FIG. 4C and D. A pair of sections farther caudal shows the passage of myelinated pallidothalamic fibers through the degenerated internal capsule (Ca.i) to the fiber bundle H_2 and the preserved terminals of the afferent pallidothalamic fibers in V.o.a. This corresponds in the Nissl picture to an almost cell deprived V.o.a and far less degenerated Rt.v.o (4D).

been demonstrated so far.

A third example is the visual system: 1. The primary receptive nuclei are the layers of the lateral geniculate nucleus, six in most of the primates (three contralaterally and three ipsilaterally supplied) and five in carnivores (three contralaterally supplied layers: A, B, B_2; and two ipsilaterally supplied layers: A_1 and B_1, according to Hassler and Hajdu (22). 2. The first integrative level of the visual system is represented by the intergeniculate pulvinar nucleus (Pu.ig) in all investigated species of primates (Fig. 7A and B) and carnivores (20). In humans with complete aplasia of the eyes, optic tracts and lateral geniculate nuclei, this first integrative level is strongly hypoplastic (Fig. 8A) (approximately six times smaller) (19). 3. The second integrative level with direct visual afferents is the lateral pulvinar nucleus (Pu. l) present in all primates as well as in carnivores, but not in the insectivores, the most aboriginal

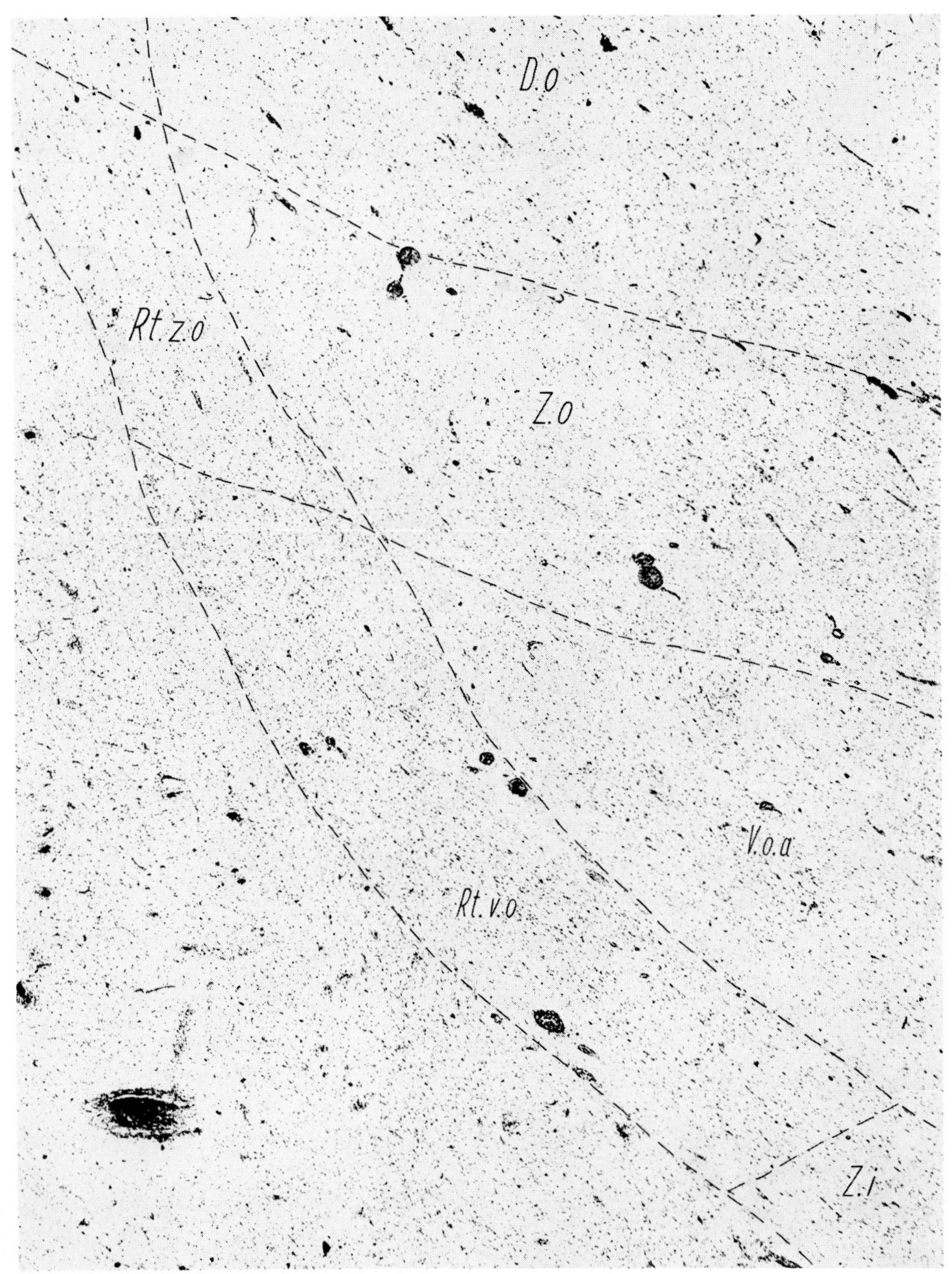

FIG. 4D

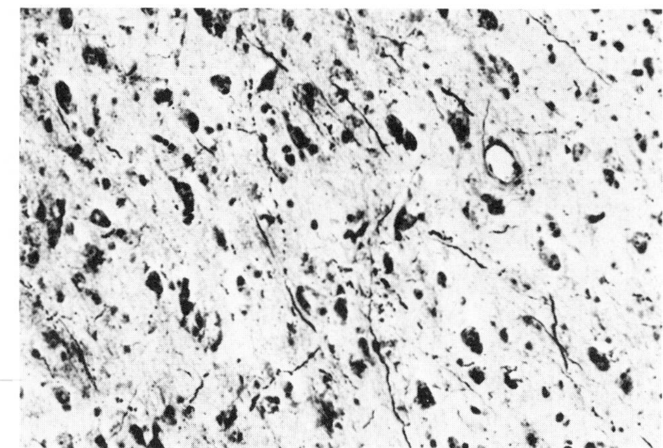

FIG. 5A. Degenerated vestibulothalamic fibers (Nauta-Gygax method) in the internal part of the ipsilateral ventro-intermediate nucleus (V.im.i) of the cat. (Grippo and Hassler 1971, unpublished).

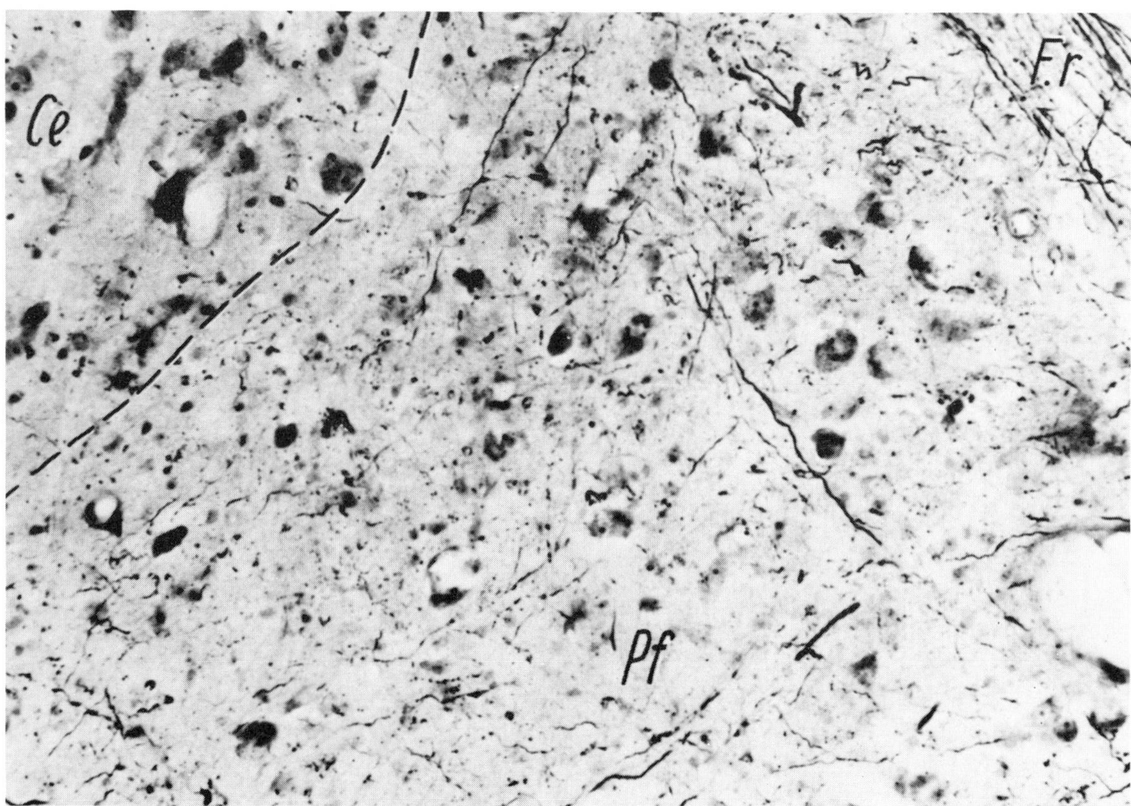

FIG. 5B. Fine degenerated vestibulothalamic fibers (Nauta-Gygax technique) in the parafascicular nucleus (Pf) after ipsilateral lesion of the vestibular nuclei. The density of degeneration is far less in the neighboring parvocellular part of central nucleus (Ce). F.r = fascicular retroflexus.

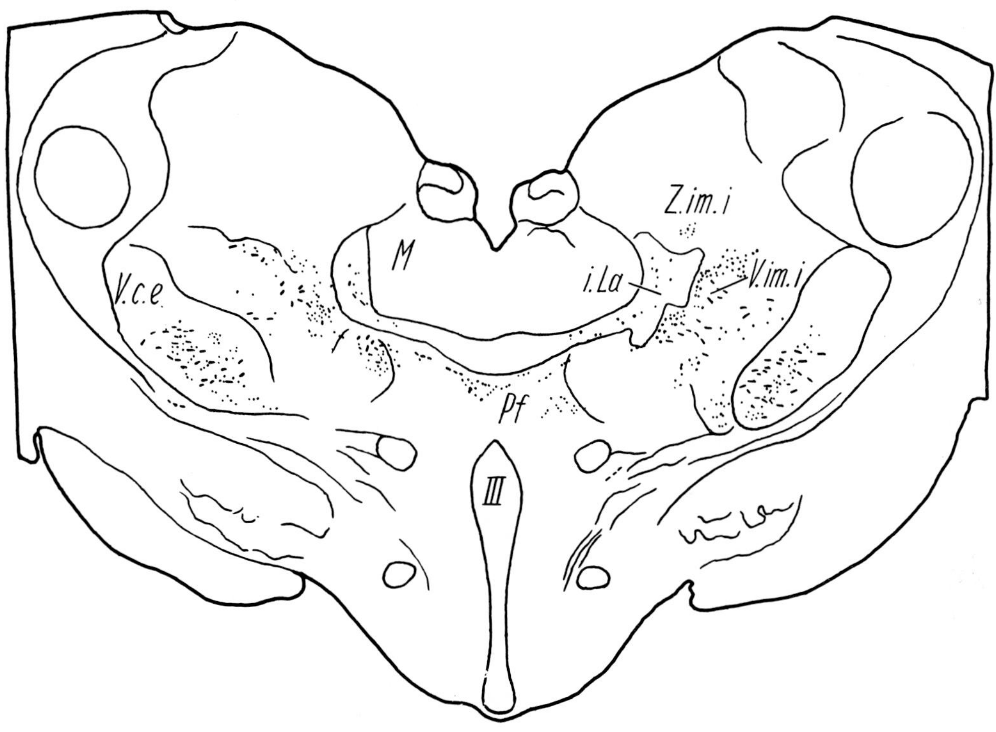

FIG. 6. Diagram of the thalamic distribution of terminal degeneration of direct vestibulothalamic fibers after vestibular nuclei lesions in the cat. On the ipsilateral (right) side the main termination is the internal ventro-intermediate nucleus (V.im.i) on the border of intralaminar nucleus (i.La), which contains sparser degenerations of vestibulothalamic fibers. Above i.La and V.im.i a smaller accumulation of terminal degenerations appears in the internal zentrolateral intermediate nucleus (Z.im.i). Except in the most rostral part of the parafascicular and central nucleus, the remaining dense accumulation of degenerated fibers does not seem to be related to vestibulothalamic fibers. (Hassler and Grippo 1971, unpublished).

mammals. This nucleus is less reduced in size in the two reported cases of human anophthalmia (Fig. 8A). 4. The multisensory termination is again represented by the magnocellular medial geniculate nucleus (G.m.mc). 5. The unspecific or truncothalamic nucleus of the visual system is the pregeniculate nucleus often referred to as nucleus geniculatus lateralis ventralis. Its projections are completely subcortical, probably to the mesencephalic reticular formation. After complete destruction of the visual cortical sphere, this nucleus is preserved and, in the rare cases of human inborn anoph-

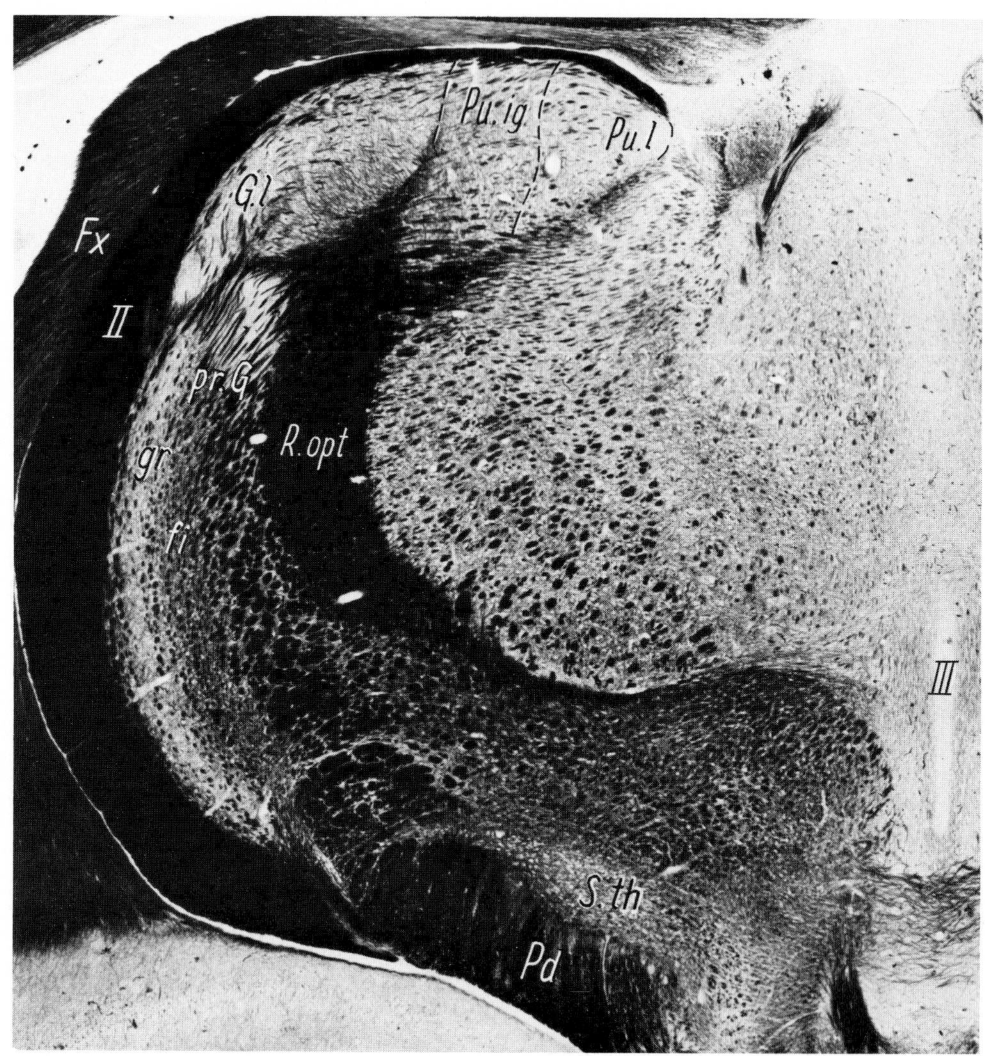

FIG. 7A and B. Cross sections through the posterior thalamus of the prosimiam Tupaia glis (tree shrew) in fiber (a) and cell staining (b); magnification 30x. Medial to the six-layered lateral geniculate (G. l) are two pulvinar nuclei, both supplied by sparse collateral degeneration of optic fibers. The intergeniculate pulvinar nucleus (Pu. ig) is directly attached to the G. l and richer in single fibers; its basal accumulation of fiber bundles enters the optic radiation (R. opt) which passes into the internal capsule. The lateral pulvinar nucleus (Pu. l) forms the medial and rostral continuation

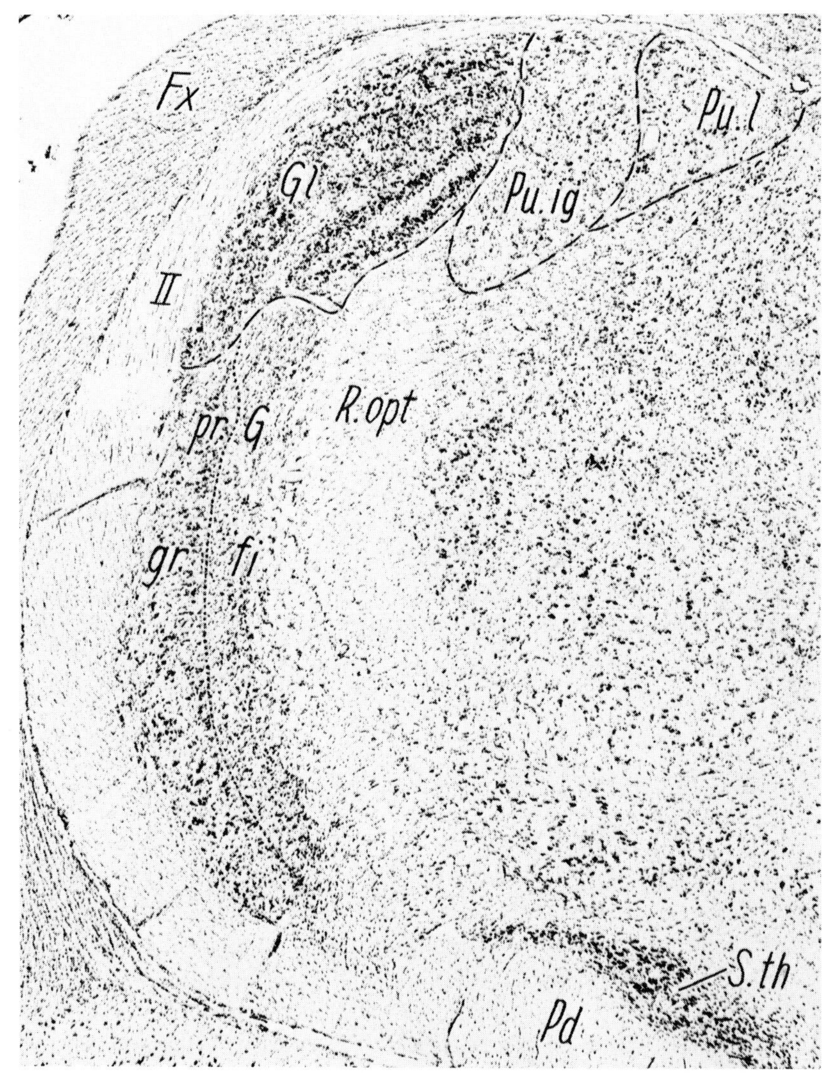

of Pu .ig and is differentiated by the lack of single fibers and a less dense cytoarchitecture. Pu .ig seems to represent the first level of integration, Pu .l the second level of integration of visual impulses. Both are covered by a prolongation of the optic tract (II). Below the lateral geniculate nucleus, the pregeniculate (pr.G) extends, divided into a gray (gr) part with larger nerve cells and a fibrous part (fi), richer in fiber bundles but with smaller nerve cells.

thalmia, is even hyperplastic (Fig. 8B; 20). 6. The primary visual projections also supply afferent fibers to the reticulate nucleus around the lateral geniculate nucleus.

After the set of thalamic terminal nuclei has been presented in detail for three

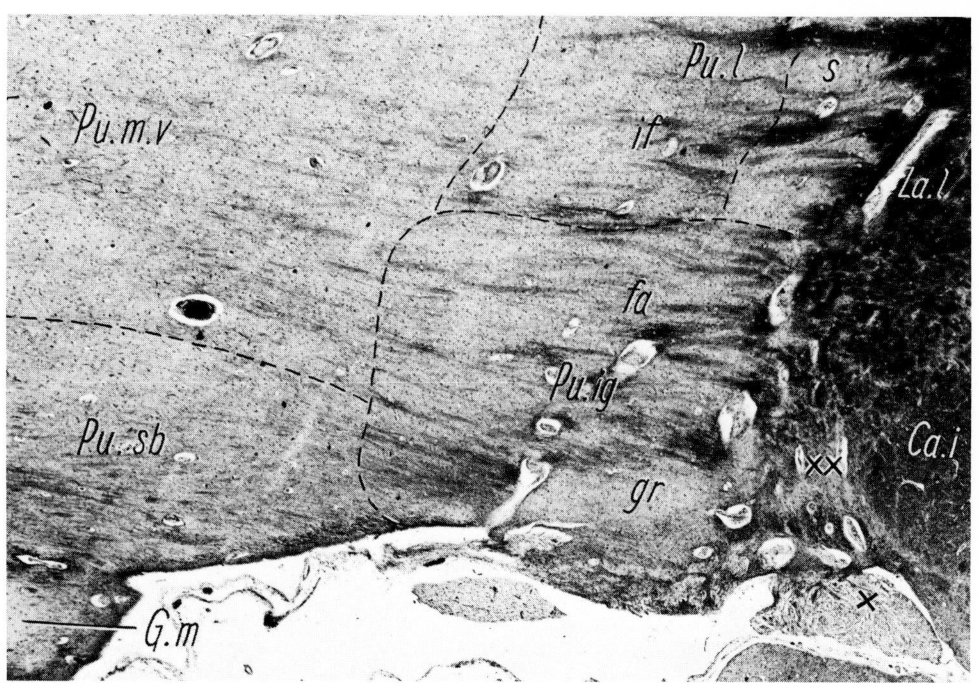

FIG. 8A. Cross section through the pulvinar of a human case of inborn anophthalmia. The optic tract and the lateral geniculate are absent and replaced by a small granulation tissue (x). Of the intergeniculate pulvinar (Pu.ig) nucleus the gray (gr) part is extremely atrophied and reduced in size, more than the fasciculosus (fa) part. Consequently their efferent fibers to the cortex are shrunken and demyelinated (xx) in the basal part of the internal capsule (Ca.i). The lateral pulvinar nucleus (Pu.l.s) is also reduced, but much less than Pu.ig. Unchanged medial pulvinar nuclei (Pu.m.v and Pu.sb). Fiber staining according to Heidenhain/Woelcke; magnification 16.5:1.

afferent systems, the question arises whether all of the 12 enumerated afferent systems have this set of six different terminations in the thalamus.

In addition to the described spinothalamic system, the two other somatosensory systems also have special relay, primary and secondary integrative, truncothalamic protopathic, multisensory and reticulate termination. This is demonstrated by experiments of Boivie (4) and our (unpublished) results for the cervicothalamic tract which represents hair movement sensation according to Horrobin (25). The primary relay nucleus is the anterior part of VPL or anterior ventrocaudal nucleus (V.c.a) which is architectonically differentiated (Fig. 3) from the posterior, as I have long emphasized.

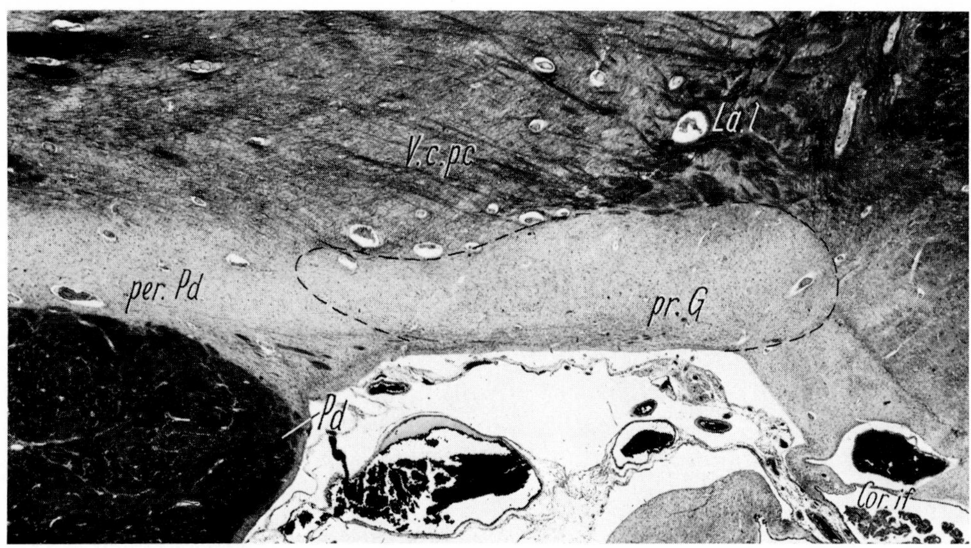

FIG. 8B. The pregeniculate nucleus (pr.G) in the same human case of anophthalmia is strongly hyperplastic (approximately nine times the usual size) although no remnant exists of the optic tract and lateral geniculate nucleus. The pregeniculate nucleus continues medially as peripeduncular nucleus (per.Pd) above the cerebral peduncle (Pd). No atrophy of the parvocellular caudal ventral nucleus (V.c.pc). Some occipito-tectal bundles (occ.-tect) are present in the medial edge. Cor.if = inferior horn of the ventricle. Fiber staining after Heidenhain/Woelcke; magnification 11.5:1.

Above the primary relay nucleus are two integrative nuclei of the cervicothalamic tract, i.e., intermediate zentrolateral and intermediate dorsal nuclei (Z.im.e and D.im.e) which are coextensive with the same nuclei of the lemniscal system. Some terminals go to the reticulate nucleus around V.c.a, while the composite nucleus, G.m.mc, also accepts some afferents. The parafascicular nucleus (Pf) is the protopathic or truncothalamic nucleus of this tract.

A set of six thalamic terminations can also be demonstrated for the lemniscal system (V.c.p, Z.c, D.im, Rt. vc, G.m.mc and i.La). The taste system has not been investigated except for its thalamic relay nucleus in the most medial point of parvocellular ventrocaudal or VPM nucleus.

In the cerebellar system, it is clear that five of the six types of terminations are realized (V.o.p, Z.o, D.o.e, Ce, Rt.v.o). Especially clear are the thin terminals for the first and second level of integration in the Marchi experiment on marmoset. The composite multisensory nucleus is probably the magnocellular part of lateropolar nucleus (L.po.mc); its cortical projection goes to the orbital cortex (27). As has previous-

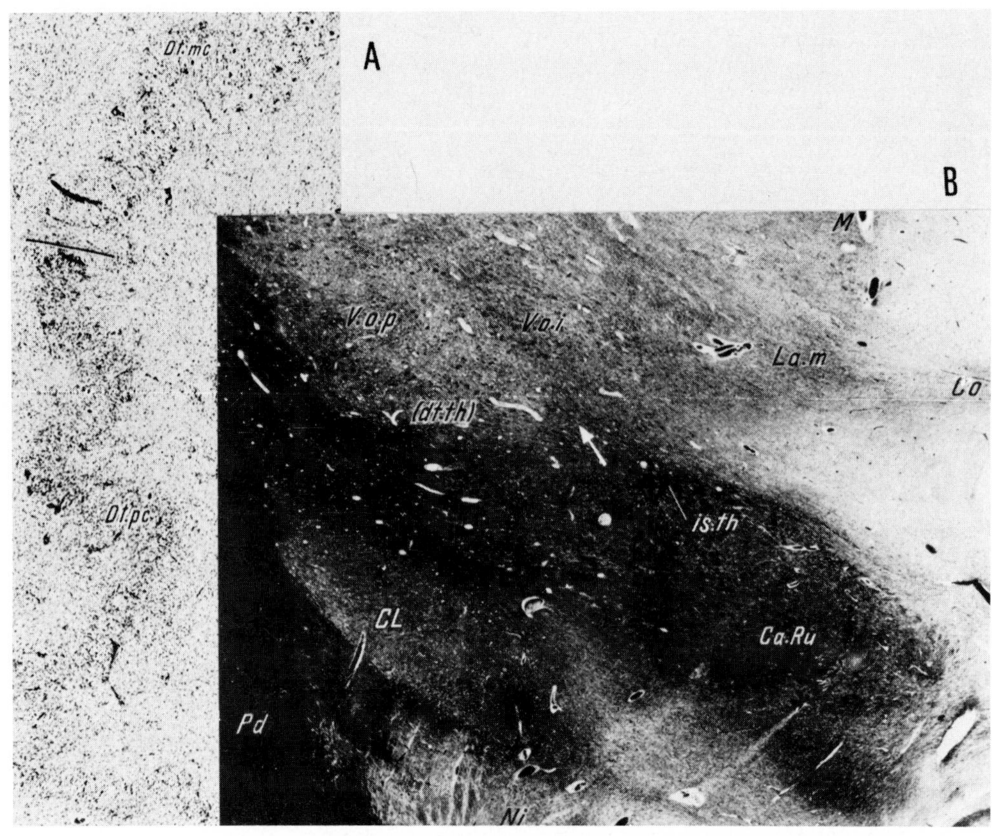

FIG. 9A and B. In a human case of iuvenile amaurotic idiocy the main (parvocellular) part of the dentate nucleus (Dt.pc) is severely degenerated and almost deprived of nerve cells whereas the magnocellular part (Dt.mc) is only slightly involved, so that most of the nerve cells are preserved (A,Nissl picture; 24:1). Consequently all dentato-thalamic fibers (dt.th) are lost in the base of their terminal nucleus V.o.p (B,fiber staining; 7,5:1) whereas the tract of interstitio-thalamic fibers (is th) are undamaged on the medial border of V.o.p at their entrance into the V.o.i nucleus (white arrow) (After Hassler 13).

ly been demonstrated in man (12) and cat (18), many cerebellar efferent fibers originating in the lateral interpositus nucleus (emboliformis) terminate in the centrum medianum nucleus (Ce). In the unique case of Bostroem and Spatz's complete dentate atrophy of idiopathic origin, in which the emboliform nucleus is spared (Fig. 10A), all cerebellar-dependent nuclei, including the red nucleus, are completely demyelinated (Fig. 10B), whereas the centrum medianum is preserved. In both pallidar systems, that from inner and outer segments, the sets of terminations are almost known: V.o.a, Z.o, D.o.e, Rt.v.o, L.po.mc and i.La (Abb. 10); and L.po.i, L.po.s, D.sf, Rt,po, L.po. mc and Co?

To date, the thalamic representations of movements in different directions which are represented in the so-called nuclei of the posterior commissure of the midbrain have been insufficiently considered and investigated. These thalamic representations are situated in the internal part of oral ventral nuclei (V.o.i: Abb. 11) whereas the locations of related secondary and protopathic nuclei are only partially known.

Thus we see that the majority of the afferent systems seem to have their own sets of six different terminal nuclei, although not all the terminations are known in every instance. This rule of a six-fold termination requires a general interpretation. Therefore I will discuss it notwithstanding that it is hypothetical or speculative.

In general, the first termination common to all afferent systems is the relay nucleus. It is, however, more than a simple relay because it has, like all cortex-dependent thalamic nuclei, complex equipment with recurrent corticothalamic fibers and the thalamo-specific small interneuron-like nerve cells, which are probably Golgi II-type.

The first integrative level, represented by the zentrolateral (Z) nuclei, is supplied by long axons from at least three systems of different modalities, and by short collaterals from the output of the ventral nucleus below it. The second integrative level, represented by the dorsal nuclei, is supplied by 1) a few direct sensory terminals, 2) collaterals of the output of the relay as well as of the first integrative nuclei and 3) recurrent information from the related reticulate nucleus and the cortical projection field.

What is the functional counterpart of each of these types of thalamic nuclei? As psychologists have known since Wernicke (1879) (41), each sensory modality excited can be experienced first as sensation; then, after a process of externalization or primary identification, as clear actual perception but as yet unidentified or unrecognized; and finally, by comparing this with earlier experiences (secondary identification) as real recognized perception which will be inserted in the treasury of personal knowledge. This stepwise building of a clearly recognized perception has its architectonic counterpart: The sensation corresponds to the sensory relay nucleus, the distinct but unrecognized perception to the first integrative level, and the identified perception to the second integrative level of each sensory input to the thalamus. Moreover, a sensory stimulus before primary and secondary identification can be experienced not only as a sensation but also as a protopathic reaction to any impact concerning the personality, known as a feeling. This is still possible after destruction of the relay and the two integrative nuclei of the same system. It corresponds therefore to the lowest unspecific truncothalamic termination responsible for the protopathic primary impression.

From the pain system we know that the cortical externalizing system for pain perception and the subcortical protopathic system for pain feeling have an antagonistic interrelation: pain feeling due to activity of the subcortical pain pathway along can be unbearable after removal of inhibitory control by the destruction of the cortical relay system for pain. That thalamic spontaneous pain is due to a disinhibition of the sub-

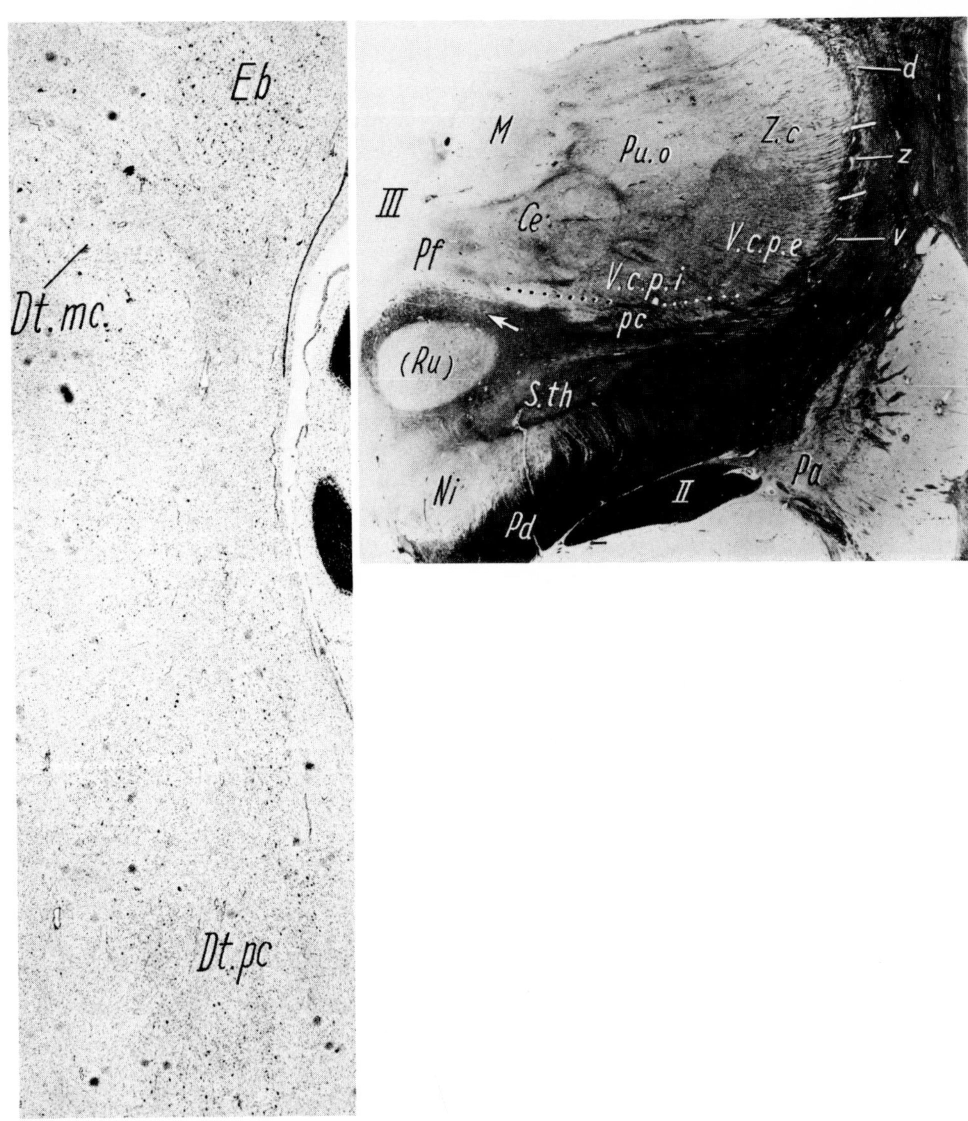

FIG. 10

cortical pain pathway is demonstrated by its relief after additional, therapeutic destruction of the truncothalamic pain nucleus, the limitans (21).

This antogonistic interrelation seems to be a general rule in the organization of thalamocortical systems. Another example is provided by those thalamic nuclei which receive inputs from the cerebellum: when the motor cortex, the effector field of the specific thalamic relay nucleus (V.o.p) of the cerebellar outflow, is removed, the result is a disinhibition of the electrical activity of the unspecific thalamic nucleus, the centre médian (CM), of the cerebellar input (28).

The antagonistic interrelation between the relay and the unspecific protopathic nuclei is also expressed anatomically in the two cases of human anophthalmia mentioned above: Whereas the visual relay nucleus, lateral geniculate, is aplastic and the first integrative level (Pu.ig) is strongly hypoplastic, the truncothalamic visual nucleus, pregeniculate, is strongly hyperplastic (approximately eight times the normal size). This is the best example and anatomical expression of the antagonism of cortical and subcortical branch of the same sensory system. The pathogenesis follows an ontogenetic rule: if one of two neighboring structures is aplastic or hypoplastic, the second is increased in size, because under normal conditions the growth factor of each structure inhibits the development of the neighboring structure (29).

The functional role of the composite multisensory areas in connection with the related thalamic afferents is not understood, unless they are responsible for the formation of the actual background of conscious experiences. The special reticulate thalamic nucleus, which belongs to a special relay or integrative nucleus, is a system of output control with feedback for the single thalamic nucleus.

What are the consequences of this complex afferent organization on the activity of the cortical motor sphere? First the motor sphere must be separated from the primarily somatosensory fields 3b, 1 and 2. Second, the motor cortex is not a unit but is composed of at least seven fields with different afferences, different structures (24) and different motor effects when locally stimulated or excited (18). The 1A spiral fiber representation, according to Oscarsson and Rosén (33) and Anderson, Landgren and Wolsk (2) lies in the ventral intermediate nucleus (V.im.e) and is projected to area 3a of the cortex.

FIG. 10. In the famous Bostroem-Spatz (3) case of brachium conjunctivum atrophy the red nucleus is completely deprived of fiber bundles, an unusual picture. This is due to the degenerative nerve cell loss of both parts of dentate nucleus (Dt.pc and Dt.mc). The nerve cell loss of the parvocellular dentate nucleus (Dt.pc) from which the dentato-thalamic fibers start is replaced by gliosis. In consequence not only the red nucleus but also the dentato-thalamic fiber bundles are demyelinated in the red nucleus capsule where the arrow points and in the neighboring V.c.pc. The consequence of the degenerative atrophy of the magnocellular dentate nucleus (without a gliosis) is the complete deprivation of the red nucleus by all bundles. In correlation to the good preservation of the fiber network of centrum medianum (Ce) the emboliform nucleus (Eb) of the cerebellum is undamaged with unreduced nerve cell content. a) Nissl picture; 12:1; b) Heidenhain picture; 3.5:1.

The area 4 γ which contains the typical giant Betz cells receives its specific afferent input from the V.o.p, i.e. the posterior basal part of VL, supplied by dentato-thalamic fibers. Stimulation of the V.o.p in unanesthetized cats elicits phasic (stimulus-synchronous) movements of the contralateral forepaw and upper extremity or of the contralateral facial muscles. The same occurs in passive human patients upon threshold stimulation; if the patient is actively moving his arm or hand or even speaking, prior to stimulation of the V.o.p, movements and speaking are accelerated; this is reproducible in 70 to 80% of the patients. This is easily explained by the artificial specific afferent excitation of area 4 γ. After high frequency destruction of the V.o.p in the human, tremor at rest and postural tremor or myoclonias are relieved. Thereafter, the most striking defects are a contralateral reduction of mimic movements, regressing ataxia and asynergia, and flaccid neglect of the contralateral extremities (17); all of which can be rapidly abolished by physiotherapy. The contralateral motor neglect can be interpreted as a release effect of the centre médian and its subcortical projection nucleus, the putamen. The centrum medianum, as an unspecific trunco-thalamic projection nucleus, belongs to the same cerebellar efferent pathway of phasic motor activity as the V.o.p. Meulders, Massion and Albe-Fessard (28) have demonstrated that the CM is disinhibited after decortication exhibiting an increased electrical activity.

There are at least four other thalamocortical motor systems for direction-selective locomotor movements and conjugated eye movements. The most thoroughly investigated system is that for ipsiversive turning movements. It is identical with the vestibulo-thalamo-cortical relay system, in that it passes (Fig. 12) through the intermediate ventral nucleus (V.im.i) presumably to the area 6aδ in the cruciate sulcus (18).

In the rostral thalamus there are also representations of rotatory and raising movements of the head, trunk and the conjugated eye apparatus. The thalamic relay nuclei belong to medial parts of the VL (V.o.i, in my nomenclature). The V.o.i is connected

---

FIG. 11. A schematic horizontal section of the diencephalon and midbrain of cat at the level of the interstitial nucleus (Nc ist) where all direction selective stimulation effects are located. All rotatory effects have black circles (●), even if they are combined with contraversive turning. They are accumulated in the anterolateral half of the Nc. ist but also along the interstitio-spinal tract (is.sp). Rostralwards they fill the base of the thalamus between the mamillothalamic (ma.th) tract and the border of the brachium conjunctivum terminals. Medialwards the rotatory effects are replaced by the "raising effects" (♂) which mostly do not transgress the line between tractus retroflexus (T.r) and mamillothalamicus (ma.th). In the reticulate nucleus of the thalamus (Rt) beneath brachium conjunctivum terminals, the rotatory stimulation effect is mostly combined with contraversive (●→) turning. While the contraversive movements are related to the efferent pallidar pathway the rotatory effect laterally belongs to the tractus interstitio-thalamicus lateralis. Behind the interstitial nucleus, most stimulation effects are lowering (♀) movements combined with ipsiversive turnings, elicited from the ipsilateral vestibulo-reticulo-thalamic pathway.

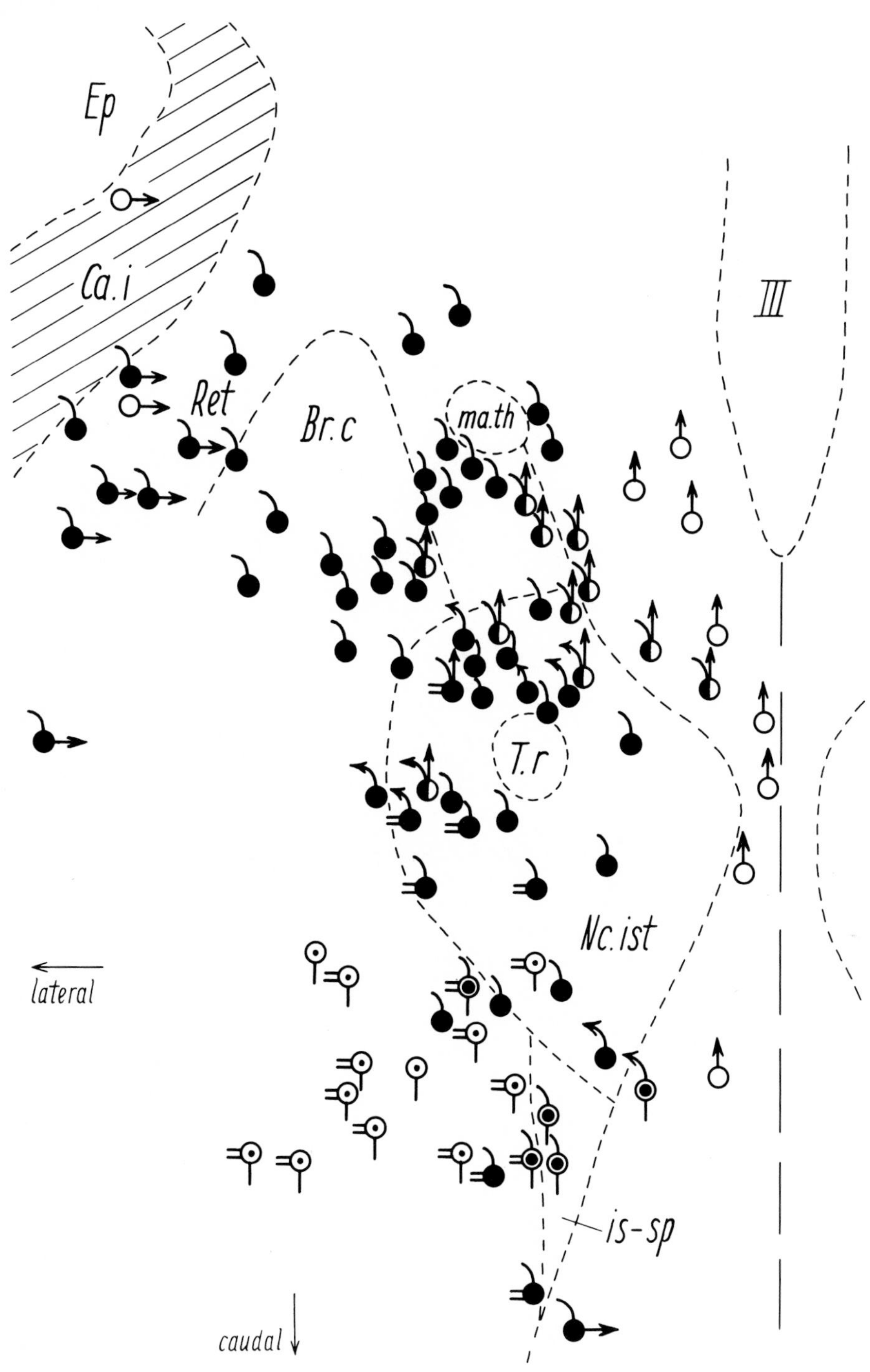

FIG. 11

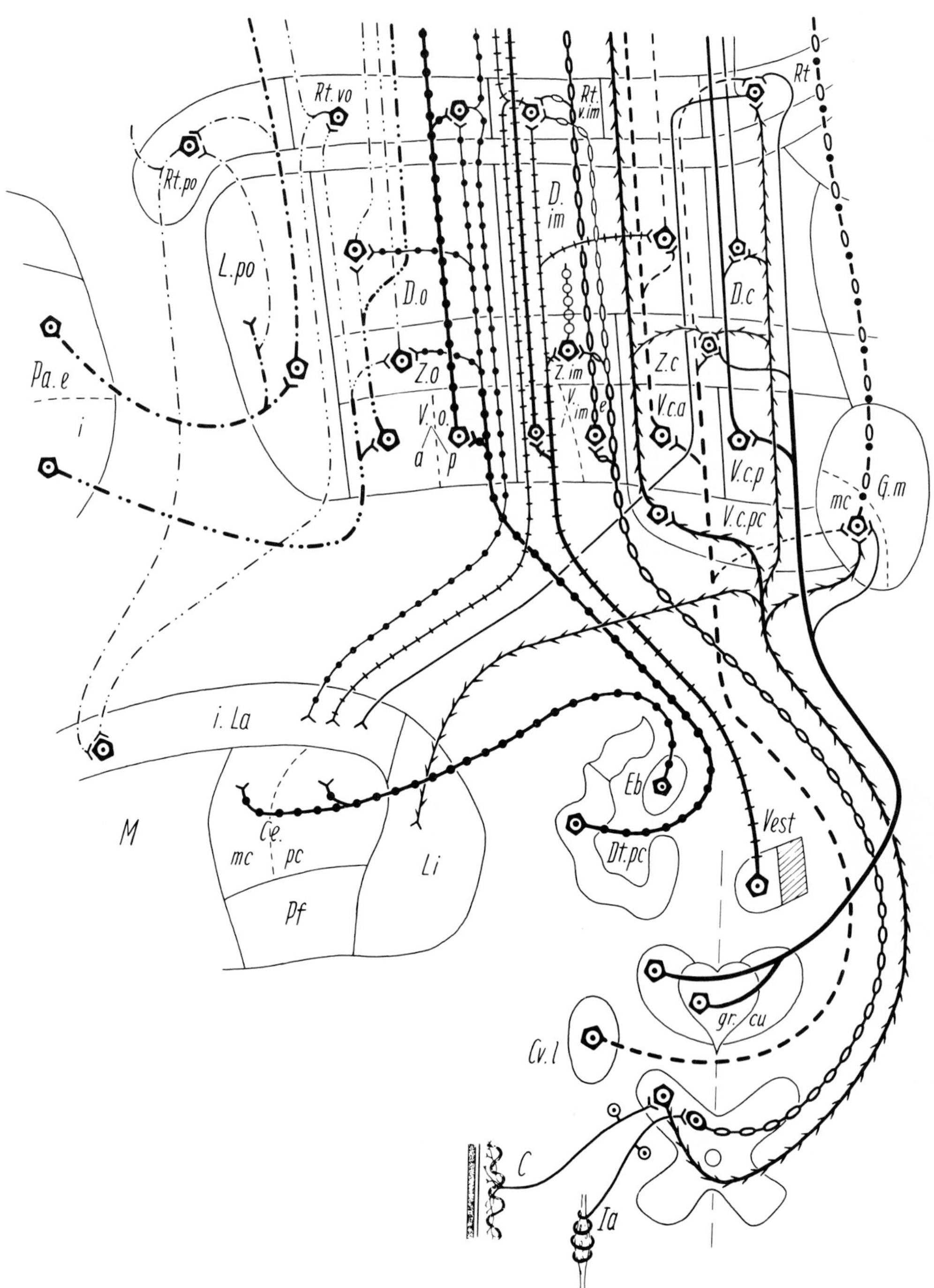

FIG. 12. Schematic drawing of the distribution of the somatosensory and coordinative afferences each to six thalamic nuclei of different functional specialization. A.

The pain pathway originating from C fibers is conducting to 1. the parvocellular ventro-caudal nucleus (V.c.pc) which projects to the cortical area 3b: 2. the caudal zentro-lateral nucleus (Z.c) above V.c.p projecting to anterior parietal lobe; 3. collaterals to the caudal dorsal nucleus (D.c) projecting to superior parietal lobe; 4. to the feed-back nucleus reticulatus ventralis caudalis (Rt.v.c); 5. the multisensory nucleus geniculatus medialis magnocellularis (G.m.mc) projecting to the preinsular multisensory area 2; and 6. the "protopathic" unspecific projecting nucleus limitans (Li). B. The medial lemniscus, originating from the dorsal column nuclei (gr.; cu) conducts to 1. Ventrocaudalis posterior (V.c.p) projecting to postcentral area 2; 2. the Zentrolateralis caudalis (Z.c) projecting to the anterior parietal lobe; 3. collaterals to the Dorsalis intermedius (D.im) projecting to the superior parietal lobe; 4. to the feed-back nucleus reticulatus ventralis caudalis (Rt.v.c); 5. the multisensory nucleus geniculatus medialis magnocellularis (G.m.mc); and 6. the intralaminar nucleus (i.La) a part of the thalamic unspecific projecting system. C. The cervicothalamic tract representing hair bending sensation, conducts to 1. the nucleus ventro-caudalis anterior (V.c.a); 2. Zentrolateralis caudalis (Z.c); 3. collaterals to nucleus dorsalis intermedius (D.im) and to the three other nuclei identical with B4, B5, B6. D. The Ia muscle spindle representation conducted from Clarke's column through the dorsolateral column terminates in 1. Ventralis intermedius externus (V.im.e) projecting to area 3a of postcentral gyrus; 2. Zentrolateralis intermedius (Z.im); 3. Collaterals to nucleus dorsalis intermedius (D.im); 4. in the feed-back nucleus reticulatus ventralis intermedius (Rt.v.im). E. The vestibulo-reticulo-thalamic tract terminates in 1. the ipsilateral nucleus ventralis intermedius internus (V.im.i); 2. the nucleus zentrolateralis intermedius internus (Z.im.i); a few collaterals terminate in the nucleus dorsalis intermedius (D.im); terminals to the reticulate nucleus are not found whereas terminals to 5. the multisensory Geniculatus medialis magnocellularis (Gm. mc) and to the parafascicular nucleus (Pf) are ascertained. F. The dentato-thalamic projection terminate in 1. Ventralis oralis posterior (V.o.p), projecting to area 4γ; in Zentrolateralis oralis (Z.o); 3. a few collaterals in Dorsalis oralis (D.o) and 4. some terminals in the nucleus reticulatus ventralis oralis (Rt.v.o); 5. in the multisensory nucleus lateropolaris magnocellularis (L.po.mc); and 6. from the emboliform nucleus the projection terminates in the centrum medianum (Ce). G. The contraversive pallido-thalamic pathway originating from the inner segment of pallidum (Pa.i) terminates 1. in the Ventralis oralis anterior (V.o.a) projecting to a special subarea of 6; 2. in the Zentrolateralis oralis (Z.o) and 3. a few collaterals in Dorsalis oralis (D.o); 4. in the nucleus reticulatus ventralis oralis (Rt.v.o); 5. in the multisensory nucleus lateropolaris magnocellularis (L.po.mc); and 6. in the intralaminar nuclei (i.La). H. The first pallido-thalamic pathway from the outer segment runs directly through the internal capsule (Ca.i) to 1. the external lateropolar nucleus (L.po.e); 2. to the superior lateropolar nucleus (L.po.s) and other to 4. the polar reticulate nucleus (Rt.po) and 6. the intralaminar nuclei (i.La).

Except the four- to six-partition of each sensory input to functionally different levels of convergence and integration this scheme also demonstrates the recurrent action of each reticulate nucleus of the thalamus by efferent pathways backwards to the intralaminar nuclei besides the collaterals to many cortical areas.

Afferent tracts	Thalamic endings					
	1. relay	2. I. integrative level	3. II. integrative level	4. composite multisensory	5. unspecific protopathic	6. reticulate feedback
visual	G.l (GLd)	Pu.ig (PUI)	Pu.l	G.m.mc	pr.G (GLv)	Rt.g
auditory	G.m.fi	G.m.fa ?	Pu.o	G.m.mc	G.m.li	Rt.pu
gustatory	V.c.i.b ? (VPMi)	?	?	?	?	-
spino-thalamic	V.c.pc (VPI)	Z.c	D.c	G.m.mc	Li + i.La	Rt.v.c
medial lemniscus	V.c.p (VPLp)	Z.c	D.im.e	G.m.mc	i.La	Rt.v.c
cervico-thalamic	V.c.a (VPLa)	Z.c	D.im.e	G.m.mc	Pf + i.La	Rt.v.c
Ia spindle afferents + Nc. cuneatus ext.	V.im.e (VIM)	Z.im.e	D.im.e	?	i.La ?	Rt.v.im
vestibulo-thalamic	V.im.i	Z.im.i	D.im.i	G.m.mc	Pf + i.La	-
efferent cerebellar system	V.o.p (VLp)	Z.o.e	D.o.e	L.po.mc (VA part)	Ce (CM)	Rt.v.o
interstitio-thalamic (direction-selective)	V.o.i	Z.o.i	D.o.i	L.po.mc (VA part)	Ce (CM)	Rt.v.o
internal pallidar	V.o.a (VLa)	Z.o.e	D.o.e	D.sf (LD)	i.La	Rt.v.o
external pallidar	L.po.e (VA part)	L.po.s (VA part)	?	L.po.mc (VA part)	Co ?	Rt.po

to the interstitial nucleus of Cajal (the interstitiothalamic tract) in the human (Fig. 9) and cat (Fig. 11) (23). Circumscribed destruction of this tract in the human patient can relieve rotatory torticollis. In the cat, this part of V.o.i projects to one or two special parts of area 6 (one is area 6 if.fu) (24), the stimulation of which elicits rotatory movements of the head and vicariously of the gaze apparatus too. Even more medial in the V.o.i nucleus is the thalamic representation of raising movements of the head, eyes and trunk (Fig. 11). It receives fibers directly from the praestitial nucleus in the rostral midbrain, which is the center of raising movements. This special part of V.o.i projects to the area 6aβ, which lies in rostral part of cruciate sulcus and the most dorsal part of the gyrus proreus (Fig. 11). Here too exists an antagonistic interrelation between the thalamocortical and the subcortical or mesencephalic systems for specific direction-selective movement.

The final but most important direction-selective neuronal system for turning and searching movements to the contralateral side (Adversiv-Bewegungen) has its most effective subcortical representation in the pallidum (32), especially in its inner segment, the cat's homologue of which is the entopeduncular nucleus. The afferent pallidothalamic fibers, also demonstrated in the cat, split up in the thalamic nucleus, V.o.a, in front of the dentatothalamic fibers with minimal, if any, overlap. Threshold stimulation of this pallidothalamic pathway, including V.o.a, in the cat, monkey and human patients induces turning of the head or the whole body to the contralateral side with dilation of the pupils and enhanced excitability (17). If these head movements are suppressed, only conjugated movements of both eyes occur. The coagulation of V.o.a is the most effective intervention to relieve parkinsonian and athetotic rigidity.

The VA nucleus also has pallidar input which originates in the outer segment and crosses the internal capsule avoiding the H_1-loop. Stimulation of the inner part of VA in the human patient elicits contraversive conjugated eye and head movements, raising of the contralateral arm and the uttering of inarticulate sounds, as from the supplementary motor area of Penfield and Welch (34).

In the human, the V.o.a nucleus projects to the cortical motor sphere, but to the most posterior part of area 6a, called 6aα. This projection is confirmed by electrophysiological investigations in the human (9) and field potential recording in the cat (6). Low frequency stimulation of the anterior part of VL (or V.o.a) evokes an augmenting response with a combination of deep and superficial thalamocortical responses, whereas stimulation of the CM evokes a superficial recruiting response only. The activator of this unspecific cortical excitation, however, seems to be the pallidum. Its threshold stimulation provokes recruiting responses mainly in the premotor area 6a. That the pallidum is the origin of this unspecific activation has been demonstrated by Dieckmann and Sasaki (6), who showed that stimulation two millimeters higher in the internal capsule failed to elicit a recruiting response. The term "unspecific," however, is not appropriate because the cortical response to stimulation of the pallidum is restricted primarily to area 6a; in those parts of area 4 which overlap area 6a, no recruiting can be established.

All the thalamic nuclei with motor afferents or motor functions discussed above project to different cortical fields in the cat situated in front of the postcruciate dimple. It is striking that even the motor cortex itself, without regard to the somatosensory fields, is not a unit, functionally or anatomically. In addition to the cortical muscle spindle representation in area 3 a and the area 4 γ, with the origin of the thickest pyramidal tract fibers it comprises at least five parts of area 6a and 8, each of which represents a special direction for locomotion, posture and eye movements while the supplementary motor area represents a special, complex psychomotor function. Further, there are special thalamocortical systems for higher integrated motor functions, such as plans to write or speak, whose loss results in different forms of apraxia as facial apraxia, constructive apraxia and agraphia.

The analysis of cortical motor functions is well behind the microphysiological analysis of the sensory systems with the complex visual neurons of Hubel and Wiesel (26) and hypercomplex tactile neurons of Sakata (36). When one speaks about the sensorimotor cortex, it must be realized that this is a huge and systematized complex of functionally different thalamocortical systems, even in the cat and much more developed in primates and man. The guiding line for research of the cortex will be the architectonic differentiation of the cortical fields, which has proven to be fruitful in the visual system. A first step will be the differentiation of the anterior part of VL (our V.o.a) which is supplied by pallidar fibers with a specific cortical projection. Another important mechanism will be the antagonistic interrelation between the cortical and subcortical systems with the same afferents.

REFERENCES

1 AGUINIS, M., Die Bedeutung des Nucleus reticulatus thalami in der stereotaktischen Parkinson-Behandlung, Acta Neurochir. 11 (1963) 151-160.

2 ANDERSSON, S.A., LANDGREN, S., and WOLSK, D. The thalamic relay and cortical projection of group I muscle afferents from the forelimb of the cat, J. Physiol. (Lond.) 183 (1966) 576-591.

3. BOSTROEM, A., and SPATZ, H. Bindearmatrophie bei idiopathischer Athetose, Arch. Psychiat. Nervenkr. 82 (1928) 271-273.

4 BOIVIE, J. The terminations of the cervicothalamic tract in the cat. An experimental study with silver impregnation methods, Brain Res. 19 (1970) 333-360.

5 BURDACH, K.F. Vom Baue und Leben des Gehirns. Bd. 2, Dyk'sche Buchhandlung, Leipzig, 1822, pp. 418.

6 DIECKMANN, G., and SASAKI, K. Recruiting responses in the cerebral cortex produced by putamen and pallidum stimulation, Exp. Brain Res. 10 (1970) 236-250.

7 FRIGYESI, T.L. and SCHWARTZ, R. Chapter in this volume.

8 GALENUS, Galeni omnia, quae extant in Latinum sermonem conversa, Venet. 1556. III. Fol.

9 GANGLBERGER, J.A. Über EEG-Veränderungen nach stereotaktischer Ausschaltung subcorticaler Strukturen bei 800 Parkinson-Kranken, Arch. Psychiat. Nervenkr. 203 (1962) 519-544.

10 GRIPPO, J. and HASSLER, R. The thalamic terminations of direct vestibular fibers in the cat (Nauta-Gygax-method). In preparation, 1972.

11 HASSLER, R. Forels Haubenfascikel als vestibuläre Empfindungsbahn mit Bemerkungen über einige andere sekundäre Bahnen des Vestibularis und Trigeminus, Arch. Psychiat. Nervenkr. 180 (1948) 23-53.

12 HASSLER, R. Anatomie des Thalamus, Arch. Psychiat. Nervenkr. 184 (1950) 249-256.

13 HASSLER, R. Functional anatomy of the thalamus, Actas y Trabajos, VI. Congr. Latinoamericano de Neurocirurgia, Montevideo, 1955, pp. 754-787.

14 HASSLER, R. Die zentralen Apparate der Wendebewegungen. I. u. II., Arch. Psychiat. Nervenkr. 194 (1956) 456-516.

15 HASSLER, R. Anatomy of the thalamus. In: Introduction to Stereotaxis with an Atlas of the Human Brain. G. Schaltenbrand and P. Bailey (Eds.), Thieme-Verlag, Stuttgart, 1959, pp. 230-290.

16 HASSLER, R. Die zentralen Systeme des Schmerzes, Acta Neurochir. 8 (1960) 353-423.

17 HASSLER, R. Motorische und sensible Effekte umschriebener Reizungen und Ausschaltungen im menschlichen Zwischenhirn, Dtsch. Z. Nervenheilk. 183 (1961) 148-171.

18 HASSLER, R. Extrapyramidal motor areas of cat's frontal lobe: their functional and architectonic differentiation, Int. J. Neurol. (Montevideo) 5 (1966) (301-316).

19 HASSLER, R. Die zentralen Systeme des Sehens. Ber. dtsch. ophthal. Ges. 66 (1965) 229-251.

20 HASSLER, R. Comparative anatomy of the central visual system in day- and night-active primates, In: Evolution of the Forebrain, R. Hassler and H. Stephan (Eds.), Thieme-Verlag, Stuttgart, 1966, pp. 419-434.

21 HASSLER, R. Dichotomy of facial pain conduction in the diencephalon, In: Trigeminal Neuralgia, R. Hassler and A.E. Walker (Eds.), Thieme-Verlag, Stuttgart, 1970, pp. 123-138.

22 HASSLER, R. and HAJDU, F. The architectonics of the terminal nuclei of primary optic fibers in the cat, Abstracts IX. Internat. Congr. Anatomists, Leningrad, 1970, p. 51.

23 HASSLER, R. and HESS, W.R. Experimentelle und anatomische Befunde über die Drehbewegungen und ihre nervösen Apparate, Arch. Psychiat. Nervenkr. 192 (1954) 488-526.

24 HASSLER, R. and MUHS-CLEMENT, K. Architektonischer Aufbau des sensomotorischen und parietalen Cortex der Katze, J. Hirnforsch. 6 (1964) 377-420.

25 HORROBIN, D.F. The lateral cervical nucleus of the cat: an electrophysiological study, Quart. J. exp. Physiol. 51 (1966) 351-371.

26 HUBEL, D.H. and Wiesel, T.N. Receptive fields and functional architecture of monkey striate cortex, J. Physiol. (Lond.) 195 (1968) 215-243.

27 IMBERT, M., BIGNALL, K.E. and BUSER, P. Neocortical interconnections in the cat. J. Neurophysiol. 29 (1966) 382-395.

28 MEULDERS, M., MASSION, J., COLLE, J. and ALBE-FESSARD, D. Effet d'ablation télencéphaliques sur l'amplitude des potentiels évoqués dans le centre médian par stimulation somatique. Electroenceph. clin. Neurophysiol. 15 (1963) 29-38.

29 MEIERHOFER, M. Enthemmtes Wachstum bei Idiotie. J. Psychol. Neurol. (Lpz.), 491 (1939) 231-274.
30 MICKLE, W.A. and Ades, H.W. A composite sensory projection area in the cerebral cortex of the cat, Amer. J. Physiol., 170 (1952) 682-689.
31 MINDERHOUD, J.M. An anatomical study of the efferent connections of the thalamic reticular nucleus. Exp. Brain Res. 12 (1971) 435-446.
32 MONTANELLI, R.P. and HASSLER, R. Motor effects elicited by stimulation of the pallido-thalamic system in the cat. In: Lectures on the Diencephalon, W. Bargmann and J.P. Schade, (Eds.), Elsevier, Amsterdam, 1964, pp. 56-66.
33 OSCARSSON, O. and ROSÉN, I. Projection to cerebral cortex of large muscle-spindle afferents in forelimb nerves of the cat, J. Physiol. (Lond.) 169 (1963) 924-945.
34 PENFIELD, W. and WELCH, K. The supplementary motor area of the cerebral cortex, Arch. Neurol. (Chic.), 66 (1951) 289-317.
35 ROSE, J.E. The cortical connections of the reticular complex of the thalamus, Res. Publ. Ass. nerv. ment. Dis. 30 (1952) 454-479.
36 SAKATA, H. Hypercomplex neurons in the anterior parietal cortex. XXV. Internat. Congress of Physiological Sciences, Affiliated Symposium on Somatosensory Mechanisms, Ulm-Reisensburg 1971.
37 SANTORINI, I.D. Observationes anatomicae, Venetiis, 1724.
38 SASAKI, K., STAUNTON, H.P. and DIECKMANN, G. Characteristic features of augmenting and recruiting responses in the cerebral cortex. Exp. Neurol. 26 (1970) 369-372.
39 SCHEIBEL, M.E. and SCHEIBEL, A.B. The organization of the nucleus reticularis thalami: A Golgi study, Brain Res. 1 (1966) 43-62.
40 SCHLAG, J. and WASZAK, M. Characteristics of unit responses in nucleus reticularis thalami, Brain Res. 21 (1970) 286-288.
41 WERNICKE, C. Lehrbuch der Gehirnkrankheiten, I-III, Theodor Fischer-Verlag, Berlin, 1881-1883
42 WILLIS, TH. Opera omnia, Genev., 1676.

DISCUSSION

GILMAN:

Did I understand you correctly, that you first coagulated the VPL nucleus, and, then, without observing the patient proceeded to coagulate the nucleus limitans? If so, how can we interpret the effects of two lesions?

HASSLER:

The patient had thalamic pain, and this thalamic pain was due to a softening in the parvocellular part of VPL. I showed this softening next to one of the coagulations. Neither of the coagulations formed a softening. The softening was due to an occlusion of the thalamogeniculate artery, and this was the reason why the patient came to us with thalamic pain. We made a pain operation, and,as we do in all pain operations, we first stimulated and then coagulated the specific pain pathways projecting to area 3 b of the cortex. But in no case is this procedure sufficient to abolish the thalamic pain, and so one must also go to the subcortical pain nucleus and destroy the nucleus limitans. And I also demonstrated that after the destruction of nucleus limitans the patient was relieved from his thalamic pain. This is the basis for the interpretation of an antagonistic interrelation of the cortical and subcortical pain pathways. After the cortical pain pathway was destroyed by the spontaneous softening in this patient, the subcortical pain pathway was disinhibited and produced spontaneous pain. That is our theory. This is in agreement with the findings of Meulders, Massion and Albe-Fessard, that there is an increased activity in the centromedian nucleus after decortications. We, thus, have the same antagonistic interrelation between the cortical pathway of the cerebellar systems through the V.o.p. to the motor cortex and the subcortical pathway from the cerebellum to the centromedian. I think it is very important for understanding thalamic function that there is an antagonistic interrelationship between the corticopetal systems of one special sensory system and the subcortical systems of the same special system.

SCHWARTZ:

The vestibular nuclei are a complex of many nuclei. It appears now that there are two ascending vestibular systems. Therefore, I would like to ask: Where is the origin of your ascending vestibular pathway?

HASSLER:

I am sorry, I don't know. We could not differentiate its origin so far.

Corticothalamic Projections and Sensorimotor Activities
T. Frigyesi, E. Rinvik, and M.D. Yahr, editors. © 1972
Raven Press, New York.

Chairman's Summary

Dominick P. Purpura

The wide range of topics covered in the preceding reports bears witness to the continuing productivity of morphophysiological studies of the thalamus and its afferent and efferent relations as well as the heuristic value of new and imaginative approaches to the analysis of cortical-subcortical interactions. Central to these problems is the necessity for a coherent plan of functional organization of the thalamic nuclei and such a plan has now been supplied by Dr. Hassler. What he has presented in his most recent formulation of the organization of thalamic nuclei is both awesome in scope and complete in detail. His search for a unifying concept on the distribution and relations of different thalamic inputs is before us for examination and appraisal. It is evident that the concept of hexapartition of thalamic inputs is not a casual interpretation of data collected over several decades. More likely it represents the culmination of a prodigious effort to reorder the wealth of information on thalamic inputs into a meaningful hypothesis concerning thalamic function.

Dr. Hassler has made a special effort to relate the specific relay nuclei to surrounding integrative nuclei and to define the manner in which these are related to cortical projection zones. The importance of the n. reticularis in his general scheme is well appreciated particularly in the light of other studies summarized in this volume. Much of the evidence brought to bear upon the hexapartition hypothesis may be subject to the criticism that it has been derived largely from neuropathological material with all the problems of interpretation this entails. However, it should be recalled here that much of what is now known about the organization of the human thalamus has resulted in large part from Dr. Hassler's previous studies. It would be remarkable indeed if the present anatomical synthesis failed to add to the current picture of this organization.

A more relevant issue concerns the extent to which Dr. Hassler is justified in proceeding from anatomical consideration of the hierarchal organization of thalamic nuclei to the functional interpretations presented. The assignment of specific steps in the perceptual process to the activities of different hierarchally arranged thalamic nuclei (and their projections) is undoubtedly a frank over-simplification. Dr. Hassler argues that sensation corresponds to the activity of the sensory relay nucleus, distinct but unrecognized perceptions to the first integrative level, and identified perceptions to the second integrative level of each sensory input to the thalamus. Further he proposes that there is an antagonistic relationship between these levels and the unspecific thalamic systems. At least from the standpoint of internuclear relations examined in the cat this antagonistic interaction has not been documented in recent intracellular investigations summarized elsewhere in this volume. But this does not contradict such assumptions insofar as they are applied to studies of thalamic pain in man and the therapeutic effects of neurosurgical lesions.

Dr. Hassler has posed a question in his report which is of general concern, i.e., "What are the consequences of this complex afferent organization on the activity of the cortical motor sphere?" While not providing a direct answer to this question, Dr. Hassler has at least indicated the necessity for caution in treating "motor" cortex areas as a unit. His identification of the functional and anatomical relations of different thalamocortical projections to different motor cortex fields emphasizes the fact that neurophysiologists have barely begun to explore the vast and complex territories of the motor cortex in their attempts to understand the thalamocortical mechanisms underlying movement control.

While it has now been established that motor cortex neurons contribute in different ways to various parameters of pyramidal tract function little information has been available on the relationship of corticofugal activities to the output functions of thalamic neurons during different types of movement activities. The report by Drs. Jasper, Lamarre and Joffrey has attempted to address this question. The salient finding in this study is the discovery that motor cortex cooling may abolish experimentally induced tremor in the monkey without affecting voluntary movements including fine coordinated movements of the fingers. Additionally, Dr. Jasper and his associates have been able to classify thalamic neuron discharges in a new manner, i.e., depending upon the responses of thalamic units to motor cortex cooling. Of particular significance has been the finding that VL units firing in bursts at the tremor frequency are altered by motor cortex cooling sufficient to arrest tremor movements. Cells have also been encountered which exhibit burst responses synchronous with tremor movements but which are uninfluenced by cortical cooling, despite arrest of tremor. Finally, neurons have been found that fire in bursts during tremorous shivering but are uninfluenced by motor cortex cooling. This study indicates that different thalamic neurons are differently organized in relation to different varieties of movements, a finding of no little importance. It will be appreciated that the results described represent the beginning of a new approach to the study of movement control systems which emphasizes cortico-subcortical rather than direct pyramidal projections as major factors in the induction of Parkinson-like tremor processes. Quite apart from this the effects of cortical cooling raise a number of questions concerning the possible morphological and physiological consequences of even short-term functional inactivation of corticofugal projections to thalamus and basal ganglia. One suspects that 20-30 minutes of cooling of cortex down to 16-18° C would lead to serious traumatic and metabolic disturbances which might conceivably be reflected in fine structural changes in corticothalamic afferents and their terminals. Considerable interest might be generated by findings of typical EM profiles of early degeneration of corticothalamic terminals without concomitant physiological abnormalities.

The remarkable synergistic effects of harmaline in facilitating tremor in animals with tegmental lesions has called attention to the complexities of brain stem interactions in systems "released" by the tegmental lesion. This is further underscored by the fact that harmaline alone can produce a higher frequency tremor which resembles shivering movements. The latter are augmented by cortical cooling. The close pursuit of the mechanisms underlying harmaline-induced tremor should provide an excellent model system for further detailed examination of brain stem-cerebellum-and spinal cord contributions to tremorogenic processes.

Few areas of neurobiological inquiry have been more intensively examined in recent years than that concerned with the morphophysiological basis of visual functions in different animal species. This subject has been considered in some detail in the studies of Dr. Holländer, Dr. Sprague and his associates and Dr. Pribram.

That the processing of visual information in different species of mammals must be different on the basis of morphology alone is evident in the findings of Dr. Holländer as well as Dr. Noback's comments pertaining to parallel and convergent evolution of visual pathways. The former has re-examined the cortico-geniculate projections in the cat and found these to be absent from area 17, in contrast to findings of others. The problem of deciding between orthograde and retrograde degeneration in experiments involving cortical lesions has been justifiably introduced as a complicating factor in interpreting findings after relatively prolonged survival times. Inadvertent damage to projections from areas outside the target zone are of course always a serious problem in lesion studies. Dr. Holländer has suggested that the introduction of labelled amino acid techniques for mapping projection pathways may help to clarify present controversies concerning cortico-geniculate relations. In this context it should be noted that axonal transport of radioactive substances as a technique for mapping neuronal connections has now been considered superior to most other methods. (Cowan, W.M., Gottlieb, D.I., Hendrickson, A., Price, J.L., and Woolsey, T.A. The autoradiographic demonstration of axonal connections in the central nervous system, Brain Research, 37 (1972) 21-51). Recently this technique has been applied to the study of discrete projections from area 17 in the rat to the lateral geniculate body with notable success (Schubert, P., Kreutzberg, G.W. and Lux, H.D. Use of microelectrophoresis in the autoradiographic demonstration of fiber projections, Brain Research, 39 (1972) 274-277). It is appropriate to mention these most recent advances in experimental neuroanatomical techniques in this Symposium since we can anticipate their wider utilization in the future to resolve many problems of current concern in the study of cortico-thalamic relations.

While it has long been known that there are reciprocal connections between visual cortical areas and superior colliculus, the report of Drs. Palmer, Rosenquist and Sprague has addressed important questions of the nature, origin and physiological significance of visual corticotectal projection systems in the cat. It is clear from their instructive review of the anatomical relations of the superior colliculus that the latter structure is a "mini-brain" in itself. Despite these complexities Dr. Sprague and his colleagues have defined a system of neurons in visual area 17 which terminate on cells in the superficial gray stratum of the superior colliculus and which have properties of complex-hypercomplex cells. These elements presumably carry visual information to the colliculus which is of critical importance in conferring properties of binocular activation and direction selectively on tectal units. Evidence is marshaled to the effect that the corticotectal projection from area 17 does not play a significant role in visual attention and orientation. To this reviewer one aspect of the study reported by Dr. Sprague deserves special attention. This is the demonstration by antidromic stimulation of corticotectal fibers in the colliculus that cells identified in visual area 17 as having projections to the superior colliculus exhibit complex-cells properties as defined by Hubel and Wiesel and P.O. Bishop and his associates. It has been known for some time that all three cortical cell types (simple, complex and hypercomplex) project axons into the corpus callosum. But it is now evident from the work of Sprague and his colleagues that complex and probably some hypercomplex cells also have axons which project to the colliculus. By definition such cells must be of the pyramidal or pyramidal-like type and not stellate or Golgi-elements. It would seem of some importance to determine whether the complex cells with direct projections to the superior colliculus receive monosynaptic connections from the geniculate in view of recent studies that have indicated monosynaptic activation of some complex cells by fast-conducting visual afferents. If such is the case it would seem plausible to consider that the parallel processing by complex cells of visual information concerning tracking of moving objects might be greatly facilitated by utilization of rapidly conducting axons in the retinogeniculate and geniculocortical projection systems.

At this juncture it is useful to remind the reader that this Summary was written several months after the manuscripts were prepared. This is pointed out not to excuse the present writer's delinquency but to explain the curious circumstance that permits the writer to include relevant new information not available at the time of the Symposium. The case in point is well illustrated by Dr. Pribram's presentation in which an hypothesis has been developed to the effect that the association cortex of the inferotemporal gyrus is a source of efferent signals, probably projecting into the basal ganglia and therefrom to the visual input system. According to Dr. Pribram the efferent signals from association cortex "increase the capability of input channels to simultaneously transit and select among different signals. Recognition, making identifications in the sensory world, depends on this motor process." Leaving aside considerations of the "motor" aspect of these efferent signals from association cortex a key feature of the hypothesis is its implication of basal ganglia structures. Obviously one test of this hypothesis would be to determine whether stimulation of the caudate or lenticular nuclei was capable of influencing visual input at relatively peripheral sites of processing of visual information. Such data have now been reported. Lenticular stimulation in lightly anesthetized or paralyzed unanesthetized cats has been shown to produce augmentation or inhibition of lateral geniculate units responding to flash stimulation. The authors of this report conclude that modification of visual signals by lenticular stimulation occurs first at the primary relay nucleus of the lateral geniculate body. (Kadobayashi, I. and Ukida, G. Effects of lenticular stimulation on unitary responses of the lateral geniculate body to light. Exp. Neurol. 33, (1971) 518-527).

While it is not the intention of the present writer to submit these data as unequivocal support of Dr. Pribram's hypothesis, on the other hand it would be foolish to suggest their irrelevancy. As Dr. Mettler has already indicated in his discussion of Dr. Pribram's report, the mass of data summarized in the latter must be treated with respect. New concepts of cortical functions are usually not received with enthusiasm especially if they threaten comfortably established albeit weakly justified "facts." If the hypothesis that the association cortex of the inferotemporal gyrus is involved in establishing a motor set which reinforces discrimination learning is correct then a major step has been taken in approaching a more adequate understanding of the role of association cortex than has been possible heretofore. Undoubtedly many details of the hypothesis will require amplification and modification as new data are obtained. But as Henle once put it, "An hypothesis displaced by new facts dies a noble death. And if it calls up for re-examination those facts by which it was displaced we owe it a debt of gratitude." Hopefully many of the hypotheses developed in this Symposium Volume may be useful enough to suffer a similar destiny.